CLINICAL CARDIOLOGY

FIFTH EDITION

made
ridiculously
simple

Michael A. Chizner, M.D. F.A.C.P., F.A.C.C., F.A.H.A.

Chief Medical Director, The Heart Center of Excellence
Director, Cardiology Fellowship Program
Broward Health
Fort Lauderdale, Florida

Clinical Professor of Medicine
University of Miami Miller School of Medicine
Miami, Florida

Clinical Professor of Medicine
University of Florida College of Medicine
Gainesville, Florida

Clinical Professor of Medicine
Dr. Kiran C. Patel College of Osteopathic Medicine
at Nova Southeastern University
Fort Lauderdale, Florida

Clinical Professor of Integrated Medical Science
Charles E. Schmidt College of Medicine at Florida Atlantic University
Boca Raton, Florida

Clinical Professor of Medicine
Herbert Wertheim College of Medicine at Florida International University
Miami, Florida

Clinical Professor of Medicine
Barry University
Miami, Florida

MedMaster, Inc., Miami

Copyright © 2019, 2018, 2017, 2016, 2015, 2014, 2013, 2012, 2011, 2010, 2009, 2008, 2007, 2006, 2004 by MedMaster, Inc. Second Printing, 2004; Third Printing, 2005; Fourth Printing, 2006; Fifth Printing, 2007; Sixth Printing, 2007; Seventh Printing, 2008; Eighth Printing, 2009; Ninth Printing, 2010; Tenth Printing, 2011; Eleventh Printing, 2012; Twelfth Printing, 2013; Thirteenth Printing, 2014; Fourteenth Printing, 2015; Fifteenth Printing, 2016; Sixteenth Printing, 2017; Seventeenth Printing, 2018

ISBN #978-1-935660-31-6

Made in the United States of America

Published by
MedMaster, Inc.
P.O. Box 640028
Miami, FL 33164

Cover and artwork by Richard March

Dedication

To my wife Susan, and our children Kevin, Ryan, and Blair,
for their enduring patience and understanding sacrifice
through the many long hours spent in the preparation of this text;

and

To my mother Sybil, and in loving memory of my father Bernard,
for their unwavering support and steadfast guidance
that inspired and nurtured me from childhood on.

I could not have accomplished this task without you.

<u>test 1</u>

pt 1 - 75 Q
pt 2 - 15mrk SA/Fill in blank
bonus - 1mrk

TEE

dipyramidol?

CV Testing - what is false

CXR will visually verify pacemaker placement - T

Pharmacology to diagnosis
└> pt has hypertension...

Valve disease

Arrhythmias

ACTs

INR

Side effects of anticoag
Preload/Afterload whats the diff?
Systolic vs Diastolic HF
JVP
Pulses, where, scale

• S4 - what makes it
• P-pulmonale
• S2 - what opens/closes
• diff resp. breathing issues
• MIBI
• Low voltage ECGs - means what
                    - what causes
• Positions of bed
• Aortic regurg - best heard
• EKGs
• Pulses - dfferons, alternons, paradoxis
• Treatments
• CP descriptions
• 3 drugs in what category

• fast HR?
• Coumadin
• BB
• anticoag
• diuretics

About the Author

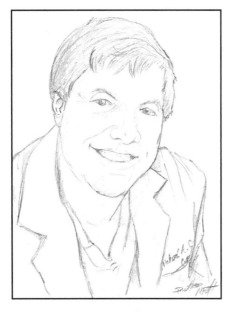

Michael A. Chizner, M.D., F.A.C.P., F.A.C.C., F.A.H.A., is a nationally renowned cardiologist, and the Founder and Chief Medical Director of The Heart Center of Excellence at Broward Health, one of the nation's largest health care systems based in Fort Lauderdale, Florida. He is a Clinical Professor of Medicine at the University of Florida College of Medicine, the University of Miami Miller School of Medicine, the Dr. Kiran C. Patel College of Osteopathic Medicine at Nova Southeastern University, the Charles E. Schmidt College of Medicine at Florida Atlantic University, the Herbert Wertheim College of Medicine at Florida International University, and Barry University. Dr. Chizner graduated with highest honors from the Weill Cornell Medical College of Cornell University where he was selected a member of the Alpha Omega Alpha National Medical Honor Society. He received his residency training in Internal Medicine at the New York Presbyterian Hospital-Weill Cornell Medical Center, and his cardiology fellowship training with legendary cardiologist, W. Proctor Harvey, M.D., at Georgetown University, where he was the recipient of the Distinguished Alumnus Award. Dr. Chizner is a board certified Diplomate of the American Board of Internal Medicine and the sub-specialty Board of Cardiovascular Disease. He is also a Fellow of the American College of Cardiology, the Council on Clinical Cardiology of the American Heart Association, and the American College of Physicians. Dr. Chizner is a highly accomplished cardiac clinician-diagnostician, widely known for his clinical skills—especially in the art of auscultation—and his

humanistic approach to patient care. Among the many awards and accolades he has received, Dr. Chizner has earned the distinction of being recognized as one of the top 1% of physicians in the nation in such prestigious publications as *America's Top Doctors, America's Top Cardiologists, America's Best Physicians, Who's Who in Medicine and Healthcare, Who's Who in America, U.S. News & World Report Top Doctors,* and *The Leading Physicians of the World.* As physician, author, editor, and teacher, Dr. Chizner has contributed greatly to the practice of cardiology and the advancement of medical education. He has written and edited numerous articles, monographs, and books in cardiology, including the best-selling *Clinical Cardiology Made Ridiculously Simple,* that have become standards in cardiovascular education, and are now being used in medical schools throughout the United States and abroad. Dr. Chizner has served on the editorial advisory boards of national cardiology journals. He has also been director, lecturer, and keynote speaker at continuing medical education conferences. Dr. Chizner has long been involved in the instruction of medical students, residents, fellows, physicians, nurses, and other healthcare professionals, and has recently been named the founding Director of the Cardiology Fellowship Program at Broward Health. In addition to the practice and teaching of cardiology, Dr. Chizner has spearheaded the establishment of The Heart Center of Excellence at Broward Health Medical Center, a world-class facility dedicated to the fight against heart disease and committed to the advancement of medical education, clinical research, and the delivery of the highest quality of compassionate, state-of-the-art patient care. As Founder and Chief Medical Director, Dr. Chizner refined the mission and vision of the heart center. He recruited an outstanding roster of cardiologists and cardiovascular surgeons, whose clinical expertise, superior outcomes, and exceptionally high performance ratings earned Broward Health Medical Center the reputation as one of the 50 Top Cardiovascular Hospitals in the nation, according to Truven Health Analytics, and the only high performing hospital for cardiology and heart surgery in the region, according to *U.S. News & World Report.* In recognition of his outstanding achievements, Dr. Chizner received a gubernatorial appointment to the Florida Board of Medicine, where he served as Chairman of the Credentials Committee, and was elected unanimously by his fellow board members as Vice Chairman and Chairman of the Board. As a result of his hard work and lifelong dedication to his profession and his patients, Dr. Chizner earned the honor of being selected as a recipient of the prestigious Marquis *Who's Who* Lifetime Achievement Award.

Foreword

One of the greatest needs in medicine and cardiology today is to teach the clinical cardiovascular evaluation of our patients on the highest level. Unfortunately, this is not being done. In fact, the situation is appalling. The technical aspects, which are the best in the world, have greatly advanced our diagnosis and treatment of heart disease. This will likely continue. However, the basic clinical evaluation has been de-emphasized to an almost unbelievable degree. We should always start and employ the clinical, so-called "five finger" approach, which is combining the findings of a complete cardiovascular evaluation. This includes a careful, detailed history and physical examination, electrocardiogram, x-ray, and simple laboratory tests. The fingers make a "fist", which is an excellent and efficient way to evaluate our patients. Here are several anecdotes to illustrate.

Recently, I examined a woman in her thirties who had the diagnosis of congenital ventricular septal defect, which had been documented by echocardiogram (echo) from a well-known hospital in Paris, France. Her husband was a diplomat in the United States Foreign Service. In fact, she had the official echo report and gave it to me. She was entirely asymptomatic, and had been advised to take antibiotic prophylaxis against infective endocarditis prior to dental procedures, operations, and other medical interventions, as previously outlined by the American Heart Association. In fact, she had already followed the instructions for some dental work in Paris. Her medical evaluation was completely normal, including the heart and cardiovascular system. Auscultation of her heart was normal. There were no murmurs; therefore, there was no ventricular septal defect. The echo was in error. The simple stethoscope quickly showed that she had been misdiagnosed. The use of this would have saved unnecessary time and expense for the patient, in addition to the mental trauma of thinking she had a heart lesion that she was born with. One sees many examples of erroneous diagnoses of the echo, which can be avoided by proper clinical auscultation. Hopefully, we won't—and do not want to—see more statements written on the request slip for an echo that says, "Rule out murmur". Don't get me wrong. The echo is a superb addition to the cardiovascular evaluation, but should be used in the total picture.

A must: Everyone evaluating patients to determine the presence or absence of heart disease should know how to tell the difference between an innocent versus a significant systolic murmur. At a recent three-day postgraduate course at the American College of Cardiology Heart House in Bethesda, Maryland, I asked a simple question before the course started. "How many of you can tell the difference between an innocent versus a significant ('guilty') murmur? Yes or No". The name of the person taking the course was anonymous, and a response system at the seat provided a quick answer of that person. At the start of the course, ninety-five percent (95%) said no, they could not. Five percent (5%) thought they could, answering yes. At the end of the course, the same question was asked. A complete reversal. Ninety-seven percent (97%) said yes, they could tell the difference, and answered in the affirmative. Three percent (3%) could not. Two previous independent post-graduate courses showed essentially the same result. Therefore, one can learn quickly. Listen to large numbers of actual patients, either in person and/or on high-fidelity tape, which provides accuracy and confidence in diagnosis.

All too often, the diagnosis of mitral stenosis was never made from the clinical exam, but from the echo and cardiac catheterization. This is appalling. In previous years, when I had the responsibility of Director of the Division of Cardiology here at Georgetown, I would have been greatly disappointed if even a second or third year medical student would miss this diagnosis. Recently, a patient with typical mitral stenosis was seen by a number of people, including students, resident staff, cardiac fellows, and others, before the diagnosis was made in the laboratory. Incredible, but true. This should not happen. One needs to listen to a large number of patients with mitral stenosis who illustrate the wide spectrum heard with our stethoscope. The confidence and accuracy of diagnosis will then result.

This book of Dr. Michael Chizner's is an excellent contribution to help reemphasize the necessity of using the "five finger" clinical method of evaluation of our patients. It is refreshing, to say the least. Make sure to pay close attention to the large number of valuable cardiac "pearls" he presents, which can be immediately applied for diagnosis and evaluation, as well as to the excellence in care for our patients. The numerous cartoons, which I like very much, represent a unique feature of this superb book, and speak of his pleasant personal humor.

One of the great pleasures of being a teacher, which I have been all of my academic life, is to see a pupil apply the knowledge learned, where at least you have had some good influence in "passing it on". Mike Chizner, a former cardiac Fellow at Georgetown, has and is doing this. He has continued along the path of excellence in his career and is now Chief Medical Director of The Heart Center of Excellence and Director of the Cardiology Fellowship Program at Broward Health, in Fort Lauderdale, Florida, and a Clinical Professor of Medicine at six universities in the state of Florida.

Thank you, Mike, for "carrying the torch". You have done it extremely well! Keep going. It will be well worth it.

W. Proctor Harvey, M.D., M.A.C.P., M.A.C.C.
Professor of Medicine (Founder and Former Director)
Division of Cardiology
Georgetown University School of Medicine
Washington, D.C.

A Tribute to W. Proctor Harvey, M.D.
(In Memoriam)

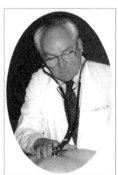

"A good teacher has the ability to take the topic that he is discussing and put it in terms so simple that everyone can understand it."

W. Proctor Harvey, M.D.

Once in a lifetime there comes an individual who leaves an indelible mark in his field. Such a man was Dr. Watkins Proctor Harvey, world renowned cardiologist, Professor of Medicine, and Founder and former Director of the Division of Cardiology at Georgetown University School of Medicine, whose lifelong dedication to the teaching and practice of clinical cardiology, earned him a legendary place in the history of cardiovascular medicine. Sadly, on September 26, 2007, at the age of 89, the world of medicine lost this much beloved and highly respected master clinician-teacher, known affectionately to his students and trainees as 'Proc'.

As one of the world's foremost cardiac clinicians and medical educators, Dr. Harvey stressed the importance of his timeless "five finger approach" to cardiovascular disease, which includes a careful, detailed history, physical examination, electrocardiogram, chest x-ray, and appropriate laboratory tests. He taught that with the intelligent use of one's senses and a stethoscope, the well trained clinician can make a rapid and accurate diagnosis, often without recourse to more costly, time-consuming, and potentially risky "high-tech" investigative methods. Indeed, Dr. Harvey's unique genius was his remarkable ability to arrive at the most sophisticated cardiovascular diagnoses from simple basic clinical examination skills. Using his teaching conferences as the theatre, the bedside as his stage setting, patients as the actors, the stethoscope as his instrument, the sounds and murmurs of the heart as the music, and his pearls of practical clinical wisdom as the lyrics, Dr. Harvey elevated the teaching and practice of clinical cardiology to an art form. The art of cardiac auscultation, as we know it today, is virtually synonymous with the name W. Proctor Harvey.

For those of us fortunate enough to have known him well, Dr. Harvey will always be thought of as a truly gifted and giving human being, mentor, and role model, whose kindness, warmth, compassion, caring, and humane concern for patients, colleagues, family, and friends, endeared him to all those with whom he came in contact. From the passion for cardiology that he instilled in us, springs the inspiration to pass along his rich legacy and to carry on the teaching tradition that is his. If we can keep the flame of his inspiration alive and burning, we will, in some small measure, repay our debt to him.

Michael A Chizner, M.D.

Preface

Cardiology has long been considered one of the most important clinical disciplines in the field of medicine. Virtually all medical students, physicians, nurses, and other health care professionals, regardless of whether they are going into cardiology or not, feel the need for at least some basic background and training in the subject matter. Although many encyclopedic reference texts are available that contain a vast amount of detailed medical information, these complex tomes often overwhelm the student of cardiology who wants to see "the forest through the trees" and becomes frustrated when there is "too much to learn and too little time to learn it".

Clinical Cardiology Made Ridiculously Simple is designed to fill this need. Now in its fifth edition, this best-selling book is tailored specifically for the medical student entering the hospital wards and clinics in the third and fourth years, as well as residents, fellows, physicians, nurses, and all other health care providers who wish to acquire a general working knowledge of cardiology and are trying to familiarize themselves with as much of the "language of the cardiologist" as possible in a relatively limited period of time. This completely revised and updated book should also be of great value to the cardiologist who wishes to "brush up", and seeks a concise but thorough overview of clinical cardiology, ranging from basic clinical evaluation skills of history taking and the cardiac physical exam, to the latest, most up-to-date "high-tech" laboratory investigations and therapeutic techniques.

This text will focus on the basics of the total clinical cardiovascular evaluation–the so-called "five finger" approach to cardiovascular disease, espoused by legendary cardiologist, Dr. W. Proctor Harvey. This orderly and systematic clinical method of evaluation includes a careful detailed history, physical examination, ECG, chest x-ray (CXR), and if needed, appropriate diagnostic laboratory tests. (**Figure P-1**)

It is a formidable task to acquire the proper knowledge and clinical skills for examining and evaluating the cardiac patient, while at the same time learn how to read and interpret ECGs and CXRs, as well as understand the mechanisms and appropriate uses for the tremendous array of cardiovascular procedures and therapeutic interventions employed in daily practice. The main aim of this unique book is to provide the reader with a clear conceptual understanding of clinical cardiology as a whole, in a simple, highly user-friendly format. With the wealth of practical clinical information provided, the reader will be able to integrate all of the clinically relevant facts obtained into an effective, individualized management plan, and thus avoid

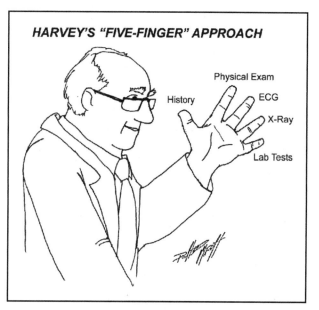

Figure P-1

the routine "cookbook" approach to patient care that often results in unnecessary, more costly, time-consuming, and potentially risky testing and/or treatment.

Despite the increasing reliance on elaborate and expensive new technology, it is still true that the great majority of patients seen for evaluation of the possibility of heart disease can and should be accurately diagnosed and treated in the office or at the bedside by employing the fundamentals of the "five finger" approach. It should be emphasized that every patient does not need every test. Skillful use of "low technology", particularly the cardiac history and physical examination, leads to intelligent, cost-effective use of "high technology" ("Hands before scans"). (**Figure P-2**)

The book is organized into three parts. The chapters in Part I explore in much detail each component of the "five finger" approach to the cardiac patient and the "keys to success" on becoming an accomplished cardiac clinician. The chapters in Part II present the reader with an overall clinical perspective on modern cardiovascular treatment, along with an in-depth discussion of the most up-to-date, pharmacological, interventional and cutting-edge surgical techniques. The chapters in Part III are designed to "put it all together", and provide the reader with a practical, "evidence-based" approach to the diagnosis and management of a broad spectrum of cardiac disease states and conditions encountered in everyday clinical practice.

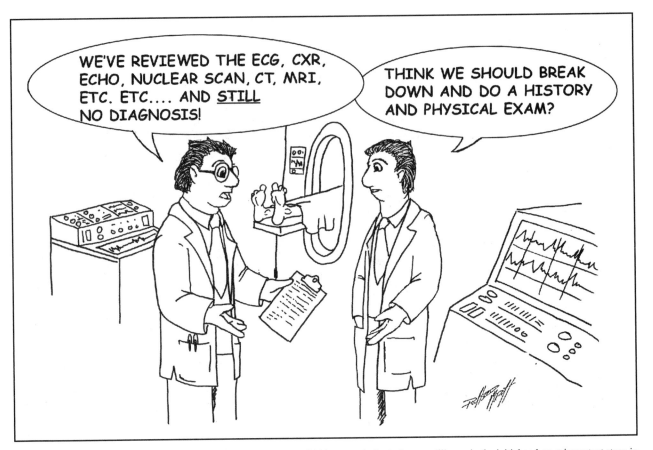

Note: Despite the growing reliance on sophisticated technology, a careful history and physical exam still remain the initial and most important steps in the clinical evaluation of the patient with heart disease. Often, by the time these simple basic steps are completed, the diagnosis has been made and treatment can begin. Remember, *simplicity is the ultimate sophistication!*

Figure P-2

This book is intended to be used as an introductory text for those new to cardiology and as a quick refresher for all others interested in updating their knowledge in this rapidly evolving field. This highly informative reference text will also serve as an invaluable study guide, packed with all the essentials of clinical cardiology one needs to know to prepare for and "ace" the board exams!

To simplify matters, the material is presented in a clear, concise, yet comprehensive manner. In addition to the written text, the numerous cardiac "pearls", schematic diagrams, summary tables, flow charts, and illustrative cartoons, interspersed throughout the book, provide a "lighthearted" approach, and serve as a visual aid to make the learning of clinical cardiology easy, memorable, and a delight rather than a drudgery. An interactive CD-ROM of heart sounds and murmurs, ECGs, CXRs, noninvasive and invasive cardiac diagnostic images, clinically oriented quizzes, and other problem solving activities, are also included to solidify key concepts, sharpen the users' cardiologic skills, and enhance one's understanding of the material presented in the text.

It is my firm belief that by learning and applying the valuable clinical information contained in this book, you can develop, over time, the magical ability to unravel and solve a multitude of mysteries in cardiology with which you may be confronted each day. The rewards are many, in particular, a feeling of great intellectual satisfaction in arriving at an accurate cardiac diagnosis and rendering appropriate treatment using your own wits and senses, what we, in the medical profession, refer to as the "art" and the "fun of medicine". In addition, you will be establishing a personal bond with your patient, the so-called "laying on of hands", which helps foster the close rapport, trust, and confidence so important to the privileged doctor-patient relationship.

It is my sincere hope that many of you will feel inspired to pick up your stethoscope, practice your techniques, perfect your skills, and thus begin the journey towards mastering clinical cardiology and becoming an *"Ace of Hearts"*.

I welcome your comments and suggestions for future editions.

Michael A. Chizner, M.D.

Acknowledgments

I would like to express my deep appreciation to the individuals whose help was invaluable in the preparation of this book.

I owe a large debt of gratitude to my mentor and role model, the late Dr. W. Proctor Harvey, one of the greatest, most influential, yet unassuming and gentle giants of American cardiology, for instilling in me a passion for clinical cardiology that has greatly enriched my professional life. Many of the graphic materials and schematic diagrams used in this book and the attached CD are adapted from the textbooks *Cardiac Pearls* by Dr. Harvey, *Clinical Auscultation of the Cardiovascular System* by Dr. Harvey and Mr. David C. Canfield, and *Classic Teachings in Clinical Cardiology, a tribute to W. Proctor Harvey, M.D.*, edited by the author. I am most grateful to Dr. Harvey and the Laennec Publishing Company for allowing me to use this material.

I particularly wish to express my heartfelt thanks to Mr. Richard March, illustrator and cartoonist extraordinaire, whose exceptional artistic skill helped to enhance the text and pictorially "bring to life" my original concepts and ideas in such a delightful and charming way. His unique creative talent was extremely valuable to this undertaking and I am indebted to him for it. I also wish to gratefully acknowledge Mrs. Dawn Burlace for her time, effort, invaluable assistance and expertise in the preparation of the graphic materials.

I would like to acknowledge the past and present members of the Board of Commissioners of the North Broward Hospital District, along with the Administration of Broward Health, whose commitment to academic excellence and the advancment of medical education is of the highest order. There is nothing more satisfying than coming to work every day surrounded by a group of amazing individuals that inspire one to reach just a bit higher. How fortunate I am to have such a team in place.

I especially wish to acknowledge my colleagues at The Heart Center of Excellence: Dr. Violeta Atanasoski-McCormack, Dr. Arnoux Blanchard, Dr. Ashok K. Sharma, Dr. John Rozanski, Dr. Kenneth Herskowitz, Dr. Frank Catinella, Dr. Andre Landau, Dr. Joel Gellman, Dr. Louis Cioci, Dr. Ahmed Osman, Dr. Hosney El Sayed, the late Dr. Harold Altschuler, Dr. Jeffrey Dennis, Dr. David Paris, Dr. Faraaz Mushtaq, Dr. Danish Sheikh, and the many other highly talented and dedicated physicians, nurses, and allied healthcare professionals with whom I have had the pleasure and privilege to work, and who have made my professional life so stimulating and rewarding.

My heartfelt thanks extends to the many medical students, residents, and cardiology fellows with whom I have had the pleasure of being associated over the years, who have been a constant source of motivation and who continue to make the learning and teaching of cardiology so meaningful and enjoyable. This book has benefited greatly from their invaluable insights.

I would also like to give special thanks and recognition to the past and present "angels" in my office: Mrs. Sandy McGarry; Mrs. Jillian Martin, RN; Ms. Linda Cupo, ARNP; Mrs. Deborah Krauser, ARNP; Mrs. Anie Geevarghese, ARNP; Mrs. Cynthia Ryan, ARNP; Mrs. Josephine March; Ms. Kasandra Aneses, PA-C; Ms. Joanne Schrager, RN; Ms. Corina Pelean-Osvat; Mrs. Julie DeLongy; Mrs. Nathalie Smith; Ms. Sandi Swift; Ms. Sherri Julius; Ms. Portia Mitchell, MA; and Mr. Osvil Zelaya, MBA, RN, whose constant encouragement, sustained enthusiasm, and unwavering support were most helpful to the completion of this project. Heartfelt thanks and deep appreciation are due Dr. S. Kimara March, one of the original office "angels," who has completed her cardiology fellowship at the Mayo Clinic in Rochester, Minnesota, and whose valuable suggestions from the fresh viewpoint of today's highly trained cardiologist have been most insightful.

I especially wish to acknowledge Mrs. Arlene Wasser and Ms. Mabel N. Nazzarri, without whose tireless efforts in the seemingly endless typing of the many drafts of this manuscript, this book would not have been possible. Special thanks and gratitude are also due Ms. Stephanie Crossley, whose unrelenting enthusiasm, dedication, and extraordinary attention to detail, were essential to bringing this newly revised and updated edition of the book to fruition. Their exceptional organizational skills, sustained loyalty, and faithful support deserve special mention, and have truly meant a great deal to me.

I owe a great debt of gratitude to Dr. Stephen Goldberg, President of MedMaster, Inc., for his meticulous review of the manuscript, and for his sage guidance and most valuable advice on how to "keep it simple". Special thanks are also due Dr. Adam Splaver, for his helpful suggestions and invaluable contributions to the book, Ms. Phyllis Goldenberg, for her detailed proofreading of the text, and Ms. Sharon Anderson, for her expertise in putting the manuscript in final form for publication.

To my devoted and loving family, my wife Susan and our children Kevin, Ryan, and Blair, and my mother Sybil and my late father Bernard, I owe more than words can ever express. I also wish to convey my deep appreciation to my sister, Ms. Joan E. Rubin, for her invaluable insight, enthusiastic support, and "100%-biased" positive feedback during the writing of this book.

I would also like to express my sincere thanks to a very important group of people who have had such a profound impact on me. These special individuals are my patients, both new and those whom I have had the distinct pleasure and privilege of knowing and taking care of through the years. They have taught me much about the privileged doctor-patient relationship, in particular, the importance of the humanistic qualities of empathy, compassion, and caring, and the immense personal satisfaction one can derive not only in the care of the patient but even more importantly in the care for the patient.

I am particularly grateful to Ms. Pamela Africk, Mr. Richard Bassett, Mr. John Bauer, Mr. T. Ed Benton, Mr. Steven R. Berrard, Mrs. Ana I. Gardiner-Bogenschutz, Mr. Charles Caulkins, the late Mr. Davis W. ("Bill") Duke Jr. the late Mr. George ("Bob") Gill; Mr. Michael S. Egan; Mr. Mark J. Grant, Mr. Robert S. Hackleman; Mr. John W. Henry; Mr. H. Wayne Huizenga; Mr. Shephard Lane; the late Mrs. Rosemary D. Larson, Mr. Joel Lavender; Senator George LeMieux; Dr. Frederick Lippman; Mr. Ralph A. Marrinson; Mr. Andrew Rosen, Dr. Richard Schulze; Dr. Kenneth Stevenson, the late Mr. Terry W. Stiles; and Mr. and Mrs. Steven and Rebecca Stoll, for their continued friendship, loyalty, and most generous support. To my dear friend, the late Mr. R. David ("Dave") Thomas, whose passing was such a great personal loss, I owe more than he would have cared to have me mention. Dave taught me, by personal example, that with hard work, perseverance, and commitment to the time-honored American values of giving back, helping others, and treating people fairly, you can reach as far as your fondest hopes and dreams will take you.

Last, but not least, I would like to express my sincere thanks and deep appreciation to all the readers who have personally commented on the merits of this book, and whose valuable suggestions and enthusiastic support have helped to make it a best-selling book in cardiology.

Writing, revising, and updating a book is truly a labor of love that makes one feel humble and grateful to countless individuals who have made it possible. I am forever grateful to those I have identified, and others too numerous to mention by name, who have made such a difference in my life, and in this effort in particular.

Michael A. Chizner, M.D.

Contents

PART I.   THE FIVE-FINGER APPROACH TO CARDIAC DIAGNOSIS

CONTENTS

PART II. CARDIOVASCULAR THERAPEUTICS

CONTENTS

PART I.   THE FIVE-FINGER APPROACH TO CARDIAC DIAGNOSIS

Despite today's advanced technology, it is still true that most cardiac patients can be accurately diagnosed by a careful history, physical examination, ECG, and chest x-ray, and only then, if necessary, by performing specialized laboratory tests (Harvey's "five finger" approach). When skillfully applied, the "five finger" approach is an efficient diagnostic method that is cost-effective and can frequently avoid invasive procedures.

CHAPTER 1.   THE CARDIAC HISTORY

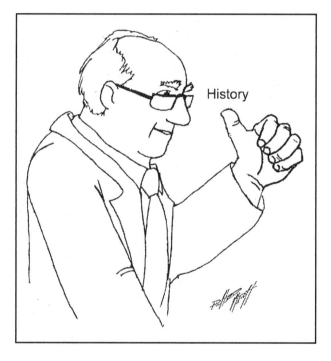

A carefully obtained clinical history is the first step in making a correct cardiac diagnosis and prescribing appropriate treatment.

Figure 1-1 summarizes the key areas to assess in the cardiac clinical history in regard to *Chief Complaint, History of Present Illness (HPI), Past Medical History, Family and Social History,* and *Coronary Artery Disease (CAD) Risk Factors.*

The information from this assessment can then be used to construct a differential diagnosis. While a single symptom may provide the clue which leads to the correct symptom may provide the clue which leads to the correct diagnosis, usually it is a combination of symptoms that most reliably suggest the diagnosis.

CHEST PAIN OR DISCOMFORT

Figure 1-2 summarizes the clinical history for chest pain. When evaluating the patient with chest pain, keep in mind the mnemonic **"OPQRST"**: **O**nset, **P**rovocation/**P**alliation, **Q**uality, **R**egion/**R**adiation, **S**everity/associated **S**ymptoms, and **T**iming.

Coronary Artery Disease (CAD)

Figure 1-3. Colorful phrases often used by patients to describe ischemic chest discomfort include: **A)** "Like an elephant sitting on my chest". **B)** "A burning sensation". **C)** "A choking feeling in my throat". **D)** "Like a toothache". **E)** "My bra is too tight".

Stable Angina Pectoris and the Acute Coronary Syndromes (Unstable Angina, Acute Myocardial Infarction)

Ischemic chest discomfort (more often than "pain") is the most frequent presenting symptom of coronary artery disease (CAD). Ischemic discomfort is deep seated rather than superficial, comes on gradually, and lasts minutes (rather than seconds)—or longer (>30 minutes) if due to evolving acute myocardial infarction (MI). It is generally felt beneath the breastbone (retrosternal), spreads across the precordium with predilection for the left side, and commonly radiates to (but on occasion may originate in) the neck, throat ("choking" sensation), upper back, interscapular area, epigastrium ("heartburn"), chest ("the flu"), shoulders ("arthritis", "bursitis"), and down the inner (ulnar) aspect of one or both arms (usually the left) to the elbows, wrists and fingers, where it is often described as a "numbness" and "tingling" ("pins and needles") sensation rather than actual pain. Some patients may even consult with their dentist initially in the mistaken belief that the cause of their jaw pain is a "toothache". It is brought on by "the four E's" (Exertion, Emotional stress, Exposure to cold and/or hot-humid weather, or after Eating a heavy meal). When symptoms last 2–15 minutes and are relieved promptly by rest and/or nitroglycerin, this is termed *"stable" angina pectoris,* which does not result in permanent myocardial damage. When angina is new in onset, increases in intensity, frequency and

---

FIGURE 1-1

**Cardiac Clinical History
A Systematic Approach**

Chief Complaint

Presenting Symptom(s) Associated with Heart Disease Listen to the patients – they will often tell you the diagnosis! (Record in the patient's own words). Include patient's age, race and sex.

- Chest pain or discomfort
- Shortness of breath (dyspnea on exertion, orthopnea, paroxysmal nocturnal dyspnea)
- Fatigue and weakness
- Cough and hemoptysis
- Palpitations
- Dizziness, near-syncope, syncope
- Weight gain, ankle swelling
- Intermittent claudication

History of Present Illness

Details of Current Symptoms

Time & Place

- Time of onset (i.e., when did the symptoms first begin? How long did the episode last? How has the condition progressed with time, etc.?)
- Mode of onset (rapid, gradual, instantaneous) and pattern (Is it continuous, or intermittent? Is it getting worse or better?)
- Location and radiation (if pain or discomfort) — Where is the pain, etc.?

Quality & Quantity

- Quality—Describe what the symptoms feel like (e.g., sharp, dull, stabbing, burning, heavy, heartburn, indigestion).
- Severity (graded mild to severe)

Provocative & Palliative

- Aggravating or relieving factors—What makes the symptoms worse? What was the setting at the time the problem arose? What makes the symptoms better?

Associated Symptoms

- Associated symptoms—Does anything else bother you, etc?
- Current treatment and drug history.

Past Medical History

- Previous CAD (e.g., angina, MI)
- Prior cardiac procedure (e.g., ECG, stress test, echocardiogram, cardiac catheterization) or intervention (PCI, CABG)
- History of rheumatic fever, heart murmurs
- Recent dental work or IV drug use
- Drugs (prescription, over-the-counter)
- Prior illness (cardiac, non-cardiac)

Family History

- MI, hypertension, cardiomyopathy, congenital heart disease, MVP, Marfan's syndrome

Social History

- Tobacco, alcohol, recreational drug use (cocaine, amphetamine)

CAD Risk Factors

- Cigarette smoking
- Hypertension
- Hyperlipidemia
- Diabetes mellitus
- Obesity
- Physical inactivity

---

duration (>20 minutes), or occurs at rest, *"unstable" angina* is said to be present and often progresses to *acute myocardial infarction* if not treated. These ischemic events are termed *acute coronary syndromes*.

Characteristically, the patient with angina pectoris stops activity and prefers to remain in the sitting or standing position to obtain relief, but may not be relieved by (and therefore resists) lying in the supine position. Redistribution of intravascular volume along with an increase in venous return in the recumbent position may increase heart size, ventricular wall tension, and myocardial oxygen de-

mand, and thus aggravate ischemic chest discomfort (*"angina decubitus"*).

Figure 1-4. The patient may have difficulty in describing the sensation of ischemic chest pain and make a clenched fist over the sternum (*"Levine's sign"*), a classic hand gesture suggesting ischemic chest pain.

Chest pain may be absent (*"silent ischemia"*) in as many as 25% or more of patients, especially in those with diabetes mellitus, in whom pain perception may be altered by neuropathy ("defective warning system"); in the elderly, where such atypical symptoms as confusion, lightheaded-

*IPPA

FIGURE 1-2

Clinical Characteristics of Chest Pain

TIME

- **Frequency**—Does the pain occur many times per day or only occasionally in response to specific precipitating factors? What has been the pattern of the episodes—more or less frequent/severe in recent days/weeks?

- **Duration**—Does the pain last for seconds, minutes, or hours? Are there quick jabs or stabs, or does the pain last for hours at a time? Is there lingering pain after the worst of the episode has cleared?

- **Course of Pain**—Does the pain remain steady or wax and wane during an episode? Does the pain begin abruptly at full intensity, or does it build up gradually? How rapidly does the pain subside?

PLACE

- **Location**—Pain may be retrosternal, diffuse across precordium, in left inframammary area, left precordial ("over the heart"), mainly in the back, shoulder(s), or subscapular area. Some cardiac pain may be felt in the epigastrium only. The consistency of the location of the pain should be determined. Pinpoint or sharply localized should be distinguished from more diffuse or generalized pain.

- **Radiation**—Are any extrathoracic sites affected? Radiation of pain to shoulders, arm, back, neck, throat, jaw or the interscapular area is not uncommon. Sensation of numbness/tingling in upper extremities may be manifestation of referred pain.

QUALITY—Pain may be described as squeezing, burning, a fullness, pressure, dull ache, sharp, gas, heartburn, indigestion, a need to belch, numbing or prickly.

QUANTITY—Rate severity on grade of 1 to 10 (10 being the worst imaginable).

PROVOCATIVE/PALLIATIVE FACTORS—Do activities such as walking uphill, hurrying, exposure to cold, emotional stress, sex, or the postprandial state bring on the pain? Is pain influenced by motion, position, respiration? Does the supine position influence the pain? Does pain come on without any precipitating factors or during sleep?

ASSOCIATED SYMPTOMS—Breathlessness, marked fatigue, diaphoresis, pre-syncope, syncope, apprehension, and sense of impending doom may occur.

---

ness, syncope, shortness of breath or gastrointestinal (GI) upset may be the presenting complaint; or in those in the perioperative state recovering from anesthesia and/or receiving analgesics. Likewise, cardiac transplant recipients do not usually feel chest pain when their coronary arteries become narrowed. Denervation of the donor heart prevents the usual symptoms of angina that signal the presence of coronary arteriopathy, a not uncommon complication. Furthermore, denial is a significant component in the presentation of chest pain caused by an acute coronary syndrome. The diagnosis may be made in retrospect by means of a routine ECG, myocardial enzyme elevations, or an echo. The presence of atypical symptoms (e.g., dyspnea, fatigue, lightheadedness, recurrent belching, or "indigestion") should not be used to exclude the possibility that an acute coronary event is occurring.

Likewise, the time of onset should not dissuade the clinician from entertaining the diagnosis of acute MI. Although most common in the early morning hours (6 am - 12 noon), acute MI can occur any time, day or night.

Women, particularly those under the age of 60, have also been reported to have a higher incidence of atypical symptoms (e.g., jaw, back, neck, shoulder or abdominal pain; shortness of breath; nausea; and fatigue). These symptoms may appear to be noncardiac in nature and often result in significant underdiagnosis and delay in receiving medical attention. Diabetes mellitus is a major risk factor for early onset of coronary atherosclerosis in women. In these atypical situations, a high index of suspicion should alert the clinician to the presence of underlying CAD.

Pertinent Past Medical History and/or Risk Factors for CAD

Many patients are capable of presenting an accurate account of their past cardiac history including the results of previous coronary angiograms and the number of arteries ballooned, stented, or bypassed. However, don't assume that you can always rely totally on the patient's description.

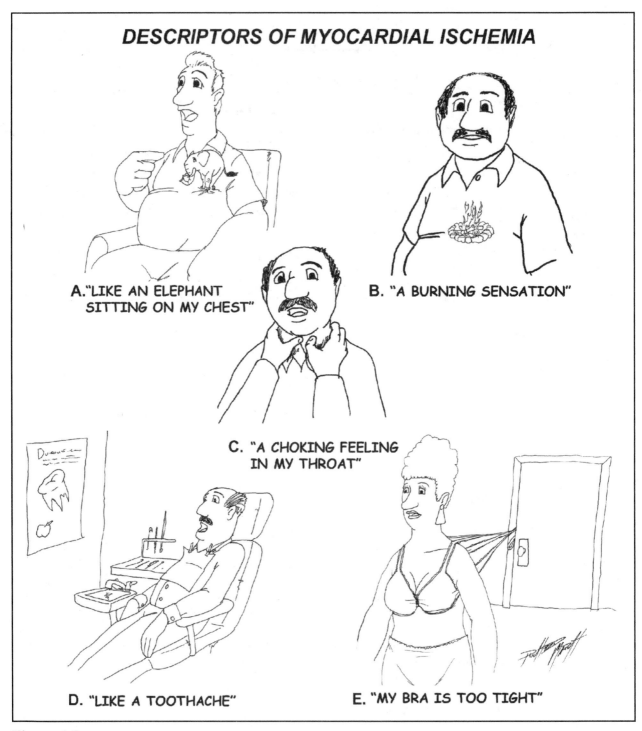

Figure 1-3

Whenever possible, obtain old records. It may be a painful step, but is well worth the effort! For example, patients may relate that they have had a past "heart attack", when in reality, they may have had an episode of noncardiac chest pain, congestive heart failure (CHF) or even an arrhythmia.

Furthermore, a patient may answer "no" when questioned about CAD risk factors, e.g., cigarette smoking. Keep in mind that being a "non-smoker" is not the same as being an ex-2 to 3 pack a day smoker for the past 20 years who gave up cigarettes one week ago!

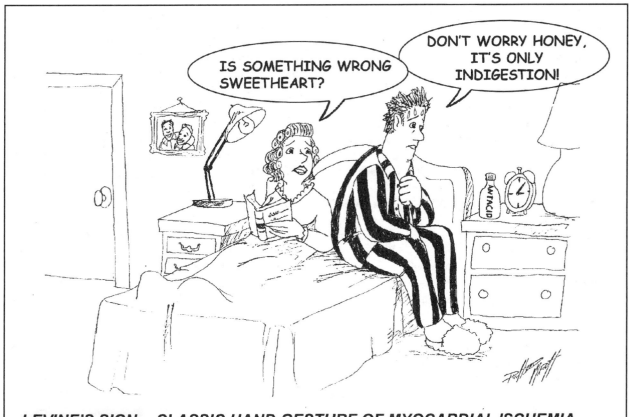

LEVINE'S SIGN -- CLASSIC HAND GESTURE OF MYOCARDIAL ISCHEMIA

Figure 1-4

Multiple risk factors for the development of CAD have been identified. Aside from cigarette smoking, the major risk factors amenable to modification include hyperlipidemia, hypertension, diabetes mellitus, lack of physical activity, and obesity (**Figure 1-1**). Risk factors that are not modifiable include advanced age, male sex, and a family history of premature CAD.

The designation of male sex as one of the major risk factors, and the observation in some studies that women with chest pain seem to have a fairly benign prognosis, have led to a failure on the part of some practitioners to appreciate the importance of chest pain in women ("*gender bias*"). Although CAD does develop about ten years later in women than men, it is highly prevalent in women, and is the most common cause of mortality (accounting for twice as many deaths as all forms of cancer).

A history of illicit drug use (e.g., cocaine, amphetamines) should also be considered a risk factor, especially in a young person (particularly a male cigarette smoker who presents with ischemic-type chest discomfort). Regardless of the route, dose, or frequency of use, cocaine can produce

a sudden increase in myocardial oxygen demand, promote coronary thrombosis, induce vasospasm, and thus precipitate an acute ischemic event (even when taken for the first time). Inquiry into the use of "over-the-counter" sympathomimetic agents and other stimulant drugs, e.g., decongestants, ephedra, Ma-huang, and sumatriptan (Imitrex - prescribed for migraine and cluster headaches) should also be made when a patient presents with chest pain. These drugs may increase myocardial oxygen demand, provoke coronary spasm, and trigger myocardial ischemia.

* * *

Ten Pearls Regarding Coronary Artery Symptoms:

1. Many patients with acute coronary syndromes do not have classic "textbook" symptoms. Variations on the theme are common. Crushing chest pain may indicate a heart attack in one patient, whereas mild shortness of breath can denote the same disease process in another (yet ignored because of its subtlety). With advancing age, chest pain declines in frequency as the presenting

symptom of acute MI, as dyspnea, syncope, acute confusion and stroke become more common. Women are more likely than men to have pain in the abdomen, back, or jaw, a feeling of indigestion or heartburn, or extreme fatigue, rather than the classic spreading chest pain. The myth that a heart attack must be a dramatic event needs to be dispelled. Remember to keep in mind that symptoms may be "atypical", e.g., nausea, vomiting, "indigestion", dizziness, the "flu", or even absent (so-called "silent ischemia"), especially in women, diabetics, or the elderly.

2. Angina does not always mean coronary artery disease. Left ventricle (LV) outflow tract obstruction (e.g., valvular aortic stenosis, hypertrophic obstructive cardiomyopathy) can also cause classic angina, as may anemia.

3. Features which make coronary pain unlikely include: stabbing pains, pains lasting < 30 seconds, localized left inframammary pain ("in my heart"), continually varying location.

4. Patients may use the word "sharp" to convey the severity of pain rather than as a description of the character of the pain.

5. Don't always assume that a change in chest pain represents unstable angina. Nitroglycerin tablets may have lost their potency. Check for associated symptoms of headache, stinging and flushing. Some patients may also be noncompliant with their medications.

6. Ongoing chest pain that has been present for an extended period of time may still represent angina. Further questioning of the patient may reveal that the pain is actually intermittent since its onset and not constant.

7. A high index of suspicion is necessary to avoid missing the diagnosis of acute aortic dissection or pericarditis. This distinction from acute MI is crucial, since thrombolytic therapy is contraindicated in these conditions.

8. Don't attribute cardiac symptoms to other chronic underlying conditions e.g., hiatal hernia, or esophageal spasm. A history of such an underlying illness does not rule out a new cardiac condition.

9. Not all patients with acute MI develop ECG changes. As many as 1/3 do not develop any changes at all, especially if the location of the MI is in electrically silent areas of the heart. (e.g., posterior) Because ECG changes are not always seen with acute MI, and serum markers may take time to evolve, the key determinant of whether or not to hospitalize a patient with chest pain remains the clinical history.

10. Although risk factors for coronary artery disease are important to keep in mind when evaluating a patient with chest pain, a significant percentage (up to 40%) of patients presenting with acute MI may have no risk factors. Their presence or absence, therefore, should not be relied upon to determine whether or not a patient who presents with chest pain should be sent home or admitted to the hospital for further work-up.

* * *

Despite the advent of chest pain centers and sensitive biochemical markers of myocardial necrosis, a number of patients presenting to the emergency department (ED) with chest pain are released after initial evaluation only to return with an acute MI within 48 hours. It is important to keep in mind that neither the ECG nor any of the current cardiac enzyme tests are perfect, and serial testing is often still necessary to rule out an acute MI. Only 50% of patients with a proven acute MI have an initial ECG indicating the disorder. Furthermore, the sensitivity of a given serum marker in detecting acute MI is dependent on the time it is measured after the onset of symptoms. Unfortunately, markers of myocardial cell injury, e.g., cardiac troponins, do not increase until 3-6 hours after the onset of chest pain. Thus, it is important to understand that not even the ECG or the most specific serum chemical marker of myocardial damage can exempt the practitioner from a careful clinical assessment of the patient who presents with chest pain. Despite its limitations, the patient's history remains the cornerstone to an initial working diagnosis and provides the basis for important triage and treatment decisions early in the course of the clinical cardiovascular evaluation.

In this modern era of reperfusion therapy and catheter-based interventions, where "every second counts" and rapid "door-to-needle" time is strongly encouraged, urgent stabilization and treatment often cannot await definitive diagnosis. The decision to introduce or withhold such life-saving treatment must be made on the basis of a careful clinical evaluation. Although the definitive diagnosis of acute MI might not be established for several hours, the patient's **H**istory, **E**CG, **A**ge, **R**isk factors, and initial **T**roponin level (so-called **HEART** score), often determines whether a patient is sent home from the ED with reassurance, or is admitted to the hospital for further evaluation and care.

Chest Pain in Other Cardiovascular Conditions

Although CAD is by far the most common cause of chest pain, chest discomfort can be a symptom of other cardiovascular conditions including valvular aortic stenosis (AS), pericarditis, aortic dissection, mitral valve prolapse (MVP), pulmonary hypertension, and hypertrophic obstructive cardiomyopathy (HOCM–a familial condition in which the ventricular and septal wall are thick and stiff, impinging on the ventricular cavity and obstructing blood outflow from the ventricle, a leading cause of sudden death in young athletes).

Pericarditis and aortic dissection are two particularly important masqueraders. A careful detailed history will assist in the diagnosis (**Figure 1-5**).

Pericarditis
The sudden onset of sharp, superficial, centrally-located chest pain radiating to the shoulders, upper back and neck (trapezius ridge) aggravated by deep breathing, coughing, twisting or turning of the torso, swallowing, lying flat in the recumbent position, are clues to acute pericarditis. The severity of pain is increased (or appears abruptly) by these

activities because they stretch the inflamed pericardium. The pain may last for hours, is usually constant in intensity, does not vary with physical exertion (as in angina pectoris), and is relieved by sitting up and leaning forward, and by anti-inflammatory agents, not nitroglycerin.

Figure 1-6. The pain of acute pericarditis–worse on inspiration and lying flat and better when sitting upright and leaning forward.

Aortic Dissection
Chest pain associated with acute thoracic aortic dissection (which occurs frequently in the setting of underlying hypertension or Marfan's syndrome) usually starts abruptly, with maximum intensity at the onset (in contrast to the pain of acute MI, which usually builds in intensity more gradually). It is excruciating, poorly relieved by narcotics, described as "ripping" or "tearing" in quality, is typically felt more severely in the chest and upper back (between the shoulder blades) and may radiate along the course of progression of

FIGURE 1-5

Differential Diagnosis of Chest Pain

Diagnosis	Onset of Pain	Quality of Pain	Relieved by
Angina pectoris	Gradual, with exertion, stress, or after large meal.	Substernal tightness, pressure, heaviness, squeezing, burning, choking, "indigestion," radiating to neck, jaw, left shoulder and arm.	Rest, nitroglycerin
Acute myocardial infarction	Sudden, may be associated with dyspnea, diaphoresis, profound weakness lightheadedness, nausea, vomiting or feeling of impending doom.	Similar to angina, but generally more severe (>30 min)	No relief with rest. Usually requires opiates or aggressive intervention (e.g., thrombolysis, angioplasty/ stenting) for relief.
Acute pericarditis	Varies, may be preceded by "flu-like" symptoms or as a sequela to another process (e.g., following acute MI).	Pleuritic, usually constant sharp pain radiating to trapezius ridge, aggravated by lying down, coughing, swallowing, and respiration, due to stretching on inflamed pericardium.	Sitting up and leaning forward, antiinflammatory agents. Not relieved by nitroglycerin. Pain does not vary with physical exertion.
Acute thoracic aortic dissection	Sudden, intense from the onset, radiates to back, may shift from upper to lower chest as dissection progresses.	"Ripping", "tearing", worst pain ever experienced, radiating to arms, neck, interscapular area, lower back, abdomen, or even lower extremities.	No relief. Requires emergent surgery (Type A—ascending aorta) and/or aggressive medical management (Type B—descending aorta).

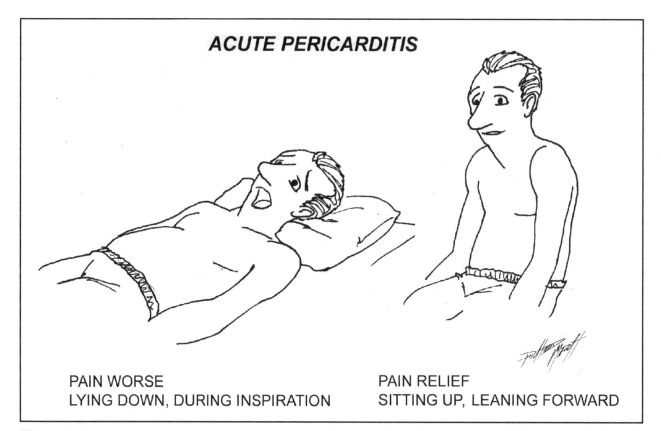

Figure 1-6

the dissection to the arms, neck, interscapular area, lower back, abdomen, and even to the lower extremities.

Figure 1-7. The pain of aortic dissection–sudden onset of severe "ripping" or "tearing" anterior chest pain radiating through to the upper back and interscapular region.

Mitral Valve Prolapse

Chest pain associated with mitral valve prolapse is usually "atypical", often described as "sharp", "sticking", or less frequently as "a dull ache", varying in location and radiation (even in the same patient), occurring at rest or during exercise, without demonstrable consistency. The pain may last for hours or even days and is unrelieved by nitroglycerin. Some attribute the association to an increased frequency of underlying psychopathology (e.g., anxiety or panic disorder) that may trigger chest pain in these patients.

Left Ventricular Outflow Tract Obstruction (e.g., Valvular Aortic Stenosis, Hypertrophic Cardiomyopathy)

In the patient who presents with typical ischemic-type (anginal) chest discomfort on exertion, the seasoned clinician should always consider the possibility of LV outflow tract obstruction, e.g., valvular aortic stenosis (AS), hypertrophic obstructive cardiomyopathy (HOCM). It is worth noting that the presence of symptoms (i.e., angina, dyspnea, and syncope) helps identify those patients with significant valvular AS who are at increased risk of death (as compared to those who are asymptomatic). This serves to underscore the importance of obtaining a careful, detailed history regarding the presence of symptoms each time the patient with known valvular AS visits the practitioner.

Pulmonary Hypertension

Severe pulmonary hypertension from a variety of causes may also be associated with exertional chest discomfort resembling angina pectoris, presumably due to right ventricular (RV) ischemia. In young, otherwise healthy appearing women (often with *Raynaud's phenomenon*—a condition in which there is intermittent digital ischemia secondary to cold or emotional stress), or in those who are obese and have taken appetite suppressing agents (e.g., Phen-fen), the presence of effort-related chest pain, along with dyspnea, fatigue, or syncope, should raise the suspicion of idiopathic (primary) pulmonary hypertension.

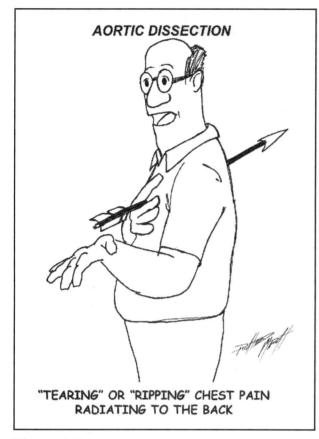

AORTIC DISSECTION

"TEARING" OR "RIPPING" CHEST PAIN
RADIATING TO THE BACK

Figure 1-7

It is important to realize that relief of chest pain must be based on an etiologic diagnosis. To simply suppress pain with analgesics or sedatives (e.g., "GI cocktail") before a diagnosis is made may hide important clues and thereby endanger the patient. The vital importance of differentiating these disorders revolves around the need to intervene promptly in some conditions (e.g., acute coronary syndromes, aortic dissection) and the fact that the beneficial treatment for one entity (e.g., aspirin, heparin, or thrombolytic therapy for acute MI) might be disastrous for the patient with another (e.g., aortic dissection, pericarditis, pericardial tamponade). (**Figure 1-5**).

SHORTNESS OF BREATH (DYSPNEA, ORTHOPNEA, PAROXYSMAL NOCTURNAL DYSPNEA)

Dyspnea, an uncomfortable, heightened awareness of difficulty breathing, is another common reason for patients to seek medical attention. It may have both cardiac and non-cardiac causes, e.g., obstructive or restrictive pulmonary disease, neuromuscular disorder, anemia, obesity, deconditioning ("couch potato"), anxiety, and is therefore nonspecific unless additional corroborating evidence of a cardiac abnormality is present.

In many ways, the approach to history-taking in dyspnea is similar to that for evaluating chest pain. The time and place, quantity and quality, provocative and palliative factors, and associated symptoms (e.g., chest pain, wheezing, cough, sputum production, anxiety) may provide clues to the underlying diagnosis. Also consider past and current use of tobacco, environmental allergies, occupational history, asthma, and a family history of lung problems.

Often, the complaint of shortness of breath is not true dyspnea but the feeling of an inability to get enough air and is characterized by deep, slow, sighing respirations due to an anxiety state. These patients complain of shortness of breath at rest, but not on exertion, and may demonstrate this type of breathing pattern as they relate their clinical history. Hysterical hyperventilation may at times be a repetitive, sighing type of breathing, and, at other times, a continued, rapid breathing pattern, accompanied by lightheadedness and a "numbness" and "tingling" feeling around the mouth and in the extremities.

When confronted with a patient complaining of dyspnea, the clinician can place the vast majority of cases into one of two broad categories: *cardiac* and *pulmonary*. Attention to the nuances of the clinical history may provide considerable insight into the cause of a patient's breathing difficulties. (**Figure 1-8**). Careful questioning about the timing of onset and pattern of dyspnea may be particularly helpful in making the diagnosis.

Figure 1-9. The New York Heart Association (NYHA) functional status classification of exercise tolerance.

Cardiac dyspnea may occur in patients with congestive heart failure (CHF) and significant LV dysfunction; it is usually characterized by rapid, shallow respiration worsened during exertion (e.g., walking short distances, climbing one or two flights of stairs, doing household chores). When dyspnea on exertion (DOE) is accompanied by *orthopnea* (inability to breathe comfortably while lying flat), and particularly *paroxysmal nocturnal dyspnea (PND)* (nighttime episodes of shortness of breath brought on by lying flat), the likelihood of CHF and underlying heart disease increases. This pattern of shortness of breath is a classic clue to the presence of excess fluid in the interstitial and/or alveolar spaces of the lungs and should lead the astute clinician to consider the various causes of pulmonary vascular congestion (e.g., CAD, hypertensive heart disease, valvular disease, cardiomyopathy). For example, a patient with a history of previous MIs who develops dyspnea, orthopnea, or PND, is likely to have decreased LV contractility as the cause, whereas a patient with a history of hypertension or heavy alcohol intake

---

FIGURE 1-8

Clinical Clues to Cardiac vs. Pulmonary Dyspnea

Cardiac Dyspnea	Pulmonary Dyspnea
Onset of dyspnea more sudden (e.g., acute CHF, myocardial ischemia)	Dyspnea tends to occur more gradually (except with pneumonitis, pneumothorax, asthma).
Associated with episodic or sudden onset chest pain (anginal equivalent or MI) palpitations (e.g., atrial fibrillation), orthopnea, and PND.	Associated with pleuritic chest pain, tachypnea, and tachycardia (e.g., pulmonary embolism) in the setting of recent surgery, malignancy, immobility, hypercoagulable state.
More commonly associated with bilateral pedal edema (e.g., left and/or right sided CHF with pulmonary hypertension).	Associated with unilateral pedal edema (e.g., deep vein thrombosis and pulmonary embolism).
History of good response to diuretic/nitrate.	History of good response to bronchodilator therapy.
Dyspnea usually not associated with sputum production.	Dyspnea often associated with sputum production and relieved by coughing up sputum.
No history of pulmonary disease.	History of chronic obstructive or other pulmonary disease.
No history of cigarette smoking.	History of cigarette smoking, exposure to noxious inhalants.

---

may have hypertensive heart disease or an alcoholic cardiomyopathy, respectively, as the etiology.

Orthopnea is due to increased venous return (preload) on lying down and is relieved by elevating the head and upper torso. The number of pillows used by the patient to prop himself or herself up at night (e.g., 2–3 pillow orthopnea) is a good way to semi-quantify the degree of breathlessness. Some patients may even have to sleep sitting up in a chair or recliner. PND, due to fluid accumulation in the lungs resulting from the reabsorption of dependent edema that has developed during the day, occurs after the patient has been asleep for a few hours. He or she suddenly awakens with breathlessness ("gasping for air"), and gets up and out of bed, often to open a window for relief. Sometimes the episode is accompanied by coughing, wheezing (*cardiac asthma*), or even a smothering sensation. Dyspnea with bending over (*bendopnea*) has also been described with CHF. A rare form of dyspnea referred to as *trepopnea* may also occur when the patient lies on his or her left side (due to distortions of the great vessels) and is relieved by turning to the right side.

DOE as a sole symptom (i.e., without chest discomfort) may signify an anginal equivalent in the patient with CAD, and, conversely, nocturnal angina (occurring alone or in association with PND) may be a manifestation of CHF. The prophylactic use of sublingual nitroglycerin often improves DOE due to ischemia, and acts as a therapeutic trial that may help establish the correct diagnosis.

Shortness of breath coincident with palpitations should direct the practitioner to search for those cardiac conditions in

---

FIGURE 1-9

New York Heart Association Functional Status Classification

Class I	No limitation to exercise tolerance. No symptoms with usual activities of daily living. (Can play singles tennis)
Class II	Mild limitation of exercise tolerance. Symptoms with ordinary exertion. (Has to play doubles tennis)
Class III	Moderate limitation of exercise tolerance. Symptoms with minimal exertion. (Can barely make it onto the tennis court)
Class IV	Severe limitation of exercise tolerance. Symptoms, e.g., chest pain or dyspnea at rest. (Has to be in bed)

---

which abnormalities in atrial contraction or rapid heart rate are hemodynamically significant. For instance, atrial fibrillation alone may be asymptomatic, but if there is a history of SOB, be alert that there may also be a noncompliant hypertrophied LV where the loss of the normal "atrial kick" of atrial contraction may decrease cardiac output (i.e., the amount of blood pumped by the ventricles each minute) as much as 30%.

Tachycardia alone normally may not produce shortness of breath but may do so in a situation, e.g. rheumatic mitral stenosis (MS), where a decreased diastolic filling time due to tachycardia also reduces cardiac output.

Some patients may not recognize, or even may misinterpret subtle manifestations of CHF. They attribute their shortness of breath and lack of stamina to "growing old" or "being out of shape". A dry, non-productive cough may be an early subtle complaint in left heart failure. A nocturnal cough, and rarely hemoptysis, mark the appearance of alveolar edema as severe CHF develops.

Cheyne-Stokes respiration, characterized by alternating periods of rapid, deep breathing and periods of slow breathing with pauses (apnea) may also occur (especially in the elderly). If the patient (especially older) is not under the influence of a sedative or narcotic and there is no significant cerebral hemisphere deficit (where Cheyne-Stokes respiration may also occur), the presence of Cheyne-Stokes respiration provides a valuable clue to advanced CHF. The patient's spouse will often observe periods of quiet breathing or even apnea and become quite alarmed and therefore may bring this to your attention. These episodes are seldom complained of by the patient. Another possibility to keep in mind is obstructive sleep apnea, often accompanied by loud snoring, with intermittent obstruction of the oropharynx by the tongue and oropharyngeal muscles. Massively obese patients may also have periodic hypoventilation followed by hyperventilation (*obesity hypoventilation syndrome*).

Some patients with CHF state that it "feels like a cold" with congestion, wheezing ("*cardiac asthma*") or coughing during exercise or even at rest. Remember the old adage that "all that wheezes is not asthma". Young patients presenting with dilated cardiomyopathy, a condition where there is ventricular dilation with little hypertrophy (commonly due to viral infection, inflammation, alcohol or other drugs, or hereditary, endocrine or neuromuscular factors) may be mistakenly diagnosed with "bronchitis" when the initial symptoms are dyspnea, wheezing and cough.

Acute pulmonary edema can develop suddenly with extreme dyspnea and pink, frothy, blood-tinged sputum. The presentation of acute CHF or "flash" pulmonary edema should initiate the search for a precipitant (e.g., acute MI, a hypertensive crisis, or acute valvular regurgitation). It is not always recognized that acute pulmonary edema may be the first manifestation of CAD (particularly in the absence of chest pain). If significant new or worsening MR is present, it is likely related to ischemic papillary muscle dysfunction and/or acute LV contractile dysfunction. A ruptured chordae tendineae or perforated mitral or aortic valve cusp (due to infective endocarditis) may also cause acute CHF or pulmonary edema. Sudden dyspnea, pleuritic chest pain,

cough, and hemoptysis can also be secondary to pulmonary emboli, which often may occur in patients with CHF.

Dyspnea (with or without fatigue, chest pain or syncope) may represent the initial clinical manifestation of idiopathic (primary) pulmonary hypertension. A high index of suspicion is essential to make this diagnosis, especially in young, otherwise healthy-appearing women (often with Raynaud's phenomenon), or in those who are obese and have taken anorexigenic agents (e.g., Phen-fen) in the past.

Taking a careful drug history may also provide valuable clues to the etiology of dyspnea. For example, the antiarrhythmic drug amiodarone may cause shortness of breath as a result of pulmonary fibrosis. Anemia, induced by GI blood loss from aspirin or non-steroidal antiinflammatory drugs (NSAIDs), can also aggravate CHF and cause symptoms of shortness of breath. Progressive dyspnea in a patient with a history of catheter ablation for atrial fibrillation may be a clue to pulmonary vein stenosis.

Other symptoms may also occur with shortness of breath and provide clues as to the origin of the problem (**Figure 1-10**). Symptoms of right heart failure occur relatively late. The patient often complains of fluid accumulation or swelling (edema) of the feet, ankles and legs ("my shoes feel too tight"), unexplained weight gain, an increase in abdominal girth (ascites), upper abdominal bloating or discomfort, and nausea (due to systemic venous congestion), extreme weakness, and a change in mental status (due to a diminished cardiac output).

Formation of increased volumes of urine during sleep when the patient is recumbent (*nocturia*) is common in early CHF due to increased preload to the heart when the patient is flat that improves cardiac output and renal perfusion. Some patients may report a decrease in urine output in the days preceding an exacerbation of CHF. Note that swelling of the ankles (peripheral edema) does not always imply right (and/or left) heart failure. More often than not, it is the result of local venous pathology (e.g., chronic venous stasis, thrombophlebitis), obesity, hepatic disease (e.g., cirrhosis) and/or renal disease (e.g., nephrotic syndrome), or a medication side effect, e.g., calcium channel blockers that may cause fluid retention.

When eliciting a history for clues to the possibility of thrombophlebitis, a simple, but rewarding trick is to misdirect your patient. For example, if while you are examining your patient's legs (for signs of heat, tenderness, erythema, and swelling), you divert attention from the fact that your fingers are palpating their calf region by asking a distracting question, and your patient stops in the middle of answering you, and says "Ouch! that hurts", this may be a clue to the diagnosis of thrombophlebitis. Conversely, had attention not been diverted, but instead focused on the palpation of the calves by

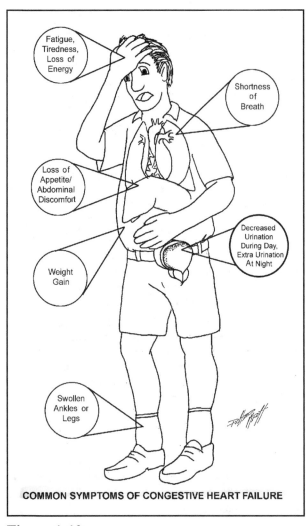

COMMON SYMPTOMS OF CONGESTIVE HEART FAILURE

Figure 1-10

your asking "does it hurt when I do this?", the answer "yes" would be more difficult to evaluate. (Likewise, when asking your patient about chest pain, it is often helpful to inquire in the reverse, i.e., "Does the pain get better when you exercise?" The answer will often be more reliable when the patient stops to think and answers: "No, in fact, it gets worse!")

Persistent edema may occur in the legs from which saphenous veins were harvested at the time of coronary artery bypass graft (CABG) surgery. When ankle swelling (classified on a scale of 1 to 4 as trace to severe) or ascites are visible manifestations of right heart failure, as much as 5 to 10 pounds of fluid may have accumulated. Ascites is especially frequent in patients with constrictive pericarditis, sometimes occurring before peripheral edema becomes apparent. Characteristically, the peripheral edema of CHF is "pitting" (i.e. an indentation may be left in the skin after

pressure is applied) and commonly occurs in the ankles and legs. The edema is exacerbated by prolonged standing (i.e., worse at the end of the day), and improves after lying down. Individuals who have been bedridden, however, may manifest edema over the sacrum and inner thighs since edema fluid tends to settle in these dependent regions under the influence of gravity.

FATIGUE AND WEAKNESS

Like effort dyspnea, fatigue and weakness are not specific for heart disease. Other possible causes include anemia, hypothyroidism, various infections, a disordered sleep pattern, medication side effects, and depression. When fatigue relates to heart disease, it is usually constant (i.e., even at rest), and may provide a clue to a depressed cardiac output state, as may be seen in patients with advanced CHF and severe mitral regurgitation (MR) with cardiac decompensation. Many patients state that they "go to bed tired and get up tired". *As CHF worsens, fatigue or decreased effort tolerance may replace dyspnea as the major complaint*. Patients with diminished cardiac output may become mentally confused and disoriented (particularly the elderly).

Fatigue, as a medication side effect, may result if vigorous diuresis (resulting in volume and/or potassium depletion) or profound hypotension occurs following treatment for hypertension and CHF. Beta-blockers and calcium channel blockers (used to treat patients with a variety of heart diseases) also may cause fatigue and lethargy. In some patients with extensive CAD, severe fatigue related to effort (perceived as a sense of weakness or heaviness in the extremities) may result from transient global myocardial ischemia (an anginal equivalent). At times, excessive fatigue and feelings of general malaise may represent premonitory clues to a future coronary event. *Fatigue can be an "anginal equivalent"*.

COUGH AND HEMOPTYSIS

Acute cough usually is caused by viral or bacterial upper respiratory infection. Chronic cough (i.e., persisting for more than 3 weeks) commonly results from asthma, gastroesophageal reflux disease (GERD), post-nasal drip, chronic bronchitis, bronchiectasis, cigarette smoking or bronchogenic carcinoma. Persistent cough may also be psychogenic. *Cough due to cardiac disease most often is dry, non-productive and is noted in the recumbent position and nocturnally*. Patients may complain of paroxysmal cough instead of the more typical symptoms of orthopnea and PND. It is often a clue to the presence of pulmonary venous hypertension secondary to left heart failure. In these patients, dyspnea often precedes the cough whereas in those with chronic pulmonary disease, cough and expectoration usually precede dyspnea. A chronic, dry non-productive cough may also be a side effect of the angiotensin-converting enzyme (ACE) inhibitor (in up to 20% of patients) being used as treatment for an underlying heart condition (e.g., hypertension, CHF). ACE inhibitor-induced cough is paroxysmal, unrelated to posture, and can vary from a mild tickle to a severe symptom. The cough generally improves within a few days after discontinuation of the drug, and a trial off ACE inhibition allows differentiation of medication side effect from worsening CHF or other causes.

Hemoptysis may accompany cough when pulmonary venous pressures are greatly elevated (as in severe left heart failure or mitral stenosis). Pink, frothy sputum may be produced during acute pulmonary edema. A myriad of pulmonary diseases e.g., chronic bronchitis, bronchiectasis, respiratory infection, and lung tumor can also cause hemoptysis, and should always be kept in mind. These problems are usually easily differentiated from cardiac disease because of their characteristic features.

PALPITATIONS

Palpitations refer to a patient's awareness of the heartbeat that occurs with sudden changes in rate, rhythm, and stroke volume (i.e., amount of blood ejected with each LV systolic contraction). Patients may sense extra, skipped, irregular, or rapid heart beats, or a "fluttering", "pounding", or "racing" sensation. Common arrhythmic causes of palpitations include premature atrial or ventricular contractions (PACs, PVCs), supraventricular tachycardia (SVT–a rapid heart beat driven by an ectopic pacemaker site above the ventricles), atrial fibrillation, ventricular tachycardia (VT), and sinus tachycardia. Although awareness of the heartbeat may suggest an abnormality of cardiac rhythm, the subjective complaint of palpitations is not always associated with an arrhythmia (as determined by ambulatory ECG monitoring).

Palpitations and the concern it evokes are a common reason for consultation. Other than atrial fibrillation, the luxury of evaluating the patient during a symptomatic episode is rarely afforded to the practitioner. Nevertheless, important clues can be obtained from the clinical history in determining the cause. The nature of onset (gradual vs. sudden), pulse rate and regularity should be specifically sought. Many patients have taken their pulse during the episode, or can characterize their rhythm (regular or irregular) and rate (rapid or slow) by tapping it out with their hand.

Figure 1-11. Palpitations described as a "*flip-flop* sensation" or a "*skip*" (something "turned over in my chest") suggest early extra heart beats, either PACs (top) or PVCs (bottom). This usually represents awareness of the more forceful beat that occurs after the pause rather than the premature beat itself. The post-extrasystolic pause may be perceived as an actual cessation of heart beat ("my heart stopped"). Premature ectopic beats occur commonly, both in the presence and absence of heart disease.

Continuous palpitation suggests paroxysmal tachyarrhythmia; *flutters* suggest atrial fibrillation, frequent extrasystoles, or a noncardiac etiology.

Placing your hand over the precordium and moving it up and down (thereby imitating the heart rate and rhythm) can often assist the patient in identifying the nature of his or her palpitation (e.g., normal rate interrupted by a "skip" and pause denotes a premature beat, very rapid rate and regular rhythm signifies paroxysmal supraventricular tachycardia, or rapid and irregularly irregular rhythm a clue to atrial fibrillation). By using this simple hand maneuver, patients can frequently identify the nature of onset and offset (gradual vs. sudden) of the arrhythmia, the rate of tachycardia, regularity or irregularity of rhythm, and the presence or absence of compensatory pauses.

Note that some patients, especially thin, tense individuals with otherwise normal hearts, or those with more severe degrees of aortic regurgitation (AR), are more likely to feel almost every premature beat they have, while others may be totally unaware of frequent or even advanced arrhythmias. Awareness of one's heart beat is most common during periods of inactivity and quiet, e.g., when first lying down at night to go to sleep (especially if lying on the left side).

Patients with more advanced degrees of AR are more likely to be aware of their arrhythmia than those with no heart disease. Patients with advanced AR become accustomed to the "bobbing" up and down of their head ("*yes-yes" sign*"), due to the marked difference between systolic and diastolic pressures. When a premature beat occurs that alters the regular prominent pulsations, the patient is immediately aware but tolerates it. However, if atrial fibrillation is present, producing irregular "bobbing", it can be very bothersome to the patient, and he or she will seek help to alleviate this sensation. Fortunately, most patients with a single aortic valvular lesion (i.e., AR and/or AS) are in normal sinus rhythm. The more advanced degrees of tricuspid regurgitation (TR) can cause systolic movement of the earlobes as well as rightward lateral movement of the head coincident with systole ("*no-no" sign*"), due to backup of venous pressure and lateral systolic distention the jugular vein. Patients are often aware of these neck pulsations (e.g., when shaving, putting on make-up) and may bring this to your attention while you are taking their history.

The slow onset of palpitations correlated with emotional stress or exercise suggests sinus tachycardia. A slow

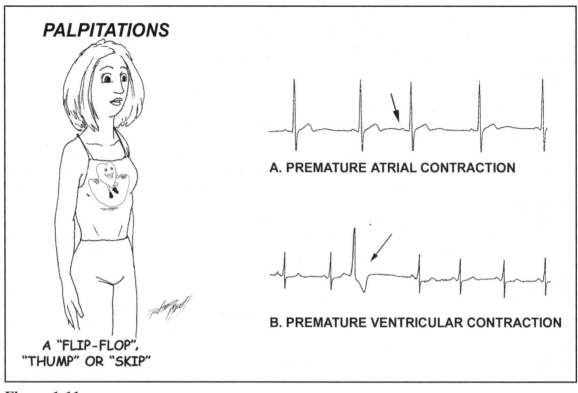

Figure 1-11

regular rhythm in a young person is consistent with sinus bradycardia but may signify acquired heart block in an elderly individual.

The sudden onset of a rapid regular rhythm ("my heart felt like it would jump out of my chest") provides a clue to the diagnosis of supraventricular tachycardia (SVT), especially if the episode can be terminated by vagal maneuvers, e.g., breath holding, inducing gagging, bearing down (Valsalva maneuver), carotid sinus massage, immersing hands in, splashing the face with, or swallowing ice water. Paroxysmal SVT often occurs in young individuals who are otherwise healthy. A history of *Wolff-Parkinson-White (WPW) syndrome* may provide a clue to SVT related to an accessory conduction pathway in the heart.

Note that chest pain may occur with an episode of tachycardia even in patients without coexisting CAD. Patients with VT, however, tend to be older and have underlying heart disease (e.g., CAD, cardiomyopathy). Although VT may or may not be associated with palpitations, prominent cerebral symptoms (e.g., pre-syncope or syncope) often occur.

Palpitations may be associated with the use of tobacco, coffee, tea, alcohol ("*holiday-heart syndrome*"), recreational and/or over-the-counter drugs (including cough and cold remedies), or may be related to hyperthyroidism or advanced pulmonary disease and its treatment.

When palpitations are associated with atypical chest pain and hyperventilation syndrome, the practitioner should consider an underlying chronic anxiety state with autonomic nervous system over-activity, or the presence of MVP. Symptoms may be particularly bothersome during introspective moments in these patients rather than during marked physical activity. Some of these patients have a normal heart rate during their complaint of palpitations. These patients may be anxious or are experiencing chest wall muscle twitching that is mistaken for the heart beat.

The consequences of an arrhythmia may differ radically in different patients. For example, an SVT in a young, healthy adult may be well tolerated, while it may precipitate syncope in a patient with valvular AS, shock in a patient with acute MI, pulmonary edema in a patient with rheumatic MS, or hemiparesis in a patient with cerebrovascular disease. Occasionally, polyuria may result (from release of atrial natriuretic peptide) during prolonged SVTs. Chronic, persistent tachycardia may even result in a dilated cardiomyopathy, often reversible if the rapid heart rate is controlled.

DIZZINESS, NEAR-SYNCOPE OR SYNCOPE

Dizziness and/or syncope can be frightening to the patient, accounting for many ED visits and about 6% of all hospital admissions. A carefully obtained history offers important clues to the proper etiologic diagnosis. (**Figure 1-12**) For example, *exertional syncope* may be the first clue to the diagnosis of LV outflow tract obstruction (e.g., severe valvular AS, HOCM), or CAD. Effort syncope in a young female (age 20's-30's) should also raise the suspicion for idiopathic (primary) pulmonary hypertension. Syncope that occurs during prolonged upright posture in a young, otherwise healthy individual may provide a clue to *neurocardiogenic (vasovagal) syncope*, where increased vagal activity causes decreased heart rate and blood pressure. Syncope during shaving, extreme head-turning, or while wearing a tight collar, lends suspicion to the diagnosis of a *hypersensitive carotid sinus*.

Stokes-Adams attacks of cardiac etiology, characterized by abrupt loss of consciousness at rest with rapid return to normal mental status, is caused by inadequate cardiac output secondary to intermittent complete heart block (failure of electrical signals to get through from the atria to the ventricles), > 5 seconds of sinus arrest (failure of the atrial pacemaker to discharge) or ventricular tachyarrhythmias.

FIGURE 1-12

Clinical Clues To Syncope

Clue	Clinical significance
Prolonged standing, following pain or emotional upset, prodrome of warmth, nausea, sweating, weakness.	Neurocardiogenic (vasovagal) syncope (with hypotension and bradycardia).
Occurring during or immediately after urination, swallowing, defecation, cough.	Situational (neurally-mediated) syncope.
Sudden onset at rest, palpitations, previous history of heart failure.	Dilated cardiomyopathy with ventricular tachycardia.
Arising from supine or sitting to upright position.	Orthostatic hypotension, e.g., from over-medication with anti-hypertensives, volume depletion, acute blood loss. Autonomic dysfunction, e.g., diabetes mellitus, multiple system atrophy (Shy-Drager syndrome).
Exercise-induced, history of angina or MI.	CAD with ventricular arrhythmia (LV aneurysm)
Occurring during or shortly after exercise. Associated with exertional related chest pain and/or dyspnea.	Valvular aortic stenosis.
Exercise-induced, family history of syncope and/or sudden death. Occurring while bearing down (Valsalva maneuver).	Hypertrophic obstructive cardiomyopathy.
Exertional-related, young female with shortness of breath, chest pain, fatigue.	Idiopathic (primary) pulmonary hypertension.
Young, anxious female with atypical chest pain, palpitations.	Mitral valve prolapse (neurocardiogenic, arrhythmic).
Occurring with shaving, tight collar, sudden head turning.	Hypersensitive carotid sinus (with bradycardia and/or hypotension).
Changing position, e.g., rolling over in bed.	Atrial myxoma (intermittent obstruction of heart valve).
After upper extremity exercise.	Subclavian steal syndrome (shunting of blood away from brain via vertebrobasilar system).

A history of dizziness or syncope occurring immediately after termination and not during the rapid palpitations, strongly suggests the *tachy-bradycardia syndrome,* where the sinoatrial node pacemaker is suppressed after a period of rapid tachycardia, causing a profound bradycardia. In *sick sinus syndrome* the SA node undergoes periods of dysfunction in which there may be syncope due to significant bradycardia. A lack of altered consciousness, though, cannot be taken as reassurance of the benignity of an arrhythmia.

The presence of an underlying disease can often serve as a clue to the nature of a rhythm disorder. A prior history of CAD, MI, dilated cardiomyopathy, or CHF of any etiology should lead the clinician to suspect a lethal ventricular arrhythmia.

A meticulous history of the patient's medications is very important. Many drugs can affect cardiac rhythm. Medications, e.g., digitalis (dig toxicity), diuretics (PVCs or VT associated with hypokalemia or hypomagnesemia), anti-arrhythmic agents, psychotropic medications, and certain antihistamines, beta agonists and theophylline can produce a variety of supraventricular and ventricular arrhythmias and should be considered in a patient who presents with palpitations and/or syncope. Administration of some pharmacological agents (e.g., digitalis, beta blockers) may evoke a profound bradycardia which presents as syncope. Nitrates or calcium channel blockers (which produce vasodilation) can aggravate vasodepressor syncope.

The common faint, often associated with fear, the sight of blood (e.g., needle sticks), pain, emotional stress and brief premonitory signs and symptoms, e.g., nausea, abdominal discomfort, yawning, sweating, pallor, diminished hearing or blurred vision, a sense of lightheadedness ("graying out") results from bradycardia and hypotension, caused by excessive vagal discharge (*vasovagal, or neurocardiogenic, syncope*), especially after prolonged upright posture (e.g., standing during religious services, or in a crowded, hot room). Often there is a long antecedent history of similar episodes, especially during adolescence and young adulthood.

Figure 1-13. Causes of neurally-mediated syncope: carotid sinus syncope occurring with **A)** shaving, **B)** wearing a tight collar, **C)** sudden turn of the head; situational syncope occurring during or immediately after **D)** urination, and **E)** vigorous paroxysms of coughing, may result in a long "pause" (ECG strip, bottom) due to transient intense vagotonia with sinus node suppression.

Syncope in the setting of any GI symptoms (e.g., nausea, abdominal cramps, diarrhea) is likely to be vagal in origin.

The long QT syndrome, while rather uncommon, is a potentially hazardous condition with a very unfavorable outcome in many patients who are not adequately diagnosed and treated. The diagnosis is relatively straightforward and does not need to be established by any sophisticated, invasive, or expensive testing. A history of unexplained syncope in a young patient or a strong family history of sudden cardiac death is a clue to the diagnosis of congenital long QT syndrome. Patients (particularly women) with congenital long QT syndrome, are at risk for developing a rapid, chaotic heart beat, a form of VT known as *torsades de pointes* ("twisting of the points"–**Figure 3-48**) and sudden cardiac death. Drugs that can prolong the ECG QT interval—certain antibiotics (e.g., erythromycin), antidepressants, antihistamines, and ironically certain antiarrhythmic drugs, as well as grapefruit juice—place the patient at risk of torsades de pointes and should be avoided.

Intermittent obstruction of a cardiac valve by an intracavitary tumor (*atrial myxoma*) is a rare cause of syncope; it may be precipitated when the patient changes position. However, many normal individuals (especially the elderly) experience transient lightheadedness with rapid changes in position, e.g., after arising from a sitting or supine position (*orthostatic hypotension*). Possible causes of orthostatic hypotension include peripheral neuropathy, autonomic dysfunction (e.g., diabetes mellitus), volume depletion and medication side effects (e.g., antihypertensive agents–particularly alpha blockers).

It is important to try to differentiate syncope (transient loss of consciousness) from seizure (convulsions). Primary fainting episodes, however, can cause convulsions in a significant number of cases. Although seizures are generally caused by abnormal bursts of electrical activity in the brain, they can also occur when the brain is starved of blood and oxygen (due to syncope). A seizure without typical postictal symptoms (confusion, disorientation, agitation) may provide a clue to hypotension caused by an arrhythmia or vasovagal syncope. A history taken from a family member or witness can help. Patients who do not respond to anti-seizure medication, therefore, should be evaluated for an alternate cardiac-related diagnosis.

Generally speaking, though, if your patient has a syncopal episode, think cardiovascular, not brain. In 50% of cases of syncope, a careful detailed cardiac clinical examination will establish the underlying cause. Cardiac causes are numerous, and include arrhythmias and/or conduction disturbances, valvular AS, HOCM, idiopathic (primary) pulmonary hypertension, atrial myxoma, etc. Investigations for neurologic causes, e.g., carotid ultrasound, EEG, CT, or MRI of the head, should not be performed routinely. Much valuable time is wasted searching for a neurologic cause which does not exist. You can usually avoid this mistake by focusing your clinical tools on obtaining an accurate history.

When the heart is structurally normal, especially in young adults, neurocardiogenic (vasovagal) syncope is

What is syncope?
What are causes?

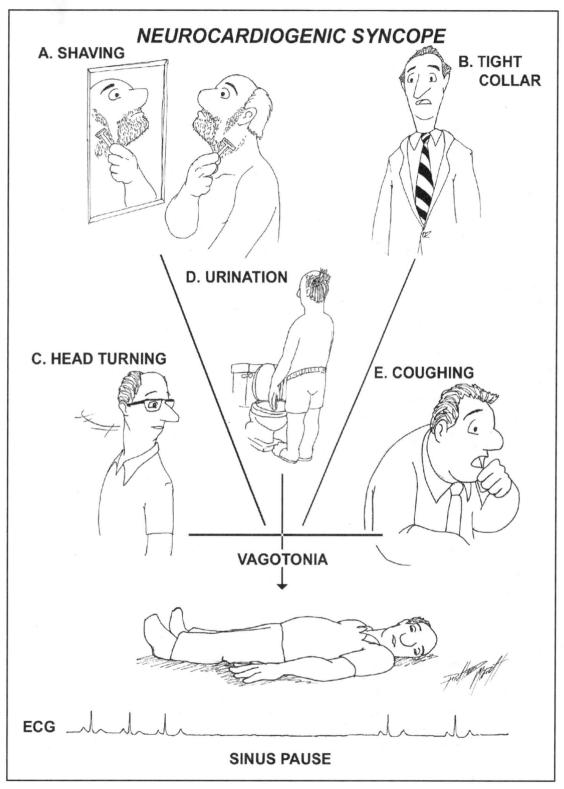

Figure 1-13

most common and almost always occurs when the patient is in the upright position. Keep in mind that the diagnosis of neurocardiogenic syncope is based on the history and the exclusion of organic cardiovascular pathology.

If the patient's symptoms appear to be postural, inquire about the use of antihypertensive or antianginal therapy and other drugs which may induce orthostatic hypotension. These iatrogenic causes of syncope can be remedied promptly without the need for exhaustive and expensive work-up or treatment. Patients have received unneeded pacemakers when a simple switch in medications instead would have sufficed.

OTHER SYMPTOMS

Fever, Chills, and Sweats

Fever, chills and sweats in any patient with a new or pre-existing heart murmur should lead one to suspect infective endocarditis. A history of valvular heart disease is not a prerequisite since previously normal valves can become infected. Regurgitant murmurs from chordal rupture or valve perforation and/or damage predominate in acute infective endocarditis and are important harbingers of CHF. A history of recent dental work, indwelling intravascular catheter, or illicit drug use (all potential causes of bacteremia) strengthens the suspicion. Fever may accompany pericarditis and on occasion an acute MI. A low-grade fever in a patient with CHF may be a sign of pulmonary emboli. Rarely an intracardiac tumor (myxoma) may produce such symptoms in the absence of infection. A profuse "cold sweat" often accompanies the early stages of acute MI. Excessive diaphoresis may also occur in patients with severe AR.

Gastrointestinal Symptoms

As previously mentioned, many patients with CAD (i.e., angina pectoris, acute MI) erroneously attribute their symptoms to the GI tract (e.g., "indigestion", "heartburn"). Conversely, pain of GI origin (e.g., reflux esophagitis, esophageal spasm, hiatal hernia) may mimic cardiac pain and may radiate from the upper epigastrium to the substernal area, the upper chest, the throat, and the arms. The discomfort with a GI etiology is worse on lying flat or on stooping, but as a general rule is unrelated to exertional activities and is not usually associated with diaphoresis or shortness of breath.

- Nausea and vomiting frequently occur during an acute MI (especially inferior).
- Anorexia, nausea and vomiting may also occur as a result of medication side effects (e.g., digitalis toxicity).

- Hepatomegaly associated with tricuspid valve disease or severe right heart failure may cause right upper quadrant and epigastric pain and fullness as well as anorexia, nausea, and early satiety.
- Abdominal discomfort due to mesenteric ischemia and/or infarction may occur in a patient with a very low cardiac output or from an embolic event.
- GI bleeding from angiodysplastic lesions (vascular malformations) of the stomach, duodenum or right colon may occur in patients with valvular AS due to mechanical disruption of von Willebrand molecules as they cross the stenotic aortic valve.

Embolic Symptoms

An embolic event may be the presenting manifestation of underlying heart disease. Blood clots may occur in the LA behind a stenotic mitral valve, within an LV aneurysm, in the ventricle of a patient with a cardiomyopathy, on a prosthetic valve, or in the leg veins and travel through a patent foramen ovale (paradoxical embolism). Emboli may also occur in atrial fibrillation. Symptoms of a *TIA or stroke* occur with emboli to the cerebral vessels; an *acute MI* may result from an embolus to a coronary artery; *hematuria and flank pain* may arise from embolization to a renal artery; and a *pale, cold, painful extremity* may result from an embolic obstruction to an arm or a leg artery. Emboli from vegetations of infective endocarditis may produce characteristic areas of necrosis in the fingers or toes. Severe extensive atherosclerosis in the abdominal aorta and iliac vessels can be responsible for showers of peripheral cholesterol emboli with multiple small reddish-blue lesions on the lower extremities, sometimes causing small areas of cutaneous gangrene ("*trash toes*"), so-called "*purple-toe syndrome*".

Intermittent Claudication

A history of pain or aching in one or both calves, thighs, or buttocks, exacerbated by walking a certain distance (*intermittent claudication*), suggests peripheral vascular disease with a poor blood supply to the affected muscles. Severe obstruction of the lower leg arteries may give rise to rest pain and skin necrosis. Claudication of calf muscles is a clue to obstruction of flow in the femoropopliteal arteries, whereas claudication in the thighs and/or buttocks suggest that aortoiliac disease is present. The most important risk factors are cigarette smoking, hyperlipidemia, and diabetes mellitus. A history of vascular disease elsewhere (e.g., CAD, cerebrovascular disease) is common.

Changes in Weight

Recent, rapid weight gain suggests fluid retention due to *CHF*. Although weight loss may be a sign of underlying malignancy, it may also reflect cardiac cachexia (related to a low cardiac output), digitalis toxicity or hyperthyroidism. Unusual weight loss, palpitations and heat intolerance suggest the possibly of thyrotoxicosis. Aggravation or precipitation of angina pectoris in patients with thyrotoxicosis is common. Often weight loss is the only symptom of hyperthyroidism in the elderly patient presenting with atrial fibrillation. Cold intolerance, fatigue and unexplained weight gain may suggest the possibility of hypothyroidism. Many overweight individuals have tried various obesity drugs, e.g., *Phen-fen,* which has been associated with pulmonary hypertension and possible valvular regurgitation (due to fibroplastic changes of valvular endocardium).

NONCARDIAC CONDITIONS AND DRUG HISTORY

Many noncardiac conditions can affect the heart, and many important clues to heart disease may be found outside the cardiovascular system. For example:

- A history of a prior malignancy, connective tissue disease, thyroid disorder, or renal failure, may explain pericarditis, a pericardial effusion, or cardiac tamponade.
- A history of treatment with chemotherapeutic agents (e.g., adriamycin) may provide an etiologic clue to cardiomyopathy and CHF, and mediastinal radiation to acute or constrictive pericarditis or coronary artery obstruction with acute MI.
- A history of human immunodeficiency virus (HIV) infection may explain the presence of a pericardial effusion, dilated cardiomyopathy, pulmonary hypertension, dyslipidemia, and accelerated CAD (which may in part be due to lipid abnormalities induced by antiretroviral therapy, particularly protease inhibitors, or by the virus itself).
- A history of anxiety and panic attacks, especially in young women, accompanied by dizziness, syncope, palpitations, "atypical" chest pain, dyspnea, chronic fatigue, and orthostatic intolerance, may provide a clue to autonomic dysfunction (dysautonomia), and the presence of mitral valve prolapse syndrome.
- A history of sudden emotional or physical stress, especially in postmenopausal women, may explain an acute reversible cardiomyopathy characterized by transient balloon-like LV apical dysfunction, typically in the absence of CAD with clinical features that mimic acute MI, known as *stress cardiomyopathy,*

broken heart syndrome, or *takotsubo cardiomyopathy* (named after the round-bottomed, narrow-necked Japanese fishing pot used for trapping octopus, that has a similar configuration to LV apical ballooning).
- Aggravation or precipitation of angina pectoris in patients with CAD is common in those patients (especially the elderly) with a history of hyperthyroidism (or in whom thyroid medication is initiated or increased). Patients with hypothyroidism, on the other hand, may present with fatigue and lethargy, along with abnormal ECG findings e.g., sinus bradycardia and low voltage (due to pericardial effusion) and significant serum lipid abnormalities.

Taking a careful drug history may also provide valuable clues:

- *Amiodarone* can cause abnormal (hyper or hypo) thyroid function as well as shortness of breath (*pulmonary fibrosis*).
- Certain agents e.g., estrogens, NSAIDs, fludrocortisone (Florinef), thioglitazones (Avandia, Actos), and minoxidil (Loniten), may cause fluid retention.
- Appetite suppressant medications e.g., Phen-fen, previously used in the treatment of obesity, may cause pulmonary hypertension, MR and AR.
- Anemia induced by GI blood loss from aspirin or NSAIDs can aggravate angina and CHF, and can accentuate the intensity of various cardiac murmurs. Remember that some of the symptoms of CHF (e.g., fatigue, shortness of breath) may also be found in the anemic patient.
- Cyclooxygenase-2 (COX-2) inhibitors, e.g., rofecoxib (Vioxx) and valdecoxib (Bextra), which have been withdrawn from the U.S. market, and celecoxib (Celebrex), used in the treatment of arthritis and pain syndromes, may have prothrombotic effects (since they decrease production of prostacyclin which has vasodilatory and antithrombotic properties) and may increase the risk of MI and stroke.
- Antiretroviral therapy, particularly protease inhibitors, used in the treatment of HIV/AIDS may be associated with dyslipidemia and the potential for accelerated CAD.
- Testosterone therapy, used in the treatment of "low T", has recently been linked to an increased risk of MI and stroke, particularly in older men and younger men with a history of cardiovascular disease.

CHAPTER 2.   THE CARDIAC PHYSICAL EXAM

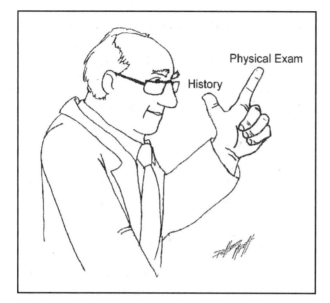

Once an initial working hypothesis has been formulated based on the clinical history, the cardiac physical exam can then be conducted to either confirm or refute the presumptive diagnosis. On occasion, a patient may be asymptomatic, and the diagnosis is made solely on the basis of the physical exam. While *auscultation* generally comes to mind first, and is immensely important, it is only one part of the complete cardiac physical examination, and is most rewarding when combined with the clues gleaned from a careful *inspection* (general appearance, jugular venous pulse*)*, and *palpation* (arterial pulse and blood pressure, precordial movements) of the cardiac patient.

   Figure 2-1 summarizes a systematic clinical method of performing the cardiac physical examination.

CARDIAC ANATOMY AND PHYSIOLOGY

A knowledge of normal cardiac anatomy and function is an essential requisite for performing and interpreting the cardiac physical examination, and for understanding the pathophysiologic alterations that can affect the heart.

   Figure 2-2. Cardiac external anatomy.
   Figure 2-3. Blood flow within the heart
   Figure 2-4. The anatomic relationship between the visceral and parietal pericardium (From Goldberg, S. Clinical Anatomy Made Ridiculously Simple, MedMaster, Inc. 2002).

External Anatomy of the Heart and Great Vessels

The heart is a four-chambered muscular organ whose function is to propel blood forward to the tissues in an amount that meets the metabolic needs of the body. It is horizontally and asymmetrically positioned in the mediastinum, between the two pleural cavities, one-third to the right and two-thirds to the left of the sternum. The top of the heart, called the base, is formed by the right and left atria. It roughly refers to the region of the great vessels (i.e., the proximal aorta and pulmonary artery) which lie just below the second rib at the upper right and left sternal borders. The tip of the heart, called the apex, is formed by the tip of the left ventricle and rests on the upper surface of the diaphragm. It is tilted forward, downward, and to the left, and can be palpated on the chest wall near the left nipple at the fifth left intercostal space in the mid clavicular line. The clinical expressions "located best at the 'apex' or the 'base'" during the cardiac physical exam refer to these areas.

   The right ventricle is the most anterior structure of the heart. It lies just below the sternum and can best be felt along the lower left sternal border. The right atrium lies superior and posterior to the right ventricle. The left ventricle is a posterolateral structure with only approximately one-fourth of the total mass visible in the anterior view. The left atrium is an entirely posterior structure and lies in front of the thoracic aorta, esophagus, and vertebral column (**Figure 2-2**).

Cardiac Chambers and Blood Flow through the Heart

The right and left atria are divided by the interatrial septum, which contains the fossa ovalis. These relatively thin-walled low pressure chambers serve as volume reservoirs that collect blood and deliver it to their respective ventricles. The right atrium receives deoxygenated blood returning from the body through the superior and inferior vena cavae, and from the heart through the coronary sinus, and then passes it along through the tricuspid valve into the right ventricle during diastole. The left atrium receives oxygen-rich blood from the lungs through the four pulmonary veins and delivers it through the mitral valve to the left ventricle. At the end of diastole, atrial contraction forcefully primes the left ventricle with up to 30% of blood for ventricular output ("atrial kick").

   The right and left ventricles serve as the main pumping chambers of the heart. They are separated from each other by the interventricular septum, which is composed of a thick muscular portion at the bottom, and a small membranous area at the top. Contraction of the right ventricle during systole propels blood across the pulmonic valve via the main pulmonary artery and its branches into the low-pressure, low-resistance pulmonary circulation and then to

FIGURE 2-1

Cardiac Physical Examination
A Systematic Approach

Basic Concepts

- Try to secure, if possible, a well-lighted, quiet, private exam area.
- Examine patient in supine, left lateral decubitus, upright, standing and squatting positions (when appropriate).
- Perform exam from patient's right side.
- Find recorded vital signs (or do them yourself - after all, they are vital!)

Inspect General Appearance of the Patient

- Overall assessment of the patient.
- Symptomatic status (does the patient look well or unwell? Check for respiratory distress, anguished facial expression, cachexia).
- State of circulation, e.g., pallor, cyanosis, clubbing (in congenital heart disease with R to L shunt), diaphoresis (sympathetic discharge), cold clammy skin, altered sensorium, dusky cyanosis (in shock).
- Body habitus, facies, gestures, skin color, and texture. Check for signs of noncardiac disease states and/or conditions, e.g., eye signs (exophthalmos, lid lag, stare) in hyperthyroidism—associated with atrial fibrillation, high output CHF; thick hide-bound skin in scleroderma— associated with cardiomyopathy, cor pulmonale; flushing attacks in carcinoid—associated with right heart valve lesions; joint manifestations of rheumatoid arthritis—associated with aortic root disease and AR; body habitus in Marfan's syndrome— associated with aortic dissection, AR, MVP; morbid obesity (Pickwickian syndrome)—associated with systemic and pulmonary hypertension.

Examination of Arterial Pulse and Pressure

- Palpate radial arterial pulse. Feel for rate and rhythm, pulse volume and contour (e.g., pulsus alternans, quick rise pulse, slow rise pulse, pulsus paradoxus). Palpate all arterial pulses (e.g., carotid, brachial, femoral, abdominal aorta, dorsalis pedis, posterior tibial). Check for radial-femoral delay (coarctation of the aorta), decreased or absent pulses (peripheral vascular disease, aortic dissection). Listen for bruits.
- Take BP measurement. Check BP in both arms (especially if dissection suspected). Evaluate for wide pulse pressure, orthostatic hypotension, pulsus paradoxus. Compare BP in arms and legs (if coarctation of the aorta or peripheral arterial disease is suspected).

Examination of Jugular Venous Pressure and Pulse

- Examine neck veins. Inspect right internal jugular vein (the external jugular can be obstructed and is unreliable). Assess JVP, normal and abnormal wave forms (a,v,x,y), positive or negative abdominojugular test. Look for change with inspiration (Kussmaul's sign).

Inspect and Palpate the Precordium

- Inspect precordium for scars, deformity, visible pulsation, and pacemakers and/or defibrillators. Check for LV apical impulse (PMI) location and character, e.g., forceful and sustained (valvular AS, hypertension), inferolaterally displaced (AR, MR), abnormal precordial pulsations, e.g., ectopic lift (ventricular aneurysm), triple ripple (HOCM), presystolic (S4) and early diastolic (S3) distention. Palpate with heel of hand for parasternal (RV) heaves, and with palm of hand for palpable thrills (loud murmurs).

Cardiac Auscultation

- Use the "inching" technique to time heart sounds and murmurs. Listen for normal and abnormal heart sounds and cardiac murmurs (systolic, diastolic, continuous), and pericardial friction rubs. Employ dynamic auscultation, e.g., effect of respiration (right-sided events), sitting, standing, squatting, Valsalva maneuver (HOCM, MVP).

Examine the Lungs

- Auscultate for rales (crackles), wheezes, decreased breath sounds (pleural effusions) - signs of CHF.

Examine the Abdomen

- Feel for palpable hepatomegaly (RV failure, and check if it is pulsatile (TR). Look for ascites, splenomegaly (infective endocarditis), and an aortic aneurysm. Listen for renal bruits (renal artery stenosis-hypertension).

Examine the Extremities

- Check for signs of peripheral vascular disease, peripheral edema, thrombophlebitis, clubbing, xanthomas, stigmata of infective endocarditis (e.g., splinter, hemorrhages, Osler's nodes, Janeway lesions) varicose veins (particularly relevant if CABG planned).

Special Examination, e.g., Eyes (fundi)

- Check for hypertensive and/or diabetic retinopathy, Roth's spots (in endocarditis), xanthelasma and corneal arcus (hyperlipidemia).

-look at pt - look
speak
breathing

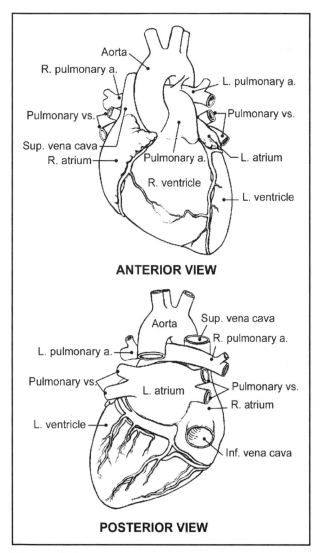

ANTERIOR VIEW

POSTERIOR VIEW

Figure 2-2

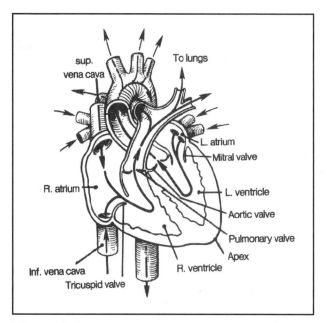

Figure 2-3

the lungs, where it absorbs ("picks up") oxygen and releases ("drops off") carbon dioxide. Contraction of the much thicker walled left ventricle pumps the oxygenated blood across the aortic valve into the high pressure, high resistance systemic circulation through the aorta and out to the rest of the body (**Figure 2-3**).

The Heart Valves

In the normal heart there are four major heart valves, attached to and supported by a fibrous cardiac skeleton, that serve as one-way doors that keep blood flowing in a forward direction, preventing backward leakage (regurgitation) from one chamber to another. These valves are divided into two main types according to their structure:

two semilunar valves (aortic and pulmonic) and two atrioventricular valves (mitral and tricuspid). They open and close in response to pressure gradients, i.e., open when pressure in the preceding chamber is higher and close when the gradient reverses. The closing of the valves creates the heart sounds heard through the stethoscope during cardiac auscultation (see below).

The funnel-shaped mitral valve (located between the left atrium and left ventricle) has two cusps or leaflets (anteromedial and posterolateral), and the tricuspid valve has three cusps (anterior, posterior, and septal). The cusps are attached to the papillary muscles in the heart wall by thin, string-like fibers called chordae tendineae. These chords of fibrous tissue descend on the papillary muscle, as if from an inverted parachute, and work together to keep the leaflets from bulging backward into the atria during ventricular contraction (systole) thereby preventing the backflow of blood.

The aortic valve (located between the left ventricle and the aorta) and the pulmonic valve (situated between the right ventricle and the pulmonary artery) each have three pocket-like cusps, but do not have chordae. The pulmonic valve is composed of an anterior, right, and left cusp, and the aortic valve, a right (coronary), left (coronary), and posterior (non-coronary) cusp that are associated with corresponding outpouchings of the aorta, called the sinuses of Valsalva. These valves open due to pressure within their respective ventricles and close due to the back pressure of blood in the great vessels, which pushes the cusps closed.

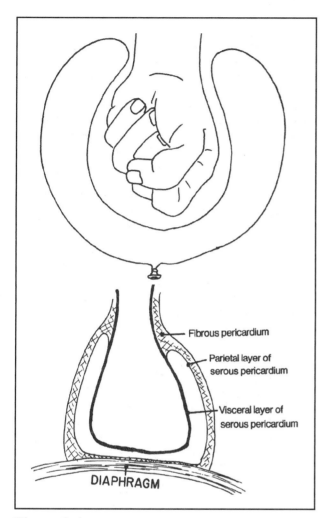

Fibrous pericardium

Parietal layer of serous pericardium

Visceral layer of serous pericardium

DIAPHRAGM

Figure 2-4

Structure of the Heart Wall

The surface of the heart valves and interior surface of the cardiac chambers are lined by a single layer of endothelial cells called the endocardium. The heart's muscular middle layer, the myocardium, has contractile properties, and makes up the largest portion of the cardiac wall. The epicardium is the outermost layer of the heart.

A fibroserous sac called the pericardium surrounds the heart and roots of the great vessels. It consists of two layers, a strong outer fibrous layer and an inner serosal layer. The inner serosal layer adheres to the outer surface of the heart and is termed the visceral pericardium (also called the epicardium). The outer parietal layer lines the inner aspect of the fibrous pericardium and is called the parietal pericardium. The parietal pericardium has attachments to the sternum, vertebral column, and diaphragm, which serve to stabilize the heart in the chest.

The relationship of the two surfaces of the pericardium can be understood by visualizing a fist thrust into a balloon filled with air (**Figure 2-4**). The surface in direct contact with the fist is analogous to the visceral pericardium, while the outer layer of the balloon is similar in position to the parietal pericardium. The pericardial space separates the visceral and parietal layers and contains a small amount (20–30 ml) of thin, clear pericardial fluid that lubricates the two surfaces and cushions the heart, thereby allowing it to move freely within the pericardial sac and easily change volume and size during contraction.

Basic Cardiac Function

In a healthy individual, the *cardiac output* (CO), the amount of blood ejected from the heart per minute, is equal to the product of the *stroke volume* (SV), the volume of blood ejected from the ventricle with each contraction, and the *heart rate* (HR) (CO = SV x HR). To maintain adequate cardiac output, the heart must adjust either frequency of beating (heart rate) or the volume ejected (stroke volume). Stroke volume is dependent on a complex interplay of three major factors: *preload* (volume of blood or pressure in the ventricles when diastole ends); *afterload,* or impedance (pressure or resistance against which the ventricle must strain to eject blood); and ventricular *contractility* (inotropic state of the myocardium). Stroke volume is calculated as the difference between the end-diastolic volume (EDV) within the left ventricle and the residual end-systolic volume (ESV) of blood within the ventricle following contraction (EDV–ESV). A comparison of stroke volume to end-diastolic volume (SV/EDV) is the fraction of blood ejected from the ventricle with each beat, known as the *ejection fraction* (normal range = 55–75%), and is the most commonly available measure of cardiac function.

INSPECTION

General Appearance

A trained observer can gain much valuable information from simple observation and often make a "spot diagnosis" even before the patient is interviewed or examined. In addition, your taking the time to make this appraisal, while greeting and shaking hands with the patient alongside the hospital bed or office examining table, conveys the impression to the patient that you are interested in him or her as a person, not just in the illness itself.

In general, the physical appearance of the cardiac patient reflects three main factors i.e., the patient's *symptomatic status,* the *state of the circulation,* as well as the

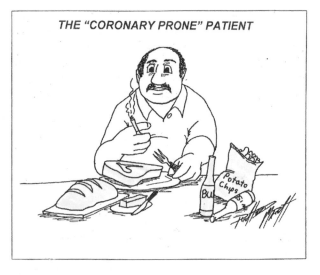

THE "CORONARY PRONE" PATIENT

Note: The typical appearance of the "coronary prone" patient is that of a sedentary, obese, bald, chain-smoking, middle-aged or older male, consuming large amounts of high fat foods, salt, sweetened beverages, and alcohol, with stigmata of underlying risk factors for CAD, e.g., nicotine-stained fingers, yellowish plaques of cholesterol deposits (xanthelasmas) around the eyelids, and a diagonal earlobe crease.

Figure 2-6

myriad noncardiac disease states and/or conditions that may involve the heart. Many valuable clues to heart disease are present in sites well removed from the cardiovascular system. Some of the more common findings that can be visualized "at a glance" are listed in **Figure 2-5.** Keep in mind that the eye often misses what's not in the observer's mind. *You see only what you look for, you recognize only what you know*.

The classic appearance of the *"coronary-prone"* individual is that of a short, balding, overweight, sedentary, chain-smoking middle-aged or older male (or post-menopausal female), consuming large quantities of high-fat, cholesterol-laden foods, with stigmata of underlying risk factors for CAD, e.g., nicotine-stained fingers or teeth (cigarette smoking); cutaneous and tendon xanthomas (especially of the fingers and Achilles tendons); xanthelasmas (yellowish plaques of cholesterol deposits) around the eyelids; and corneal arcus senilis (signs of hyperlipidemia); a diagonal earlobe crease (except in Native and Asian Americans); and perhaps an aggressive, highly-competitive and/or hostile (so-called "type A") personality **(Figure 2-6)**.

In this age of electronic medical records, look at the patient, not just the computer! Watching a patient's body language may impart more information than the actual words he or she speaks. For example, *Levine's sign* **(Figure 1-4)** is a classic and common hand gesture whereby the patient clenches his or her fist over the substernal area to graphically depict the constrictive nature of ischemic chest

discomfort. This so-called "language of the hands" provides a valuable non-verbal clue to the presence of CAD.

The patient with an acute MI may appear restless, anxious, and agitated, often thrashing about in bed in an effort to find a more comfortable position. In contrast, those with exertional-related angina pectoris tend to remain quiet, and sit or stand still in an effort to obtain relief, recognizing that movement may enhance chest pain.

The patient may appear ashen, pale, and profusely diaphoretic with cool and clammy skin (even in the absence of shock) due to vasoconstriction resulting from an intense reaction to increased catecholamine levels. Respiratory distress, characterized by dyspnea, orthopnea, dry nonproductive cough, and wheezing (*"cardiac asthma"*), may dominate the clinical picture when ischemic LV dysfunction and/or significant MR is present. The person may appear tachypneic, sitting bolt upright in bed, gasping and struggling for breath, coughing up frothy pink sputum if acute ("flash") pulmonary edema ensues. Some patients with severe CHF and a poor cardiac output, especially those who are older with underlying cerebrovascular disease (particularly during sleep and/or sedation), manifest a cyclic breathing pattern characterized by hyperpnea alternating with apnea (*Cheyne-Stokes respiration*).

Cardiogenic shock may be the predominant feature, due to extensive impairment of LV function (involving 40% or more of the myocardium) and/or one of the mechanical complications of acute MI, e.g., ventricular septal defect (VSD) or papillary muscle rupture. Then, signs of a low cardiac output and decreased peripheral perfusion, e.g., cold and clammy skin, marked facial pallor, cyanosis of the lips and nail beds, and bluish-red mottling of the extremities, may become evident. The individual may have an altered sensorium resulting from cerebral hypoperfusion.

The practitioner with a trained eye can quickly distinguish between myocardial ischemic pain and musculoskeletal pain and make the diagnosis "at a glance". Chest wall pain, as occurs with anxiety, costochondritis (*Tietze's syndrome*) is a frequent cause of chest pain. Patients usually use a finger to point to the pain of musculoskeletal disorders. The pointing finger of localized left costochondral junction pain or fleeting, inframammary chest pain, coupled with the deep, sighing respiration of emotional distress often provide the clues that the patient's chest pain is noncardiac in origin. Don't forget the nerve root pain of herpes zoster (*shingles*), which may occur before (or even without) a rash. In many cases, this diagnosis is only made in retrospect.

Deviations from the patient's normal mental status should always be aggressively investigated. In the patient

FIGURE 2-5

Clinical Clues to Heart Disease from Inspection

Clue	Clinical significance
Apprehensive, diaphoretic, with clenched fist ("Levine's sign"), and sudden labored respirations	CAD and acute LV failure
Sitting upright, leaning forward, unable to lay flat due to chest pain	Pericarditis
Tall, thin, myopic, with wide arm span, long "spider-like" fingers, high arched palate, hyperextensible joints	Marfan's syndrome—associated with aortic dilatation, dissection and regurgitation, MVP
Morbidly obese (particularly male), with loud snoring, daytime hypersomnolence, prolonged periods of apnea	Pickwickian (sleep apnea) syndrome—associated with systemic and pulmonary hypertension, cor pulmonale, RV and LV failure, cardiac arrhythmias
Thin with quick "bird-like" movements, exophthalmos, lid lag, stare, tremor	Hyperthyroidism—associated with hypertension, supraventricular tachyarrhythmias (e.g., rapid atrial fibrillation), angina, high output heart failure
Lethargic, slow-moving; with dull face; hoarse voice; periorbital puffiness; loss of outer third of eyebrows; dry, brittle hair, thick, sallow skin	Hypothyroidism—associated with sinus bradycardia, pericardial effusion, low voltage on ECG, hyperlipidemia, CHF
Young, slender, anxious (particularly female), with straight back, pectus chest deformity, hypomastia	Mitral valve prolapse—associated with chest pain, arrhythmias, shortness of breath, and mitral regurgitation
Cheyne-Stokes respiration, cachexia, ascites, peripheral edema or cyanosis	Advanced heart failure
Xanthelasma, xanthomas, corneal arcus senilis	Hyperlipidemia—associated with CAD

Head bobbing:
  up and down ("yes-yes" sign)
  side-to-side ("no-no" sign) with pulsatile earlobes
	Aortic regurgitation
	Tricuspid regurgitation

Conjunctival petechiae, subungual "splinter" hemorrhages, Osler's nodes, Janeway's lesions, Roth spots	Infective endocarditis—associated with fever, heart murmur, bacteremia
Central cyanosis (including conjunctiva and mucous membranes) with or without clubbing of fingers and toes	Congenital heart disease (right-to-left shunt), e.g., ASD, VSD. If toes cyanotic and fingers pink ("differential cyanosis") – PDA.
Peripheral cyanosis	Congestive heart failure (low cardiac output), peripheral vascular disease
Firm, taut, shiny, hide-bound skin; tightening of skin and mouth; tapered and contracted fingers with ischemic ulcers	Scleroderma—associated with systemic and pulmonary hypertension, Raynaud's phenomenon, myocardial and pericardial disease
Blue sclera	Osteogenesis imperfecta—associated with aortic dilatation, dissection and regurgitation, mitral valve prolapse
Facial and neck flushing, violaceous hue	Carcinoid syndrome—associated with tricuspid and pulmonic stenosis and/or regurgitation, right heart
Straight back ("poker spine")	Ankylosing spondylitis—associated with aortic regurgitation and complete heart block
Abdominal obesity	Metabolic syndrome—associated with hypertension, glucose intolerance, and atherogenic dyslipidemia (low HDL cholesterol, elevated triglycerides, and small dense LDL particles)

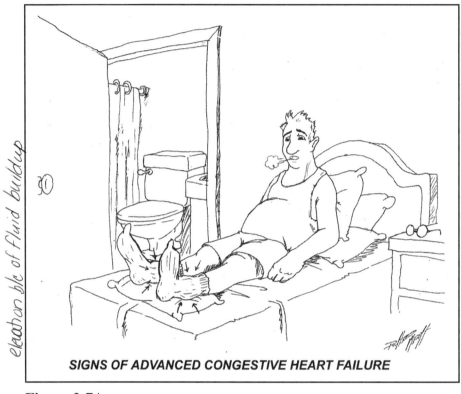

elevation 3/c of fluid buildup

SIGNS OF ADVANCED CONGESTIVE HEART FAILURE

Figure 2-7A

receiving thrombolytic therapy, especially those older females who are hypertensive, or who are also receiving adjunctive anticoagulation therapy, the sudden onset of lethargy or mental obtundation should alert the clinician to the possibility of intracranial bleeding. It should be realized, however, that acute confusion and altered mental status is a common atypical presentation of acute MI (especially in the elderly) and this, in and of itself, may deter the practitioner from administering fibrinolytic therapy.

The cachectic patient (i.e., those with severe weight loss, muscle wasting) with elevated neck veins, edematous legs, a distended abdomen (ascites), and peripheral cyanosis (due to a low cardiac output) may be suffering from the ravages of chronic ("end-stage") CHF.

Figure 2-7A. A patient with CHF. He is dyspneic, sitting upright with 2–3 pillow orthopnea, has distended neck veins, a protuberant abdomen (ascites), and pitting peripheral edema. Patients with CHF often have to get up in the middle of the night to urinate (nocturia) as well. The clinical appearance may resemble that of constrictive pericarditis. Distended neck veins and ascites, disproportionate to edema, may also be a clue to constrictive pericarditis.

Gynecomastia may be seen in patients receiving digitalis or spironolactone.

The distressed individual leaning forward, taking shallow, splinting respirations while complaining of chest pain, lends suspicion to the presence of acute pericarditis.

Figure 2-7B. A middle-aged markedly obese man with obstructive sleep apnea (*Pickwickian syndrome*). The patient may present with daytime hypersomnolence and/or loud snoring. His partner may be concerned that he stops breathing frequently during sleep. These patients often have systemic and pulmonary hypertension, heart failure, and cardiac arrhythmias, e.g., sinus bradycardia, sinus arrest, asystolic episodes, PACs, atrial fibrillation, PVCs, or VT. Sleep apnea is reversible with administration of continuous positive airway pressure (CPAP) therapy.

The patient with severe COPD, tachypneic at rest, using the accessory muscles to aid in respiration, may also have co-existing right heart failure and pulmonary hypertension (*cor pulmonale*).

Figure 2-8. *Marfan's syndrome* characteristically is associated with abnormally wide arm span and long tapered hyperextensible ("spider-like") fingers (*arachnodactyly*) (top) with thumb extensible beyond the ulnar aspect of the hand ("*thumb sign*") (bottom) in a thin, highly myopic individual. It is said that Abraham Lincoln may have had Marfan's syndrome, and that patients with Marfan's syndrome may

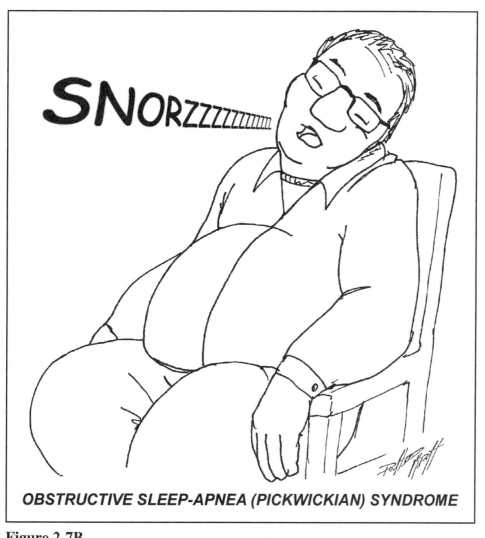

OBSTRUCTIVE SLEEP-APNEA (PICKWICKIAN) SYNDROME

Figure 2-7B

resemble him. The condition is often associated with aortic root disease (e.g., AR, aneurysm, dissection) and/or MVP.

Pulsation of the sternoclavicular joint may be a rare clue to aneurysm of the ascending aorta.

A lethargic, slow-moving person, who has a hoarse, raspy voice, coarse thick hair, periorbital puffiness and sparse eyebrows (loss of the outer third), may have advanced *hypothyroidism (myxedema)* with coexisting hyperlipidemia (due to decreased cholesterol and triglyceride clearance), sinus bradycardia, and low voltage on the ECG (due to pericardial effusion).

A thin individual who is often hyperkinetic, with fine, silky hair, warm, salmon-colored skin, excessive perspiration, quick "bird-like" movements, bulging eyes (exophthalmos) with lid lag, stare, goiter, and a fine resting tremor, may have *hyperthyroidism* and present with increased blood pressure (BP), rapid atrial fibrillation, sinus tachycardia, and/or CHF.

The young, slender female with a straight back, pectus chest deformity (**Figure 2-9**) and hypomastia, complaining of atypical chest pain, palpitations, shortness of breath, lightheadedness, fatigue, anxiety and panic attacks, should alert the practitioner to the possibility of underlying *mitral valve prolapse.*

An abnormal gait (often with other signs of neurologic impairment, e.g., facial droop, hemiparesis, may be the first sign of a stroke secondary to an embolic event, which may occur in the setting of atrial fibrillation, prior acute MI, infective endocarditis, prosthetic valve disease, atrial myxoma, or other valvular and/or myocardial disease.

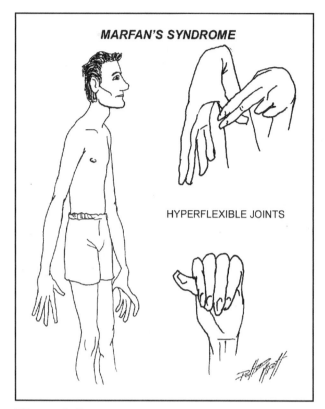

MARFAN'S SYNDROME

HYPERFLEXIBLE JOINTS

Figure 2-8

Cutaneous Manifestations (Skin Color, Temperature, Texture)

The astute clinician should also be on the lookout for specific abnormalities in skin color and texture, which may provide the first clue to cardiovascular disease. *Chronic pallor* (as may be seen by inspecting the conjunctiva or palmar lines of the patient's hand), for example, is a clue to underlying anemia (which may precipitate ischemic chest pain and/or CHF in a patient with heart disease). *Acute pallor* in a person with ischemic chest pain, on the other hand, may be a sign of angina or acute MI (due to peripheral vasoconstriction and increased systemic vascular resistance).

Cyanosis is an abnormal bluish discoloration of the skin that generally reflects an arterial oxygen saturation of ≤ 85% (normal being ≥ 95%). Cyanosis of the buccal mucosa, conjunctiva, and nail beds (with or without associated clubbing of the fingers and toes) may provide a clue to congenital heart disease, e.g., atrial or ventricular septal defect (ASD, VSD) and pulmonary hypertension with a reversed (right-to-left) shunt (Eisenmenger syndrome), which allows poorly oxygenated blood from the right side of the heart to flow to the left side, bypassing the lungs. Cyanosis and clubbing of the toes, with pink, nonclubbed fingers ("differential cyanosis") is a clue to patent ductus arteriosus (PDA). Peripheral cyanosis (seen on the tip of the nose, ears, and distal extremities) along with cool, pale skin indicates reduced blood flow to the limbs due to systemic vasoconstriction and may be evident in severe circulatory failure with a low cardiac output (cardiogenic shock).

Sudden pallor or cyanosis of the fingers or toes associated with small, tender areas on the skin, are clues to the presence of systemic emboli (from atherosclerotic lesions in the aorta, atrial myxoma, intracardiac clots or vegetations). A bluish-gray color of the skin, hands, and nose may occur in patients receiving amiodarone antiarrhythmic therapy. The brick-red color of *polycythemia* may be evident in a patient with hypertension, vascular thromboses, and acute MI. *Ecchymoses* may be present in patients receiving antiplatelet agents (e.g., aspirin, clopidogrel) and/or anticoagulant therapy (e.g., warfarin). *Petechiae* and subungual *"splinter" hemorrhages*, and rarely *Osler's nodes* (painful, tender erythematous nodules on the fingers and toes), *Janeway lesions* (non-tender, hemorrhagic macular lesions on the palms and soles), and *Roth spots* (retinal hemorrhages with white center) often support a diagnosis of *infective endocarditis*, especially in association with fever and a heart murmur.

Clubbing of the digits may also be seen in patients with lung cancer and may provide a clue to the presence of pericardial metastases and effusion and/or atrial arrhythmias.

Close inspection of the skin for scars, e.g., sternotomy (previous CABG, valve surgery), clavicles (pacemaker/ICD), or legs (saphenous vein harvest for CABG) may provide valuable clues to heart disease.

Cutaneous scarring along the course of the antecubital veins (needle puncture "track-marks") is a clue to IV drug use, an important underlying cause of infective endocarditis of the tricuspid valve.

Rheumatoid arthritis, along with its typical hand deformity (subluxation of the metacarpophalangeal joints, ulnar deviation of the digits), may be seen with pericardial, valvular, or myocardial disease.

Jaundice, a yellowing of the skin and sclera (best noted using natural light) can be seen in patients with right-sided heart failure with hepatic impairment. Prosthetic heart valve-induced hemolysis is an uncommon cause of jaundice.

A specific diagnosis can sometimes be made by inspecting the face, its appearance giving a clue to the likely diagnosis. A *malar flush* (pinkish-purple patches) over the cheeks (due to dilatation of the malar capillaries) may be seen with long-standing rheumatic MS (*mitral facies*) associated with pulmonary hypertension and a low cardiac output. A *butterfly rash* across the nose and cheeks may be a clue to *systemic lupus erythematosus,* associated with verrucous endocarditis, myocarditis, or pericarditis.

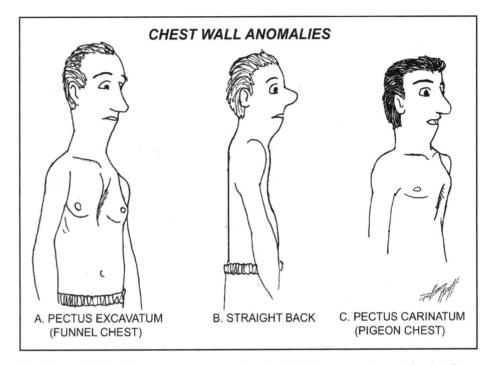

CHEST WALL ANOMALIES

A. PECTUS EXCAVATUM
(FUNNEL CHEST)

B. STRAIGHT BACK

C. PECTUS CARINATUM
(PIGEON CHEST)

Note: Chest wall deformities, e.g., pectus excavatum (or carinatum) with a narrow anteroposterior chest diameter, and a straight thoracic spine may be seen in patients with mitral valve prolapse and Marfan's syndrome.

Figure 2-9

Raynaud's phenomenon affects mostly women between the ages of 15–40 (in men it occurs later in life). Episodes are characterized by triphasic color changes (white, blue, red) as follows: On exposure to cold (or strong emotion) the blood vessels in the hands and feet of these patients first go into spasm and turn chalky *white*. They may also sting or become cold and numb. If a patient complains of arm pain while driving an automobile in the winter (before the heater has warmed up the car) suspect Raynaud's disease. Such pain can be an early symptom and at first may be erroneously diagnosed as ischemic heart disease. The skin may then turn *blue* (cyanosis) and then bright *red* (due to reperfusion) upon return to a warmer environment before normal color returns. Raynaud's phenomenon may occur as an isolated entity (~20% of patients) or be a clue to the presence of other conditions, e.g., Prinzmetal's angina (a peculiar angina variant in which spasm occurs without obvious atherosclerotic lesions), idiopathic pulmonary hypertension, connective tissue diseases, various drugs and toxins. Primary Raynaud's disease is a benign condition, with treatment emphasizing protection from cold exposure and other vasoconstrictive influences.

Voice

Close observation of the patient's voice may provide valuable clues to heart disease. As previously mentioned, a husky, low pitched voice may give a clue to hypothyroidism (myxedema), but more commonly suggests laryngitis, vocal cord nodule, or carcinoma. A hoarse voice may also indicate pressure on the left recurrent laryngeal nerve from an aortic arch aneurysm, a dilated pulmonary artery, or an enlarged left atrium.

Jugular Venous Pressure (JVP) and Pulse

Estimating JVP

The internal jugular vein acts as a manometer of right atrial pressure. Elevation of JVP contributes supporting evidence to the presence of right heart failure due to primary or secondary pulmonary hypertension of lung disease (cor pulmonale), left-sided heart failure that backs up to result in high right-sided filling pressures, RV infarction, tricuspid valve disease, constrictive pericarditis or cardiac tamponade. The backup of blood in these conditions increases the central venous pressure, as noted by estimating the pressure in the internal jugular vein.

In determining the jugular venous pressure the most important first step is to place the patient in the proper position. The patient should be comfortably supine but without a pillow, which can create a sharp angle. The object is to measure the highest point of pulsation of the internal jugular vein. If the JVP is high, i.e., the venous pulsations are too high in the neck to be seen, the patient should be placed in a more upright position to facilitate easier observation of the venous waves. If the JVP is low, and the height of the pulsation of the internal jugular vein is too low to be seen, the patient should be lying more flat. Jugular venous pulsations ascend with CHF and may even reach the earlobes, causing them to pulsate. Venous pulsations become less visible when the internal jugular veins are tensely distended from the very high venous pressure of CHF or constrictive pericarditis.

Figure 2-10. Inspection of the neck veins. Look for the right internal jugular vein (which has no valves and is a more direct route to the right atrium), which passes just medial to the clavicular head of the sternocleidomastoid up

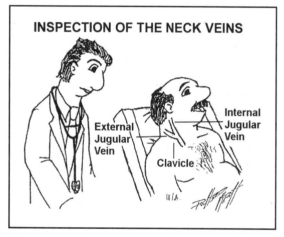

Figure 2-10

behind the angle of the jaw to the ear lobes. Do not rely on the external or left internal jugular vein because the left internal JVP can be elevated from partial obstruction of the left innominate vein by an unfolded aorta (especially in the elderly). You should observe two features: the *height,* i.e. jugular venous pressure (JVP), and the *wave form* of the

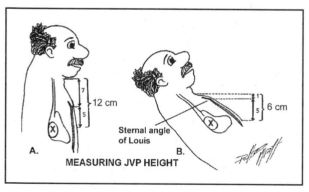

Figure 2-11

pulse. The examiner should be on the patient's right side, with the patient's head turned slightly away toward the left. A source of light (e.g., pocket flashlight) that strikes the neck at an angle may be used to cast shadows and enhance visualization of the neck veins.

Figure 2-11. Determining the height of the JVP. The middle of the right atrium (x) lies about 5 cm below the sternal angle of Louis, regardless of the patient's body position. One may measure the distance (in cm) from the sternal angle to the top of the venous column (internal jugular vein) and add

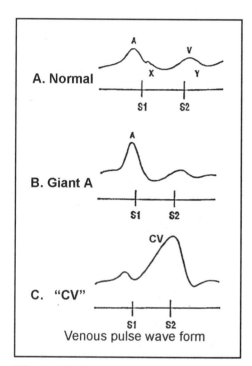

Figure 2-12

5 cm to obtain the JVP in cm of water. The normal mean JVP is approximately 7 cm. **A)** Patient with markedly elevated JVP (12 cm); **B)** Patient with normal JVP (6 cm).

Figure 2-12. Determining the wave form of the pulse. **A)** Normal wave form. The A wave, corresponding to atrial contraction (see **Figure 2–36** for explanation of the A and V waves as part of the cardiac cycle), is normally the dominant wave. **B)** Large "giant" A waves (occurring during atrial contraction) as may be seen in patients with pulmonary hypertension. **C)** Large V (CV) waves (occurring during the period of ventricular contraction) may occur in patients with tricuspid regurgitation (look for movement of the ear lobes. Note that since the A wave corresponds to atrial contraction, there are no A waves in atrial fibrillation).

It is important to emphasize that many patients who have pulmonary crackles or rales (or peripheral edema) are not in CHF. Too often the emphasis is on rales, yet these are the least reliable signs of heart failure. Furthermore, in chronic heart failure, increased lymphatic clearance can result in the absence of pulmonary rales or even markedly elevated pulmonary wedge pressures (the pressure measured when a catheter is passed up the pulmonary artery to record pressure backing up from the left atrium). The absence of rales (or edema), therefore, is an insensitive sign of heart failure that may mislead the clinician away from making the proper diagnosis. *Elevated JVP (and an S3 gallop, an auscultatory finding that commonly arises with LV systolic dysfunction—discussed below in the auscultation section) are the most valuable and specific findings of heart failure and are virtually diagnostic in patients with compatible symptoms.*

Peripheral edema is not a specific sign of heart disease. More often than not, it is a result of local venous disease (especially when unilateral), noncardiac conditions (e.g., kidney or liver disease), or even a drug side-effect (e.g., calcium channel blockers). Measurement of the JVP remains the "gold standard" in defining a cardiac cause for edema. *Except in patients who have recently received diuretics, the finding of a normal JVP virtually "rules out" backward failure of the right heart.*

Abdominojugular Test
Examination for jugular venous distention at rest or inducible by the abdominojugular (*hepatojugular reflux*) test is an extremely useful, highly sensitive and specific (~80%) clue to identifying patients with chronic CHF who have elevated left and right heart pressures. The use of abdominal

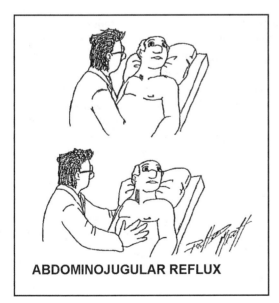

ABDOMINOJUGULAR REFLUX

Figure 2-13

or hepatic compression to "bring out" latent or borderline elevation of the JVP is an easily mastered technique for showing pulmonary venous hypertension and an elevated pulmonary capillary wedge pressure in patients with chronic left heart failure.

Figure 2-13. Method of eliciting positive abdominojugular (hepatojugular) reflux. Steady pressure is applied with the palm of the examiner's hand over the upper abdomen for 10 seconds or more while carefully observing the jugular venous pulsation. The normal response is a brief rise and a decline in the mean JVP while pressure is applied. An abnormal result consists of a progressive and sustained rise in the mean venous pressure during the course of applying pressure. The most common cause of a positive test is right heart failure secondary to elevated left heart filling pressures. Thus, the abdominojugular test is invaluable in diagnosing and monitoring patients with actual or suspected CHF. *All too often daily chest x-rays are ordered to follow the progress of a hospitalized patient with CHF when an accurate and less costly approach is a careful daily clinical evaluation of the JVP and the response to the abdominojugular test.*

Worthy of mention, RV infarction with diminished RV compliance is one condition that will produce a positive abdominojugular test without elevation of the pulmonary wedge pressure. With inspiration, mean venous pressure normally falls as the blood is drawn into the heart by the negative pressure of inspiration. When the right heart cannot accept the normal increase in venous return that occurs with inspiration, mean venous pressure *rises*. An inspiratory rise in mean JVP (*Kussmaul's sign*) is a sign of decreased RV compliance as seen in patients with right-sided heart failure and/or RV infarction, or in constrictive pericarditis (due to a rigid pericardial shell that inhibits inspiratory augmentation of RV filling) (**Figure 2-14**). Kussmaul's sign is rarely seen in patients with cardiac tamponade (since inspiratory augmentation of RV filling is not inhibited until late).

Abnormalities of the Venous Wave Form
Assessment of the contour of the pulse wave is an important aspect of the examination of the jugular venous pulse. Underlying structural, functional, or electrical abnormalities of the heart often cause the neck veins to pulsate abnormally, and impart flicking movements which correlate with the A and V waves, thereby allowing for accurate diagnostic inferences "at a glance".

Giant A waves occur whenever it is more difficult for the contracting RA to empty into the RV. Recognition of giant A waves raises the possibility of increased RV end-diastolic pressure due to pulmonary hypertension from any cause (e.g., LV failure, MS, pulmonary emboli, COPD) or

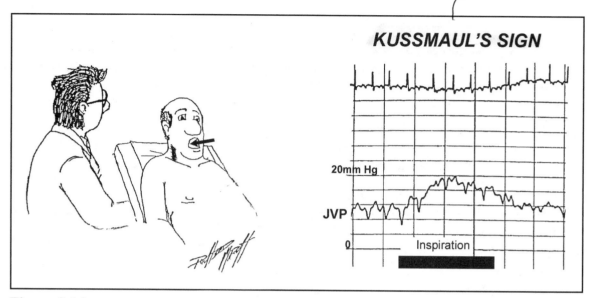

what is it?

Figure 2-14

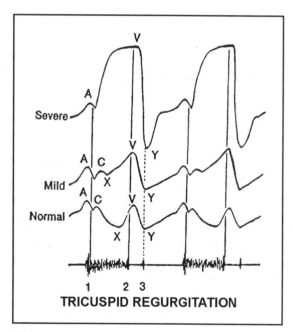

Figure 2-15

Figure 2-15. Tricuspid regurgitation. Note that the systolic regurgitant V (CV) wave produced by the leak of the tricuspid valve becomes higher and broader during atrial filling as TR increases in severity. When atrial fibrillation is also present, no atrial (A) wave is demonstrated. (Courtesy of Dr. Jonathan Abrams).

The large systolic expansion of the internal jugular vein in TR may cause lateral movement of the patient's head from side to side coincident with systole ("*no-no*" *sign*). When TR is severe, one may see systolic movements of the patient's earlobes (or eyeballs), as the large V waves cause them to "dance" with each pulsation. Prominent V waves, equaling the A waves in amplitude, are also noted in patients with an atrial septal defect (ASD). The skilled examiner may appreciate the markedly distended neck veins with brisk, very prominent negative waves ("X" and "Y" descents) in a patient with constrictive pericarditis.

Figure 2-16. Constrictive pericarditis. Note the classic M or W-shaped pulse, the elevated mean level of venous pressure and the X and Y descents (caused by a fall in venous pressure with atrial relaxation [X] and opening of tricuspid valve/atrial emptying [Y] respectively). (From Ronan JA, Jr. and Gordon, MA. Cardiol in Pract, 1984, Le Jacq Communications, Inc., with permission).

In pericardial tamponade, the "Y" descent is blunted, due to the high pericardial pressure that compresses the RV and impairs RA emptying.

The simultaneous use of two senses (e.g., seeing and feeling, or seeing and listening) often dulls the perceptiveness

pathology resulting in significantly diminished RV diastolic compliance, e.g., RV hypertrophy, pulmonic stenosis (PS) or an increase in resistance to RV filling at the level of the tricuspid valve (e.g., tricuspid stenosis, RA myxoma). Abnormal systolic V waves are a hallmark of significant TR.

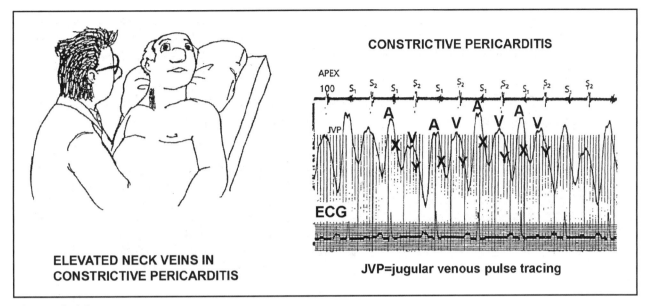

Figure 2-16

of either sense. For example, the best way to detect and time the specific waves of the jugular venous pulse in the neck is to look for both the venous and carotid arterial pulsations in the same localized area (i.e., concentrate solely on the visual). The venous pulsation is lateral and the arterial is medial. If you detect a venous pulsation just before the carotid, it is an A wave. When both the arterial and venous waves occur simultaneously, it is a V wave. Although timing may also be accomplished by palpating the carotid artery pulsation or listening to the first and second heart sounds and correlating it with the jugular venous pulse, concentrating on one sense at a time is best.

Although the ECG is the most important aid and final arbiter for definitive diagnosis of arrhythmias and/or electrical conduction disturbances, valuable clues may be obtained by close inspection of the jugular venous pulse (along with careful palpation of the arterial pulse — see next section). For example, the venous A wave completely disappears with atrial fibrillation or atrial standstill. Cannon A waves are large intermittent A waves resulting from RA contraction against a closed tricuspid valve. Intermittent cannon A waves serve as a clue to forms of atrioventricular (AV) dissociation and may occur with PVCs, VT, complete heart block, and with electronic RV pacing.

Figure 2-17. Intermittent cannon A waves in a jugular venous pulse (JVP) tracing, resulting from premature ventricular contractions (PVCs). Cannon A waves occur when the atrium contracts against a tricuspid valve that is closed by a PVC. The cannon wave is much higher than the other A waves. (From Ronan JA, Jr. and Gordon, MA. Cardiol in Pract, 1984, Le Jacq Communications, Inc., with permission).

Figure 2-18 summarizes clinical clues to heart disease from jugular venous pulsations and pressure.

PALPATION

Blood Pressure and Arterial Pulse

Practitioners need to know not only how to measure the BP (**Figure 2-19**), but also the limitations of the BP readings, including under and over estimates. When measuring the blood pressure, use the appropriate size cuff. The cuff bladder should nearly encircle the patient's arm. If the cuff is too small for the arm, an erroneously high pressure may result. If the cuff is too large for the arm, a false low pressure may result.

Abnormalities of Blood Pressure
Hypertension affects about 100 million Americans. Approximately 95% of patients have "essential" (idiopathic or primary) hypertension.

Clues, in the history and physical, to a secondary cause of hypertension include:

• A history of the use of birth-control pills
• Steroidal and nonsteroidal anti-inflammatory drugs (NSAIDs)

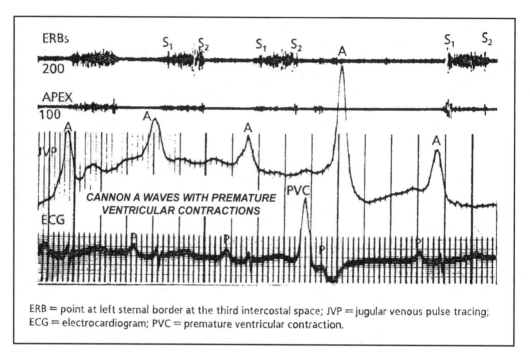

ERB = point at left sternal border at the third intercostal space; JVP = jugular venous pulse tracing; ECG = electrocardiogram; PVC = premature ventricular contraction.

Figure 2-17

FIGURE 2-18

Clinical Clues to Heart Disease from Jugular Venous Pulsations and Pressure

Clue	Clinical Significance
Large A waves	Pulmonary hypertension, decreased RV compliance, RV hypertrophy
Cannon A waves	Complete heart block, VT, PVCs, electronic RV pacing (AV dissociation)
Absent A waves	Atrial fibrillation or atrial standstill
Large V waves ("no-no" sign)	Tricuspid regurgitation
Rapid X and Y descents ("M" or "W" shaped)	Constrictive pericarditis
Blunted Y descent	Cardiac tamponade, tricuspid stenosis
Elevated jugular venous pressure	Right heart failure, RV infarction, constrictive pericarditis, cardiac tamponade
Kussmaul's sign	Right heart failure, RV infarction, constrictive pericarditis
Positive abdominojugular (hepatojugular reflux) test	Left and right heart failure, RV infarction

---

- Cold, allergy and sinus medications; nasal decongestants
- Diet pills
- Cyclosporine, erythropoietin, cocaine, amphetamines, or the ingestion of large amounts of licorice (containing glycyrrhizic acid, a salt-retaining compound)
- Diminished or delayed femoral pulse (so-called radial or brachial-femoral lag) in coarctation of the aorta (particularly in younger patients)

FIGURE 2-19

Proper Blood Pressure Technique

- Patient should be in a relaxed and comfortable (supine or sitting) position.

- Recent caffeine intake, cigarette smoking, adrenergic stimulants (e.g., phenylephrine in nasal decongestants) exposure to cold, bladder distention, or tight clothing can affect blood pressure.

- Use cuff size appropriate to upper arm diameter to avoid false readings. The bladder should nearly encircle the patient's arm ~ 20% wider than arm diameter.
  —Undersized cuff causes falsely elevated pressures (e.g., normal cuff on obese arm).
  —Oversized cuff causes falsely low values (standard cuff on thin arm).
  —Loosely applied cuff causes falsely high readings.

- Do not check blood pressure through clothing.

- Have arm well supported at heart level.

- Palpate arterial pulse and inflate cuff 20 to 30 mmHg above disappearance of pulse - to avoid "auscultatory gap" (disappearance and reappearance of Korotkoff sounds).

- Deflate the cuff slowly (~2 to 3 mmHg/second).

- Record both systolic and diastolic blood pressures. Systolic blood pressure is recorded as the pressure at which Korotkoff sounds appear (phase I, which reflects the force of LV contraction).

- Use Korotkoff phase V (complete disappearance of sounds) for diastolic blood pressure. Although diastolic BP usually correlates more with the disappearance of the sound, phase IV Korotkoff (when the sound becomes muffled) is a more accurate indication in severe AR.

- For diagnosis, obtain three sets of readings at least one week apart. A single elevated BP does not necessarily indicate hypertension.

- Recheck blood pressure after 5 minute rest or at end of examination if abnormally high (anxiety can transiently elevate blood pressure ["white coat" hypertension]).

- Initially, check blood pressure in both arms and use higher reading. Normally, there is up to 5-10 mmHg difference in systolic blood pressure and 5 mmHg difference in diastolic blood pressure.

- Failure to wait 2 minutes between inflations of cuff can result in falsely high diastolic readings.

- Check for 2 minute orthostatic drop (> 10 mmHg in systolic or 5 mmHg in diastolic) in blood pressure (in patients with dizziness or syncope on assuming upright posture), particularly in the elderly or diabetics or those receiving antihypertensive therapy.

- Thin skin, truncal obesity, buffalo hump, hirsutism, abdominal striae, and rounded facial changes (moon facies) in Cushing's syndrome

- A history of the "Ps" in **p**heochromocytoma (i.e., **p**aroxysmal hypertension with **p**ostural hypotension, head **p**ain, **p**alpitations, **p**allor and **p**erspiration) in a thin, anxious, hypermetabolic person (remember there are "no fat pheos").

- A history of loud, nocturnal snoring with daytime somnolence in a markedly overweight male with sleep apnea syndrome (due to increased sympathetic nervous system activity and endothelium-derived constricting factors released in response to hypoxemia during apnea).

- Abdominal or flank bruit in renal artery stenosis. The sudden onset of severe, worsening or resistant hypertension should alert the clinician to search for the bruit of renal artery stenosis.

- Coarctation of the aorta and atherosclerotic peripheral arterial disease (PAD) can result in a lower BP in the legs than in the arms. (Normally, the BP in the legs is 10–20 mmHg higher than in the arms.) The ratio of the ankle to the brachial systolic BP, termed the *ankle-brachial index* (ABI), is a useful tool in assessing the presence and severity of PAD (ABI < 0.9 = mild PAD; < 0.4 = severe PAD).

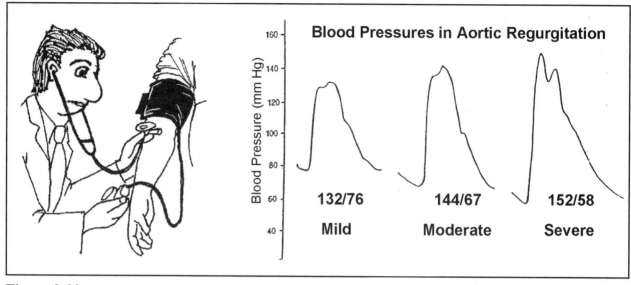

Figure 2-20

Elevated systolic pressure with normal diastolic pressure may be present in the elderly who have generalized severe arteriosclerosis with decreased elasticity of the aorta and peripheral vessels. Systolic hypertension also frequently accompanies thyrotoxicosis. Spurious elevations under stress or in the practitioner's office (so-called "*white-coat*" hypertension) sometimes occur (more so in women than in men), especially in those who are anxious.

It is helpful to check for postural hypotension (particularly in patients receiving diuretics, antihypertensive drugs or nitroglycerin), by measuring blood pressure in the standing position after 1–3 minutes. In older patients, postural or orthostatic hypotension (secondary to autonomic dysfunction as may occur in diabetes) can be associated with falls and syncope.

Abnormalities of blood pressure are an important feature of several types of heart disease: In AR there may be a wide pulse pressure, with increased systolic pressure and decreased diastolic pressure to 60 mmHg or less, depending on severity. Wide pulse pressure may also be found with the inelastic aorta in the elderly and with arteriovenous fistula.

Figure 2-20. The arterial blood pressure in aortic regurgitation. There is little alteration in the arterial blood pressure in mild aortic regurgitation. With increasing reflux across the aortic valve, systolic blood pressure increases and diastolic blood pressure decreases, resulting in widening of the pulse pressure (Modified from Abrams J. Prim Cardiol 1983, with permission).

Abnormalities of Arterial Pulse
Palpation of the radial and carotid pulse can provide useful information. After you greet and shake hands with the patient, it is easy and natural to feel the radial pulse, which is readily accessible (even when the patient is partly dressed) and is often reassuring to the apprehensive and nervous patient by virtue by the "laying on of hands". It is important to palpate all the arterial pulses in examining the cardiac patient (**Figure 2-21**). Findings on palpating the pulse include:

- Slow heart rates are found in sinus bradycardia and complete heart block.
- Regular rhythm tachycardia is found in sinus tachycardia and supraventricular tachycardia.
- A "*regularly* irregular" rhythm is commonly found with premature atrial or ventricular contractions and other cardiac conduction disturbances.
- An "*irregularly* irregular" rhythm, accompanied by a pulse deficit (i.e. apical heart rate is greater than peripheral pulse rate) suggests atrial fibrillation. (In atrial fibrillation, in those beats where diastole is too short for adequate filling of the heart, too small a volume of blood is ejected during systole for a pulse to be palpated consistently at the wrist, thereby creating the pulse deficit.)

Figure 2-22:
A) Normal pulse

B) A brisk, *quick-rising* ("flip") pulse suggests AR (*water hammer* or *Corrigan pulse*), HOCM, severe MR, VSD, or PDA. In advanced AR there may even be an up and down bobbing of the head (*de Musset's* or *"yes-yes" sign*) with each heart beat.

C) *Pulsus alternans* (alternating pulse amplitudes) denotes LV systolic dysfunction. It is best palpated in the

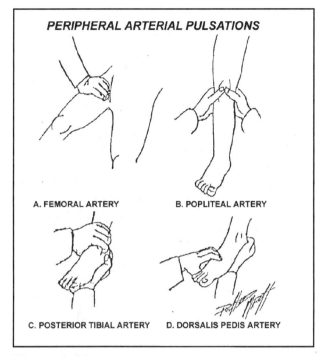

PERIPHERAL ARTERIAL PULSATIONS

A. FEMORAL ARTERY   B. POPLITEAL ARTERY

C. POSTERIOR TIBIAL ARTERY   D. DORSALIS PEDIS ARTERY

Figure 2-21

radial or femoral arteries. A sensitive way of detecting it is to use a blood pressure cuff, lowering the pressure slowly to just below the systolic level. On auscultation, pulsus alternans is heard as alternating louder and fainter sounds, or by a sudden doubling of the heart rate as the cuff pressure is further lowered. Pulsus alternans is often palpable transiently after premature ventricular contractions, and may be sustained when significant LV systolic dysfunction is present.

D) A *small, weak (hypokinetic) pulse* suggests a low cardiac output state and decreased LV function.

E) A *paradoxical pulse* (>10 mmHg inspiratory decrease in BP–**Figure 2-23**) raises the concern for cardiac tamponade (less commonly constrictive pericarditis, and severe asthma and COPD). Actually, the name "pulsus paradoxus" is a misnomer since it is an exaggeration of the normal phenomenon of decreased BP with inspiration. A quick bedside test to check for the presence of pulsus paradoxus consists of feeling the pulse and noting whether or not it diminishes (or even disappears) during inspiration. A normal volume pulse during inspiration reduces the likelihood of cardiac tamponade. (With severe LV systolic dysfunction and shock, though, where the pulse as a whole may be very weak, the pulsus paradoxus may be relatively diminished and difficult to detect.)

A slowed upstroke of the femoral artery pulse with a noticeable delay in the arrival of the femoral pulse beat compared with the radial pulse (*radiofemoral delay*) is an important clue to coarctation of the aorta (**Figure 2-24**). *Disparity in amplitude* between major arterial pulses may provide a clue to the presence and location of aortic dissection.

A slow-rising, small, late-peaking plateau pulse ("*pulsus parvus et tardus*") is characteristic of valvular AS, whereas a quick-rising, twin peaking ("*spike and dome*") pulse is characteristic of HOCM. (**Figure 2-25A**). On BP testing, a narrow pulse pressure is usually a late finding in

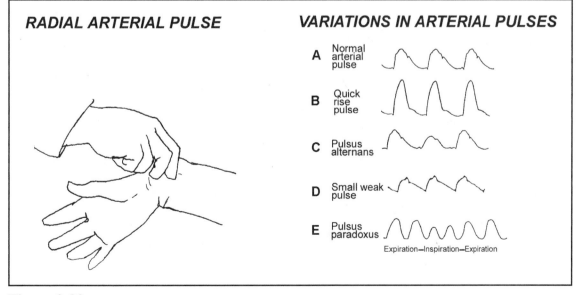

RADIAL ARTERIAL PULSE

VARIATIONS IN ARTERIAL PULSES

A Normal arterial pulse

B Quick rise pulse

C Pulsus alternans

D Small weak pulse

E Pulsus paradoxus

Expiration–Inspiration–Expiration

Figure 2-22

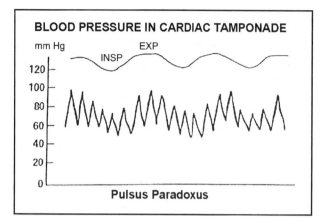

BLOOD PRESSURE IN CARDIAC TAMPONADE

Pulsus Paradoxus

Figure 2-23

patients with severe valvular aortic stenosis. In healthy older adults, though, decreased compliance and increased arterial stiffness may result in an increase in arterial pulse amplitude and wider pulse pressure, which can mask the typical small amplitude arterial pulse contour of valvular aortic stenosis.

Figure 2-25B. Carotid arterial pulse tracing in aortic regurgitation. Note the rapid initial upstroke and a bifid (bisferiens) or twin-peaked pulse, best detected using light finger pressure over the carotid arteries. (Modified from Abrams J: Prim Cardiol, 1983.)

Clues to peripheral vascular disease and a blocked artery include the 6 "P"s: *pulseless, pallor, pain, paralysis, paresthesia,* and *poikilothermia* (coolness). The most common cause of a small, weak arterial pulse is a low cardiac output state.

Figure 2-26 summarizes clinical clues to heart disease from blood pressure and arterial pulse.

Precordial Movements and Palpation

Careful inspection and palpation of the precordium (the area over and around the heart) may yield a large number of valuable clinical clues to the existence of heart disease. Abnormal palpation may arise from:

- LV hypertrophy and/or dilation
- LV wall motion abnormalities (fixed or transient)
- Increased force of left atrial contraction
- Accentuated diastolic rapid filling
- Anterior thrust of the heart from severe mitral regurgitation
- RV hypertrophy and/or dilatation
- Loud murmurs (thrills)
- Loud heart sounds (normal and abnormal)
- Dilated or hyperkinetic pulmonary artery
- Dilated aorta

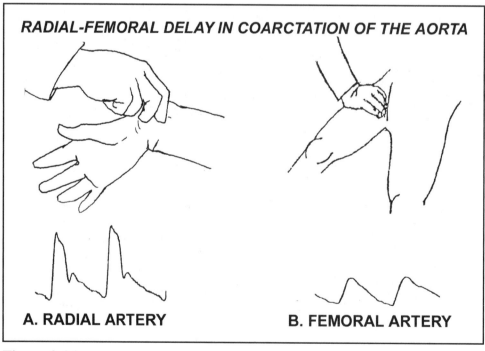

RADIAL-FEMORAL DELAY IN COARCTATION OF THE AORTA

A. RADIAL ARTERY

B. FEMORAL ARTERY

Figure 2-24

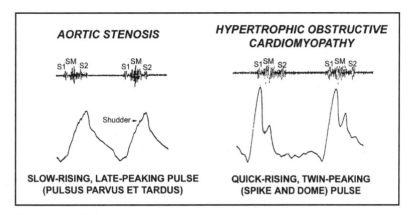

Figure 2-25A

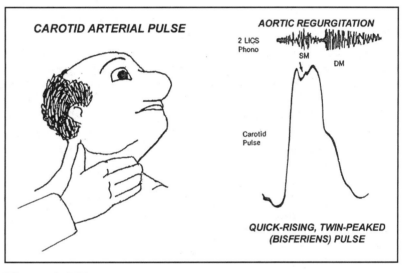

Figure 2-25B

FIGURE 2-26

Clinical Clues to Heart Disease from Blood Pressure and Arterial Pulse

Clue	Clinical Significance
Pulsus alternans	LV systolic dysfunction
Pulsus paradoxus	Cardiac tamponade, constrictive pericarditis, severe CHF
Slow-rising, late-peaking pulse ("pulsus parvus et tardus")	Severe valvular aortic stenosis
Rapid or quick-rise ("flip") pulse	AR, HOCM, severe MR, patent ductus arteriosus
Radial or brachial-femoral delay	Coarctation of the aorta
Small, weak, low-volume pulse	Low cardiac output (eg. decreased LV function)

Figure 2-27. Schematic diagram illustrating areas to be inspected and palpated for abnormal precordial pulsations. **A)** aortic area; **B)** pulmonic area; **C)** RV (left parasternal) area; **D)** LV (apical) area; **E)** ectopic area. Impulses at the aortic and pulmonic areas are usually due to a dilated aorta or pulmonary artery respectively. Impulses at the left sternal border are usually caused by RV contraction in patients with pressure and/or volume overload of the RV, and those at the apex relate to LV contraction. Impulses in the ectopic area are usually due to LV aneurysm and/or dyskinesis (paradoxical outward motion of the heart wall, e.g., due to anterior wall MI).

Precordial palpation is best performed with the patient supine or in the left lateral decubitus position. The latter position may be necessary to palpate the apical impulse, often referred to as the point of maximal impulse (PMI), in a patient with a thick muscular chest or large breasts. This shifts the heart and apex beat leftward, however, and must be taken into consideration when evaluating the location of precordial pulsations. The clinician should stand to the patient's right side with the right hand over the patient's lower left chest wall, fingertips over the cardiac apex, and palm over the right ventricle. Localized impulses are best felt with the under-surface of the fingertips, whereas murmurs (thrills) are most easily perceived by palpation with the palmar surface of the hand.

Figure 2-28. Left. Palpation of the precordium. **Right.** Major types of LV precordial motion. **A.** *Normal* precordial motion. **B.** *Hyperkinetic* precordial motion, e.g., volume overload states (AR, MR). **C.** *Sustained* precordial motion, e.g., pressure overload states (hypertension, AS), ischemic LV dysfunction, and/or non-ischemic cardiomyopathy. Note palpable presystolic (S4) and early diastolic (S3) gallops. (Courtesy of Dr. Jonathan Abrams).

The apical (LV) impulse is an excellent indicator of heart size and cardiac activity. It is examined for *location, duration,* and *character.* The apical impulse normally is felt over a small area (2–2.5 cm in diameter, about the width of one intercostal space), *location* being at the fifth left intercostal space at or medial to the midclavicular line. Its *duration,* extends through only the first part of systole. The normal apical impulse *character* is appreciated as a brief outward movement in early systole (produced as the LV strikes the chest wall) without palpable diastolic movements. Normally, there is a zone of "septal" retraction medial to the impulse. (**Figure 2-29**). This may be absent, however, when the RV occupies the apex (e.g., in rheumatic MS).

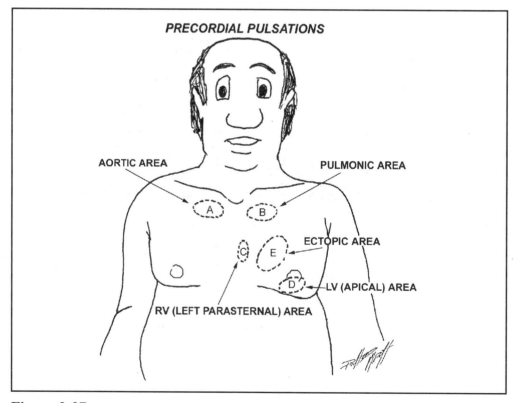

Figure 2-27

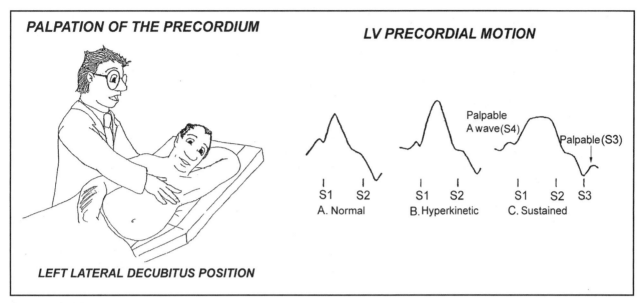

Figure 2-28

Abnormal Location:

- As the LV enlarges with CHF (e.g., dilated cardiomyopathy) or volume overload (e.g., AR, MR), the apical impulse is displaced downward and to the left of the midclavicular line; the impulse may enlarge to >3cm in diameter.
- Ventricular aneurysms, as well as localized myocardial dysfunction, may result in a sustained systolic precordial impulse in the apical or so-called "*ectopic*" areas of the precordium.
- *Parasternal* impulses may be felt when the heel of the hand is rested just to the left of the sternum with

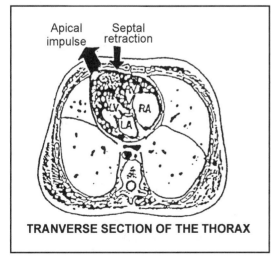

Figure 2-29

the fingers lifted just off the chest and may provide a clue to RV hypertrophy or volume overload. (However, a palpable RV impulse is considered normal in children and slender adults.)

- Severe MR may produce a more forceful, brisk left parasternal thrust or lift, predominantly in late systole, as a result of a recoil phenomenon related to the regurgitant jet of blood into the left atrium pushing the heart forward against the chest wall ("*left atrial rock*").
- Aortic aneurysm may cause pulsation in the right upper chest (just lateral to the sternum) or at the right sternoclavicular joint.
- In CAD, an "ectopic" systolic impulse (bulge) may be palpated (transiently with angina or over a long period of time with acute MI) in the third and fourth intercostal spaces between the lower left sternal border and cardiac apex. This represents a dyskinetic segment of myocardium expanding paradoxically during systole, and it may be a clue to the presence of a ventricular aneurysm (**Figure 2-30**).
- Right-sided filling sounds, i.e., S3 gallops (resulting from beginning of right ventricular diastolic filling) and S4 gallops (resulting from end of right ventricular diastolic filling during right atrial contraction) may also be palpated at the left sternal border and are augmented during inspiration when right heart filling is enhanced. (See **Figure 2-36** for explanation of the S3 and S4 sounds).

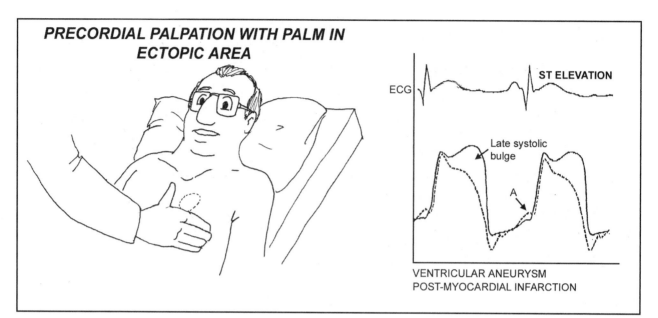

PRECORDIAL PALPATION WITH PALM IN ECTOPIC AREA

Figure 2-30

Abnormal Duration:

- A sustained (throughout systole), forceful, slow apical lift may occur with *LV hypertrophy* due to increased pressure load (e.g., AS, hypertension). When the thickening of the myocardium grows inward rather than outward, the apex beat usually occupies its normal position.

Character:

- Double or bifid apical impulses can occur when an outward movement during systole, due to LV dilatation or hypertrophy, is associated with a palpable pre-systolic (S4) distention (reflecting forceful LA contraction into a noncompliant LV) or early diastolic (S3) component. A palpable S4 may feel like the apical impulse has a "break on the upstroke". The patient may need to be in the left lateral decubitus position to feel this. At times, evidence of a gallop (S1–S2–S3 or S4–S1–S2) rhythm can be seen and felt even when not well heard.
- *Hypertrophic obstructive cardiomyopathy* can produce a pre-systolic, along with a double systolic outward thrust, resulting in a characteristic three-component apical impulse ("*triple ripple*"). The first component is due to presystolic distention of a poorly compliant left ventricle. The second component is the systolic ejection movement, and the third component is the obstruction that is experienced during ejection due to the HOCM.
- Observation of the location of retraction (**Figure 2-29**) relative to the outward thrust of the cardiac apex may help to determine which ventricle occupies the apex (retraction medial to the PMI suggests the LV; retraction lateral to the PMI suggests the RV).

The chest x-ray is commonly used as a reliable method of detecting cardiomegaly. However, precordial palpation may be superior to the chest film (or ECG), especially in detecting LV hypertrophy where the hypertrophy extends inward toward the ventricular space rather than outward.

When palpating the precordium, you should use both hands, which will enable you to feel both sides of the chest (and thus exclude an unsuspected dextrocardia).

Turbulent blood flow, which causes heart murmurs, may sometimes be palpable, where the grade is 4/6 or more (**Figure 2-31**). These palpable murmurs are called *"thrills"* and are a clue to an organic lesion. Innocent murmurs do not present with a thrill. The vibrations of the thrill are best detected by the palmar surface rather than the tips of your fingers, which generally are best to detect impulses, localized precordial movements, or arterial pulses.

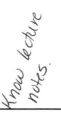
Know lecture notes.

FIGURE 2-31

Grading of Murmurs (Levine-Harvey)

Grade 1 Faintest murmur heard only with special effort (concentration or "tuning in" required)

Grade 2 Faint murmur but heard immediately

Grade 3 Moderately loud murmur

Grade 4 Loud murmur associated with a palpable thrill

Grade 5 Very loud murmur heard with part of stethoscope touching chest wall

Grade 6 Loudest murmur heard with stethoscope removed from chest wall

---

- A systolic thrill over the aortic area directed toward the right clavicle is most consistent with valvular AS. A diastolic thrill felt in the aortic area is consistent with aortic regurgitation. These may best be appreciated with the patient sitting and leaning forward.
- A systolic thrill over the pulmonic area directed toward the left clavicle suggests pulmonic stenosis.
- A systolic thrill over the left lower sternal border directed towards the right chest, suggests a VSD.
- An apical systolic thrill is consistent with MR, whereas an apical diastolic thrill raises the suspicion of MS.
- An abnormal pulsation of the sternoclavicular joint in a patient with chest pain may be an early clue to aortic dissection.

Figure 2-32 summarizes the kinds of abnormal precordial movements that can be detected.

FIGURE 2-32

Clinical Clues to Heart Disease from Precordial Movements and Pulsations

Clue	Clinical Significance
LV thrust or heave	LV hypertrophy (e.g., valvular aortic stenosis, hypertension, hypertrophic cardiomyopathy)
Early diastolic impulse (S3) and inferolateral displacement of LV impulse	LV dilatation and/or failure (e.g., dilated cardiomyopathy), volume overload (e.g., severe aortic regurgitation, mitral regurgitation)
Pre-systolic impulse (S4)	Pressure or resistant loads (e.g., valvular aortic stenosis, hypertension), coronary artery disease (diastolic dysfunction)
Pre-systolic and double-systolic impulse ("triple-ripple")	Hypertrophic obstructive cardiomyopathy
"Ectopic" systolic bulge (above and medial to cardiac apex)	Coronary artery disease (LV dyskinesis, LV aneurysm)
Parasternal lift	
Early	RV hypertrophy or dilatation (e.g., pulmonic stenosis, pulmonary hypertension)
Late	Mitral regurgitation ("left atrial rock")
Thrills	
Aortic area	Valvular aortic stenosis
Pulmonic area	Valvular pulmonic stenosis
Left sternal border	Ventricular septal defect
Cardiac apex	Mitral regurgitation

From class know sound pitch quality timing

The first heart sound, second heart sound, and an ejection sound (see next section for a description of ejection sounds) may also be palpable. When these sounds are palpable, it usually implies increased intensity (e.g., a palpable S1 should raise the suspicion of mitral stenosis, and a palpable P2 may be the initial clue to pulmonary hypertension).

AUSCULTATION

Auscultation of the heart has long been considered the centerpiece of the cardiac physical exam. Despite its long and rich tradition in clinical cardiology, the cardiac stethoscopic examination is now at risk of becoming a lost art. Emphasis away from the essentials of cardiac auscultation has been a growing trend, reinforced by enthusiasm for newer, more sophisticated imaging techniques, e.g., portable echo (**Figure 2-33**). Sophisticated high technology, however, should aid and not replace a solid foundation in cardiac auscultation. When used properly, the stethoscope is a most reliable and cost-effective clinical tool, often allowing the experienced clinician, skilled in the art of auscultation, to arrive at a rapid and accurate cardiac diagnosis and render appropriate treatment, often without the need for additional laboratory tests. (**Figure 2-34**). The following section reviews the fundamental techniques of cardiac auscultation, emphasizing the diagnostic importance and practical implementation of this venerable, but virtually vanishing, clinical art (**Figure 2-35**).

The Cardiac Cycle

Effective auscultation of the heart requires a basic understanding of the cardiac cycle.

Figure 2-36. Diagram of the cardiac cycle. (From Goldberg, S. Clinical Physiology Made Ridiculously Simple, MedMaster, Inc., 2001)

- In the ECG line (also written "EKG") at the top of **Figure 2-36,** the P wave of the ECG represents the electrical depolarization of the atrial myocardial cells. The QRS represents the depolarization of the myocardial cells of the ventricles and the T wave the

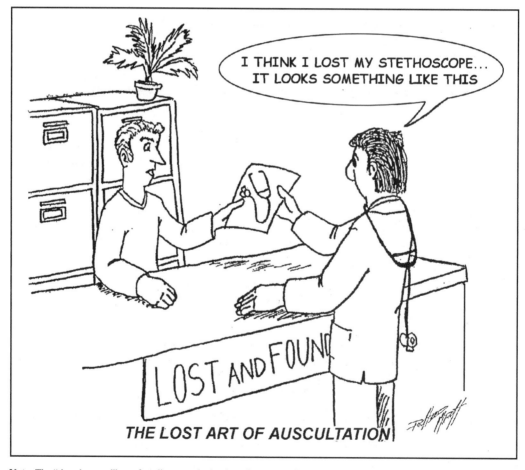

Note: The "time-honored" art of cardiac auscultation is an important clinical skill that is being lost amid growing reliance on newer, more sophisticated technology and the time constraints of clinical practice.

Figure 2-33

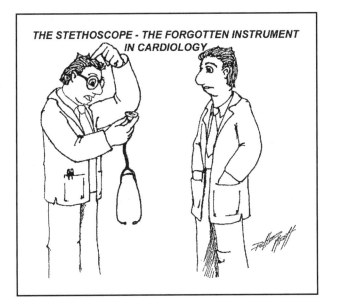

Note: Despite advances in technology, the stethoscope, when used properly, still remains a valuable and cost-effective diagnostic tool in the evaluation of patients with heart disease.

Figure 2-34

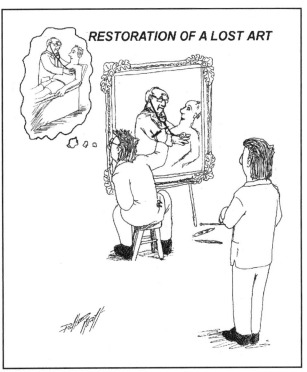

Note: Cardiac auscultation, once the hallmark of a master clinician, is rapidly becoming a lost art. Restoration of the lost art requires commitment, proper training, and repeated practice. Listening to large numbers of patients enables one to gain skill, confidence, and accuracy in diagnosis.

Figure 2-35

repolarization of the ventricles. Note that the actual contractions of the atria and ventricles follow slightly *after* their respective depolarizations. (**Figure 2–36** diagrams events on the left side of the heart; a similar diagram applies for the right side as well.)

- The first and second heart sounds (S1 and S2) reflect valve closure. Normally, valve opening is not heard.
- When the left ventricle contracts (systole), the mitral valve closes (S1 sound) before the aortic valve opens. This avoids backflow into the left atrium during ventricular contraction. Physiologically, this occurs because the pressure in the aorta is greater than that in the left atrium, so it is harder to open the aortic valve than to close the mitral valve.
- When the left ventricle relaxes (diastole), the aortic valve closes (S2 sound) before the mitral valve opens because of the relatively high pressure in the aorta. So the aortic valve is last to open and first to close.
- There are two phases to (ventricular) diastole. The first phase consists of the rapid *passive* flow of blood from the left atrium into the left ventricle when the ventricle expands and in a sense "sucks" blood from the left atrium (the S3 sound). The second phase of (ventricular) diastole is *active,* consisting of the contraction of the left atrium, giving an extra "*atrial kick*", pushing blood from the left atrium into the left ventricle (the S4 sound). If the left atrium is diseased and not contracting (e.g. in atrial fibrillation), this kick may be absent, but the

heart may still be able to function efficiently. However, the patient may be symptomatic on exercise or with dysfunction of the left ventricle, e.g. in situations where there is stiffness and decreased compliance of the left ventricular wall. The S3 and sometimes the S4 sounds may at times be heard normally in young people, athletes or in hyperkinetic cardiac states (e.g. hyperthyroidism, third trimester of pregnancy), but when they are heard in older people they typically represent cardiac pathology.

- There is an "*A" wave* toward the end of ventricular diastole, representing the brief pressure rise in the atrium from its late contraction in ventricular diastole. This occurs in both the right and left atria, but is only shown for the left atrium in **Figure 2-36.** The A wave can be transmitted back from the right atrium to the internal jugular vein, where it can be observed during the cardiac exam. The A wave will not be present in cases where there is no atrial contraction, e.g. atrial fibrillation. The A wave may be gigantic where there is resistance to atrial contraction, as in pulmonary hypertension and states of right ventricular stiffness and decreased compliance.

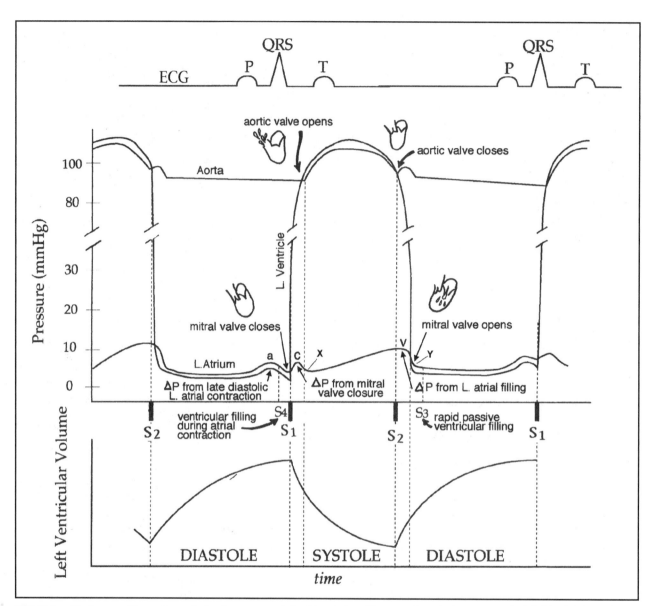

Note: Schematic diagram of the cardiac cycle showing pressure relationships, timing of heart sounds, and other events on the left side of the heart. Systole refers to the phase of ventricular contraction; diastole refers to the phase of ventricular relaxation and filling.

Figure 2-36

- The is also a *"C" wave* representing increased pressure in the atrium from closure of the AV valves at the onset of ventricular systole and a *"V" wave* representing atrial filling at the end of ventricular systole. The "X" in the diagram represents the descent of the A wave (atrial relaxation), while the "Y" represents the descent of the V wave (atrial emptying). These may be evaluated by a skilled examiner on observing the jugular venous pulse (**Figure 2-16**).

* * *

Mnemonic:

"A" wave = **A**trial contraction raises right atrial pressure.

"C" wave = **C**losure of tricuspid valve in early ventricular systole raises pressure in right atrium.

"V" wave = **V**entricular systole nearly o**V**er (right atrial filling occurring and pressure rises in right atrium).

* * *

- Normally, closure of the heart valves produces an audible sound, but opening does not, unless there is an abnormality such as a valve stenosis, congenital bicuspid aortic valve, or dilatation of one of the great arteries, in which case opening of the valve results in an ejection sound.

- S1 is the sound of closure of the mitral and tricuspid (AV) valves at the start of ventricular systole.
- S2 is the sound of closure of the aortic and pulmonic valves at the start of ventricular diastole.
- S3 is the sound of rapid filling of the ventricles during the early, passive phase of ventricular diastole.
- S4 is the sound of ventricular filling during the late, active ("atrial kick") phase of ventricular diastole.
- The S4 is heard commonly with diastolic (4 syllables in word) dysfunction and a "stiff" left ventricle (e.g., due to ischemia or hypertrophy) and is heard as an S4 gallop (S4–S1–S2). The S3 may be heard wherever there is ventricular systolic (3 syllables in word) dysfunction, due to poor contractility (e.g. acute MI, dilated cardiomyopathy) or when there is increased volume of ventricular flow (e.g. MR, AR, VSD, PDA), and is heard as an S3 gallop (S1–S2–S3). As mentioned, S3 and S4 may also be heard normally in young people, athletes or in hyperkinetic cardiac states (e.g. hyperthyroidism, third trimester of pregnancy).
- Murmurs are sounds that last a while within systole and/or diastole. (The term "systole" implies "contraction" while the term "diastole" implies "filling". In general, when the term "systole" or "diastole" are used alone in this text, they will refer to *ventricular* systole and diastole, rather than *atrial* systole and diastole). Murmurs are always abnormal when occurring in diastole or throughout systole (*holosystolic* murmurs). However, when they are midsystolic and of crescendo-decrescendo form, they may be normal in young people or in hyperdynamic states, and are flow murmurs due to strong efficient ventricular contraction. However, the same murmur may be abnormal in an older person. The innocence or pathology of such murmurs has to be judged not just on how it sounds but in the context of other clinical findings. Such murmurs would be considered normal in a young person with no other signs or symptoms of cardiac pathology and would then not be grounds for further diagnostic tests.
- The S1 sound is the combination of the sounds of the mitral and tricuspid valves closing. Normally, these sounds are so close together that they may be heard as one.
- The S2 sound is the combination of the sounds of the aortic and pulmonic valves closing. Since the pressure in the aorta is significantly higher than that in the pulmonary artery, the aortic valve normally closes first; A2 normally precedes and is louder than P2 (due

to the relatively high pressure in the aorta). S2 may thus be heard as a split sound on inspiration, since inspiration increases venous return to the heart and prolongs flow through the pulmonary artery, delaying closure of the pulmonary valve still further. Inspiration also reduces blood return to the left atrium and ventricle so that there is less pressure in the left ventricle, allowing the aortic valve to close sooner.

Use of the Stethoscope

A variety of stethoscopes are available for cardiac auscultation. Many have a separate diaphragm and bell.

Figure 2-37. The varying heads of the stethoscope are designed for optimal listening to different kinds of sounds, usually with a double head or triple head (Harvey) stethoscope. **A)** Flat diaphragm. **B)** Corrugated diaphragm. **C)** Bell.

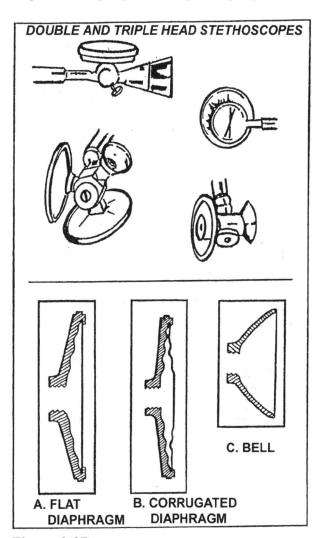

DOUBLE AND TRIPLE HEAD STETHOSCOPES

A. FLAT DIAPHRAGM   B. CORRUGATED DIAPHRAGM   C. BELL

Figure 2-37 (Courtesy of W. Proctor Harvey, M.D.)

- As a rule, firm pressure on the *diaphragm* is best for detecting faint high-frequency sounds such as the diastolic murmur of aortic regurgitation, systolic clicks, ejection sounds and most systolic murmurs.
- Light pressure on the *bell* is best for detecting faint, low-frequency gallop sounds (S3 and S4) and/or diastolic rumbles.
- A third chest piece (the *corrugated diaphragm*), present on the triple-headed ("Harvey") stethoscope, provides an "overview" of the cardiac auscultatory events, and is especially good for picking up low-frequency gallop sounds and murmurs (e.g., diastolic rumbles).

Remember to use all chest pieces on each patient. Of note, some stethoscopes have a single head (the *tunable diaphragm*) that enables the examiner to listen to both low frequency sounds (light pressure) and high frequency sounds (firm pressure) without rotation of the chest piece. Keep in mind, however, that to become proficient at cardiac auscultation, it takes more than just a good stethoscope—it's what's between the ears that counts! (**Figure 2-38**) Auscultatory findings should always be judged in the context of the "company they keep", namely the other important components of the cardiac physical examination.

Some general rules in applying the stethoscope:

1. Make sure that the room is quiet and free of distracting noise. This may be difficult to accomplish in an emergency department setting or in a hospital room with other patients and their visitors. By simply closing the door, turning off the television, and requesting that all conversation be terminated (if possible), you can vastly improve the results of your auscultation. **Note:** Modern electronic stethoscopes are now available that have the ability to amplify heart sounds, while at the same time filter out distracting background noise.

2. Resist all temptation to examine a patient who is still fully dressed. For maximal auscultatory yield, your stethoscope should be touching his or her bare skin, not clothes (**Figure 2-39**).

3. To ensure patient comfort, warm the diaphragm of your stethoscope with your hand before you proceed.

4. Use an examining table or bed so that your patient can be examined in various positions, e.g., supine, sitting upright, or turned to the left lateral decubitus position. In the upright position, the patient may be uncomfortable with legs extended straight. It is natural and more comfortable for the patient to sit with knees bent and legs dangling over the side.

5. When listening to a large-breasted woman, the left breast may need to be displaced away from the area of auscultation. You may find it helpful to ask your patient to lift her breast upward and to

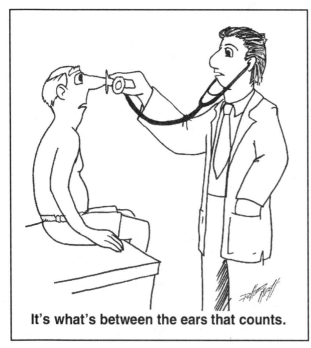

It's what's between the ears that counts.

Figure 2-38

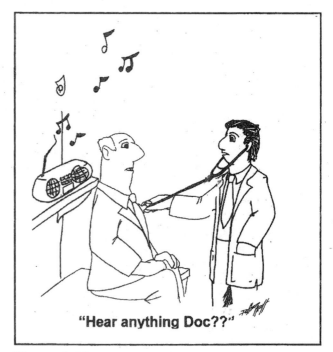

"Hear anything Doc??"

Figure 2-39

the left or you can use your non-dominant hand to do so.

6. Most practitioners conduct the examination from the right side of the patient and begin with the patient reclining in the *supine position*.

7. The examiner listens over the patient's second right intercostal space (*aortic area*) and slowly moves ("inches") (**Figure 2-40**) the stethoscope across to the second left intercostal space (*pulmonic area*), downward along the left sternal edge to the lower left sternal border (*tricuspid area*), and then laterally to the cardiac apex (*mitral area*), using *both the*

diaphragm and bell chest pieces. Although some practitioners prefer to reverse this sequence, it is important for the examiner to adopt a systematic method of auscultation, beginning in one area and then carefully exploring all areas in an orderly and unhurried fashion, so that nothing is overlooked.

8. **Figure 2-41:** Next, the patient is turned to the *left lateral decubitus position* while the clinician "tunes in" to *low-frequency sounds and murmurs* (e.g., S4 and S3 gallops, diastolic rumble of mitral stenosis) using the *bell* of the stethoscope applied lightly to the chest wall at the cardiac

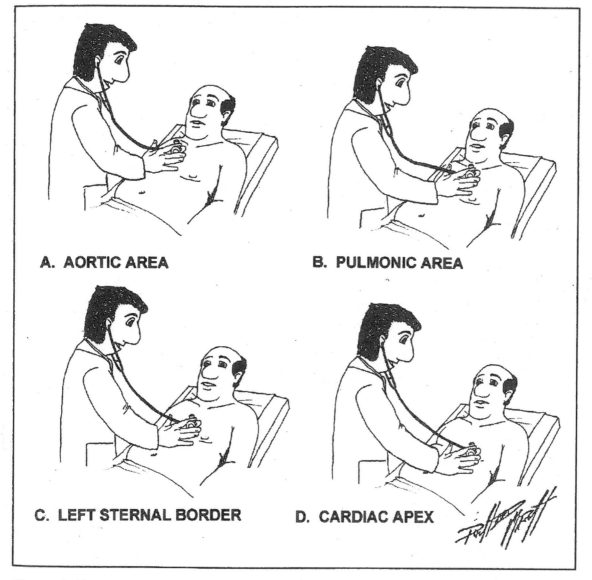

A. AORTIC AREA

B. PULMONIC AREA

C. LEFT STERNAL BORDER

D. CARDIAC APEX

Figure 2-40

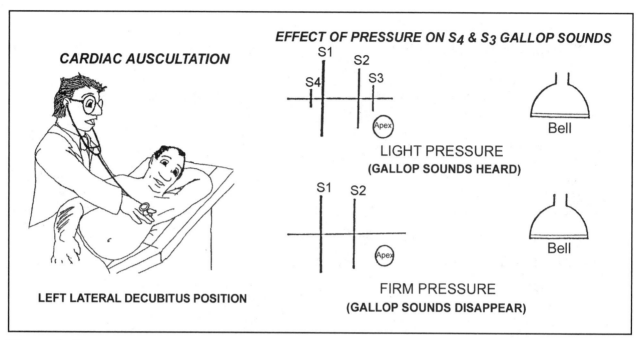

Figure 2-41 (Courtesy of W. Proctor Harvey, M.D.)

apex, barely making an air seal. Light pressure is essential, since heavy pressure stretches the skin and converts the bell into a diaphragm, and thereby diminishes or eliminates ("filters out") these low-frequency events.

9. **Figure 2-42:** Then, with the patient in the *sitting position, leaning forward with the breath held in deep expiration*, the examiner listens over the base of the heart (right and left 2nd intercostal spaces) or left sternal border, to detect *high-pitched sounds and murmurs,* e.g., diastolic murmur of AR, pulmonary hypertensive regurgitation (*Graham Steell murmur*), pericardial friction rub. Use the diaphragm chest piece pressed firmly enough against the chest wall to leave a temporary imprint (after-ring) on the skin.

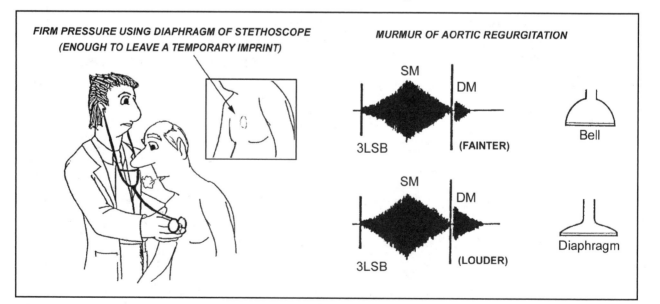

Figure 2-42 (Courtesy of W. Proctor Harvey, M.D.)

10. Not everyone has the same capacity to hear sound. The ability to hear the faint high-frequency diastolic murmur of AR may be lost to those who are aging or even to the young who have listened to loud music for prolonged periods of time. It is possible to hear better by "selective listening". That is, "tune in" to what you are listening for and block all other sounds and murmurs from your consciousness.

11. At times, accurate and efficient auscultation over the chest and neck is accomplished by having the patient stop breathing. In this way, breath sounds are not interfering with your ability to hear. You should also stop breathing. This will remind you when to tell your patient to resume breathing.

Figure 2-43. *Inching technique* for determining S1 and S2. The second heart sound (S2) is normally louder than the first (S1) over the aortic area (ao), a point that can be helpful in distinguishing which sound is S1 and which is S2. If you keep S2 in mind as a reference as the stethoscope is moved or "inched" from the aortic area to the apex, any sound or murmur you hear before S2 will be systolic in timing, and after S2, diastolic. This point can be helpful when there is a rapid cardiac rhythm and it is uncertain which sound is S1 and which is S2.

Figure 2-44. The inching technique in a patient with an S4 gallop. Inching from the aortic area (AO) to the apex identifies the extra sound as an S4 gallop occurring before the first heart sound (S1). In this instance S1 (which is louder than S2 at the apex) often serves as an even better reference than S2 when inching.

Figure 2-45. The inching technique in a patient with an S3 gallop. Inching from the aortic area (AO) to the apex

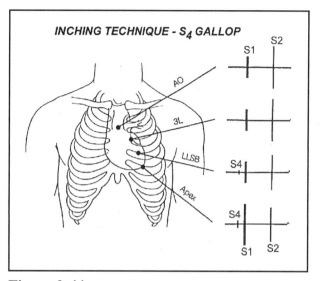

Figure 2-44 (Courtesy of W. Proctor Harvey, M.D.)

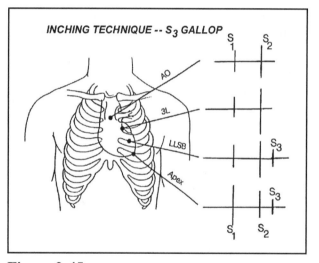

Figure 2-45 (Courtesy of W. Proctor Harvey, M.D.)

identifies the extra sound as an S3 gallop occurring after the second heart sound (S2).

In clinical practice, it is customary to listen for specific heart sounds and murmurs over the traditional so-called "valve" areas, which are points over the precordium where events originating in each heart valve are best transmitted and heard (**Figure 2-46**).

- Sounds and murmurs of the aortic valve and aorta, for example, are well heard at the second right intercostal space (*aortic area*).
- Sounds and murmurs from the pulmonic valve and pulmonary artery are usually heard best at the second left intercostal space (*pulmonic area*) or (mid) left sternal border.

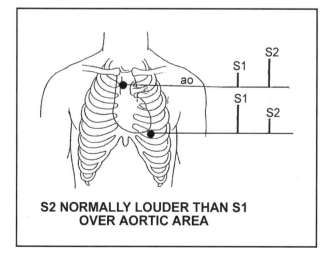

Figure 2-43 (Courtesy of W. Proctor Harvey, M.D.)

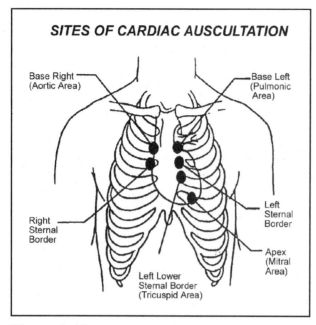

SITES OF CARDIAC AUSCULTATION

Base Right (Aortic Area)

Base Left (Pulmonic Area)

Right Sternal Border

Left Sternal Border

Apex (Mitral Area)

Left Lower Sternal Border (Tricuspid Area)

Figure 2-46 (Courtesy of W. Proctor Harvey, M.D.)

- The *mid-left sternal border* is usually the best site to detect the diastolic murmur of AR (blood rushes back into the left ventricle).
- The *lower left sternal border* (*tricuspid area*) is the customary location for evaluation of the first heart sound, systolic clicks, right-sided S4 and S3 gallops, and tricuspid valve sounds and murmurs. The characteristic increase in intensity of the holosystolic murmur of TR with inspiration (*Carvallo's sign*) is best appreciated at this site. (In general, murmurs originating on the right side of the heart increase with inspiration.) The holosystolic murmur of VSD, often accompanied by a palpable thrill, is also located over the tricuspid area.
- The apex (*mitral area*) is usually best for identification of left-sided S4 and S3 gallops and murmurs of mitral valve origin. Aortic ejection sounds and murmurs, however, are often well heard in this location as well.

Important findings may also be present in other locations :

- Neck—transmitted systolic ejection murmur of valvular aortic stenosis along the aortic branches, bruit of carotid arterial occlusive disease
- Clavicle—bone transmission of valvular aortic stenosis
- Supraclavicular fossa—continuous murmur of jugular venous hum heard in children (normal),

thyrotoxicosis, anemia, pregnancy, or in any hyperkinetic state
- Left axilla and posterior lung base—"band-like" radiation of holosystolic murmur of chronic MR
- Right sternal border—so-called "right-sided" diastolic murmur of the special type of AR due to aortic rightward displacement with aortic root pathology e.g., aortic dissection, aneurysm, Marfan's syndrome. (The *valvular* type of aortic regurgitation is best heard along the *left* sternal border.)
- Abdomen—bruit of renal artery stenosis
- Over scars—continuous murmur of arteriovenous fistula, which can result in high-output heart failure

Certain heart sounds and/or murmurs may be faint and difficult to hear over the precordium, and, therefore, can be overlooked, especially in a patient with chronic obstructive pulmonary disease and an increase in anterior-posterior chest diameter. This is true if one listens over the usual areas of the chest. Listening over the xiphoid area or epigastrium (with the patient in the upright position), however, may help you detect these sounds more easily. Also, keep in mind that although mitral stenosis can at times be "silent" (with no murmur present), in most of these cases, the bell of the stethoscope is not properly placed over the point of maximum impulse, a localized spot (which may be the size of a quarter) where the diagnostic diastolic rumble may be heard. The murmur can be missed unless the stethoscope is placed exactly over this small area.

Dynamic Auscultation

Changes in body position and bedside physiologic maneuvers (*dynamic auscultation*) may help in the evaluation of heart sounds and murmurs (**Figure 2-47**):

- *Squatting* (compresses veins in the legs and abdomen) causes the venous return to the heart to increase and also increases peripheral vascular resistance. As a result, it brings out the murmurs of AR, MR and VSD. With prompt squatting, the *left ventricular volume temporarily increases*. The mitral valve is then less redundant. This results in a *delay* of the click and murmur of *mitral valve prolapse* to a later point in systole as well as a shorter murmur of decreased volume. (As a *mnemonic*, think of squatting as moving the murmur of MVP toward the "rear", i.e., closer to diastole.) Squatting similarly decreases the intensity of the murmur of HOCM, because the outflow obstruction created by movement of the anterior mitral leaflet toward the ventricular-impinging hypertrophic septum (Venturi effect) is

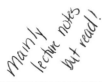

FIGURE 2-47

Clinical Response of Auscultatory Events to Physiologic Interventions

Auscultatory Events	Intervention and Response
Systolic murmurs	
Innocent systolic murmur	Louder with supine position; fainter with sitting or standing
Valvular aortic stenosis	Louder following a pause after a premature beat.
Hypertrophic obstructive cardiomyopathy.	Louder on standing, during Valsalva maneuver; fainter with prompt squatting.
Mitral regurgitation	Louder on sudden squatting or with isometric handgrip.
Mitral valve prolapse	Midsystolic click moves toward S1 and late systolic murmur starts earlier on standing; click may occur earlier on inspiration; murmur starts later and click moves toward S2 during squatting.
Tricuspid regurgitation	Louder during inspiration.
Ventricular septal defect (without pulmonary hypertension)	Louder on sudden squatting or with isometric handgrip.
Diastolic murmurs	
Aortic regurgitation	Louder with sitting upright and leaning forward, sudden squatting, and isometric handgrip.
Mitral stenosis	Louder with exercise, left lateral decubitus position, coughing. Inspiration produces triple sequence of A2-P2-OS ("trill").
Continuous murmurs	
Patent ductus arteriosus	Diastolic phase louder with isometric handgrip.
Cervical venous hum	Disappears with direct compression of the jugular vein.
Extra heart sounds	
S3 and S4 gallops	Left-sided gallop sounds: accentuated by lying in left lateral decubitus position; decreased by standing or during Valsalva. Right-sided gallop sounds usually louder during inspiration, left-sided during expiration.
Ejection sounds	Ejection sound in pulmonic stenosis fainter and occurs closer to the first sound during inspiration.
Pericardial friction rub	Louder with sitting upright and leaning forward, and with inspiration.

---

relieved temporarily by the increased ventricular volume. While squatting *decreases* the murmur intensity of HOCM, it *increases* the murmur of aortic stenosis due to the increased left ventricular stroke volume. Thus squatting can help distinguish HOCM from aortic stenosis, since it decreases the murmur volume in HOCM (as it does in MVP) but increases the murmur volume in aortic stenosis. *Standing* (pools blood in the lower extremities) decreases venous return and ventricular filling. As a result, it decreases the intensity of all murmurs except HOCM and MVP. The squatting maneuver is ideally performed if the practitioner remains comfortably seated, and listens for any subtle auscultatory changes while the patient squats and stands.

(*Mnemonic*: the large heart of HOCM "squashes", i.e., reduces, the murmur during squatting.)

Figure 2-48. Effect of squatting on the murmur of mitral valve prolapse. When the patient moves quickly from standing to squatting the click(s) move closer to the second heart sound (S2) and the murmur gets shorter and fainter. Standing causes the click(s) to move closer to the first heart sound (S1) and the murmur gets longer and louder.

Figure 2-49. Effect of squatting on the murmur of HOCM. The murmur decreases on squatting.

- The *Valsalva maneuver* (increases intrathoracic pressure) and *standing* (pools blood in the legs) have the opposite effect of squatting. They decrease

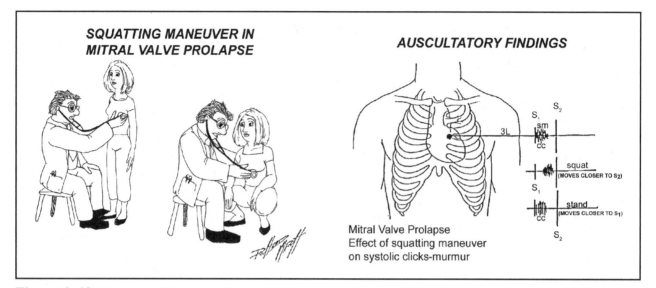

Figure 2-48 (Courtesy of W. Proctor Harvey, M.D.)

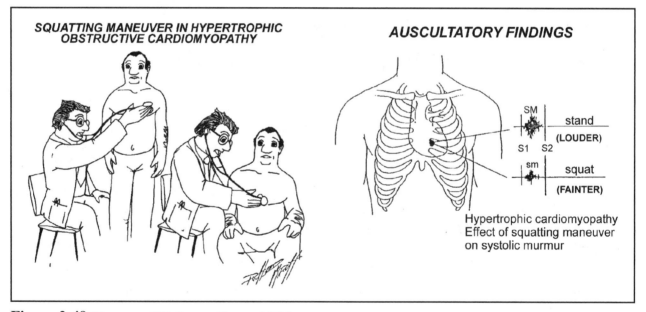

Figure 2-49 (Courtesy of W. Proctor Harvey, M.D.)

venous return to the heart and *decrease left ventricular volume*. The systolic click and murmur of MVP moves *earlier* in systole and the sounds become more accentuated, since the valves are more redundant in the smaller ventricle cavity and flop and move sooner back into the left atrium. The systolic murmur of HOCM *increases* (increased obstruction with reduced ventricular volume), while

the systolic murmur of aortic stenosis *decreases* (less forceful ventricular contraction with decreased ventricular volume).

• *Isometric hand grip exercise* (or transient arterial occlusion of both arms with two blood pressure cuffs) increases peripheral vascular resistance (i.e., the afterload) and *increases* the murmurs of MR (more blood goes back into the left atrium), VSD

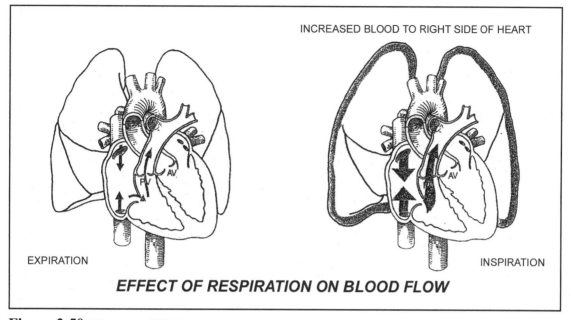

INCREASED BLOOD TO RIGHT SIDE OF HEART

EXPIRATION

INSPIRATION

EFFECT OF RESPIRATION ON BLOOD FLOW

Figure 2-50 (Courtesy of W. Proctor Harvey, M.D.)

(more blood goes from left ventricle into right ventricle), and AR (more blood goes back into the ventricle). (*Mnemonic:* Your regurgitation would increase, too, if you were squeezed.)

The click and murmur of mitral valve prolapse may be masked or disappear altogether with the increased blood volume and ventricular dimensions during pregnancy, returning after delivery in the postpartum state. Likewise, beta blocking agents (frequently used to treat these patients) decrease heart rate and contractility and increase ventricular volume (allowing more time for ventricular filling) and may attenuate or abolish the classic findings of MVP. These auscultatory phenomena, therefore, may help explain why patients with mitral valve prolapse may have no acoustic findings on one occasion yet prominent findings on another.

Noting the *effect of respiration* on hearts sounds and murmurs can provide important diagnostic clues:

Figure 2-50. Inspiration increases the venous return to the right side of the heart, causing a delayed pulmonic valve (PV) closure because the right ventricle requires a little longer to pump this normal increase in the amount of blood. Also, there is earlier closure of the aortic valve (AV) with inspiration, since less blood returns to the left side of the heart, there is less pressure in the left ventricle, and the aortic valve can close more quickly against this reduced pressure. Shaded areas indicate expansion with inspiration, and arrows denote blood flow.

Figure 2-51. Effect of respiration on the splitting of the second heart sound (S2):

A. Normally, S2 is split on inspiration due to the relative delay in closure of the pulmonic valve (P2).

B. In paradoxical splitting (in LBBB, AS, hypertension) the split becomes more noticeable during expiration, since the pulmonic valve in the resting state closes before the aortic valve in these conditions. (In LBBB the left ventricle doesn't contract fast enough; in AS and hypertension it takes longer for blood to be ejected from the left ventricle against resistance.)

C. In ASD (where blood generally shunts from left to right atrium, but may do the reverse in severe pulmonary vascular disease, resulting in cyanosis), the splitting is fixed in inspiration and expiration, since the shunt equilibrates the pressure differential between left and right atrium during respiration. (To make this diagnosis, there needs to also be a systolic murmur of ASD; without the murmur, ASD is not likely.)

D. In RBBB and pulmonary stenosis (PS), splitting widens on inspiration but is also heard in expiration, since the pulmonary valve is even further delayed in its closure. In RBBB the delay is due to a slowly contracting right ventricle; in PS the delay in pulmonic valve closure is due to delay of blood flow through the stenotic pulmonary valve.

E. In pulmonary hypertension the splitting is narrow and the P2 component of the S2 is particularly loud due to loud closure of the pulmonic valve resulting from the pulmonary hypertension.

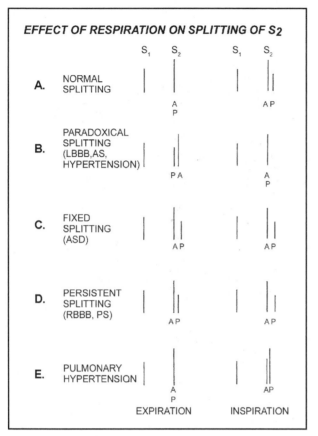

Figure 2-51

- *All right-sided heart sounds and murmurs,* (with the exception of the pulmonic ejection sound of pulmonic stenosis*) increase in intensity with inspiration* because inspiration increases the venous return through the right side of the heart and the murmurs increase with the increased blood flow. (The pulmonic ejection sound does not increase with inspiration in pulmonic stenosis, and, in fact, decreases, because the higher pressure in the right ventricle gets the valves starting to move upward even before right ventricular systole; thus, there is a less of a valve excursion and less sudden thrusting open of the valves when systole occurs.)

Figure 2-52. Inspiration *decreases* the left-sided murmur of mitral regurgitation (decreased blood volume and flow on the left side during inspiration), but *increases* the right-sided murmur of tricuspid regurgitation (increased blood volume and flow on the right side during inspiration).

Figure 2-53. Sometimes a pause in the ECG after a premature beat or in a paused interval of atrial fibrillation may change the quality of a murmur and provide further clues as to the differential diagnosis. For instance, the systolic murmur (SM) of mitral regurgitation remains relatively unchanged in intensity after a pause (since the LV to LA pressure gradient is minimally affected by alterations in cycle length). In contrast, the systolic (ejection) murmur (SM) of aortic stenosis is louder after a pause (prolonged

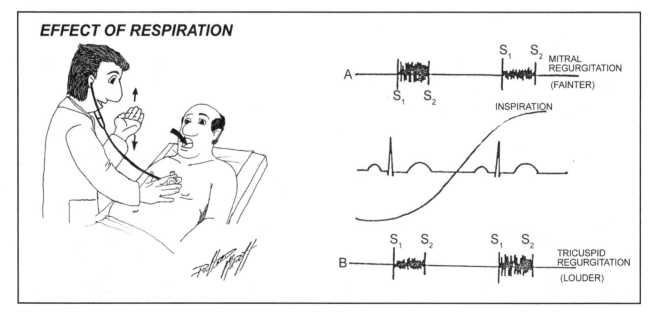

Figure 2-52 (Courtesy of W. Proctor Harvey, M.D.)

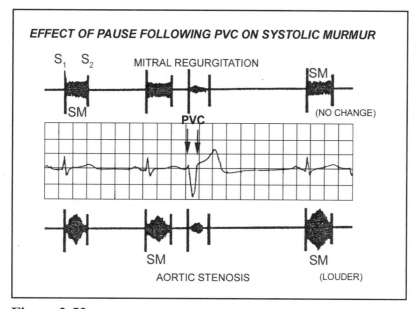

Figure 2-53 (Courtesy of W. Proctor Harvey, M.D.)

diastole results in greater filling of the left ventricle, along with an increase in stroke volume, and greater flow of blood across the narrow aortic valve).

When evaluating the effect of respiration, a helpful technique is to have the patient follow your free hand, and breathe in when your hand moves upward, and breathe out when it moves downward.

Heart Sounds: Normal and Abnormal

First and Second Heart Sounds (S1 and S2)
Please see attached CD for an interactive overview of heart sounds and murmurs-the so-called *"music of the heart"*.

Figure 2-54 reviews the proper cardiac auscultatory technique in listening for abnormal sounds and murmurs.

When performing auscultation it helps to focus on one aspect of the cardiac cycle at a time rather than trying to hear everything at once, and to have a set sequence of listening. For instance, focus on S1, then on S2, then on systolic sounds and murmurs, then on diastolic sounds and murmurs. Paying close attention to their *timing* (location within the cardiac cycle), *intensity* (loud, normal or faint), *frequency* (high, medium, low-pitched), *tonal quality* (sharp, dull, muffled, snapping, tambour), may provide valuable clinical clues to underlying heart disease.

Figure 2-55 summarizes clinical clues to heart disease from auscultation of heart sounds and murmurs.

Auscultation of S1 ("Lub")

Pay attention to the intensity of S1 (faint or loud). Most clinically significant abnormalities of S1 are of intensity rather than split-ting. Since S2 is normally louder than S1 at the aortic area, the clinician may identify a loud S1 if it is equal to or louder than S2 over the aortic area.

Loud S1

The intensity of S1 is augmented by any condition that increases the force of ventricular contraction and the rate of pressure development in the ventricle in systole, or brings the heart closer to the chest wall. Thus, S1 is physiologically louder in children and young adults, in patients with a thin chest wall, and in hyperkinetic states (e.g., exercise, tachycardia, anemia, hyperthyroidism, fever, pregnancy, excitement). In the presence of a normal ventricular rate, however, a loud S1 should provide a clue to the possibility of a cardiac problem:

- A loud S1 is heard in *rheumatic mitral stenosis*. In mitral stenosis with mobile cusps, the loud S1 relates to the high left atrial pressure (from blood that couldn't get through to the ventricle), which causes the valve to remain open more widely until a very sharp high-velocity closing movement is produced by ventricular contraction. In fact, unless the mitral valve is immobilized by calcific deposits, an increase in intensity of S1 can be considered an auscultatory hallmark of mitral stenosis.
- A loud S1 occurs with a *short ECG PR interval* (the time required for conduction of the electrical impulse through the atria to the ventricles up to the time of ventricular depolarization), since the valve

---

FIGURE 2-54

Proper Cardiac Auscultatory Technique

- Room should be quiet.
- Time heart sounds and murmurs by "inching" technique (or by palpation of carotid artery or apical impulse).
- The bell of the stethoscope is best for low-frequency sounds and murmurs (e.g., S4 and S3 gallops, diastolic rumbles).
- The diaphragm of the stethoscope is best for high-frequency sounds and murmurs (e.g., aortic regurgitation).
- Listen with bell lightly applied at cardiac apex, with patient turned to left lateral decubitus position, for S4 and S3 gallops and/or rumble of mitral stenosis.
- Listen with diaphragm firmly applied over the left sternal border with patient sitting forward, during held expiration for diastolic blowing murmur of aortic regurgitation, and/or pericardial friction rub.
- Listen individually to S1 and S2.
  —Are both S1 and S2 present?
  —Is either sound loud, normal, or faint? Does splitting of S2 widen, remain "fixed", or reverse with inspiration?
- Listen for extra sounds in systole (e.g., mitral clicks, aortic or pulmonic ejection sounds) or diastole (e.g., S4 and S3 gallops, pericardial knock sound, mitral opening snap, "tumor plop").
- Listen for murmurs.
  —Systolic (early, mid, late, holosystolic)
  —Diastolic
  —Continuous
  —Where is the murmur heard and radiate?
  —Does the murmur change with body position, respiration, certain maneuvers (e.g., Valsalva)?
- Listen for pericardial friction rubs or prosthetic valve sounds

---

leaflets are in a wide open position at the onset of ventricular contraction and close more forcefully.

- When a loud S1 is heard along with a holosystolic murmur of mitral regurgitation, the clinician should always consider the diagnosis of *mitral valve prolapse*. There, the loud S1 may be due to an increased amplitude of leaflet excursion beyond the line of closure and/or the merging of S1 with the systolic click of mitral valve prolapse (see below).

Faint S1

- A faint S1 may accompany a *prolonged PR interval on the ECG* (0.20 - 0.24 seconds), as occurs in first degree AV block (i.e., where there is slowing of the electrical communication to the ventricles and a delay in ventricular contraction), since the mitral leaflets are almost in a closed position by the time ventricular contraction begins.
- In *acute, severe aortic regurgitation,* a sudden volume overload in the left ventricle from the regurgitation results in a markedly elevated end-diastolic pressure, which may lead to premature closing of the mitral valve and therefore reduce the intensity of S1. The faint S1 is an important clue to this urgent diagnosis, where early surgical intervention can be life-saving.
- S1 may be diminished in *mitral regurgitation* by thickening, fibrosis, calcification and shortening of the valve apparatus, resulting in ineffective valve closure and loss of mobility.
- Body build, chest configuration (e.g., emphysema with an increased anteroposterior chest diameter) and other extracardiac factors (e.g., obesity, large breasts, increased chest wall thickness, and pericardial effusion) may also play a role in diminishing the intensity of S1.

Variable Intensity of S1

- A variation in the intensity of S1 may be detected during atrioventricular dissociation (the atria and ventricles do not contract in a coordinated manner) due to varying PR intervals (e.g., heart block), and

FIGURE 2-55

Clinical Clues to Heart Disease from Auscultation of Heart Sounds and Murmurs

Clue	Clinical Significance
• **First heart sound (S1)**	
Loud S1	Short PR interval, mitral stenosis, (holosystolic) MVP, hyperkinetic states; normal in children, young adults, patients with thin chest wall and narrow A-P diameter.
Changing intensity of S1	AV dissociation (varying PR intervals), e.g., complete heart block, VT; atrial fibrillation.
Faint S1	Long PR interval (first-degree AV block) decreased LV contractility (congestive heart failure, acute myocardial infarction, cardiomyopathy); severe aortic regurgitation, mitral regurgitation; increased tissue, air or fluid between heart and stethoscope (e.g., emphysema, obesity, large breasts, thick chest wall, increased A-P diameter, pericardial effusion).
Wide splitting of S1	RBBB, PVCs. VT, ASD
• **Second heart sound (S2)**	
"Fixed" split S2	Atrial septal defect
Paradoxically split S2	Severe valvular aortic stenosis, hypertrophic obstructive cardiomyopathy, left bundle branch block, severe LV systolic dysfunction (e.g., acute MI)
Wide "physiologic" split S2	Mitral regurgitation, large ventricular septal defect, pulmonic stenosis, RBBB
Loud "tambour" A2	Severe hypertension, aortic dilatation
Faint A2	Valvular aortic stenosis
Loud P2	Pulmonary hypertension
Faint P2	Pulmonic stenosis
• **Third heart sound (S3 gallop)**	LV or RV systolic and/or diastolic dysfunction, mitral regurgitation, aortic regurgitation, VSD, PDA (due to large volume of ventricular flow)
	Physiologic in healthy child or young adult, athlete, hyperkinetic state or 3rd trimester of pregnancy
• **Fourth heart sound (S4 gallop)**	LV or RV diastolic dysfunction (CAD, systemic or pulmonary hypertension, LV or RV hypertrophy, valvular AS, PS, dilated, restrictive or hypertrophic obstructive cardiomyopathy, aging), pulmonary hypertension
	Normal in some apparently healthy older persons
• **Extra heart sounds**	
Opening snap	Mitral stenosis (pliable)
Ejection sounds	
Aortic	Bicuspid aortic valve, dilated aortic root (aneurysm, hypertension, valvular aortic stenosis, aortic insufficiency)
Pulmonic	Pulmonic stenosis, dilatation of pulmonary artery
Pericardial knock	Constrictive pericarditis
Pericardial friction rub	Pericarditis
• **Systolic murmurs**	
Early-mid	"Innocent" systolic murmur, aortic sclerosis, valvular AS, PS, HOCM
Holosystolic	MR, TR, VSD
Late systolic	MVP, papillary muscle dysfunction, calcified mitral annulus
• **Diastolic murmurs**	
Early (high frequency)	AR, pulmonic regurgitation
Mid-late (low frequency)	Mitral stenosis, flow rumble in severe MR, AR
• **Continuous murmurs**	Patent ductus arteriosus, jugular venous hum, arteriovenous fistula

with changes in cycle lengths (e.g., atrial fibrillation), since there is variation in position of the mitral leaflets at the time of ventricular contraction. The finding of a slow heart rate (~ 40 beats/min), accompanied by a varying intensity of S1, is an auscultatory clue to the clinical diagnosis of complete heart block (where there is no effective electrical communication between atria and ventricles and both contract independently in an uncoordinated fashion).

- Ventricular tachycardia is also marked by a changing intensity of S1.

Wide splitting of S1 can be observed sometimes in conditions where there is a significant delay in right ventricular contraction (or where there is early left ventricular contraction), resulting in a late closure of the tricuspid valve in relation to the mitral valve (e.g. RBBB, PVCs, ventricular tachycardia, atrial septal effect). Wide splitting of S1 should be distinguished from other sounds that can simulate a split S1, e.g., S4 gallop, ejection sound, early systolic click (see below) .

Auscultation of S2 ("Dub")

S2 is normally higher in pitch, shorter and sharper than S1. A2 is normally louder and earlier than P2, and can be heard well over the entire precordium. P2 is normally heard over the pulmonic area and mid-left sternal border, and does not radiate to the apex, except in young, thin individuals (with a narrow anteroposterior chest diameter) or when pulmonary hypertension is present.

Intensity and Splitting of S2

Note whether S2 is faint or loud and particularly note the effect of respiration on the splitting of S2 into A2 and P2 components, which can provide significant diagnostic information (**Figures 2–51 and 2–56**).

In many normal older patients (> 50 years of age), splitting of S2 may be less discernible to the examiner, with

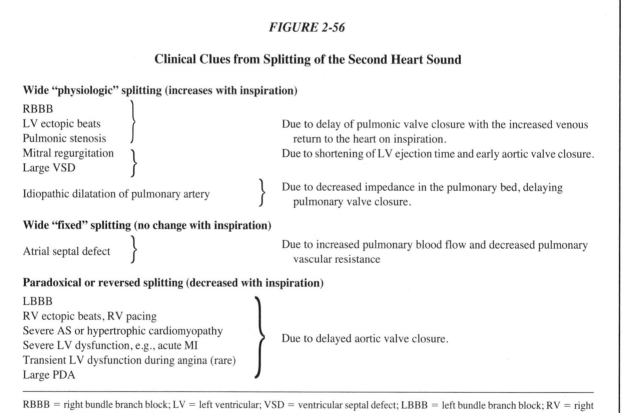

FIGURE 2-56

Clinical Clues from Splitting of the Second Heart Sound

Wide "physiologic" splitting (increases with inspiration)

RBBB
LV ectopic beats
Pulmonic stenosis } Due to delay of pulmonic valve closure with the increased venous return to the heart on inspiration.

Mitral regurgitation
Large VSD } Due to shortening of LV ejection time and early aortic valve closure.

Idiopathic dilatation of pulmonary artery } Due to decreased impedance in the pulmonary bed, delaying pulmonary valve closure.

Wide "fixed" splitting (no change with inspiration)

Atrial septal defect } Due to increased pulmonary blood flow and decreased pulmonary vascular resistance

Paradoxical or reversed splitting (decreased with inspiration)

LBBB
RV ectopic beats, RV pacing
Severe AS or hypertrophic cardiomyopathy
Severe LV dysfunction, e.g., acute MI } Due to delayed aortic valve closure.
Transient LV dysfunction during angina (rare)
Large PDA

RBBB = right bundle branch block; LV = left ventricular; VSD = ventricular septal defect; LBBB = left bundle branch block; RV = right ventricular; AS = aortic stenosis; PDA = patent ductus arteriosus.

a single audible S2 on inspiration and expiration. This results from a delayed A2 (e.g., from left ventricular dysfunction or aortic stenosis) and earlier P2, secondary to decreased pulmonary "hang-out" time (decreased compliance in the pulmonary vascular bed). An inaudible P2 may also exist in older adults with increased anteroposterior chest diameter. This may result in a single S2 heard during both expiration and inspiration (or single during inspiration but split on expiration, leading to the false impression of paradoxical splitting of S2; the A2 and P2 do not in that case fuse during inspiration, but rather the P2 just can't be heard due to the increase in AP chest diameter on inspiring).

A loud S2 will result from elevation of pressure in either of the great vessels, causing a forceful valve closure sound. Hence:

- In systemic arterial hypertension there is a loud "tambour" (ringing, musical) A2.
- In pulmonary hypertension there is a loud P2. As mentioned, P2 is not normally heard at the apex, except in young thin individuals. If it is heard at the apex (along with A2), consider pulmonary hypertension.
- In aortic stenosis, there is a faint A2.
- In pulmonic stenosis, there is a faint P2.

Sounds in Systole
Ejection Sounds and Systolic Clicks

Normally, the opening of the aortic or pulmonic valves is acoustically silent. In certain cardiac conditions, brief, sharp and high-pitched sounds in early systole, occurring shortly after S1, may be heard and are referred to as *aortic or pulmonic ejection sounds*. They occur at the *onset* of ventricular ejection and systolic flow into the great vessels. They are heard best with the diaphragm chest piece, and frequently are close enough to S1 to simulate splitting. They are usually the result of "doming" of the maximal opening motion of a congenitally stenotic, but mobile and compliant, aortic or pulmonic valve.

Figure 2-57. The mechanism of the aortic valvular ejection sound (E.S.) in aortic stenosis. When the valve moves from closed (in diastole) to open (in systole), a "*doming effect*" occurs because of restriction to complete opening. The ejection sound occurs when the valve is checked at its maximally distended position. The intensity of the ejection sound correlates directly with the valve's mobility and becomes faint or disappears with calcific fixation of the aortic valve. Ao, aortic valve; S.M., systolic murmur. (Courtesy of Dr. James A. Ronan, Jr.).

Aortic ejection sounds are widely transmitted over the precordium, but are best heard at the aortic area and the

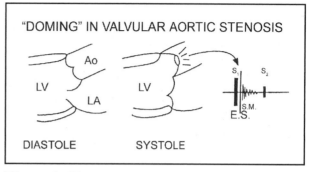

Figure 2-57

cardiac apex (where they may even be loudest). The ejection sound of pulmonic stenosis is similar, but, unlike the aortic ejection sound (which remains unchanged in inspiration and expiration), it decreases in intensity during inspiration (since the inflow of blood to the right ventricle moves the stenotic pulmonic leaflets upward to a more open position, resulting in less systolic excursion). Also, the pulmonic ejection sound is not heard at the apex (it's heard best at the base over the second left intercostal space [pulmonic area] or mid left sternal border).

Figure 2-58. Decrease in the intensity of the ejection sound of pulmonic stenosis with inspiration, in comparison with the lack of change in aortic stenosis.

In other cases, ejection sounds are due to abrupt "checking" of the rapid initial systolic distention of a dilated ascending aorta (e.g., aneurysm, hypertension), or main pulmonary artery (vascular, rather than valvular, origin). They may also occur with forceful LV ejection (e.g., thyrotoxicosis, anemia, pregnancy, exercise, high cardiac output states). Ejection sounds also occur with prosthetic (mechanical) aortic valve opening.

It is important that the clinician becomes adept in the detection of ejection sounds, as they often serve as one of the first clues to the diagnosis of these conditions.

Systolic clicks are discrete high-frequency sounds caused by *prolapse of the mitral valve* leaflets into the left atrium during systole. Prolapse may also occur in the tricuspid valve. Isolated tricuspid valve prolapse, however, occurs only rarely, and when it does it usually accompanies mitral valve prolapse. Systolic clicks may be single or multiple. They are heard best at the cardiac apex or lower left sternal border, and are usually mid to late systolic, although occasionally they occur sufficiently early to simulate an ejection sound. They are thought to be generated by the sudden tensing of the redundant mitral valve leaflets and elongated chordae tendineae when the mitral leaflet is checked at the farthest extent of its valve motion.

Figure 2-59. There can be a wide spectrum of auscultatory findings in mitral valve prolapse, even in the same

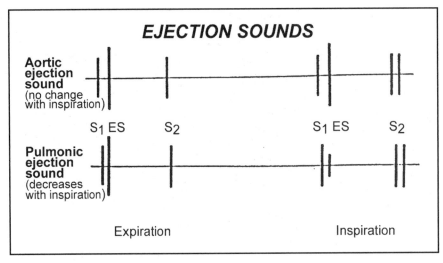

Figure 2-58

patient. Sometimes, no click or murmur is present. At other times, an isolated systolic click (or clicks) with or without a mid to late systolic (crescendo-decrescendo, or crescendo) or holosystolic murmur, or musical "whoop" or "honk" of MR may be audible. One negative examination does not exclude the diagnosis. **A)** single click, **B)** multiple clicks, **C)** click-systolic murmur.

Careful examination with a stethoscope remains a most valuable and cost-effective means of diagnosing MVP. The di-

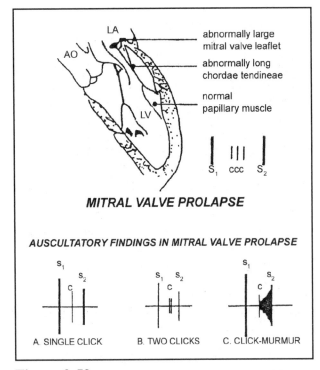

Figure 2-59 (Courtesy of W. Proctor Harvey, M.D.)

agnostic acoustic hallmark, the systolic click, may even be heard in patients with no evidence of MVP on echo (or angiography). These clicks, however, are often overlooked when the clinician does not properly time them or listen specifically for these high-pitched sounds in systole. As a rule, the findings are best detected using the diaphragm of the stethoscope. The auscultatory phenomena described usually occur in otherwise healthy asymptomatic individuals, often young women. However, a variety of symptoms and associated complications may occur, e.g., atypical chest pain, dyspnea, palpitations (attributed to arrhythmias), chronic anxiety, panic reactions, fatigue, autonomic nervous system dysfunction, high adrenergic tone, orthostatic hypotension, dizziness, syncope, transient cerebral ischemic attacks, progressive mitral regurgitation, ruptured chordae tendineae, infective endocarditis, and, rarely, sudden death. Infective endocarditis may occur on the mitral valve, even when only a click (or clicks) and no murmur is detected. It is particularly rare for sudden death to occur in patients with an isolated click. It ususally occurs in symptomatic individuals with a click, murmur, and thickened valve leaflets on echo.

Idiopathic MVP (*myxomatous degeneration*) has proved to be the most common basis for systolic clicks. Other heart diseases, however, have been associated with systolic clicks, including Marfan's syndrome, ostium secundum atrial septal defect, papillary muscle dysfunction secondary to coronary artery disease, and cardiomyopathy.

Sounds in Diastole
Third and Fourth Heart Sounds (S3 and S4)

The S3 is the sound of early diastolic passive ventricular filling, and the S4 is the sound of late active ventricular filling as the atrium contracts. An S3 or an S4 can be either left-sided or right-sided, reflecting a problem either with the left or right side of the heart. An

S3 commonly is normal (*physiologic S3*) in a healthy child or young adult, athlete, hyperkinetic states, or third trimester of pregnancy. It diminishes with age as the ventricles become less compliant, and usually disappear by age 20–30 years except in those in good athletic shape. The S3 is an abnormal sound (*pathologic S3 or S3 "gallop"*) in heart failure and/or cardiomyopathy with LV or RV systolic and/or diastolic dysfunction, and MR, AR, VSD, or PDA due to large volume of ventricular flow.

The S3 or S4 is heard as an S1–S2–S3 or S4–S1–S2 gallop rhythm (like the canter of a horse), or as a *quadruple rhythm* (S4–S1–S2–S3). The S3 and S4 are best heard with the bell of the stethoscope applied lightly to the apex point of maximum impulse with the patient turned to the left side (for left-sided gallops) or tricuspid area or xiphoid process (for right-sided gallops). Right-sided gallops increase with inspiration due to increased venous return and increased blood flow in the right ventricle, while left-sided gallops are heard best on expiration due to the narrower diameter of the chest.

S3 gallops are generally particularly faint sounds. Most S3 gallops are usually heard every third or fourth beat rather than with every beat. On the other hand, an S4 gallop is more likely to be heard with almost every beat.

In rapid tachycardias the S3 and S4 can sometimes occur so close to one another as to fuse in a *"summation" gallop,* which may be louder than both the S1 and S2.

The *S4 gallop,* in particular, is a hallmark of myocardial infarction, or conditions where there is decreased ventricular compliance (*diastolic dysfunction*), which necessitates a more forceful atrial contraction for completion of ventricular filling. This change in compliance may be related to ventricular hypertrophy, ischemia, infarction, fibrosis or an increased afterload, e.g., elevated aortic or pulmonary artery pressure resulting in ventricular hypertrophy and stiffening of the ventricular wall. The detection of an S4 gallop and a loud "tambour" second heart sound (A2) are the earliest auscultatory findings detected in hypertensive heart disease, often preceding ECG and other signs of LV hypertrophy or symptoms of cardiac decompensation.

S4 gallops are also commonly heard in patients with *acute* severe MR (e.g., ruptured chordae tendineae, papillary muscle rupture following an acute MI), reflecting the presence of vigorous left atrial contraction resulting in acceleration of blood flow into the LV. This contrasts sharply with the absence of an S4 gallop in *chronic* MR, since the left atrium is large in chronic MR, dilated and unable to generate much contractile force. The presence of an S4 gallop in conjunction with the murmur of MR is, therefore, an important clue alerting you that the valve leak is acute or of recent onset.

An *S3 gallop* (a sign of *systolic dysfunction*) is heard predominantly in dilated hypocontractile left ventricles and results from the sudden cessation of early, rapid LV filling impelled by high LA pressure. It can also be heard in diastolic dysfunction, and a variety of conditions, *not necessarily implying a failing ventricle.* If blood rapidly accelerates into the ventricle because of an *increased volume of flow,* an S3 may also occur (e.g., MR, AR, VSD, PDA). Left-sided S3 gallops, though, do commonly suggest a loss of LV function, along with an elevated LA and LV filling pressure, particularly when accompanied by pulsus alternans and alternation of intensity of heart sounds and/or murmurs. A patient with hypertension may have an S4, known for many years and without cardiac decompensation; however, once systolic heart failure occurs, the S3 gallop may be noted for the first time.

An S3 would not be expected in tight mitral stenosis. In fact, an audible S3 in isolated mitral valve disease virtually excludes the diagnosis of severe mitral stenosis.

An S4 gallop may be detected, if carefully searched for, in almost all patients with an acute MI due to the presence of a stiff, noncompliant, ischemic LV; it may become louder during the early phase of infarction or during an episode of angina pectoris. The S4 gallop may therefore provide a useful clue if it appears intermittently during attacks of chest pain suspected of being ischemic in etiology. Likewise, since the S4 gallop appears almost universally in patients with acute MI, its absence should raise serious doubts as to the diagnosis. It is most unusual not to hear an S4 gallop in those patients who are in normal sinus rhythm and have had a prior myocardial infarction. It may occur with or without clinical evidence of CHF.

Since an S4 relies on atrial contraction, it is not present during atrial fibrillation. An S3 may still persist.

Right-sided S3 gallops are present in patients with dilated right ventricles and elevated right heart pressures. These sounds, therefore, may even be heard over the cardiac apex when the dilated right ventricle occupies it. They are commonly heard in those patients with RV failure, TR, pulmonary hypertension, cor pulmonale due to pulmonary emboli or pulmonary parenchymal or vascular disease.

In the middle-aged and older adult (age >50) an S3 (which was normal in youth) may now afford one of the earliest clues to the presence of volume overload (e.g., MR, AR) or cardiac decompensation (due to LV systolic dysfunction). The S3 thus can have great diagnostic and prognostic value. An S3 in an asymptomatic young person with otherwise normal cardiac examination, ECG, and CXR (i.e., physiologic S3) has a meaning entirely different (normal) from an S3 in a patient with shortness of breath, pulsus alternans, pulmonary rales, and cardiomegaly.

To distinguish an S4 from a split S1 or ejection sound, note that alternating the pressure with the bell causes the S4 gallop to fade in and out, but will not obliterate a split S1 or ejection sound. Also, to distinguish from an aortic ejection sound, note that an S4 usually is not heard over the aortic area.

Ejection sounds may be difficult to differentiate from a split S1. However, the separation of S1 from an ejection sound or an early systolic click is generally wider than the separation in a split S1. Pay careful attention to location (aortic ejection sounds are loudest at the aortic area and apex, pulmonic ejection sounds are loudest at the pulmonic area, split S1 is loudest at the tricuspid area and occasionally the apex, but not over the aortic or pulmonic areas). Also note variation in intensity with inspiration (aortic ejection sounds do not vary with respiration).

If you hear what appears to be a loud S1 in the aortic or pulmonic area, while remembering that S2 is normally louder than S1 in this location, the loud S1 in these areas should be an immediate clue that this represents an ejection sound, unless the patient has an unusually loud S1 at the apex, as may occur with mitral stenosis or short PR interval. One should not confuse the tricuspid closure sound (T1) with the pulmonic ejection sound, since the intensity of T1 tends to increase rather than decrease during inspiration (while the intensity of pulmonic ejection sound decreases with inspiration).

The timing of a systolic click is usually later (mid to late systole), and if early, will vary in position with various maneuvers that alter ventricular volume (standing will cause the click to occur earlier in systole and closer to S1; squatting will cause the click to occur later in systole and closer to S2). These maneuvers, therefore, are helpful in distinguishing the systolic click of MVP from aortic and pulmonic ejection sounds. The ejection sound is relatively fixed in timing in early systole, compared with the first heart sound, despite maneuvers that alter the ventricular volume.

The S4 gallop also occurs when there is prolongation of the PR interval with first-degree heart block (due to the delay in AV conduction that separates atrial contraction from ventricular contraction).

Other Diastolic Sounds

In addition to the S3 and S4, other sounds that may be heard in diastole include:

- *Opening snap* of *mitral stenosis*
- *Pericardial knock sound* of *constrictive pericarditis*
- *"Tumor plop"* of *atrial myxoma*
- *Opening sound of mechanical prosthetic mitral valve*

These are further differentiated on the attached CD on "Heart Sounds" and in **Figure 2-60.**

Figure 2-60. Timing of heart sounds in systole and diastole. Note that S1 and P2 are accentuated with mitral stenosis. With constrictive pericarditis, a pericardial knock sound (K) occurs slightly later in diastole than the opening snap (OS) of MS, since mitral valve opening precedes early LV filling, and earlier than an S3, because LA pressure is

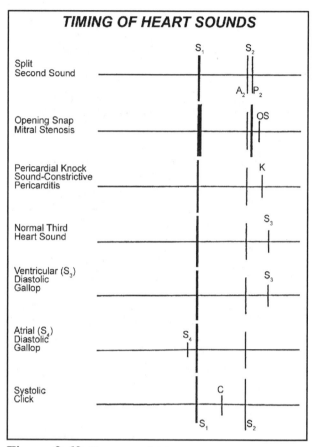

Figure 2-60 (Courtesy of W. Proctor Harvey, M.D.)

higher and LV filling is more rapid with constriction than with heart failure. An S4 occurs as a result of forceful LA contraction prior to the next systole. Non-ejection sounds (i.e., clicks) from MVP occur in mid systole.

The pericardial knock can occur with or without pericardial calcification. The more severe the constrictive process, the earlier and louder the knock sound. Following successful surgery, the sound becomes later and fainter. Because of its characteristic higher frequency, the pericardial knock sound may be mistaken for an opening snap. The presence of this early diastolic heart sound, however, in association with an elevated JVP increasing during inspiration (*Kussmaul's sign*) and in the absence of a loud S1 and diastolic rumble of mitral stenosis, should provide the clinician with an immediate clue to the diagnosis of constrictive pericarditis. Nowadays, one should specifically search for these findings in the patient who presents with unexplained heart failure (especially right-sided) following cardiac surgery.

Figure 2-61. "Doming" of the stenotic mitral valve at the onset of left ventricular (LV) filling. **Left.** In the normal mitral valve the anterior mitral leaflet (AML) and posterior mitral leaflet (PML) open widely and no sound is produced. **Right.** In mitral stenosis the free edges of the

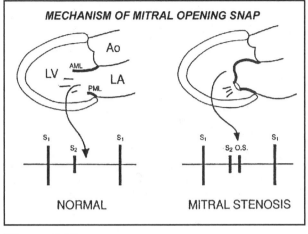

Figure 2-61

two leaflets are bound together but the belly domes forward. When it reaches its limit, the opening snap (O.S.) occurs. The closer the O.S. is to S2 (the higher the LA pressure) the more severe the degree of stenosis. (Courtesy of Dr. James A. Ronan, Jr.).

Figure 2-62. The pericardial knock sound in a patient with early, or mild, constrictive pericarditis. Note pericardial knock sound (K) is heard only on inspiration. S1, first heart sound; S2, second heart sound. The knock is due to sudden restriction of blood flow by the constricting pericardium during diastolic filling of the ventricles.

Heart Murmurs: Systolic, Diastolic, and Continuous

Heart murmurs are a series of audible vibrations that result from turbulent blood flow through the cardiac chambers, valves, and great vessels. Their timing in the cardiac cycle (systolic, diastolic, or continuous), intensity, duration, configuration, quality, location, radiation, and response to dynamic maneuvers, are all important clues in identifying their origin and significance.

Heart murmurs can be heard in many individuals, both with and without cardiac disease. In the last few decades, the prevalence of cardiac diseases that cause the most common heart murmurs heard in clinical practice has changed. With the declining incidence of acute rheumatic fever, the most common conditions include aortic sclerosis of the elderly (which recently has been linked to atherosclerosis and an increased risk of acute MI and stroke, but in itself may not be dysfunctional), valvular AS, MR due to MVP, papillary muscle dysfunction (as seen in ischemia, acute MI, cardiomyopathy, or LV failure from any cause), calcified mitral annulus (especially in elderly females), and hypertrophic cardiomyopathy. Recent onset of a heart murmur may provide a clue to infective endocarditis (e.g., acute MR, AR) or a serious complication in a patient with acute MI (e.g., acute VSD, MR).

Figures 2–63 and **2–64** summarize the major systolic, diastolic, and continuous murmurs.

Systolic Murmurs: Innocent vs. Significant ("Guilty")

It is particularly important to be able to distinguish between an innocent and a significant murmur. Early and mid systolic murmurs less than grade 3 (**Figure 2-31**) may be "innocent" or "significant" (when accompanied by other signs of cardiac pathology). Loud systolic murmurs (grade 3 or greater) are more likely to be hemodynamically significant and due to underlying heart disease. The loudness of a murmur, however, while commonly correlating with the severity of the underlying abnormality, does not always

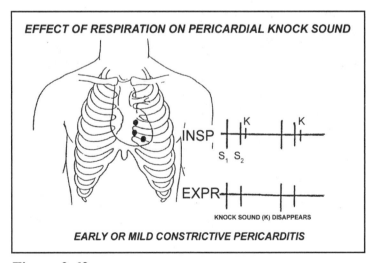

Figure 2-62 (Courtesy of W. Proctor Harvey, M.D.)

SYSTOLIC MURMURS*

	AUSCULTATION	HEARD BEST	COMMENT
EARLY-MIDSYSTOLIC Innocent murmurs	S1 S2 S1		Typically early to midsystolic, stopping before S2. Heard best in 2nd to 4th left interspaces, but may also be heard at apex and aortic areas. Typically grade 1 or 2 intensity. May have a musical, vibratory or buzzing quality (Still's murmur). Normal splitting of S1 and S2 and no abnormal extra heart sounds or murmurs. Commonly diminishes in intensity or disappears when sitting. Heard best with **diaphragm**, patient supine.
Aortic stenosis	S1 S2 S1 / S1 S2 S1 — Peaks later with increased severity		May include an S4 and aortic ejection sound. Heard in the aortic area, neck along the carotids, clavicles, and may also be transmitted to apex, where it may be musical (Gallavardin phenomenon). Murmur may decrease with severe stenosis and low cardiac output. Best heard with patient sitting forward. Paradoxical splitting of S2 due to delay in closure of aortic valve. Heard best with **diaphragm**.
Pulmonic stenosis	S1 S2 S1		May be accompanied by a pulmonic ejection sound early in systole, as well as an S4. May radiate toward left clavicle. Wide splitting of S2 (splitting noted on both inspiration and expiration) due to delayed closure of pulmonic valve. Found particularly in children as a congenital condition. Similar murmur may be found in high flow across pulmonary valve, e.g. with atrial septal defect. Heard best with **diaphragm.**
Hypertrophic obstructive cardiomyopathy — S1 S2 S1 Supine	S1 S2 S1 Dec on Squatting / S1 S2 S1 Inc on Standing or Valsalva		May radiate to apex, but not neck. Systolic murmur decreases with squatting, increases with standing or Valsalva maneuver. May include an S4 or S3. Quick carotid pulse rise (distinguishes it from aortic stenosis, where carotid pulse is diminished and slow to rise); palpable "triple ripple" at LV apex. Paradoxical splitting of S2 and a systolic murmur of mitral regurgitation at the cardiac apex may occur. Best heard with **diaphragm**.
Atrial septal defect	S1 S2 S1 Expiration / S1 S2 S1 inspiration (fixed split)		Early to midsystolic murmur, wide "fixed" splitting of second heart sound, best heard with **diaphragm** over pulmonic area &/or 3rd ICS. If significant, an additional tricuspid diastolic flow rumble may be heard, best heard with **bell** along lower left sternal border.
Systemic hypertension	S1 A2 S1 AORTIC AREA / S1 S2 S4 S1 APEX		Auscultatory findings in a patient with long standing systemic arterial hypertension. Loud ("tambour") second heart sound (heard best with **diaphragm**) due to accentuated aortic valve closure (A2) and a short early to mid systolic murmur (SM) at the aortic area. An S4 gallop (heard best with **bell**) due to diastolic dysfunction can also be heard over the apex.
HOLOSYSTOLIC Mitral regurgitation	S1 S2 S1 Mild / S1 S2 S1 Moderate / S3 S1 S2 S1 Severe — S3 Flow rumble		Blowing holosystolic fixed amplitude murmur. In mitral valve prolapse, may be late systolic, since LV must first achieve a critically small size before the mitral valve actually prolapses. Radiates from lower LSB and apex to the axillary lines and posterior lung-base. May include an S3 and, if severe, an S3 and diastolic flow rumble. Wide-splitting S2 due to early closure of aortic valve. Murmur of chronic MR generally decreases with inspiration (in contrast to TR which increases). Systolic murmur best heard with **diaphragm**. (S3 and flow rumble best heard with **bell** at apex.)
Tricuspid regurgitation	S1 S2 S1 Expiration / S1 S2 S1 Inspiration		Holosystolic blowing murmur heard best in tricuspid area. Murmur may increase on inspiration (unlike chronic mitral regurgitation, where murmur decreases on inspiration). May include an S3, as in more advanced mitral regurgitation. Murmur best heard with **diaphragm** along lower LSB.
Ventricular septal defect	S1 S2 S1		Murmur results from flow from left ventricle to right ventricle. Holosystolic high pitched, often very loud, murmur (accompanied by palpable systolic thrill). Usually heard louder along the lower left sternal border than at the apex. Best heard with **diaphragm**.
LATE SYSTOLIC Mitral valve prolapse — S1 S2 S1 Click-murmur (supine)	S1 S2 S1 Squatting / S1 S2 S1 Standing		Murmur crescendos in late systole. Squatting pushes the click &/or murmur closer to S2. Standing moves click &/or murmur closer to S1. Best heard with **diaphragm**.

*Note: Systolic murmurs begin with or after S1 and end with or before S2. They are classified based on timing as early-mid systolic, holosystolic, or late systolic. Systolic murmurs arise when turbulent blood flow occurs across a normal cardiac structure (i.e., innocent murmur); forward flow occurs across a narrowed valve (e.g., AS, PS) or outflow tract (e.g., HOCM); increased flow occurs across a pulmonary trunk (e.g., ASD) or into a dilated aortic root (e.g., systemic hypertension); backward flow occurs through an incompetent valve (e.g., MR, TR); or blood is shunted from a high to a low pressure area through an abnormal opening (e.g., VSD).

Figure 2-63

DIASTOLIC & CONTINUOUS MURMURS*

	AUSCULTATION	HEARD BEST	COMMENT
EARLY (High frequency) Aortic regurgitation			High-pitched, blowing diastolic murmur. May radiate to the apex or RSB if loud. Sit patient upright, leaning forward, and holding breath in deep expiration with the **diaphragm** of the stethoscope firmly applied to the chest wall. When heard louder on right 3rd & 4th interspace, suggests aortic root disease (e.g. dissection) rather than aortic valvular disease (Harvey's sign). May include an S3 or S4 (with **bell** over apex). Austin-Flint (AF) murmur may mimic mitral stenosis, but without opening snap.
Pulmonic regurgitation			Usually low or medium frequency murmur in congenital low pressure state, beinning after a pause following S2. Murmur of pulmonary valve insufficiency with pulmonary hypertension may be the same as AR, but often has stigmata of pulmonary hypertension, like loud P2, pulmonic ejection sound, and abnormal RV lift (RV hypertrophy), distinguishing it from AR. Best heard with **diaphragm** in pulmonic area and mid LSB.
MID/LATE (Low frequency) Mitral stenosis			Loud S1, opening high-pitched snap, middiastolic low-pitched murmur with late presystolic accentuation. Early to middiastolic part due to rapid ventricular filling; presystolic accentuation due to atrial contraction. Use **diaphragm** of stethoscope at lower left sternal border and apex for S1 and OS. For diastolic rumble (usually preceded by an opening snap in diastole), turn the patient to the left, **bell** of the stethoscope lightly and precisely over PMI. Heard better in expiration and after exercise.
Tricuspid stenosis			Mid-late diastolic rumbling murmur heard during inspiration; may disappear on expiration. Heard best at LSB (tricuspid area) with **bell**.
CONTINUOUS Patent ductus arteriosus			Continuous "machinery" murmur, peaks at and envelopes S2. Best heard with **diaphragm** at pulmonic area.
Jugular venous hum			Frequent in children and young adults, especially during pregnancy, and in thyrotoxicosis or anemia. Use **bell** over the supraclavicular fossa, especially on the right side, with the patient's head turned and stretched to the opposite direction; hum eliminated by gentle pressure over the vein. Louder during diastole
Coronary arteriovenous fistula			Loud, continuous murmur tends to crescendo-decrescendo both in systole and diastole, the diastolic component being louder. listen over 3rd and 4th intercostal space of left sternal border.
MISCELLANEOUS Pericardial friction rub			To and fro noises differentiated from systolic and diastolic heart murmurs by rough, scratchy, leathery, creaking, superficial quality and having at least 2 or 3 components (ventricular systole and early and late ventricular diastole). Best heard with patient leaning forward with breath held in deep expiration and with **diaphragm** of the stethoscope firmly over the left mid precordium. Generally increases with inspiration.

*Note: Diastolic murmurs begin with or after S2 and end with or before S1. They are classified by timing as early diastolic or mid/late diastolic. Diastolic murmurs are pathologic and can be regurgitant (e.g., AR, PR) or stenotic (e.g., MS, TS). Continuous murmurs begin with S1 and continue through S2 into part or all of diastole. Except for the jugular venous hum, they are pathologic and are caused by continuous flow from a vessel with high pressure into a vessel with low pressure (e.g., PDA, AV fistula). Pericardial friction rubs may be mistaken for both systolic and diastolic murmurs, however, they are transient in nature, and have a superficial and scratchy quality.

Figure 2-64

correlate. For example, flow across a small ventricular septal defect (VSD) is frequently associated with a loud murmur because of the turbulence, whereas the systolic murmur of severe AS may lessen in intensity or even be inaudible with CHF. The length of a murmur is often more indicative of the severity of a lesion than its intensity. *Holosystolic, late systolic and diastolic murmurs virtually always signify an abnormality of cardiac structure or function.*

The recognition that a systolic murmur is "significant" rather than "innocent" often rests on associated clinical findings (i.e., the "company it keeps"), rather than on the characteristics of the murmur itself. The presence of symptoms suggestive of cardiovascular disease and/or associated abnormal cardiac physical, ECG and chest x-ray findings, may increase the likelihood that the murmur is significant. Certain abnormal heart sounds that reflect cardiac pathology may all serve as immediate clues to the presence of a "significant" murmur. These abnormal sounds include persistent ("fixed") splitting of S2 in atrial septal defect, ejection sound in congenital bicuspid aortic valve or pulmonic valvular stenosis, systolic click in MVP, loud "tambour" A2 in systemic hypertension, loud, closely split or single (fused) S2 with an accentuation of P2 in pulmonary hypertension. Unfortunately, it is easy to overlook the presence of these abnormal heart sounds unless one listens specifically for them.

In contrast, the "innocent" systolic murmur that can be found in children, young adults, athletes, pregnant women and those with a hyperkinetic circulatory state (as brought on by fever, anemia, exercise, excitement, hyperthyroidism), is a faint (Grade 1–2/6), early to mid-systolic, crescendo-decrescendo murmur, often with a musical, vibratory or buzzing quality (*Still's murmur*), that diminishes with sitting, standing, or the Valsalva maneuver. It is heard best over the pulmonic area or mid left sternal border, but may be heard at the apex and aortic areas as well. It is characteristically accompanied by normal respiratory splitting of S2, a physiologic S3 at the cardiac apex, waxing and waning with respiration, a jugular venous hum heard best with the bell placed over the right supraclavicular fossa with the head turned ("on a stretch") to the opposite direction, and the absence of abnormal heart sounds (e.g., ejection sounds, clicks, gallops), or other systolic or diastolic murmurs. When heard in the asymptomatic individual without any clinical manifestations of heart disease (along with a normal ECG and CXR), the "innocent" systolic murmur can be diagnosed with a high degree of certainty, without the need for more specialized imaging techniques (e.g., echo).

Figure 2-65. Systolic murmurs can be divided into *ejection* murmurs and *regurgitant* murmurs. **Left.** The classic holosystolic (pansystolic) murmur of mitral regurgitation begins with the first heart sound (S1) and continues up to and through the aortic component of the second heart sound (S2), since left ventricular (LV) pressure continues to exceed left atrial (LA) pressure. **Right.** The classic mid systolic ejection murmur occurs during the period of LV ejection. It begins after S1, is crescendo-decrescendo in nature, and stops before S2.

Early-mid Systolic (Ejection) Murmurs

- *Ejection murmurs* (e.g., innocent systolic murmur, aortic sclerosis, valvular AS, PS, HOCM) are crescendo-decrescendo and reflect turbulent flow across the aortic or pulmonic valve or outflow tract.
- A short, early or mid-systolic crescendo-decrescendo murmur heard best at the right or left second intercostal space or left sternal border is common in children and young adults and is considered an *"innocent"* (or physiologic) *systolic murmur* (**Figure 2-66**).
- Significant systolic murmurs (e.g., mild bicuspid aortic valve stenosis, HOCM, atrial septal defect), however, may present as a systolic murmur of similar character, length, and configuration. The judgment that cardiac pathology is present, therefore, is often based not only on the presence of the murmur, but also on additional clinical information. For example:
- *Aortic valve stenosis*—an ejection sound is heard over the precordium from aortic area to apex, the AS murmur is harsh in quality, may have S4 gallop, paradoxically-split S2, and other signs on physical exam (delayed arterial pulse, palpable systolic thrill). (*Gallavardin phenomenon* is a musical quality to the AS murmur at the apex). Aortic stenosis may also be accompanied by symptoms of chest pains, SOB or fainting spells.
- *Pulmonary valve stenosis/artery dilatation*—wide physiologic splitting of S2 on inspiration and expiration; may have an ejection sound (that decreases on inspiration) and a right-sided S4 (that increases on inspiration).
- *Hypertrophic cardiomyopathy*—decreased systolic murmur with squatting and increased with standing and/or Valsalva maneuver; may have an S4 or S3 or paradoxical splitting of S2. The patient may also have a history of syncope, chest pain, or symptoms of left heart failure, coupled with the

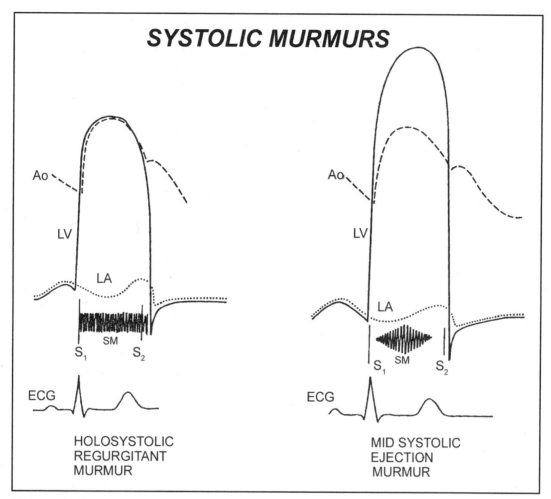

Figure 2-65

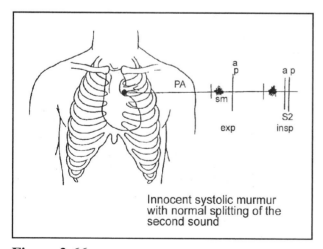

Figure 2-66 (Courtesy of W. Proctor Harvey, M.D.)

presence of a quick rising ("flip") arterial pulse and a presystolic and double systolic apical impulse ("*triple ripple*"—see "Precordial Movements and Palpation" section of this chapter).

Remember, all diastolic murmurs, holosystolic murmurs, and late systolic murmurs should be considered pathologic, whereas early or mid-systolic murmurs may be functional.

Aortic sclerosis is common in elderly patients; 25% of those > 65 years of age are affected. The condition is often diagnosed when a short early to mid-systolic murmur, with no ejection sound, is detected in an otherwise asymptomatic patient during a routine physical. When a systolic murmur becomes prolonged (i.e., occupies more and more of systole) the likelihood of organic heart disease increases.

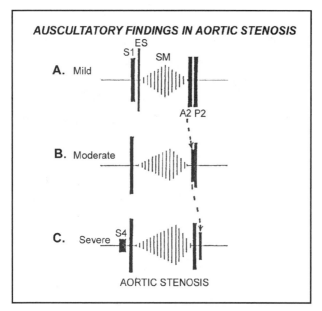

Note: The systolic murmur of severe aortic stenosis is long, late peaking, ends with a faint A2 or paradoxically split S2, is preceded by an S4 gallop, and is accompanied by a slow rising carotid arterial pulse. With progression of the disease, the ejection sound becomes faint or absent.

Figure 2-67

Figure 2-67. Auscultatory findings in mild, moderate and severe aortic stenosis.

A. *Mild aortic stenosis:* An aortic ejection sound (E5) follows the first heart sound. A midsystolic ejection murmur (SM) ends before the normal aortic component (A2) of the second heart sound. **B.** *Moderate aortic stenosis:* With progression of the disease, the systolic ejection murmur peaks later in systole and splitting is minimal since the faint aortic component is synchronous with the pulmonic component (P2). The ejection sound becomes faint or absent as the valve becomes less mobile. **C.** *Severe aortic stenosis:* A fourth heart sound or atrial gallop (reflecting decreased LV compliance), along with an even later peaking systolic ejection murmur, and a paradoxically split second heart sound are heard. The faint aortic component of S2 is delayed, occurring after the pulmonic component, and the splitting at the pulmonic area is wider on expiration than inspiration.

In general, all forms of obstruction to left or right ventricular outflow (e.g., valvular AS, PS) result in the presence of a systolic ejection murmur. As a rule, the more severe the degree of obstruction, the longer the corresponding murmur, peaking later in systole. The location of maximal intensity and the direction of radiation of the murmur (aortic area to right shoulder for valvular aortic stenosis, pulmonic area to left shoulder for pulmonic valve stenosis), like the thrill noted on palpation, provide important clues to the site of obstruction.

The murmur of aortic stenosis can also radiate to the apex, where it may assume a more musical quality (Gallavardin phenomenon). Remember to also listen over both clavicles; since bone is such a good transmitter of sound, the murmur of AS may even be louder here than in the neck. *If you hear a high-frequency musical systolic murmur at the apex, always rule out aortic stenosis.* The patient is usually an elderly man, who has an increase in the anterior-posterior diameter of the chest (due to emphysema). Late-systolic murmurs of *mitral valve prolapse* (MVP) can also assume a musical character (*"systolic whoop"*, or *"precordial honk"*). They are among the most striking of auscultatory findings, and are usually heard along the left sternal border or at the cardiac apex.

In *hypertrophic obstructive cardiomyopathy* (HOCM) (**Figure 2-49**) the systolic flow murmur through the aortic valve during ventricular contraction *increases* on standing (SM) and *decreases* on squatting (sm), because the outflow obstruction created by movement of the anterior mitral leaflet toward the ventricular-impinging hypertrophic septum (Venturi effect) is relieved temporarily by the increased ventricular volume in squatting. Additional auscultatory findings may include a paradoxical splitting of S2 (delayed closure of the aortic valve) and a systolic murmur of MR at the cardiac apex (the HOCM may cause MR by distorting the mitral valve area). The murmur of HOCM can be increased by a Valsalva maneuver, such as putting the finger in the mouth and blowing; this reduces venous return, reduces the size of the left ventricle, thereby increasing the obstruction to blood flow by the impinging hypertrophic ventricle wall.

In *atrial septal defect* (**Figure 2-63**) there is wide "fixed" splitting of S2 (A2, P2) and a systolic murmur (SM).

Figure 2-68. Auscultatory findings in a patient with long-standing *systemic arterial hypertension*. Note the loud (*"tambour"*) second heart sound due to accentuated aortic valve closure (A2) and a short early to mid-systolic murmur

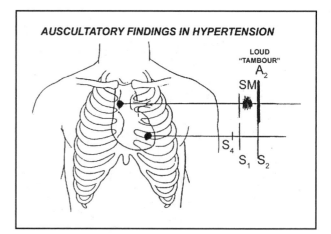

Figure 2-68 (Courtesy of W. Proctor Harvey, M.D.)

(SM) resulting from ejection of blood into a dilated aorta, heard best at the aortic area. An S4 gallop due to diastolic dysfunction can also be heard over the apex.

Holosystolic Murmurs

The character of the murmur of MR depends on:

- whether the MR is *acute* or *chronic*
- whether the MR is *mild, moderate* or *severe*
- whether it is the *anterior* or *posterior leaflet* that is involved

Figure 2-69. Chronic vs. acute mitral regurgitation. In *chronic* MR, the left atrium has enlarged and is more compliant. LA pressure is normal or only slightly elevated and pulmonary congestive symptoms are less common if LV contractile function is intact. In *acute* MR, the left atrium is normal in size and is non-compliant. LA pressure rises markedly (diamond-shaped holosystolic murmur decreasing in late systole), and pulmonary edema may result.

Figure 2-70. Mild, moderate, and severe mitral regurgitation. Trivial MR (not shown) is usually manifested by a late systolic murmur, and significant MR by a holosystolic murmur (the longer the murmur, the more significant). In general, however, the severity of MR is not reflected in the intensity of the systolic murmur, but by the accompanying diastolic events. *Mild* MR is characterized only by a systolic murmur, *moderate* MR adds an S3 gallop, and *severe* MR

adds a diastolic flow rumble to that, which results from the great volume that has to be expelled from the left atrium.

Figure 2–71. Mitral regurgitation, anterior versus posterior leaflet involvement. With *anterior leaflet* involvement, the murmur radiates toward the axilla and back. With *posterior leaflet* involvement, the murmur radiates toward the aorta and base of the heart. When the murmur radiates up to the base of the heart, it can be confused with the murmur of aortic stenosis (which also radiates to the right shoulder). The second heart sound (S2), in both MR and mild to moder-

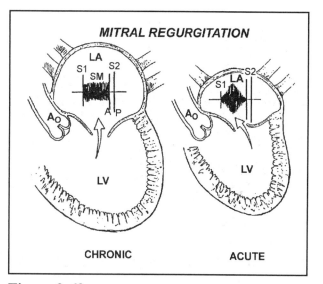

Figure 2-69 (Courtesy of W. Proctor Harvey, M.D.)

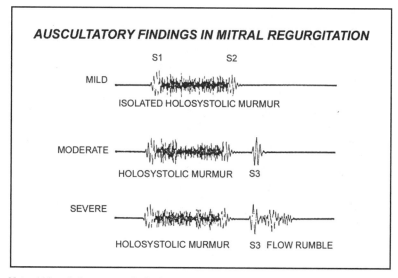

Note: Although the murmur of mitral regurgitation is heard in *systole*, its severity is judged by listening for the presence of an S3 gallop and a flow rumble in *diastole*.

Figure 2-70

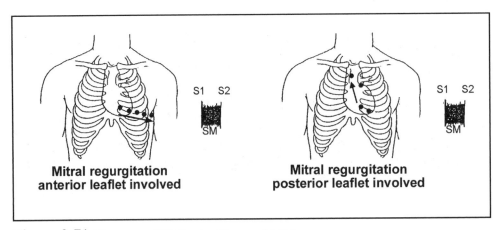

Figure 2-71 (Courtesy of W. Proctor Harvey, M.D.)

ate AS, splits over the pulmonic area (ap), and widens on inspiration (severe AS may have paradoxical splitting of S2).

If a murmur extends throughout all of systole (holosystolic murmur), think of three possibilities: MR, TR, VSD. MR is the most common of the three. The location of maximal murmur intensity, radiation, and, in the case of TR, inspiratory increase in murmur intensity, all help to determine which of the three entities is present.

Figure 2-72. If there is a holosystolic murmur, think of either MR, TR or VSD:

A. Chronic mitral regurgitation is best heard at the apex and may radiate to the axilla and back (anterior leaflet involvement) or to the aorta and base of the heart (posterior leaflet involvement) (**Figure 2-71**).

B. The holosystolic murmur (SM) of TR is heard best at the lower left sternal border and increases in intensity during inspiration (*Carvallo's sign*) exp = expiration; insp = inspiration.

C. The holosystolic murmur of acute VSD secondary to rupture of the interventricular septum in a patient with an acute myocardial infarction is heard better along the LSB than at the apex.

At times, it may be difficult to differentiate between the murmur of valvular aortic stenosis and mitral regurgitation. A valuable clue is to listen specifically to the murmur after a pause (with a premature beat or atrial fibrillation). The murmur of AS increases in intensity whereas the murmur of MR shows little change. Keep in mind that most patients with isolated aortic valve disease are in normal sinus rhythm. The presence of atrial fibrillation in and of itself may provide a clue to mitral valve disease. Also, aortic valve disease is more common in men, whereas mitral valve disease is more common in women.

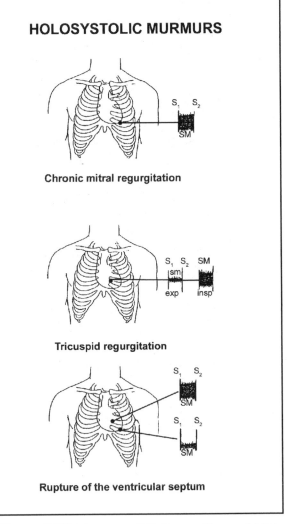

HOLOSYSTOLIC MURMURS

Chronic mitral regurgitation

Tricuspid regurgitation

Rupture of the ventricular septum

Figure 2-72 (Courtesy of W. Proctor Harvey, M.D.)

Late Systolic Murmurs

As mentioned, *mitral valve prolapse* can present with just a single systolic click, multiple clicks, or a click(s) along with a late systolic (or sometimes holosystolic) murmur (**Figure 2-59**). The murmur may be due to a mild degree of mitral regurgitation, and the patient may or may not be symptomatic. Papillary muscle dysfunction may also present with a holosystolic, mid or late systolic murmur of MR.

Figure 2-73. For practice, it is a good idea to sketch out the murmurs that you hear as you hear them:

A) Short systolic murmur in midsystole with normal aortic and pulmonic components of second heart sound, consistent with innocent murmur.

B) Prolonged diamond-shaped or "kite-shaped" systolic murmur with S4 and ejection sound present, typical of bicuspid valvular aortic stenosis of increasing severity.

C) Midsystolic murmur, wide "fixed" splitting of second heart sound (atrial septal defect).

D) Crescendo-decrescendo systolic murmur, not holosystolic, with S4 and S3 gallops, consistent with mitral systolic murmur (a variant of mitral regurgitation) heard with congestive cardiomyopathy or CAD with papillary muscle dysfunction and cardiac decompensation.

E) Late apical systolic murmur of hemodynamically insignificant MR in mitral valve prolapse.

F) Systolic click-late apical systolic murmur in mitral valve prolapse.

G) Holosystolic murmur consistent with MR, TR, VSD.

H) Holosystolic murmur peaking in midsystole, also consistent with MR, TR, VSD.

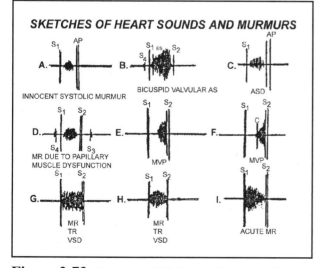

SKETCHES OF HEART SOUNDS AND MURMURS

A. INNOCENT SYSTOLIC MURMUR
B. BICUSPID VALVULAR AS
C. ASD
D. MR DUE TO PAPILLARY MUSCLE DYSFUNCTION
E. MVP
F. MVP
G. MR TR VSD
H. MR TR VSD
I. ACUTE MR

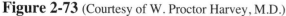

Figure 2-73 (Courtesy of W. Proctor Harvey, M.D.)

I) Holosystolic murmur decreasing in the latter part of systole, as seen in acute MR (e.g., ruptured chorda tendineae).

Figure 2-74. Left. Schematic diagram of a Starr-Edwards (ball and cage) prosthetic valve. **Right.** A patient with significant aortic regurgitation. A systolic murmur (SM) is due to flow, not aortic stenosis. Before surgery, the "to and fro" systolic and diastolic murmurs (SM, DM) are heard. After surgery, several systolic prosthetic valve sounds (xx) are heard over the pulmonic area (pa) produced by the prosthetic ball "jiggling" and striking the top of the cage. A mid-systolic murmur (sm) also is present. These are normal findings in a patient with a Starr-Edwards valve.

Figure 2-75. Left. Schematic diagram of a porcine valve. **Right.** Auscultatory findings in an elderly man with severe aortic stenosis and advanced heart failure. A loud, long, harsh aortic systolic murmur (sm) is heard. The second heart sound (S2) is faint. Atrial fibrillation also is present. Note that after a pause, the murmur increases in intensity (second beat, top sketch). After surgery (post-op) a faint grade 2–3/6 systolic murmur (SM) is heard, which is a normal finding for a porcine valve.

Diastolic Murmurs

All diastolic murmurs are pathologic. They include:

- Early diastolic murmurs (*aortic* and *pulmonic regurgitation*)
- Mid/late rumbling murmurs (*mitral* and *tricuspid stenosis*)
- Combined systolic/diastolic murmurs (*With the exception of the jugular venous hum, all continuous murmurs heard over the thorax are abnormal*). Examples are:

   Patent ductus arteriosus (PDA)
   Jugular venous hum
   Coronary arteriovenous fistula
   Pulmonary arteriovenous fistula
   Ruptured sinus of Valsalva aneurysm

Early Diastolic Murmurs

Aortic or pulmonic regurgitation results in an early diastolic murmur. In the case of AR, the murmur is of high frequency, decrescendo in configuration, and "blowing" in character. Most commonly, it is loudest along the left sternal border and aortic area (**Figure 2-76**). When heard best along the *right* sternal border in the third and fourth intercostal spaces (so-called "right-sided" diastolic murmurs), consider unusual causes of aortic regurgitation due to *aortic root pathology* (e.g., dissection, aneurysm) (**Figure 2-77**).

Figure 2-76. A patient with a congenital bicuspid aortic valve and aortic regurgitation. Note the high frequency

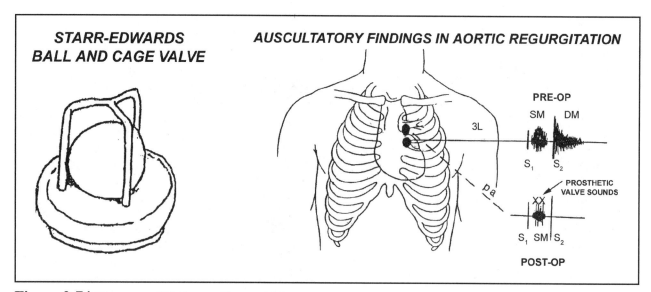

Figure 2-74 (Courtesy of W. Proctor Harvey, M.D.)

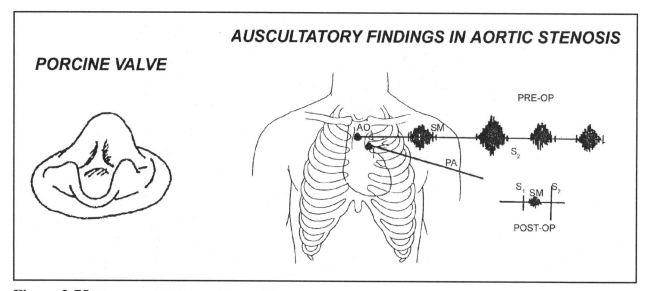

Figure 2-75 (Courtesy of W. Proctor Harvey, M.D.)

diastolic murmur (DM), heard along the third left sternal border (3L) and the aortic ejection sound (e), the hallmark of such a valve, which can be heard at the apex as well as over the aortic area. A faint, grade 1–2/6 murmur of AR is often commonly missed because its frequency closely approximates ambient room noise (e.g., air conditioning). A careful search is often needed to properly elicit the murmur, with the patient sitting upright and leaning forward, with the breath held in full expiration, and the examiner applying firm pressure on the diaphragm of the stethoscope, enough to leave an imprint on the skin. If the murmur is overlooked, one may miss the opportunity to provide antibiotic therapy for a diseased aortic valve in infective endocarditis, or

diagnose a paravalvular leak from dehiscence of a prosthetic aortic valve. You may previously have suspected its presence because of an aortic ejection sound, an abnormal right second interspace lift (suggesting aneurysmal dilatation of the aorta), or a history of previous hypertension, current chest or interscapular back pain, and unequal upper extremity pulses suggesting aortic dissection.

A poorly appreciated and seldom used maneuver for auscultation of the diastolic murmur of AR is to have the patient lying on his or her stomach, propped up on the elbows. This position moves the heart closer to the chest wall and is also especially useful to detect a pericardial friction rub, and enhance the intensity of heart sounds and murmurs

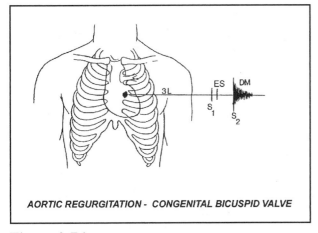

Figure 2-76 (Courtesy of W. Proctor Harvey, M.D.)

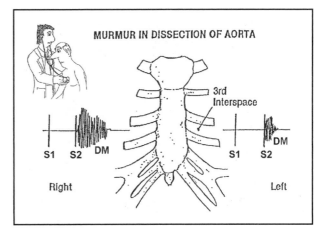

Figure 2-77 (Courtesy of W. Proctor Harvey, M.D.)

in some patients having a pericardial effusion. Keep in mind that patients having a slight leak of the aortic valve can be completely asymptomatic. It is only when the leak becomes significant that the murmur, being louder, is heard, and other symptoms and signs occur.

The clinical presentation of a regurgitant pulmonary valve varies depending on whether pulmonary artery pressure is normal or elevated. Pulmonary valve insufficiency with normal pulmonary artery pressure is usually the result of congenital valve insufficiency, in association with idiopathic dilatation of the pulmonary artery. The murmur is usually of low or medium frequency, best heard at the second left interspace or left sternal border. It starts at some interval before or immediately after P2, and most often has a crescendo-decrescendo configuration. In the congenital variety, all clinical parameters other than the murmur may be normal.

When pulmonary valve insufficiency occurs along with pulmonary hypertension, the diastolic murmur may assume the same high frequency, decrescendo character as that noted in aortic valve regurgitation. However, there are often stigmata of pulmonary hypertension, such as a loud P2, a pulmonic ejection sound, and an abnormal RV lift (RV hypertrophy) to help distinguish it from AR.

Figure 2-77. *Dissection of the aorta.* Auscultation of the diastolic murmur of aortic regurgitation with the patient in the sitting position, leaning forward with breath held in deep expiration. The diastolic murmur (DM) of aortic regurgitation is heard louder at the 3rd *right* intercostal space, rather than the left, affording an immediate clue to aortic root disease (e.g., dissection) rather than aortic valvular disease (*Harvey's sign*).

Figure 2-78. Severe chronic aortic regurgitation. Note the typical "to and fro" systolic and diastolic murmurs (SM, DM) of advanced degrees of aortic regurgitation best heard along the mid left sternal border. If, when taking the blood pressure, the patient has a very wide pulse pressure (e.g.,

160–170/40 down to 0), the presence of a loud aortic systolic murmur (even with a palpable thrill) represents flow, not aortic stenosis. Also note the *Austin-Flint rumble* at the apex, both in the mid as well as late portion of diastole (presystole), accentuating up to the first heart sound (S1). The Austin-Flint murmur implies significant aortic regurgitation.

Middiastolic and Presystolic Murmurs

Murmurs resulting from turbulent flow across the mitral or tricuspid valve tend to be of low frequency and thus are best heard with the bell of the stethoscope lightly applied at the cardiac apex with the patient in the left lateral position. *Mitral Stenosis* (MS) results in a diastolic rumbling murmur, usually preceded by an opening snap. In normal sinus rhythm, a presystolic crescendo murmur up to S1 is common (**Figure 2-79**). Similar murmurs may be heard with obstructing atrial myxomas, but the latter commonly fluctuate with the patient's position, as the tumor moves toward or away from the mitral valve opening.

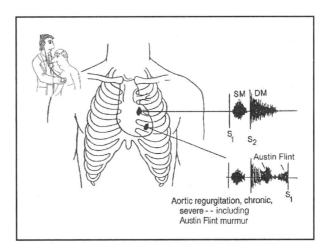

Figure 2-78 (Courtesy of W. Proctor Harvey, M.D.)

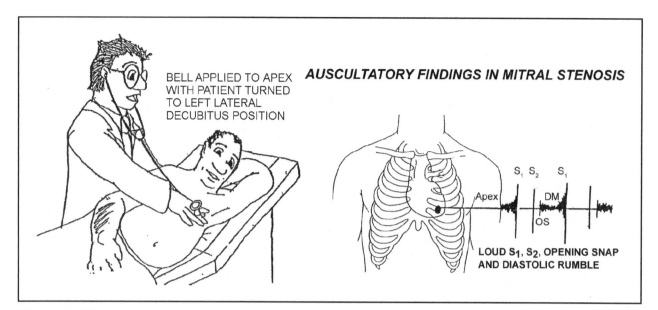

Figure 2-79 (Courtesy of W. Proctor Harvey, M.D.)

Figure 2-79. Left. Auscultatory findings in mitral stenosis. Note the loud first heart sound (S1), second heart sound (S2), and opening snap (OS) followed by the typical rumbling diastolic murmur (DM) with presystolic accentuation. The murmur is best heard over the cardiac apex using light pressure on the bell of the stethoscope with the patient turned to the left lateral decubitus position.

The murmur of MS is often missed. Improper positioning and/or use of the bell of the stethoscope are important reasons. Frequently, the murmur is confined to a very small area (the size of a quarter) over the cardiac apex, and the bell of the stethoscope must be applied over this small area with the patient turned to the left. The position brings the apex closer to the chest wall and overlying stethoscope, which increases the audibility of the low intensity murmur. Appreciating a loud S1, OS and P2 are helpful clues. Always keep in mind, if you hear a loud S1 search for the diastolic rumble of MS.

Tricuspid valve events, in contrast to the mitral valve, are usually best appreciated along the lower left sternal border rather than the cardiac apex. Tricuspid valve obstruction, although rare, results in a rumbling diastolic murmur similar to that noted in MS. As a right sided event, inspiratory augmentation in intensity of the murmur helps to distinguish its tricuspid valve origin.

In severe AR, the regurgitant jet from the aorta into the LV may strike the ventricular surface of the anterior mitral leaflet, moving it toward a more closed position. At the same time, blood flow from the LA to the LV tends to move the anterior leaflet to a more open position. The relative narrowing of the effective mitral valve orifice results in a diastolic rumbling murmur at the cardiac apex *("Austin-*

Flint" murmur) which may mimic the murmur of MS (although there is no opening snap). The Austin-Flint murmur is present only when the degree of AR is moderate or severe. (**Figure 2-78**).

Continuous Murmurs
Continuous murmurs last throughout all of systole and continue into at least early diastole. Continuous *jugular venous hums* are frequently heard in children and young adults, especially during pregnancy (along with the mammary soufflè–a systolic/diastolic murmur heard over the breast in late pregnancy and lactation), and in thyrotoxicosis or anemia. Venous hums are best heard over the right internal jugular vein at the base of the neck with the patient's head turned to the opposite direction ("on a stretch"), but occasionally may be loud enough to be transmitted to the upper chest. They are generated by continuous flow from a vessel or chamber with high pressure into a vessel or chamber with low pressure.

Figure 2-80. Technique to elicit a jugular venous hum, best heard with the bell of the stethoscope over the right supraclavicular fossa with the patient's head turned upward and to the left ("on a stretch"). Gentle pressure over the jugular vein generally eliminates the hum, as does turning the patient's head to the forward position.

Causes of a continuous murmur include *PDA, coronary arteriovenous fistula, pulmonary arteriovenous fistula,* and *ruptured sinus of Valsalva aneurysm* into the right heart. Many of these murmurs do not actually occupy the total cardiac cycle. Characteristically they begin in systole and spill over into diastole. The recognition of the exact cause of the continuous murmur is aided by the location

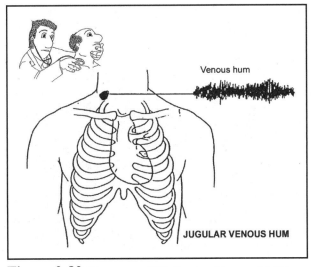

Figure 2-80 (Courtesy of W. Proctor Harvey, M.D.)

of its maximal intensity (murmur peaking at the second heart sound, murmur peaking in both systole and diastole, or murmur accentuated in diastole alone or systole alone). The typical continuous "*machinery*" murmur of PDA, for example, is maximal at the first and second left intercostal spaces, and *peaks and "envelops" S2* (**Figure 2-81**). The continuous murmur in coronary AV fistula tends to crescendo-decrescendo both in systole and diastole, the diastolic component being louder. The murmur of a venous hum and ruptured sinus of Valsalva both peak in diastole, not over S2.

Figure 2-81. Patent ductus arteriosus (arrow on left). Note the continuous murmur heard over the pulmonic area

that envelops the second heart sound (S2). If the murmur does not envelop S2, although sounding continuous, it may be a clue to a cause other than patent ductus.

Miscellaneous

Pericardial Friction Rubs

Figure 2-82. A typical three-component pericardial friction rub (as, vs, vd) which generally gets louder with inspiration. To detect the rub, listen along the left sternal border, exerting firm pressure on the diaphragm of the stethoscope with the patient sitting upright, breath held in deep expiration. The components represent friction during the different parts of the cardiac cycle–atrial systole, ventricular systole, and ventricular diastole. These noises may be mistaken for both systolic and diastolic heart murmurs, but can be differentiated by their rough, scratchy, leathery, creaking, superficial quality and by the fact that they have at least two or three components (systolic, diastolic, presystolic). The transient nature of the sounds also provides a clue to their pericardial origin. They occur in patients with acute pericarditis, after acute MI, cardiac surgery, chest injury, and in association with uremia, malignancy or connective tissue diseases. Rubs generally become louder with inspiration and may occur even with a large pericardial effusion.

* * *

Pearls:

- An S4 gallop is pathologic and can indicate LV diastolic dysfunction, LV hypertrophy, or acute myocardial ischemia.
- An S3 can be physiologic and present in athletes, pregnant females, and healthy young individuals. A

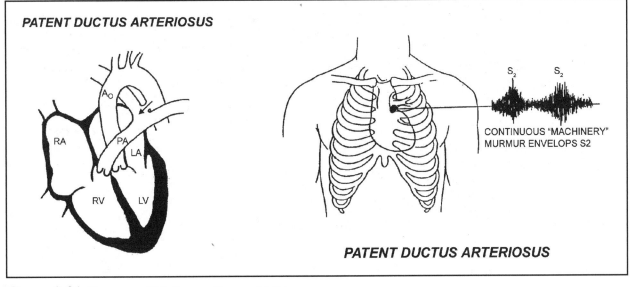

Figure 2-81 (Courtesy of W. Proctor Harvey, M.D.)

pathological S3 gallop may be heard in both systolic and diastolic LV dysfunction. When accompanied by pulsus alternans, an S3 gallop is an indicator of LV systolic dysfunction and is associated with an elevated LV filling pressure, a reduced ejection fraction, and an elevated brain natriuretic peptide level.

- Innocent murmurs are faint (grade 1-2/6) and early-mid systolic in timing. All diastolic, holosystolic, late systolic, or continuous murmurs should be considered pathologic.
- If a holosystolic murmur is heard, think of 3 conditions: MR, TR, and VSD.
- A murmur that is only late systolic in timing argues against severe MR. When MR is severe, the murmur is accompanied by an S3 gallop and a diastolic "flow rumble" at the apex. When the anterior leaflet is involved the murmur radiates to the back. When the posterior leaflet is involved the murmur radiates to the base. The murmur of both VSD and TR are best heard along the left lower sternal border. The murmur of TR increases with inspiration. A JVP that mimics a carotid pulse (large V waves) is a clue to TR.
- The auscultatory findings that correlate with severe AS include a harsh late peaking systolic ejection murmur, an absent or paradoxically split S2, and an S4 gallop. A normal A2 excludes severe AS.
- The diastolic murmur of AR is louder along the *right* sternal border if the etiology is aortic *root* dilatation (e.g., dissection, aneurysm). If valve *leaflet* pathology is the cause then the murmur is louder at the *left* sternal border.
- The Austin Flint murmur is a diastolic rumble at the cardiac apex heard with severe AR and is caused by the AR jet striking the anterior mitral leaflet. Unlike MS, there is no opening snap.
- The murmur of AR may become musical when the aortic cusps are everted or perforated (e.g., infective endocarditis).
- A systolic click along with a mid to late systolic murmur or musical "whoop" or "honk" of MR are classic auscultatory findings of MVP.
- The earlier the OS, and the longer the diastolic rumble, the more severe MS is due to higher LA pressures forcing the valve open in early diastole.
- A loud P2 or closely split S2 heard over the cardiac apex implies significant pulmonary hypertension.

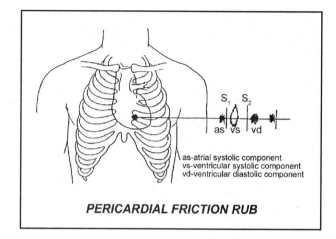

PERICARDIAL FRICTION RUB

as-atrial systolic component
vs-ventricular systolic component
vd-ventricular diastolic component

Figure 2-82 (Courtesy of W. Proctor Harvey, M.D.)

- Loud heart sounds are usually due to mild-moderate stenotic lesions, while faint heart sounds are usually due to regurgitant or severe stenotic lesions.
- All right-sided heart sounds and murmurs increase with inspiration except the systolic ejection sound of PS, which decreases with inspiration.
- The murmur of an ASD is a systolic crescendo-decrescendo murmur heard at the pulmonic area due to increased pulmonary flow. It is accompanied by fixed splitting of S2.
- The murmur of a PDA at the pulmonic area is continuous throughout systole and diastole.
- The systolic murmur of HOCM can be mistaken for the murmur of AS or MR. Certain maneuvers, however, e.g., standing and Valsalva, will increase the obstruction and make the murmur louder, whereas squatting will decrease the obstruction and make the murmur fainter. In contrast to AS, the systolic murmur of HOCM does not radiate to the carotids.
- The pericardial friction rub can be evanescent. Repeated auscultation may be needed to detect it. Unless 2 or 3 components are heard, however, the diagnosis of a pericardial friction rub should not be made since most 1 component sounds are usually scratchy systolic murmurs.

* * *

Note: Please refer to the attached CD for an interactive overview of heart sounds and murmurs.

CHAPTER 3. ELECTROCARDIOGRAM

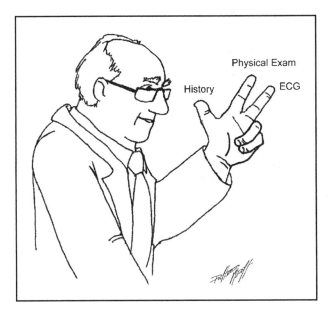

The electrocardiogram (ECG) is the most commonly used noninvasive test in cardiology. The ECG is a simple, inexpensive, and useful clinical tool in assessing cardiac arrhythmias, myocardial ischemia and/or infarction, pericarditis, cardiac chamber enlargement and hypertrophy, metabolic and electrolyte imbalances, drug-induced effects, and electronic pacemaker function. Indeed, it is considered the procedure of "first choice" in the evaluation of patients with chest pain, dizziness, or syncope.

BASIC ELECTROCARDIOGRAPHY

Cardiac Electrical Activity and the ECG

The ECG records cardiac electrical activity from different angles of view. It records two basic electrical processes:

1. *Depolarization* (the spread of electrical current through the heart muscle) producing the P wave from the atria and the QRS from the ventricles.
2. *Repolarization* (the return of the stimulated muscle to the resting state), producing the ST segment, T wave and U wave. (**Figure 3-1**).

The ECG provides three pieces of information about the electrical activity generated by the heart during the cardiac cycle: *duration, amplitude,* and *direction* (electrical axis).

The *duration* is the time required to depolarize (or repolarize) various structures. At a standard paper speed of 25 mm/sec, each small box (1 mm) horizontally on the ECG

paper represents 0.04 seconds and each large box (5 mm) represents 0.20 seconds. (**Figure 3-1**) Abnormal duration may indicate impairment of electrical propagation.

The *amplitude* of the electrical activity is expressed in millivolts and is measured by the vertical markings on the ECG paper; when the ECG machine is set at "standard" each millimeter of amplitude equals 0.1 mV (10 mm = 1 mV). Voltage is determined in part by the size of the cardiac chambers as well as the body habitus and various pathological conditions.

The *direction* of electrical activity refers to the overall vector direction of electrical depolarization of the ventricular myocardium. Many abnormalities affect the direction of electrical activity produced by depolarization as well as repolarization.

Standard ECG Leads

The "standard" ECG consists of 12 different leads used to provide a complete panoramic picture of the heart's electrical activity as seen from different angles.

Figure 3-2. Attachments and viewing angles of the limb and chest leads. (From Goldberg, S. Clinical Physiology Made Ridiculously Simple, MedMaster, Inc., 2002)

- Six leads are called *extremity* or *limb leads:* 3 bipolar leads (I, II, and III), and 3 unipolar augmented leads (aVR, aVL, and aVF), which register the direction, amplitude and duration of the heart's electrical activity, as seen from 6 different positions in the frontal plane (picture a flat plane lying on the patient's chest).
- The 6 remaining leads are called *precordial* or *chest leads* (V1 to V6). These leads provide information about the heart's electrical activity in the horizontal plane (picture a flat plane crossing through the patient's chest).

Each ECG lead provides a view of the heart's electrical activity between two points or poles (a positive pole and a negative pole). The direction in which the electric current flows determines how the waveforms appear on the ECG tracing:

- The 3 bipolar limb leads I, II, and III record the difference in electrical potential between the right arm (−) and left arm (+) for lead I; right arm (−) and left leg (+) for lead II; and left arm (−) and left leg (+) for lead III. (**Figure 3-2**). An electrode is also attached to the patient's right leg, but this serves only as an electrical ground and is not an active recording site.

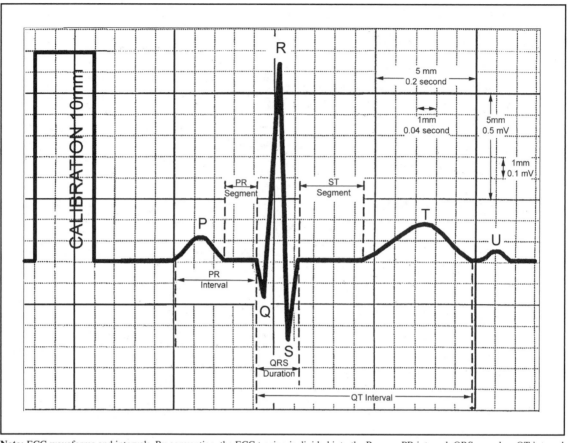

Note: ECG waveforms and intervals. By convention, the ECG tracing is divided into the P wave, PR interval, QRS complex, QT interval, ST segment, T wave, and U wave.

Figure 3-1

• The 3 unipolar limb leads (aVR, aVL, aVF) are devised by connecting all three extremities to a "central terminal" which serves as the reference electrode. (**Figure 3-2**). If a wave of depolarization is moving toward a positive electrode, this is reflected in a positive (upward) movement of the wave on the ECG recording. If the wave of depolarization is moving away from a positive electrode, this results in a negative (downward) deflection of the wave on the ECG recording.

Figure 3-3. The 6 unipolar precordial leads are placed as follows: V1, the fourth intercostal space to the right of the sternum; V2, the fourth intercostal space to the left of the sternum; V3, midway between leads V2 and V4. Lead V4 is placed in the fifth intercostal space at the midclavicular line, V5 is placed between V4 and V6, and V6 is placed at the midaxillary line at the level of lead V4. V1 and V2 lie medially and are good leads for examining right-sided abnormalities, e.g. right bundle branch block (RBBB) and anteroseptal MI, whereas V5 and V6 are situated more laterally and are good leads for examining more lateral

abnormalities, e.g., left bundle branch block (LBBB) and anterolateral MI. Leads V3 and V4 overlie the interventricular septum and the anterior wall of the left ventricle.

In certain circumstances, additional chest leads not part of the "standard" 12 lead ECG may be used to view specific areas of the heart. Right-sided chest leads (particularly V4R), placed in a "mirror image" pattern to the normal left-sided leads, can provide clues to RV infarction. Posterior chest leads (V7, V8, and V9), placed in the posterior axillary, mid scapular, and left paraspinal lines, respectively, can help confirm the diagnosis of posterior MI.

APPROACH TO ECG INTERPRETATION

There are several general approaches to interpreting ECGs. One is the pattern recognition method, where the interpreter commits all possible patterns to memory, and then studies each ECG for the presence of these patterns. If the practitioner has perfect memory, and is always presented with classic ("textbook") ECGs, this approach may be reasonable. However, many patients "don't read the textbook". Another perhaps

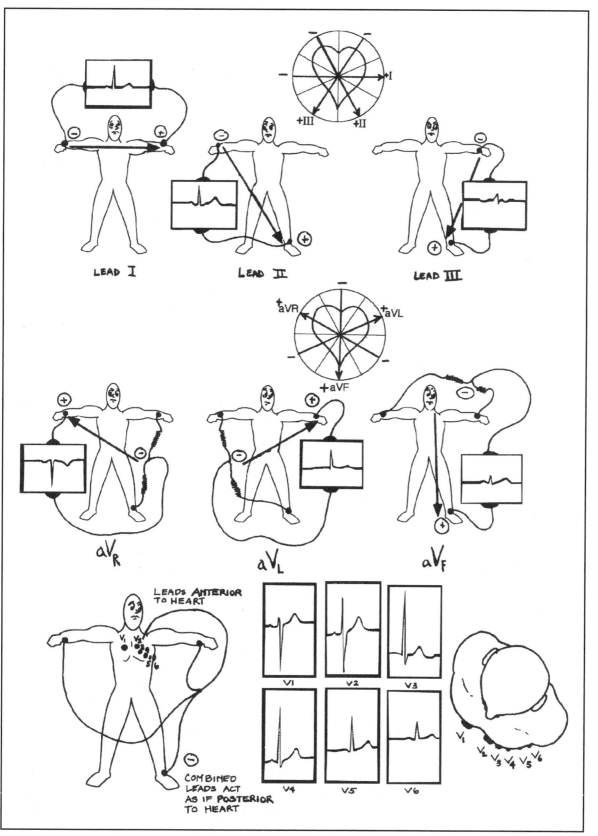

Figure 3-2

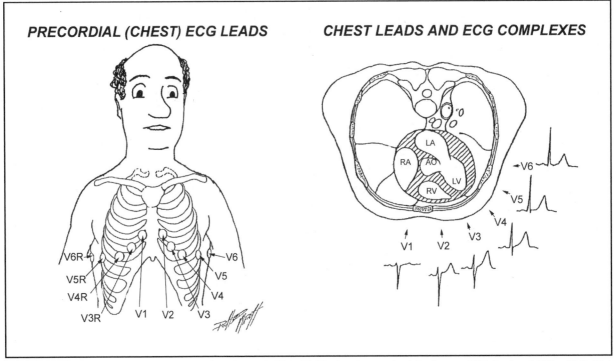

PRECORDIAL (CHEST) ECG LEADS

CHEST LEADS AND ECG COMPLEXES

Note: Right-sided chest leads (particularly V4R) mirror the standard left-sided leads and are used to help diagnose RV infarction. Additional left-sided leads (V7, V8, and V9) placed at the posterior axillary, mid scapular, and left paraspinal lines, respectively, may help diagnose a true posterior MI.

Figure 3-3

more practical and logical method is to take a "step-by-step" approach, so that nothing is overlooked, as follows:

- First check the *voltage calibration* of the ECG machine.
- Determine the *heart rate and rhythm*.
- Examine each wave or complex (*P, QRS, ST, and T*) and *interval (PR, QRS, QT)*.
- Determine the mean directional electrical *QRS axis*.
- Put this information together and assess it for signs of conduction disturbances, hypertrophy, myocardial ischemia and/or infarction, as well as drug effects and electrolyte abnormalities, interpreting them in light of the clinical context (i.e., patient's age, presenting complaint, and additional relevant clinical history).

With repeated practice, you may begin to master the essentials of ECG interpretation.

The P-QRS-T complex of the normal ECG represents electrical activity over one cardiac cycle.

Figure 3-4. The cardiac conduction system. An electrical impulse begins in the sinoatrial (SA) node, the heart's primary pacemaker (at a rate of 60–100 beats per minute). The impulse travels to atrial myocardial muscle cells by way of internodal tracts in the right and left atria, causing a

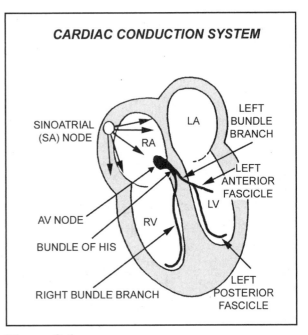

CARDIAC CONDUCTION SYSTEM

Figure 3-4

wave of atrial muscle cell depolarization. The electrical impulse briefly slows at the AV node, delaying ventricular activity and allowing blood from the atrial contraction to fill the ventricles. From the AV node, the impulse passes extremely rapidly through the bundle of His to the right and left bundle branches and to the Purkinje fibers, which trigger ventricular muscle cell depolarization and then contraction of the ventricles. The electrical activity of the AV node, bundle of His and Purkinje fibers does not show up on the ECG. Rather, it is the actual depolarization of myocardial fibers that shows up. In the absence of an SA node, the AV node will drive the heart beat, albeit at a slower rate than normal (40–60 beats per minute). In the absence of the SA and AV node functions, a slower ventricular rhythm will prevail (20–40 beats per minute). These backup mechanisms help ensure that the ventricles will continue beating in the presence of defects to SA and/or AV nodal discharges.

Figure 3-5. The overall direction of ventricular myocardial cell depolarization normally spreads inferiorly and to the (patient's) left and is referred to as the axis of depolarization. The axis may point outside the patient's lower left quadrant in different pathological states, either to the patient's right side (right axis deviation) or the patient's left upper quadrant (left axis deviation). (From Goldberg, S. Clinical Physiology Made Ridiculously Simple, MedMaster, Inc., 2002).

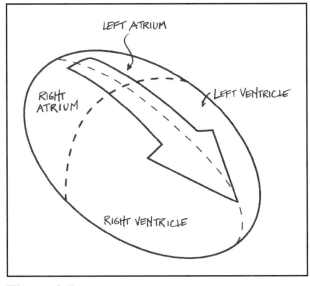

Figure 3-5

- The *P wave* indicates atrial depolarization.
- The *QRS complex* indicates ventricular depolarization.
- The *T wave* represents ventricular repolarization
- A *U wave* (not always seen), follows the T wave and indicates poorly understood ventricular afterpotentials.

- The *PR interval* is the time between the beginning of the P wave and the beginning of the QRS. It is the time between the onset of atrial depolarization and the onset of ventricular depolarization. It is commonly used as an estimation of AV nodal conduction time, since most of this interval is spent in the delay traversing the AV node.
- The *ST segment* is the segment between the *end* of the QRS interval and the *beginning* of the T wave. It is the pause between the end of ventricular depolarization and the beginning of ventricular repolarization.
- The *QT interval* (the time between the *beginning* of the QRS and the *end* of the T wave) represents the total duration of both ventricular depolarization and repolarization. (**Note:** A "segment" is a stretch of baseline. An "interval" includes at least one wave.)

Figure 3-6. The Normal 12 Lead ECG consists of the following waves, segments and intervals:

- The P wave, a record of atrial depolarization, is upright in lead I, II, aVF, typically inverted in aVR, and may be inverted or biphasic in III, aVR, V1 and V2.
- The PR interval, the interval from the beginning of the P wave to the beginning of the QRS complex, is normally 0.12–0.20 seconds. It reflects the time required for conduction of the impulse through the atria, AV node, bundle of His, and bundle branches up to the time of ventricular depolarization.
- The QRS interval, the interval from the beginning of the Q wave to the end of the S wave, is usually 0.06–0.10 seconds. It reflects ventricular depolarization. The precordial transition zone (midpoint between negative and positive deflections) usually occurs between V2 and V4.
- Q waves are typical in leads aVR, V1 and V2. However, small q waves (<0.04 seconds in duration and height <25% of R wave) are common in most leads and should not be confused with old MI. The ST segment, the segment between the end of the QRS interval and the beginning of the T wave, is usually isoelectric. It may vary from 0.5 mm below to 1 mm above baseline in the limb leads. Up to 3 mm concave upward (valley-like) elevation in precordial leads may be seen ("early repolarization").
- The T wave reflects ventricular repolarization. It is upright in leads I, II, V3–V6; typically inverted in aVR and V1; may be variable (upright, flat, inverted, or biphasic) in III, aVL, aVF, V1 and V2. T wave inversion in V1–V3 may be seen in healthy young adults ("persistent juvenile pattern").

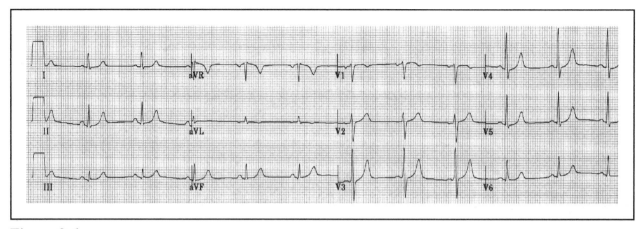

Figure 3-6

- The QT interval, the interval between the beginning of the QRS and the end of the T wave, represents the duration of ventricular electrical activity, and corrected for heart rate (see below) is usually ≤0.44 seconds (in men) and ≤0.46 seconds (in women). It varies inversely with heart rate. (Roughly, if the heart rate is between 60 and 100, the QT interval should be less than 1/2 of the R-R interval).
- The U wave is a small deflection following the T wave. It is usually, but not always, observed in the precordial leads, and may be due to repolarization of the bundle branches and Purkinje fibers.

Note: The rectangular upward deflection at the beginning of the ECG tracing is the voltage calibration signal (10 boxes =1 mV). Each small box on the ECG grid = 0.04 seconds.

A patient's ECG can tell the practitioner much about the heart's depolarization-repolarization cycle:

Rate and Rhythm

A normal cardiac rhythm (normal sinus rhythm, NSR) is present if the heart rate is between 60 and 100 beats per minute and if every P wave is followed by a QRS, every QRS is preceded by a P wave, the P wave is upright in leads I, II and III (indicating that the P wave is originating from the sinus node), and the PR interval is >0.12 seconds. The heart rate can be estimated in several ways:

- Find an R wave that lands on a heavy black line. Then count the number of large boxes to the next R wave. Count "300-150-100" and then "75-60-50" as each large box goes by until you get to the next R wave, thus providing an estimate of the heart rate

(**Figure 3-7**). Alternatively, you may divide 300 by the number of large boxes (or divide 1500 by the number of small boxes) between R waves.
- If the heart rate is less than 60, the above method may not be accurate. In that case, count the number of R waves in a 6-second strip and then multiply by 10. This method is also useful if there is an irregular rhythm, where the distances between R waves may vary and one needs a number of R waves to average out the measurement.

Figure 3-7. Estimating heart rate on the ECG. Count the number of QRS complexes between 3 markers (6 seconds) and multiply by 10. A similar rate is obtained using the "(300-150-100)(75-60-50)" method. In this case, the ventricular rate, as measured by the QRS complexes, is about 60–70.

Figure 3-8. A. Normal sinus rhythm. **B.** A sinus rhythm that is slow (<60 beats/min) is a *sinus bradycardia*. **C.** A sinus rhythm that is fast (>100 beats/min), is a *sinus tachycardia*. **D.** If the SA node fails, a backup pacemaker may arise in the AV node or proximal bundle of His, conducting at about 40–60 beats/min. This is termed a junctional escape rhythm, or *idiojunctional rhythm*. There may not be a visible P wave or there may be an inverted P wave either before or after the QRS complex, reflecting retrograde conduction of the P wave. **E.** Failing that, the rhythm may be paced by the ventricles at about 20–40/min, termed a ventricular escape rhythm, or *idioventricular rhythm*. Note the wide QRS arising from a pacemaker focus in the myocardium.

The term *supraventricular tachycardia* refers to tachycardias that are "above the ventricles", i.e. that are not ventricular in origin. They include atrial tachycardias as well as those originating within the AV node.

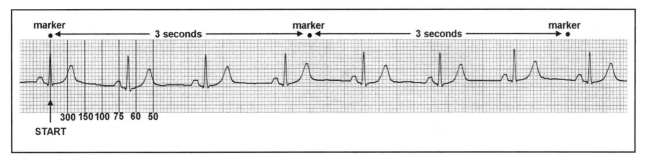

Figure 3-7

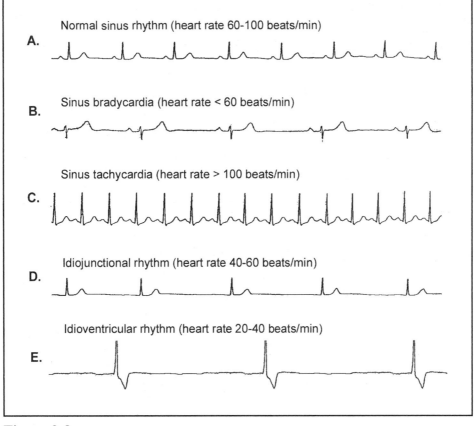

Figure 3-8

In normal sinus rhythm, the distance between the QRS complexes varies somewhat with respiration, the rate increasing slightly with the effort of inspiration and decreasing with the passive process of expiration (*sinus arrhythmia*).

Rhythms other than NSR are termed "arrhythmias". Some arrhythmias are regular rhythms, but just slow (<60 beats/min) or fast (>100 beats/min), where the QRS complexes appear at regular intervals. Some rhythms are regularly irregular (e.g., Wenckebach phenomenon, where the QRS complexes get progressively farther apart, skip a beat and then start all over closer together), while others are irregularly irregular (e.g., atrial fibrillation, where the distances between QRS complexes has no regularity). It is important to ascertain whether an arrhythmia originates from the atria, ventricles or conduction system that connects the atria and ventricles. This can make an important difference in understanding the underlying pathology and planning a therapeutic approach.

Diagnosing the origin of an ECG rate and rhythm often depends on a careful analysis of the individual ECG components, which will be discussed below in the section on arrhythmias.

The P Wave

P wave morphology is best assessed in leads V1 and II. A small upright rounded P wave (as seen in lead II) represents normal atrial depolarization. P wave abnormalities may deviate from the normal with respect to their location, amplitude (voltage), duration, positive or negative deflection, or contour (configuration).

Figure 3-9. In right atrial enlargement, the P wave in lead II is tall (>2.5 mm) and pointed, and the amplitude of the right atrial component of the P wave in lead V1 is increased ("P pulmonale"), seen as an enlargement of the first part of the curve (in lead V1), since right atrial depolarization slightly precedes left atrial depolarization. In left atrial enlargement, the P wave in lead II is broad and notched, and the terminal downward deflection of the biphasic P wave in lead V1 is increased in amplitude and duration (>1 mm wide and >1 mm deep) ("P mitrale"), reflecting the later depolarization of the left atrium.

	Lead II	Lead V$_1$
NORMAL		
RA enlargement ("P Pulmonale")	Tall P Wave (>2.5mm)	Tall P Wave
LA enlargement ("P Mitrale")	Broad & Notched P Wave	Wide & Deep Biphasic P Wave

Figure 3-9

If the P wave is negative in leads I or II, the practitioner should keep in mind three possibilities: inadvertent limb lead reversal, dextrocardia, and junctional rhythm (where the AV node pathologically is the pacemaker and impulses spread backwards from the AV node to depolarize the atria).

The QRS

The Q wave is the first downward deflection of the QRS complex. It is followed by an upward R wave, and then a downward S wave. This total QRS complex represents the electrical activity of ventricular depolarization. The normal QRS complex is predominantly positive (above the baseline) in leads that "look" at the heart from the left side (I, aVL, V5–V6) and in leads that "look" at the inferior sur-

face of the heart (II, III, aVF). It is negative (below the baseline) in leads that "look" at the heart from the right side (aVR, V1–V2). The QRS complex is biphasic (part above and part below the baseline) in leads V3–V4. If there is only a single downward deflection with no R wave, then you cannot know whether to call the deflection a Q wave or an S wave, so it is termed a "QS" wave.

The QRS *width* (interval) normally is 0.10 seconds or less and should be examined for possible conduction abnormalities. The ECG demonstrates widening of the QRS and other changes representing interference with conduction when there is a block of conduction in either the right or left bundles. It is better to evaluate QRS width in the limb leads than in the chest leads, since the amplitude of the QRS is generally higher in the chest leads, and a lag in ability of the ECG pen to write quickly may artifactually widen the QRS in the chest leads.

In *right bundle branch block* (RBBB), there is blockage of transmission of electrical information through the right bundle branch to the right ventricle myocardium. As a result, information has to take a divergent route from the left side of the heart to the right side, resulting in a delay of appearance of the right ventricle QRS. The QRS complexes of the right and left ventricles normally overlap to form a single QRS, but in RBBB the right ventricle QRS appears slightly after the start of the left ventricle QRS, resulting in an abnormally widened QRS (>0.12 sec) with two R wave peaks (seen best in lead V1). In *left bundle branch block* (LBBB) there is a similar widening of the QRS, but it is the left ventricular QRS that occupies the later part of the abnormally widened QRS. It, too, is often, but not always, notched at the top.

Figure 3-10. Top. Right bundle branch block (RBBB). Note that the QRS is prolonged (>0.12 seconds) and the terminal positive wave is inscribed in lead V1 (rSR'–"rabbit ear" pattern), since V1 lies on the right side and "sees" the RBBB delay moving toward it. Conversely, in lead V6, the delay is moving away from the electrode, producing a terminal wide negative S wave. **Bottom.** Left bundle branch block (LBBB). Note the QRS is prolonged with a slurred upright R wave in lead V6 (the delay is moving toward the electrode), whereas the right precordial leads (V1) have a deep negative wave (the delay is moving away from the electrode). Since normal left to right septal activation does not occur in LBBB, the normal septal q wave in lead V6 is lost. Furthermore, because the QRS from the left ventricle is delayed in LBBB, the left side of the LV QRS fuses with the QRS of the right ventricle, masking the Q wave and also (often, in V5 or V6) producing a notch in the LBBB R wave in V6 which may also be seen. Also note prominent repolarization abnormalities (ST-T changes in V6).

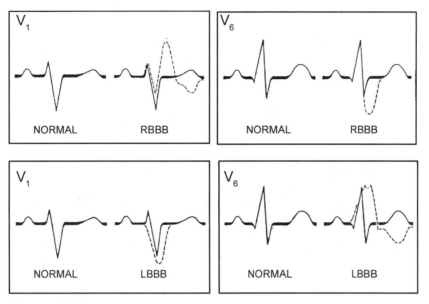

Figure 3-10

Figure 3-11. Right bundle branch block. V1 typically is triphasic with the initial r of lesser amplitude than the subsequent R'. V6 has a terminal s that is widened and of less amplitude than the initial R.

Figure 3-12. Left bundle branch block. V1 has a small R and a deep S with a rapid downslope. A broad slurred monophasic R wave is present in lead V6 (and a notch in V5). In LBBB there is a broad usually notched R (the notch indicating the two asynchronous R waves, one from the right ventricle and the later one from the left ventricle) in leads I, V5–V6, and aVL. Because of abnormal septal depolarization, there is a marked loss of initial R wave voltage in precordial leads V1–V3, and absence of a small Q wave normally seen in V6.

The QRS may also be prolonged in other cases where there is aberrant conduction through ventricular myocardial tissue. For instance, a ventricular contraction resulting from an abnormal ectopic discharging focus in the ventricle, such as a premature ventricular contraction (PVC) characteristically results in a widened QRS of abnormal shape (**Figure 3-8**).

The QRS interval can also be increased (0.12 seconds or more) in ventricular hypertrophy and severe hyperkalemia.

The QRS *height* should be measured for possible ventricular hypertrophy. The normal QRS complex in the precordial leads is less than 25 mm high. *Left ventricular hypertrophy* is suggested with an S wave in V1 + R wave in V5 or V6 ≥35 mm, or R wave in aVL >11 mm, or R wave in lead I > 15 mm in height. *Right ventricular hypertrophy* is suggested with an R wave height >S wave in V1, with the R wave becoming progressively smaller on proceeding from V1 to V6, along with right axis deviation (see below under "Axis").

Figure 3-13:

Left ventricular hypertrophy (top) resulting in a tall R wave in lead V6 and a deep S wave in lead V1. When the sum of the S wave in V1 and the R wave in V5 or V6 is ≥35 mm in the age group over 45 years, a voltage criterion for LV hypertrophy is present. In addition to voltage, changes suggesting LV hypertrophy include left axis deviation (**Figure 3-18**), prolongation of the QRS interval, along with ST segment depression and T wave inversion (as seen in lead V6) which suggests LV "strain" (**Figure 3-16F**). Large P waves due to left atrial enlargement may also be present.

Right ventricular hypertrophy (bottom). Since the right ventricle is to the right of and anterior to the left ventricle, right ventricular hypertrophy results in increased anterior forces (tall R waves) in the right precordial leads (V1) and a deep S wave in lead V6. The R/S ratio in lead V1 is ≥1, and the R/S ratio in lead V6 is ≤1. Right axis deviation (**Figure 3-18**) along with ST segment depression and T wave inversion in the right precordial leads (V1) suggest RV strain.

The QRS should be assessed for the presence of normal or abnormal Q waves. A normal Q wave should have a width of ≤0.04 seconds and a height <25% that of the QRS complex. While small negative initial deflections (Q waves) are normal, large Q waves can be due to an electrically unexcitable area just under the recording electrode and frequently indicate a past MI.

- Changes in QRS morphology thus can provide an important clue to underlying heart disease (e.g., conduction defect, MI, ventricular hypertrophy).

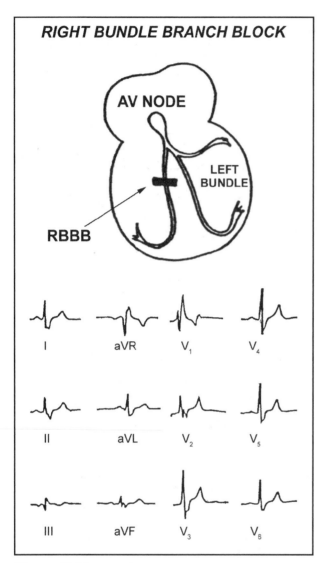

Figure 3-11

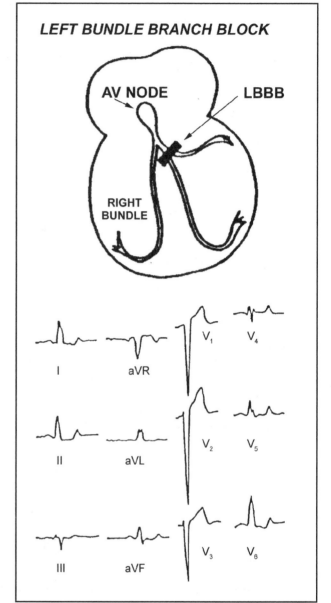

Figure 3-12

Low voltage QRS complexes (< 5 mm in limb leads and/or < 10 mm in precordial leads) are commonly present in COPD, obesity, hypothyroidism, pericardial effusion, extensive MI, myocardial fibrosis, or infiltrative cardiomyopathy (e.g., amyloid).

Normally, the R wave becomes progressively taller as one progresses from V1 to V6 (**Figure 3-3**). A number of conditions, however, may be associated with "poor R wave progression" in leads V1 to V3–V4: LV hypertrophy, RV hypertrophy, chronic pulmonary disease, anteroseptal MI, conduction defects, e.g., LBBB, left anterior hemiblock (blockage of the left anterior fascicle of the conduction system), cardiomyopathy, chest wall deformity, *normal variant*, and lead misplacement. Incorrect lead placement can lead to misdiagnosis and makes comparisons with previous ECGs difficult.

The T Wave

Many factors can influence the T wave (e.g., metabolic disturbances, drug effect, autonomic stimuli, myocardial hypertrophy, bundle branch block, ischemia, or inflammation. **Figure 3-14.** Electrolyte imbalances affecting the T wave.

The U Wave

A *U wave,* which follows the T wave, indicates poorly understood ventricular afterpotentials. Lead II and a slow heart rate provide the best opportunity to observe a U wave

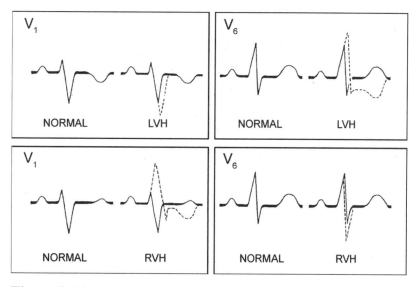

Figure 3-13

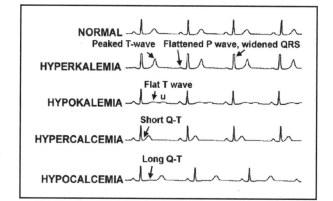

*Note: In severe hyperkalemia, a "sine wave" pattern is present.

Figure 3-14

in the normal ECG tracing. In addition to bradycardia, *positive* U waves may occur with central nervous system disease, antiarrhythmic medication, electrolyte disturbances (e.g., hypokalemia, hypomagnesemia). Causes of a *negative* U wave include LV hypertrophy and ischemia.

The PR Interval

The PR interval, QRS duration, and QT interval are measured from the limb leads (I, II, III, aVR, aVL, aVF).

The *PR interval* (normally = 0.12–0.20 seconds) can be shorter than normal if the impulse originates in an ectopic site close to or in the AV junction (*junctional rhythm*) and in preexcitation syndromes, where the electrical impulse is conducted faster than normal through an accessory pathway that bypasses the AV node and bundle of His.

The PR interval may be longer than normal if the electrical impulse is abnormally delayed traveling through the AV node (e.g., first degree AV block–**Figure 3-51**). Common causes of first degree AV block include normal variant, athletic conditioning, high vagal tone, medications, e.g., digitalis, beta blockers, rate-slowing calcium channel blockers (verapamil, diltiazem), and certain antiarrhythmic agents (e.g., amiodarone), and a diseased AV node.

The ST Segment

While the ST segment is usually flat and at the baseline (isoelectric), small deviations are not always pathological (e.g., non-specific ST changes). As part of a complete ECG interpretation, the *ST segment* is assessed for deviations.

Figure 3-15. The normal ST segment and its variations in early repolarization, ischemia and infarction. Note the ST segment is normally isoelectric (flat, at the baseline) from the J point (junction of the QRS complex and the ST segment) until it gradually slopes into the shoulder of the T wave. Many healthy young individuals have slightly elevated concave upward ST segments (like a "smile"), particularly in the precordial leads (so-called "*early repolarization*"). During spontaneous angina pectoris or an exercise stress test, the ST segment is horizontal and depressed (*ischemic pattern*). When ischemia progresses to a transmural MI, convex ST segment elevation (like a "frown") occurs ("*injury*" pattern).

Although convex upward ("domed") ST elevation is usually the earliest change noted in acute MI, it is not

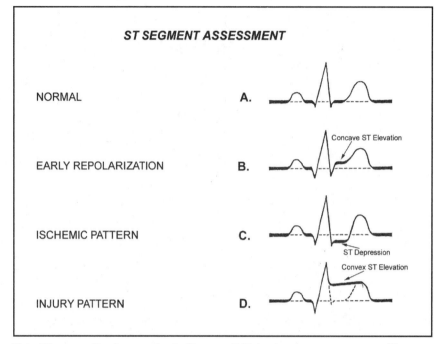

Note: ST segment elevations associated with myocardial injury have a convex appearance (like a "frown"), while ST segment elevations in early repolarization (or pericarditis) tend to be concave (resemble a "smile").

Figure 3-15

pathognomonic, and may be seen in other forms of myocardial injury, including Takotsubo (stress) cardiomyopathy and variant (*Prinzmetal's*) angina (from coronary artery vasospasm), and as a stable change with ventricular aneurysm (persisting for months to years). In *pericarditis,* the elevated ST segment tends to be *concave* upward, but can easily be differentiated from acute ST segment elevation MI by its presence throughout all of the leads (except aVR, V1). (**Figure 3-16D).** As mentioned, sometimes the ST segment may be slightly elevated above the baseline in perfectly healthy people as a normal variant (i.e., *early repolarization pattern*), especially in young males, and resembles closely the concave upward ST elevation pattern of acute pericarditis.

Reciprocal ST depression in opposite ECG leads is highly characteristic of acute MI.

Figure 3-16. ST and T waves configurations in a variety of cardiac disease states and conditions.

A. Hyperacute peaked T wave in early acute MI.

B. Typical convex upward ST segment elevation, along with Q wave and inversion of the T wave (discussed below) in acute MI. If ST segment elevation persists, it may be a clue to LV aneurysm formation.

C. T wave inversion in myocardial ischemia or non-ST elevation (non Q-wave) MI. *Subendocardial infarction* is a type of non Q wave infarction in which the infarct involves only the subendocardial part of the myocardium (which lies near the ventricular cavity), rather than the

full-thickness of the myocardium. The subendocardial region is the most susceptible part of the myocardium to infarct. In this type of non Q wave MI, the ST segment is depressed, rather than elevated. ST depression also occurs in ischemia (short of infarction) as in an abnormal stress test (see **G**).

D. Concave upward ST segment elevation along with PR segment depression in acute pericarditis.

E. Concave upward ST segment and J point elevation in early repolarization.

F. Downsloping ST segment merging into T wave inversion (so-called "strain pattern") in LV hypertrophy.

G. Horizontal ST segment depression in myocardial ischemia, or non-ST elevation (non Q-wave) MI or subendocardial infarction (see C).

H. Transient ST segment elevation in variant or Prinzmetal's angina and Takotsubo ("stress") cardiomyopathy.

I. Horizontal ST segment depression and low voltage with non specific ST-T changes often seen in CAD.

J. Downward coving (valley-like) ST segment seen with digitalis effect (*mnemonic:* "dig" a valley).

K. Coved ST segment elevation and RBBB morphology in Brugada syndrome.

L. J or Osborne wave simulating ST segment elevation in hypothermia.

Although ST depression is most often associated with myocardial ischemia, other common causes include LV and

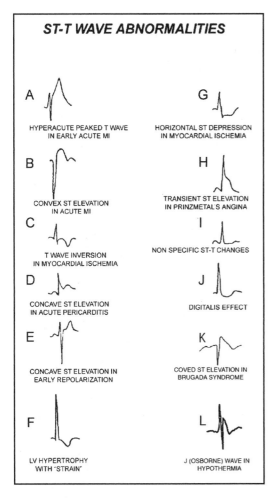

ST-T WAVE ABNORMALITIES

A — HYPERACUTE PEAKED T WAVE IN EARLY ACUTE MI

B — CONVEX ST ELEVATION IN ACUTE MI

C — T WAVE INVERSION IN MYOCARDIAL ISCHEMIA

D — CONCAVE ST ELEVATION IN ACUTE PERICARDITIS

E — CONCAVE ST ELEVATION IN EARLY REPOLARIZATION

F — LV HYPERTROPHY WITH "STRAIN"

G — HORIZONTAL ST DEPRESSION IN MYOCARDIAL ISCHEMIA

H — TRANSIENT ST ELEVATION IN PRINZMETAL'S ANGINA

I — NON SPECIFIC ST-T CHANGES

J — DIGITALIS EFFECT

K — COVED ST ELEVATION IN BRUGADA SYNDROME

L — J (OSBORNE) WAVE IN HYPOTHERMIA

Figure 3-16

RV hypertrophy, dilated and hypertrophic cardiomyopathies, LBBB, RBBB, hypokalemia, and certain medications, e.g., digitalis, which causes a characteristic sagging ("scooped-out") appearance (**Figure 3-16J**). In addition, many individuals have resting ECG tracings with minor degrees of ST depression and/or T wave changes, which in the absence of other objective findings, should not lead the practitioner to the mistaken diagnosis of heart disease.

The QT Interval

The QT interval varies normally with heart rate (the faster the heart rate, the shorter the QT). It is measured from the start of the QRS to the end of the T wave. The corrected interval is obtained by dividing the measured QT interval in seconds by the square root of the R-R interval (in seconds). The normal corrected QT interval is ≤0.44 seconds (in men) and ≤ 0.46 seconds (in women). A quick determination can be done if the heart rate is between 60 and 100 beats per minute by noting that the normal QT interval in

that setting should measure less than one-half of the R-R interval. If the QT interval is more than one-half of the R-R interval, it is prolonged. With faster rates it may become slightly longer than half of the R-R interval, but this "rule of thumb" is sufficient for most purposes.

A long QT interval can be congenital or acquired as a result of toxic drug effects (certain antiarrhythmic agents), tricyclic antidepressants, phenothiazine, hypokalemia, and hypomagnesemia) and may predispose an individual to the development of a specific type of polymorphic VT called *"torsades de pointes"* (**Figure 3-17**).

Figure 3-17. ECG manifestations of the long QT syndrome (LQTS). In LQTS, the time it takes the heart muscle to recharge (the QT interval) is prolonged (usually >0.44 sec), leaving the individual susceptible to an unstable, dangerously rapid heart rhythm referred to as polymorphic ventricular tachycardia ("torsades de pointes").

QRS Axis

Figure 3-18. The mean QRS axis (the overall direction of the wave of myocardial cell depolarization passing through the myocardium) normally falls between -30° and +90°. An analysis of the direction of the QRS complexes in leads I and II may provide the information for a qualitative assessment of the axis. If the complexes in leads I and II are both predominantly positive, the axis is normal. If the complex is negative in lead I and positive in lead II, right axis deviation is present. (*Mnemonic*: visualize the numbers I and II written on the patient's chest so that I is on the patient's right side and II is on the patient's left. In right axis deviation, I, on the right, is negative; in left axis deviation, II, on the left, is negative.) If the complex is positive in lead I and negative in lead II, left axis deviation is present, and if the complex is negative in both leads I and II, extreme axis deviation is present. (Try to fix in mind **Figure 3-18** for easy recall of these criteria).

Left axis deviation can occur in LV hypertrophy, inferior wall MI (MI on the diaphragmatic surface of the heart often in-

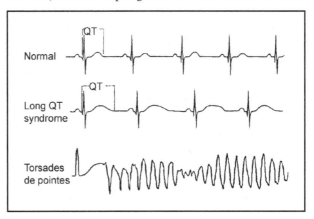

Normal

Long QT syndrome

Torsades de pointes

Figure 3-17

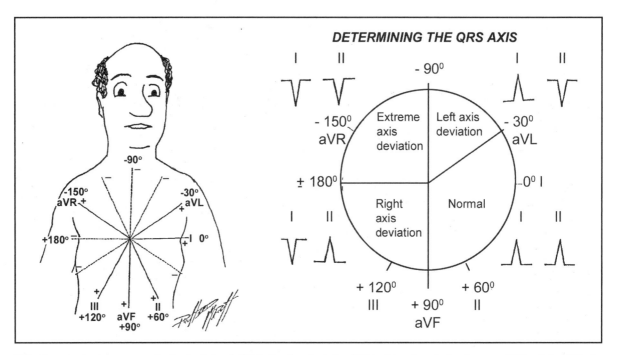

DETERMINING THE QRS AXIS

Note: Some textbooks recommend using leads I and aVF (rather than leads I and II) to determine whether the mean QRS axis is within the normal range (-30° to +90°). However, using leads I and aVF can erroneously classify a mean QRS axis between 0° and -30° as "abnormal".

Figure 3-18

cluding the right ventricle), and left anterior fascicular block (conduction block in the anterior division of the left bundle, which produces unopposed, delayed depolarization upward and to the left of the anterior portion of the left ventricle).

Right axis deviation can occur in RV hypertrophy, acute right heart strain (massive pulmonary embolism), left posterior fascicular block (conduction block in the posterior division of the left bundle, which produces unopposed, delayed depolarization downward and to the right of the posterior portion of the left ventricle), lateral wall MI, and left and right arm lead reversal (look for an inverted P wave in lead I). The axis tends to point *toward* ventricular hypertrophy and *away* from infarction.

Deviation of the electrical axis in the presence of BBB (particularly RBBB) is often a clue to more extensive disease of the conduction system (e.g., block of the left anterior or posterior fascicle in addition to RBBB) - termed "bifascicular block").

MAJOR ECG ABNORMALITIES: DIAGNOSTIC CLUES AND CLINICAL CORRELATIONS

Myocardial Ischemia and Infarction

When a patient presents with chest pain or palpitations, try to obtain an ECG during the episode, because the discomfort and/or arrhythmia may be transient. If you wait until a

more detailed history has been taken, the opportune time might be missed. The ECG during chest pain usually demonstrates evidence of ischemia (classically, ST segment depression). Remember, however, that the resting ECG can be normal even in the presence of significant coronary artery disease, and up to 20% of patients with ischemic episodes do not demonstrate ECG changes with pain.

Figure 3-19. Patterns of ECG abnormalities during ischemia. Ischemia denotes temporary, reversible reduction of blood supply with deprivation of oxygen to the heart muscle. Myocardial ischemia is present when 1 mm or more horizontal or downsloping ST segment depression is present. Transient (horizontal or downsloping) ST segment *depression* during an episode of chest pain provides a clue to myocardial ischemia due to fixed *obstructive* CAD (where there is a fixed narrowing of the vessel lumen). Transient T wave inversion

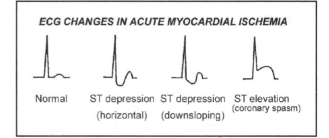

ECG CHANGES IN ACUTE MYOCARDIAL ISCHEMIA

Normal — ST depression (horizontal) — ST depression (downsloping) — ST elevation (coronary spasm)

Figure 3-19

is also a sign of myocardial ischemia. Transient ST segment *elevation,* though, suggests variant or Prinzmetal's angina and provides a clue to underlying *coronary artery spasm.*

Figure 3-20. ECG tracing from a young female with migraine headaches and variant (Prinzmetal's) angina. At the onset of chest pain, there is marked ST segment eleva-

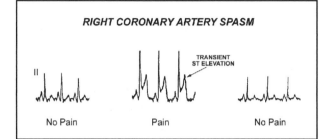

RIGHT CORONARY ARTERY SPASM

No Pain   Pain   No Pain

Figure 3-20

tion in lead II (due to spasm of the right coronary artery). Note that as the pain subsides several minutes later, ST segment elevation returns to baseline and the ECG is normal.

Profound ST segment elevation or depression in multiple leads usually indicates very severe ischemia. It is important to realize, however, that the resting ECG may be entirely normal between episodes of angina pectoris (i.e., when no symptoms and no ischemia are present) in ~50% of patients with significant CAD without a history of previous MI. Furthermore, some episodes of transient myocardial ischemia, particularly those associated with disease in the left circumflex coronary artery (**Figure 3-23**), do not lead to overt abnormalities on the ECG.

With *injury,* which refers to (early) infarction in cardiology, there is prolonged (but potentially reversible) reduction in blood supply to the myocardium along with ST segment elevation. Q waves are a sign of (late) *infarction,* i.e., irreversible death of heart muscle due to prolonged coronary artery occlusion. In time, the ST elevation may disappear, but the Q wave remains as an indicator of previous MI (**Figure 3-21**).

Figure 3-21. *Acute MI* characteristically produces a sequence of changes in the ECG that involve both the QRS and the ST-T complexes. This figure depicts ECG evolution in acute ST elevation (Q-wave) myocardial infarction. Note that the ST segment elevation (convex upward, domed) occurs prior to the formation of the Q wave. During these early hours, PCI/thrombolysis is often undertaken to reverse the process. As time passes the Q wave forms, the ST segment becomes less elevated, and the T wave inversion reverts to upright again. The final outcome of what the ECG looks like varies greatly, depending on the amount of myocardial damage. If successful early reperfusion is achieved, the elevated ST segment returns to baseline without subsequent T wave inversion or Q wave formation.

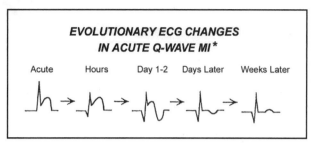

EVOLUTIONARY ECG CHANGES IN ACUTE Q-WAVE MI*

Acute   Hours   Day 1-2   Days Later   Weeks Later

Figure 3-21 (*also termed acute ST elevation MI)

Figure 3-22. Schematic representation of a non ST segment elevation myocardial infarction as recorded in a lead overlying the left ventricle at that location. Non ST segment elevation MIs (non Q wave MIs) represent incom-

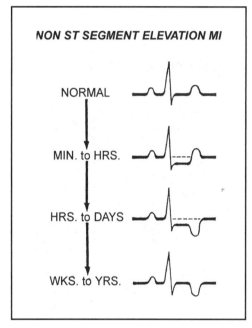

NON ST SEGMENT ELEVATION MI

NORMAL

MIN. to HRS.

HRS. to DAYS

WKS. to YRS.

Figure 3-22

plete infarcts that selectively affect the subendocardial part of the myocardium.

In the case of acute chest pain syndromes, an early ECG may provide evidence of tall positive (hyperacute) T waves over the ischemic zone (**Figure 3-16A**) and convex upward (domed) ST segment elevation, with reciprocal (in opposite leads) ST depression, a reasonably specific sign that helps to confirm the clinical suspicion of an acute MI.

Figure 3-23. The coronary arteries. Note that the left main coronary artery bifurcates into the left anterior descending (LAD) and left circumflex coronary arteries.

- The *LAD* provides blood supply to the anterior wall and interventricular septum, and the left circumflex to the lateral wall.

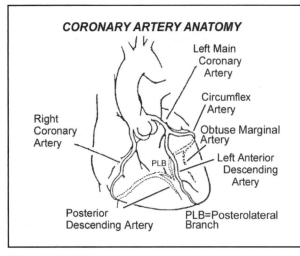

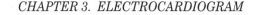

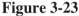

Figure 3-23

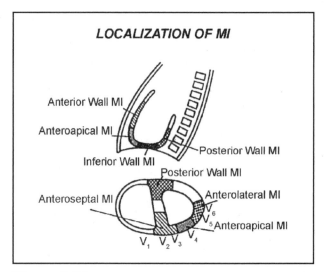

Figure 3-24

- The right coronary artery (*RCA*) provides blood to the inferior (diaphragmatic) wall of the left and/or right ventricle, the sinus node in ~55% and AV node in ~90% of cases. (At other times the left circumflex artery supplies the SA or AV node.) Sudden total occlusion of the RCA results in an acute inferior MI (leads II, III, aVF) and/or right ventricular (RV) MI (right sided ECG lead V4R). Sinus bradycardia (from SA nodal involvement) and first, second, or third degree heart block (from AV nodal involvement) may occur (**Figure 3-51**).
- Sudden occlusion of the left main coronary artery leads to extensive anterior MI (leads V1–V6, I, aVL), pump failure, and sudden death. ST elevation in lead aVR greater than in lead V1 may be a useful clue.
- Sudden occlusion of the LAD coronary artery leads to anterior MI (leads V1–V6) with LV failure, atrial and ventricular arrhythmias, bundle branch block and Mobitz type II (fixed PR interval with abrupt dropped beat–**Figure 3-51**) second degree AV block due to involvement of the conduction system in the interventricular septum.
- Sudden occlusion of the left circumflex coronary artery leads to acute lateral MI (leads I, aVL). In ~10-20% of patients, this artery (rather than the RCA) also supplies the inferior and posterior walls of the LV. The standard 12 lead ECG does not have electrodes to look at the posterior surface of the LV (or RV). Posterior MI is manifest reciprocally (tall R waves with ST depression) in leads V1-V3 ("mirror image"). Posterior chest leads (V7-V9) help confirm the diagnosis.

Figure 3-24. Schematic diagram showing the locations of myocardial infarctions. Although the right ventri-

cle may become infarcted, infarction usually involves only the left ventricle.

The ECG taken during pain frequently identifies the specific area of infarct:

- *Anteroseptal* [V1-V4]
- *Anterolateral* [V5-V6, I, AVL]
- *Lateral* [I, AVL]
- *Inferior* [II, III, AVF]
- *True posterior* (tall broad R waves with ST depression V1-V3 -mirror image)

Figure 3-25 summarizes the areas of the heart affected by MI, and their corresponding arteries and ECG leads.

Pathologic Q waves develop in leads II, III, aVF (in inferior MI), V1-V3 and sometimes V4 (in anteroseptal MI), I and aVL (in high lateral MI), and an increase in R wave (reciprocal of the Q wave) in V1-V2 in true posterior MI. (**Figures 3-26 through 3-29**). A prominent R wave in V1, however, is not pathognomonic of true posterior MI, since similar changes are sometimes seen with RV hypertrophy, WPW syndrome, counterclockwise rotation of the heart, and RBBB.

Figure 3-26. 12 lead ECG tracing in a patient with acute *inferior MI*. Note that the ST segment elevation in the inferior leads (II, III, and aVF) results in reciprocal ST segment depression in leads I and aVL.

Figure 3-27. Acute *lateral wall MI*. Note the ST segment elevation in leads I and aVL, with reciprocal ST segment depression in the inferior leads II, III and AVF.

Figure 3-28. *Anteroseptal MI*. Note the prominent Q waves with ST segment elevation and T wave inversion in leads V1-V4.

Review

FIGURE 3-25

**ECG Clues to the Location of Myocardial Infarction
and Coronary Artery Involved**

LOCATION OF INFARCTION	ECG LEADS		CORONARY ARTERY
Anterior			
• Extensive anterior	V1-V6, I, AVL	Left:	Left main* Proximal LAD
• Anteroseptal	V1-V4	Left:	LAD
• Anterolateral	V5-V6, I, AVL	Left:	LAD
• Apical	V5, V6, I, II, AVF	Left: Right:	LAD (usual) PDA
High lateral	I , AVL	Left:	OMB of CFA Diagonal of LAD
Inferior (diaphragmatic)	II, III, AVF	Right: Left:	PDA (80%) CFA (20%)
Right ventricular	Right precordial leads e.g., V4R, V1-V2	Right:	(proximal)
True posterior	Tall, broad R waves with ST depression V1-V3 (mirror image) Posterior chest leads e.g., V7-V9	Left: Right:	CFA PL branch

LAD = left anterior descending; CFA = circumflex artery; PDA = posterior descending artery;
OMB = obtuse marginal branch; PL = posterolateral branch
*Note: Widespread ST depression along with ST elevation in lead aVR >VI may be a useful clue to left main coronary artery occlusion.

Figure 3-29. Acute *posterior MI*. Q waves and ST elevation are represented reciprocally ("mirror images") as tall R waves with ST segment depression in leads V1- V3. The inferior and/or lateral leads are often involved in the infarction process.

Figure 3-30. Typical evolutionary ECG changes of an *anterior wall MI* (seen through lead V1) compared with those of a posterior wall MI (seen through lead V1). The changes in the anterior wall MI are typical (as noted in **Figure 3-21**). However, since there are no posterior leads in a standard 12 lead ECG, a posterior MI is reflected by changes in the precordial leads that are the inverse ("mirror image") of what one would see in leads overlying the posterior myocardium, i.e., ST segment depression (inverse of the current of injury) and a tall R wave (inverse of a Q wave).

Figure 3-31. Classic evolutionary ECG changes in acute *anterior MI*. **A.** Hyperacute ST segment elevation and peaking of T waves. **B.** Marked ("tombstone") ST segment elevation in leads V1-V6, I and aVL. Multifocal premature ventricular contractions are also present. **C.** Development of more pronounced Q waves and T wave inversion with re-

gression of coved and convex upward (domed) ST segment elevation. Persistent ST segment elevation suggests LV aneurysm formation.

Figure 3-32. Classic evolutionary ECG changes in acute *inferior MI*. **A.** Hyperacute ST segment elevation and peaking of T waves. **B.** Marked ("tombstone") ST segment elevation in leads II, III, aVF with "reciprocal" ST segment depression in precordial leads. **C.** Loss of R waves, development of pathologic Q waves, T wave inversion and return of ST segment elevation toward baseline.

ST segment elevation in lead III greater than in lead II is a useful clue to occlusion of the proximal-mid right coronary artery. The occurrence of ST segment elevation and loss of R waves in right-sided chest leads (particularly V4R), in association with an inferior or posterior MI are sensitive clinical clues to an *RV infarction*. (**Figure 3-33**).

Figure 3-33. Left. Location of right-sided precordial ECG leads (V1R-V6R). **Right.** ECG tracing demonstrating acute *inferior wall MI* with *RV infarction*. Note ST segment elevation in leads II, III, aVF, along with ST segment elevation in leads V4R–V6R.

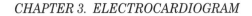

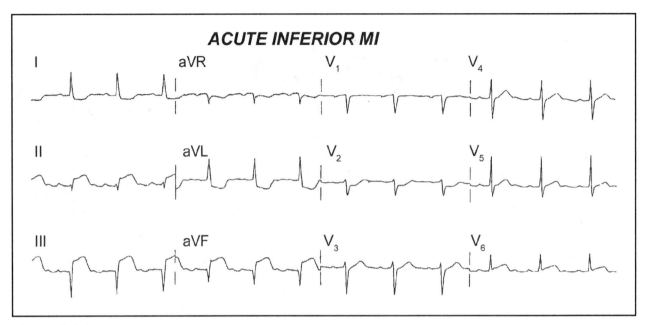

Figure 3-26

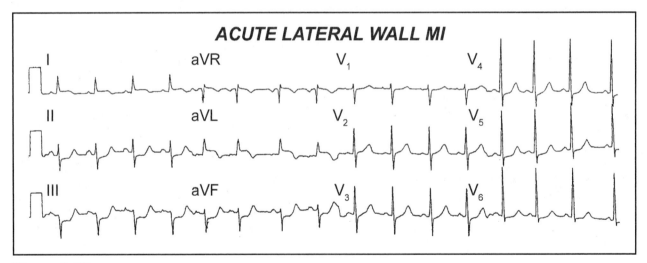

Figure 3-27

Combined with the patient's history and physical examination, the 12-lead ECG is the major determinant of eligibility for PCI/thrombolysis. The two key ECG findings are new ST segment elevation (not disappearing rapidly as in Prinzmetal's angina) in two or more anatomically contiguous leads, or new (or presumably new) LBBB (especially if the ST segment changes are concordant or excessively discordant with the QRS). These suggest that the damage may involve recent thrombosis and that the patient may be a candidate for reperfusion therapy. No evidence of benefit from emergent reperfusion is found in patients with ischemic chest pain who lack either appropriate ST segment elevation or new LBBB. Unlike patients with ST segment elevation MIs, those with non ST segment elevation MIs (non Q wave MIs) do not benefit from thrombolytic therapy.

In general, the larger the MI, the greater the mortality reduction with reperfusion therapy. The size of an MI is reflected by either the absolute number of leads showing ST segment elevation on the ECG, or a summation of the total ST segment deviations from the baseline (i.e., both ST

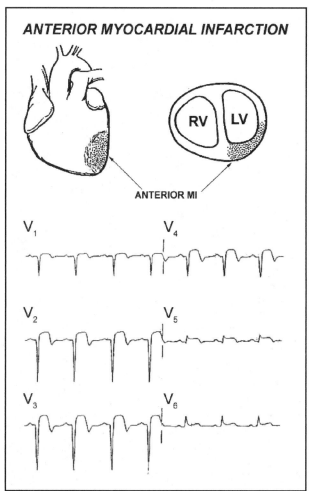

ANTERIOR MYOCARDIAL INFARCTION

ANTERIOR MI

V_1 V_4

V_2 V_5

V_3 V_6

Figure 3-28

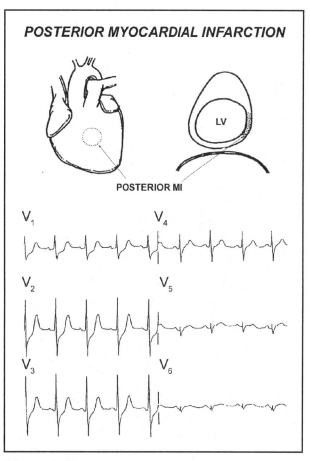

POSTERIOR MYOCARDIAL INFARCTION

POSTERIOR MI

V_1 V_4

V_2 V_5

V_3 V_6

Figure 3-29

segment depressions and elevations). Patients who present with ischemic chest pain and deep T wave inversions in multiple precordial leads (e.g., V1-V4), with or without cardiac enzyme elevations, typically have a high-grade stenosis in the proximal LAD coronary artery ("*Wellens pattern*"). If untreated, these patients may go on to develop an extensive anterior MI within a few weeks to months.

Figure 3-34. Clinical markers of reperfusion. **A.** Serial ECG recording (leads V1-V3) in a patient with acute anterior MI treated with thrombolytic therapy. Note the ST segment elevation begins to decrease rapidly and falls by more than 50% over the next half hour. During this time, the patient reported rapid and complete relief of chest pain. **B.** The appearance of accelerated idioventricular rhythm (AIVR–a rhythm paced by a ventricular focus, rather than the SA node) often provides additional evidence of reperfusion.

While its clinical importance is beyond question, the ECG has many limitations: The initial ECG may remain normal for hours after an acute MI and it may be diagnostic in only 50-60% of patients. Furthermore, although the presence of Q waves suggests prior MI, their absence is not helpful in excluding significant CAD. An MI may occur without diagnostic ECG changes (there may be only slight or even absent ST-T changes), depending on the extent, location, and associated ECG abnormalities (e.g., left bundle branch block, electronic ventricular pacemaker). In left ventricle infarct with LBBB, it is difficult to identify Q waves since the left ventricle depolarizes later than the right ventricle and the Q wave part of the left ventricle QRS is buried within the preceding right ventricle depolarization. Since the ECG taken during the early stages of an acute MI, when the patient is most susceptible to primary ventricular fibrillation, may appear normal (in as many as 20% of cases), if the clinical suspicion is high, the normal ECG should not be considered evidence against the diagnosis. All too often a patient is sent home inappropriately from the emergency department with an acute MI because of an over-reliance on the ECG (**Figure 3-35**).

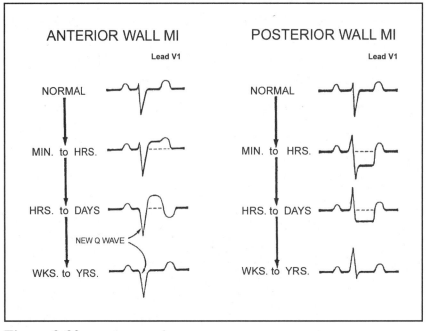

Figure 3-30

Figure 3-35. Lesson of the normal ECG. Note that leads V1–V3 from a 12 lead ECG taken in the Emergency Department in a patient who presented with chest pain were entirely normal. Fortunately, the patient was appropriately admitted to the coronary care unit based on the clinical history despite the normal ECG. Note that ST segment elevation and T wave peaking (so-called "hyperacute change") appeared 2 1/2 hours later when chest pain intensified and clinical appearance worsened.

Despite sophisticated laboratory tests, including new cardiac serum markers (e.g., troponins) and imaging techniques, and the limitations cited above, the ECG still remains the most reliable inexpensive tool for the rapid confirmation of acute MI, dictating appropriate triage and prompt treatment with life-saving reperfusion therapy.

Whenever possible, a prior ECG should be obtained to help determine if abnormalities seen on a current tracing are new or old. Without previous tracings, any ECG finding that cannot be proved to be old must be assumed to be new. On occasion, a new ECG abnormality can "erase" a previously existing one. Complete normalization of the ECG following a Q wave infarction is uncommon, but may occur particularly with smaller infarcts. Serial ECGs permit evaluation of the response to therapy and of progression, remission, or persistence of an abnormality noted on the baseline tracing. For example, the ECG may be used to assess the response to a thrombolytic agent or to anti-ischemic therapy. Complete resolution of ST segment elevation promptly following thrombolytic therapy (or after PCI) is a specific, although not sensitive, marker of successful reperfusion (**Figure 3-34**).

It is important not to over-interpret the ECG. A patient may have serious underlying heart disease with little or no abnormality on the ECG, or no detectable heart disease, but an abnormal ECG tracing. Reliance on computer-generated ECG interpretation can also result in potential mischief (i.e., incorrect, over- and/or under-diagnoses), occasionally with devastating clinical consequences. The computer analysis must be carefully reviewed and edited to avert misdiagnosis before a final interpretation is made. The range of normal is broad, and clinical circumstances should dictate the importance of a particular ECG observation. Examples:

- The presence of Q waves and a pseudo-"infarct" pattern on the ECG (e.g., in WPW syndrome) does not always reflect CAD (**Figures 3-36** and **3-37**). The presence of delta waves helps distinguish WPW.

Figure 3-36. 12 lead ECG tracing in a patient with *WPW syndrome* simulating anteroseptal MI (due to delta waves distorting the QRS complexes in the anterior leads).

Figure 3-37. 12 lead ECG tracing in a patient with *WPW syndrome* mimicking inferior MI. This asymptomatic patient had a "routine" ECG and was told he had evidence of a "heart attack". Note prominent Q waves in leads III and aVF that could easily be misinterpreted as an inferior MI (due to delta waves distorting the QRS complexes in the inferior leads).

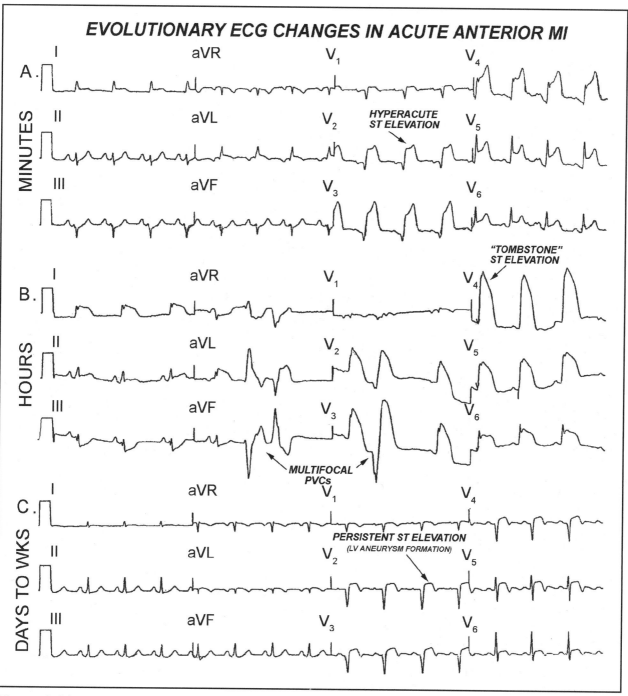

Figure 3-31

- Pathologic Q waves may be seen in patients with non-ischemic cardiomyopathy, either idiopathic or secondary (e.g., sarcoid, amyloid, tumor, scleroderma), caused by infiltration and/or replacement of the myocardium.
- Pathologic Q waves, ST segment elevation, negative T-waves, and QT prolongation may be seen in the absence of fixed CAD in patients with *stress (tako-tsubo) cardiomyopathy* (due to coronary vasospasm or neurogenic myocardial stunning).
- Patients with hypertrophic cardiomyopathy also frequently have abnormal Q waves (caused by septal hypertrophy) in the inferior and lateral leads that mimic MI along with LV hypertrophy.

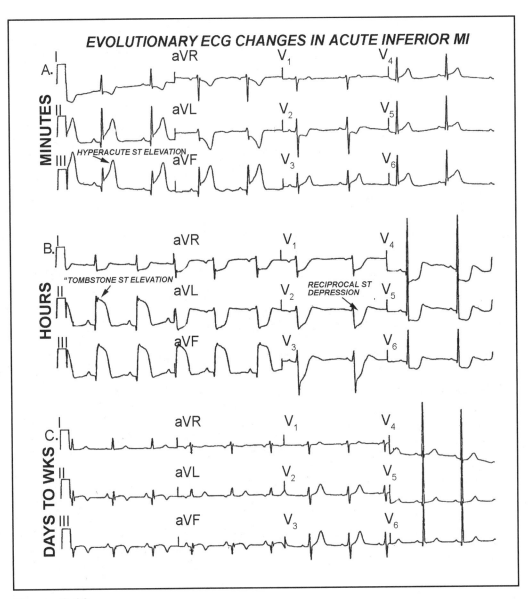

Figure 3-32

- Giant negative (inverted) T waves in the precordial leads provide clues to the presence of a variant form of hypertrophic cardiomyopathy localized principally to the apex. *The ECG is a very useful tool in screening for hypertrophic obstructive cardiomyopathy since a normal tracing almost rules out this diagnosis.*

Cardiac Chamber Enlargement and Hypertrophy

Perhaps the least reliable of anatomic diagnosis based on ECG criteria is that of ventricular hypertrophy or enlargement. Very significant degrees of anatomic RV hypertro-

phy can exist with little or no detectable change in the ECG. In addition, considerable LV hypertrophy can occur with only slight enhancement of the normal LV dominance. Nevertheless the ECG may offer supporting evidence of RV or LV hypertrophy though it is a relatively insensitive method of detecting it:

- For RV hypertrophy, a combination of right axis deviation with an R/S wave ratio in V1 > 1 and deep S waves in V6 are valuable clues.
- For LV hypertrophy, increased voltage amplitude (particularly in the precordial leads, e.g., SV1 + [RV5 or RV6] > 35 mm; or [RV5 or

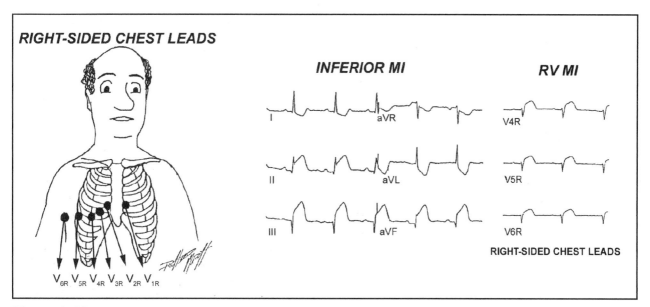

Figure 3-33

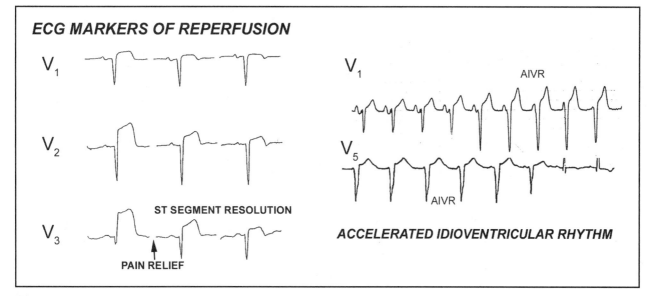

Figure 3-34

RV6] > 25 mm), or in the limb lead R aVL > 11mm, is the most sensitive (and least specific) of all ECG criteria. Of equal value is evidence ST-T abnormalities (LV "strain" pattern, i.e., ST segment depression and T wave inversion in the left precordial leads V4-V6) reflecting secondary repolarization changes, in the absence of ischemia or digitalis.

• Voltage criteria for LV hypertrophy, along with ST-T wave changes ("LV strain" pattern) may also provide clues to target organ damage from long-standing hypertension, as well as dilated and/or hypertrophic cardiomyopathy (**Figure 3-38**).

Figure 3-38. 12 lead ECG tracing in a patient with poorly controlled hypertension. Note the increased QRS voltage in the precordial leads with ST depression ("strain pattern"), left atrial abnormality (biphasic P wave in lead II suggesting atrial enlargement) and left axis deviation, all

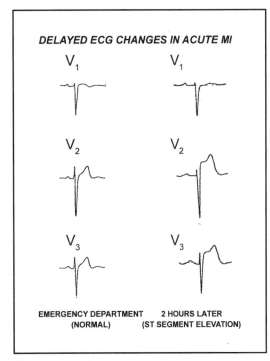

Figure 3-35

characteristic features of LV hypertrophy. Although the QS pattern (a single negative wave with no R wave to distinguish whether the deflection is Q or an S wave) in the right precordial leads raises the possibility of anteroseptal MI, it is not unusual for LV hypertrophy by itself to present this way.

- Valvular heart diseases with resultant pressure (stenosis) or volume (regurgitation) overload of the LV can also produce ECG evidence of LV hypertrophy. In valvular aortic stenosis, signs of LV hypertrophy on the ECG may serve as a clue to a significant degree of outflow tract obstruction. Tall positive T waves may also be seen in LV volume loads due to MR or AR.
- RV hypertrophy can result from a number of conditions, e.g., congenital heart disease, pulmonic valve stenosis, ostium secundum ASD (associated with incomplete or complete RBBB patterns), rheumatic MS, pulmonary hypertension, and lung disease (**Figure 3-39**).

Figure 3-39. 12 lead ECG tracing from a woman with severe pulmonary hypertension. Note the large prominent R wave in lead V1 along with persistent precordial S waves and extreme right axis deviation seen with RV hypertrophy.

- ECG findings of acute RV overload, e.g., right axis deviation, *S1Q3T3 pattern* (deep S wave in lead I, Q wave in lead III and T wave inversion in lead III), along with sinus tachycardia, in patients with *pulmonary embolism* provide clues to obstruction of >50% of the pulmonary arterial bed and significant pulmonary hypertension (**Figure 3-40).**

The ECG is not sensitive for the detection of small degrees of LV hypertrophy. Evidence of LV hypertrophy

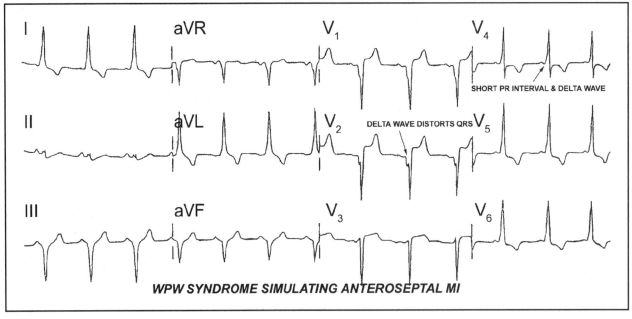

Figure 3-36

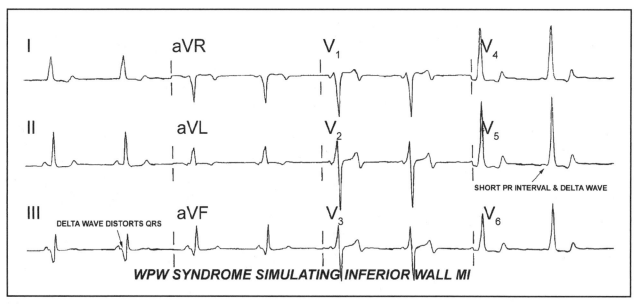

Figure 3-37

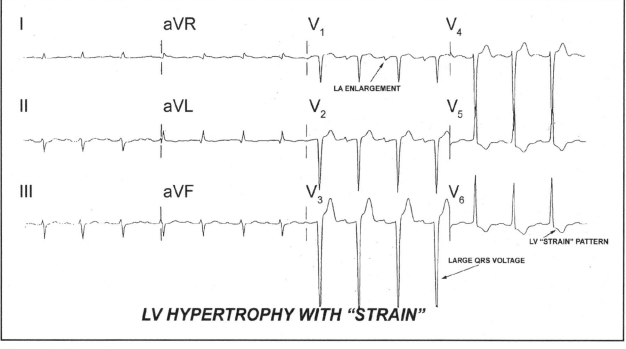

Figure 3-38

(particularly when associated with ST segment depression) and chamber enlargement on the ECG, however, usually signifies an advanced stage of disease (i.e., chronic conditions such as hypertension and severe AS that impose prolonged pressure loads on the heart), with a poorer prognosis.

Note that effective treatment of systemic arterial hypertension reduces ECG evidence of LV hypertrophy and decreases the associated risk of cardiovascular mortality.

Remember that an "abnormal looking" ECG does not necessarily mean that the patient has CAD or even

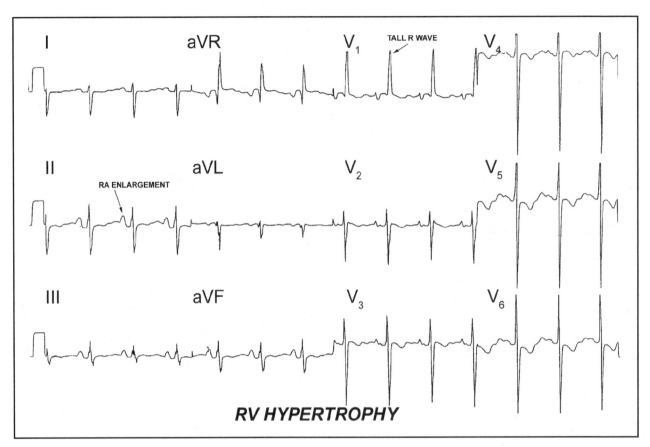

Figure 3-39

an abnormal heart. Mimics of an "MI, age indeterminate" include:

- Incorrect chest lead placement
- Normal variant (e.g., QS pattern in leads V1 and V2 even with correct lead placement)
- LV hypertrophy with poor R wave progression in leads V1-V3, mimicking anteroseptal MI
- Incomplete LBBB
- Cor pulmonale secondary to COPD with poor R wave progression or a QS pattern in the precordial leads
- WPW syndrome with pseudo-Q waves mimicking inferior or anterior MI
- HOCM with Q waves in the inferolateral leads
- Involvement of the heart by amyloid, sarcoidosis, scleroderma, neoplasm, or neuromuscular disease
- A misdiagnosis of an old anteroseptal MI (due to "poor R wave progression") can be made in a patient with a long asthenic chest build, and a "teardrop" heart. Electrode placement, even though in the correct interspace, is the culprit. You should place the chest leads one or two interspaces lower,

and the normal progression of R wave (rather than slow) may result.

In addition, don't be disappointed when an ECG tracing is returned with an interpretation of "non-specific ST-T changes". To suggest that such changes always represent "ischemia" significantly overstates the accuracy of the test and can lead to serious consequences. For example, T wave inversions in leads V1-V3 are more likely to represent a normal variant in a healthy young female (*juvenile T wave pattern*) than the same findings in a middle-aged or older male with chest discomfort and risk factors, where it may represent a clue to underlying CAD.

Miscellaneous Patterns

Figure 3-41. Diffuse concave upward (valley-like) ST segment elevation (in all leads except aVR and V1), along with PR segment depression may provide helpful clues to the diagnosis of *pericarditis*.

Figure 3-42. Low voltage and total *electrical alternans* (alternating ECG complex heights) of the P, QRS, and T waves (due to the swinging motion of the heart) strengthens

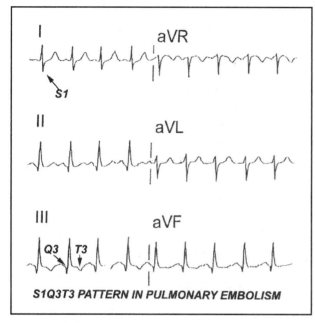

Figure 3-40

the clinical suspicion of *pericardial effusion with tamponade,* as seen in precordial leads V2-V4 in this 12 lead ECG.

Figure 3-43. In *early repolarization* in healthy, asymptomatic, young individuals, concave upward ST segment elevation (most often seen in the precordial leads) along with notching of the J point (the junction of QRS with the beginning of the ST segment) can mimic acute MI or pericarditis. This is generally a "benign" variant, especially in African-American males and trained athletes, as seen in this 12 lead ECG. Notching in the J point (lead V4) and upward concavity ("smile"-like) of the ST segment favor early repolarization pattern ("fishhook appearance").

Note: A "malignant" variant of early repolarization has been described in which notching of the J point in the inferolateral leads may be associated with an increased risk of VF, but the absolute risk is low. A convex elevation of the J point (J wave or Osborne wave) may also be seen with profound hypothermia. The height of the Osborne (J) wave is proportional to the degree of hypothermia.

Figure 3-44. LV aneurysm. This patient had a previous anterior MI. Persistence of *both* Q waves and ST segment elevation in the anterior leads several weeks or more after an MI may provide a clue to an *LV aneurysm.*

There are many causes of ST segment and T wave abnormalities that can mimic those of ischemia (e.g., LV hypertrophy and electrolyte, metabolic and drug-induced effects). The clinician should also be aware of the wide spectrum of normal variations, especially pertaining to repolarization patterns, and not falsely label a healthy patient as having heart disease on the basis of a non-specific finding (e.g., "persistent juvenile pattern" T wave inversion, a common normal variant), which may be of no significance, and lead to unnecessary anxiety and potential harm. ST and T wave changes are the most common and sensitive of the ECG abnormalities but are also the least specific.

Arrhythmias and Conduction Disturbances

The sensitivity and specificity of ECG changes for cardiac rhythm and conduction abnormalities are relatively high and provide clues to the origins of palpitations, dizziness, or syncope such as:

- Atrial and/or ventricular extrasystoles
- Significant tachy or bradyarrhythmias
- Mobitz type I (Wenckebach) second degree AV block (gradually increasing PR interval with eventual dropped beat–**Figure 3-51**)

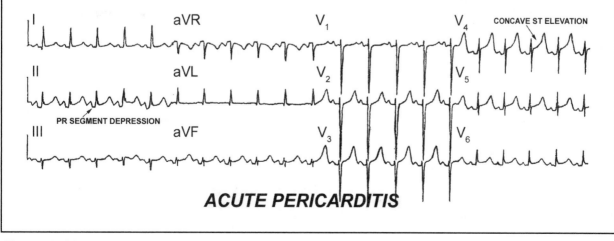

Figure 3-41

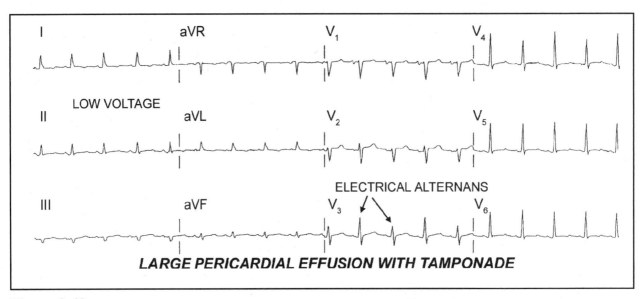

Figure 3-42

- Mobitz type II second degree AV block (fixed PR interval with abrupt dropped beat–**Figure 3-51**)
- Complete heart block (changing PR intervals with complete lack of communication between P and QRS)
- Right or left bundle branch block
- Wolff-Parkinson-White (WPW) syndrome
- Long QT interval (e.g., resulting from antiarrhythmic agents, hypokalemia, hypomagnesemia, tricyclic antidepressants) with its attendant risk of

polymorphic ventricular tachycardia ("torsades de pointes")

In general, it is first helpful to note whether there is a bradycardia or a tachycardia. Bradycardias may originate from an overactive parasympathetic system, a sick sinus node, or a defect in the conduction of impulses from the atria to the ventricles. Tachycardias may originate from an overactive sympathetic system, hyperactivity of the SA node, ectopic atrial pacemakers, hyperactive cardiac con-

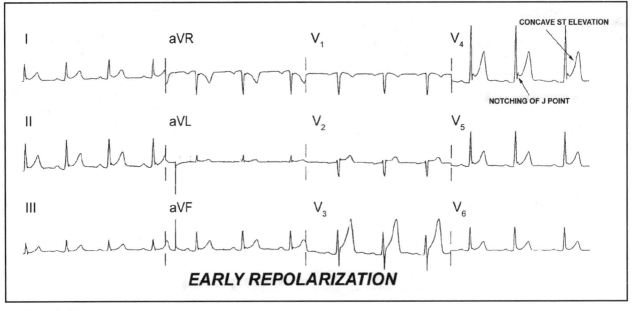

Figure 3-43

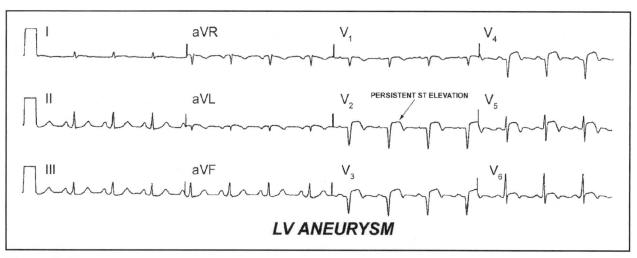

Figure 3-44

duction system (e.g., irritable focus in the bundle of His) or irritable focus in the ventricular myocardium. Sympathetic stimulation, hyperthyroidism, digitalis toxicity, caffeine, ethanol, amphetamines, cocaine, and, to some degree, low O_2 can cause irritability of the atrial and conduction system foci. Anoxia and low potassium are more likely causes of ventricular irritability, but adrenergic stimulants can also irritate ventricular foci.

It is helpful to note whether the arrhythmia involves a normal narrow QRS complex or a wide QRS complex. Nar-row complex arrhythmias imply that the problem is not in the ventricular myocardium, since abnormal discharges there result in bizarre wide QRS complexes. Wide QRS complexes imply that the atria are not the sole origin of the arrhythmia; there is some other deficit, whether in the conduction system, involving a blockage somewhere in the conduction system (e.g., RBBB or LBBB) or an aberrant reentry circuit, or an abnormal focus in the ventricular myocardium.

Figure 3-45. Mechanisms of various supraventricular tachyarrhythmias and their corresponding ECG features.

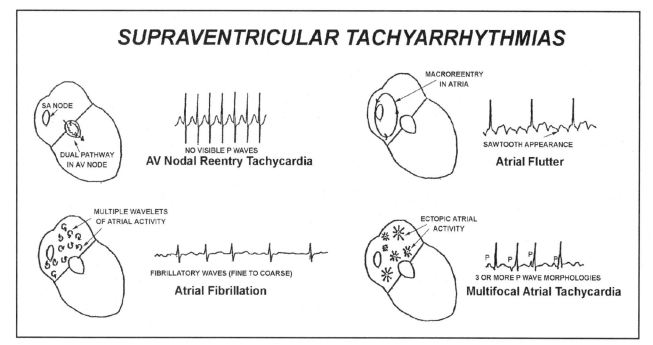

Figure 3-45

Left Top. In *AV nodal reentry tachycardia,* the QRS complexes are regular and the P waves are usually buried in or distort the terminal portion of the QRS. Reentry occurs using dual pathways in the AV node. **Left Bottom.** In *atrial fibrillation,* the QRS complexes are irregularly irregular, and no organized P waves are seen. Multiple reentry sites ("wavelets") in the atria fire impulses in an uncoordinated fashion down the AV node. **Right Top.** In *atrial flutter,* the contractions of the atrium are more coordinated, involving macroreentry (a larger reentrant circuit) in the right atrium, and the heart rhythm tends to be regular. The "sawtooth pattern" of flutter waves is best seen in the inferior leads. **Right Bottom.** In *multifocal atrial tachycardia,* 3 or more P waves of differing morphologies are present. There is increased automaticity at multiple sites in the atria and the rhythm is irregular.

In most cases, logical reasoning should enable you to determine whether the arrhythmia originates in the atria, ventricles or conduction system.

Figure 3-46. Atrial arrhythmias:

A. *Premature atrial complex.* Early beat originates in atria not in sinus node, resulting in a short PR interval, since a number of potential atrial ectopic foci lie around the coronary sinus, the myocardial venous drainage channel, which empties into the right atrium and lies near the AV node. Sometimes there may be a slight widening of the QRS (PAC with aberrancy), if one of the bundle branches is not yet repolarized when the atrial impulse gets through. The most common unexpected pause is due to a non-conducted PAC.

B. *Atrial escape beat.* Occurs when the sinus node is firing so slowly that an ectopic focus in the atrium acts to fill in a beat.

C. *Ectopic atrial rhythm.* The rhythm originates from an ectopic focus in the atrium, resulting in a short PR interval, since the ectopic focus is closer to the AV node. (Note that the P wave may not be upright in lead II in ectopic atrial rhythm.)

D. *Wandering atrial pacemaker.* The atria are activated by multiple foci, resulting in changes in P waves on the ECG. The rate is typically less than 100 beats/min. When it exceeds that, it is called *multifocal atrial tachycardia (MAT),* which is not uncommon in chronic obstructive pulmonary disease (COPD).

E. *Multifocal atrial tachycardia.* Note more than 3 different P wave morphologies and varying PR intervals due to each complex originating from different foci in the atria. A flat isoelectric baseline between the P waves distinguishes MAT from atrial fibrillation.

F. *Atrial flutter* with 4:1 AV conduction. Note the "sawtooth" pattern of flutter waves due to continuous circus movement of the electrical wave form (macro-reentry)

within the atrium. Typical atrial firing rates in atrial flutter are 250-350/min with varying ventricular responses.

G. *Atrial fibrillation.* An irregularly irregular rhythm with no organized atrial activity and no effective mechanical atrial contraction. Note irregular fibrillatory waves arising in atria. Typical atrial firing rates in atrial fibrillation are 350-600/min with varying ventricular responses. When atrial fibrillation is detected on the ECG the clinician should consider the possibility of mitral valve disease, hyperthyroidism, pericardial disease, or atrial septal defect.

H. *Atrial tachycardia (AT).* A rapid, regular atrial rhythm, generally originating from an ectopic atrial focus.

I. *Atrial tachycardia (AT) with block.* The atrial firing rate may be so fast that not every impulse can get through to the ventricles (commonly seen in the presence of digitalis toxicity). In this case there are 2 P waves for every QRS complex.

Figure 3-47. *Sick sinus syndrome.* The ECG tracing may show severe *sinus bradycardia* (top) or prolonged *sinus pauses* (middle). ECG strip of a patient with *tachy-brady syndrome* (bottom). Note the tachycardia component is paroxysmal atrial fibrillation and the bradycardia component is a long pause that is followed by a junctional escape beat. Symptoms may include lightheadedness, fainting spells, fatigue, and palpitations.

Figure 3-48. Ventricular arrhythmias:

A. *Unifocal premature ventricular complex (PVC).* Early beat is wide with full compensatory pause between narrow beats.

B. *Ventricular escape beat.* Accommodates for too long a delay in receiving an impulse through the conduction system.

C. *Ventricular bigeminy.* Fixed coupling of independently firing atrial and ventricular complexes. The pattern may also be that of trigeminy (2 normal QRS complexes for every ectopic one) and quadrigeminy (3:1 ratio) with increasing ratio of normal to abnormal QRS complexes.

D. *Ventricular parasystole.* An automatic ventricular focus with entrance block (i.e., the focus is "protected" and is not depolarized by the natural pacemaker or other outside impulses), creating an independent ectopic ventricular rhythm occurring alongside the native dominant rhythm. All interectopic intervals are a multiple of a constant shortest ventricular interectopic interval.

E. *Multifocal PVCs* occurs when there are more than one irritable foci. The PVCs are of different shape.

F. *Accelerated idioventricular rhythm.* Idioventricular rhythm is that paced by the ventricle at 20-40 firings/min, in the absence of input from the SA node. When the rhythm is greater than 40/min, it is termed an accelerated idioventricular rhythm. Note fusion beat (second complex) (signifying a P wave that got through the AV

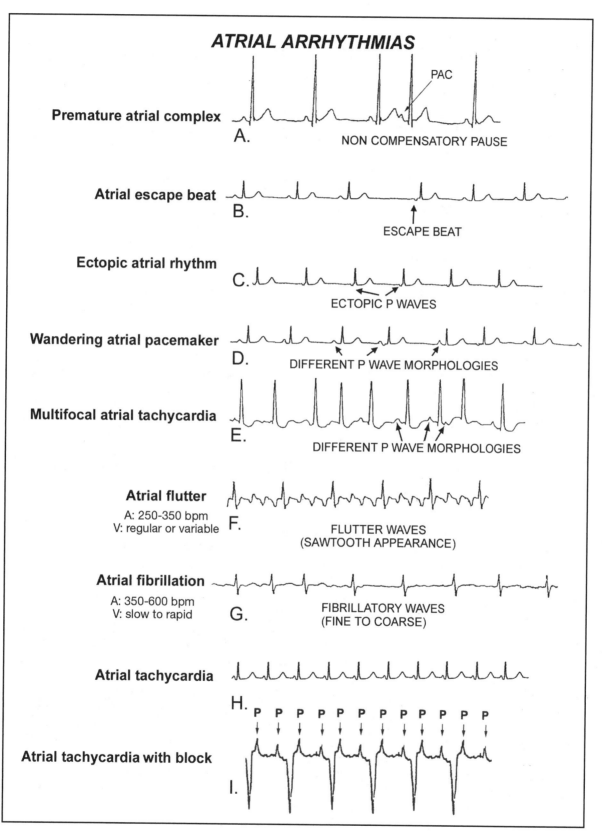

Figure 3-46

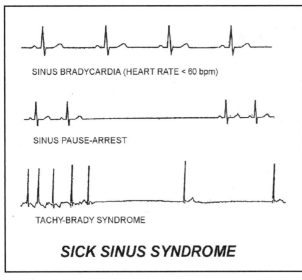

Figure 3-47

node to generate part of a normal QRS complex that fuses with an abnormal ventricular complex).

G. Sustained *monomorphic ventricular tachycardia*. A rhythm that originates in the ventricle, either from an ectopic focus or reentry in the ventricle. Note the rapid succession of wide QRS complexes at rates of 150-250/min. Ventricular flutter (rates of 250-350/min) can look like a very fast ventricular tachycardia and commonly degenerates into ventricular fibrillation.

H. *Polymorphic ventricular tachycardia* with long QT interval ("*torsades de pointes*"). A form of ventricular tachycardia in which the QRS complex twists around the baseline. Note alternating negative and positive deflections. This patient had *long QT syndrome,* which predisposes to this arrhythmia. Note that a premature ventricular complex occurring in the T wave provokes the arrhythmia. Initiation of torsades de pointes follows a "long-short" interval.

I. *Ventricular fibrillation*. A catastrophic dysrhythmia categorized by total disorganization of electrical activity in the heart, resulting in cardiac arrest. There are no identifiable ECG wave forms and the baseline is undulating and wavy due to deflections (fibrillatory waves) that vary in amplitude and morphology.

Figure 3-49. ECG tracing demonstrating ventricular tachycardia. Note capture beat (3rd complex) and fusion beat (4th complex) characteristic of this dysrhythmia. A capture beat is a normal QRS complex arising when an atrial impulse succeeds in getting through the AV node to accompany the abnormal PVC-type complexes of a ventricular tachycardia. A fusion beat occurs when the impulse that got through fuses with a PVC type complex of the ventricular tachycardia to form a hybrid.

Figure 3-50. Top. ECG tracing showing monomorphic ventricular tachycardia in a patient with CAD. All the QRS complexes have the same configuration. Note that the 2nd beat is a fusion beat. **Bottom.** ECG tracing (lead V1) demonstrating wide complex tachycardia with dissociation of the P waves from the QRS complexes which strongly suggests the diagnosis of VT. Arrhythmias may also originate in the conduction system:

Figure 3-51. Heart blocks at the AV node:

A. *First degree AV block,* where there is excessive delay at the AV node, resulting in a prolonged, constant PR interval ≥0.20 sec.

B. *Mobitz type I second degree AV block.* Note 3:2 "*Wenckebach*" pattern, i.e., PR interval gets progressively longer until P wave isn't conducted. The sequence is then repeated.

C. *Mobitz type II second degree AV block.* Fixed PR interval with some non-premature P waves not conducted (dropped QRS beats, 3:2 block in this case).

D. *Third degree (complete) AV block.* Varying PR intervals; i.e., atria and ventricles are contracting independently of each other.

Figure 3-52. Arrhythmias originating from junctional (AV nodal) irritability:

A. *AV junctional escape beat or rhythm.* An escape beat that originates in the AV node secondary to depression of the higher sinus pacemaker. The QRS may be slightly prolonged in cases where a bundle branch is not completely repolarized at the time the premature impulse comes through the bundle of His.

B. *Premature junctional beat.* A premature, ectopic supraventricular impulse that originates from the area in and around the AV node. A visible P wave may or may not be present. If visible, the P wave commonly occurs just before (short PR interval) or just after the QRS complex and is inverted in leads II, III, and aVF.

C. *AV nodal reentry tachycardia* (at rates of 150-250/min) looks similar on ECG to that of paroxysmal junctional tachycardia. It is driven by a reentry circus loop within the AV node. P waves may not be seen, or they may be inverted (before or after the QRS) due to retrograde transmission to the atria.

D. *Paroxysmal (AV) junctional tachycardia* occurs when a tachycardia is driven by an irritable focus within the AV node. P waves may not be seen, or they may be inverted (before or after the QRS) due to retrograde transmission to the atria.

Figure 3-53. Arrhythmias seen in digitalis toxicity.

Figure 3-54. Left. Schematic illustration of typical mechanism of supraventricular tachycardia due to AV nodal reentry using dual pathways in the AV node. α fibers = slow

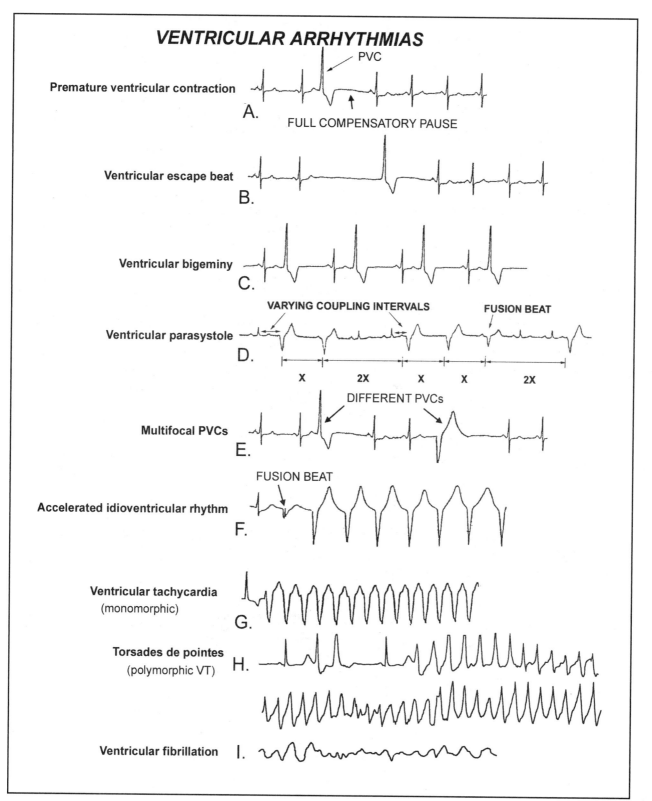

Figure 3-48

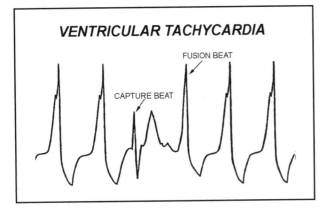

Figure 3-49

pathway, β fibers = fast pathway that was previously blocked. It is a rapid and regular heart rhythm that begins and ends abruptly. Heart rate may be 150-250 beats/min.

A rapid PAT may also look like a paroxysmal junctional tachycardia (no P waves seen), but the treatment of the two is similar.

Figure 3-55. *Wolff-Parkinson-White (WPW) syndrome.* Conduction occurs through an accessory pathway between the atria and ventricles as well as the normal pathway via the AV node. The accessory pathway starts stimulating the ventricle early (*preexcitation*) and the combination

of accessory and normal pathways results in a widened QRS and a shortened PR interval. Note the short PR interval, due to rapid conduction through the accessory pathway, slurred upstroke of the QRS complex (*delta wave*), and prolonged QRS secondary to slow ventricular activation. There may also be an inverted T wave. WPW may also present as a tachycardia, with a reentry circuit loop. Whether the reentry tachycardia is associated with a narrow (normal) or a wide QRS complex is determined by whether antegrade conduction is through the AV node (normal QRS width) or through the accessory pathway (widened QRS complex due to the aberrant route though the ventricles). The latter arrhythmia is difficult to distinguish from VT.

Figure 3-56. ECG tracing of atrial fibrillation conducted down an accessory pathway in a patient with preexcitation (WPW) syndrome. The presence of a ventricular rate >200 beats/min in the setting of atrial fibrillation provides a clue to WPW and a bypass tract that circumvents the AV node since it is unlikely that the AV node will conduct more than 200 impulses per minute. This arrhythmia can degenerate into ventricular fibrillation if AV nodal blocking agents (e.g., digoxin, verapamil, beta blockers) are administered, which block the AV node and allow more conduction through the bypass tract.

Figure 3-57. Top. Schematic representation of rapid atrial fibrillation in preexcitation (WPW) syndrome. Note

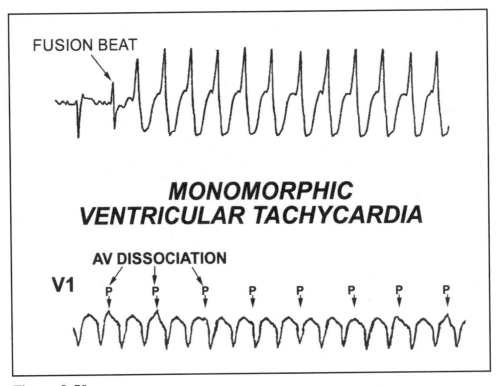

Figure 3-50

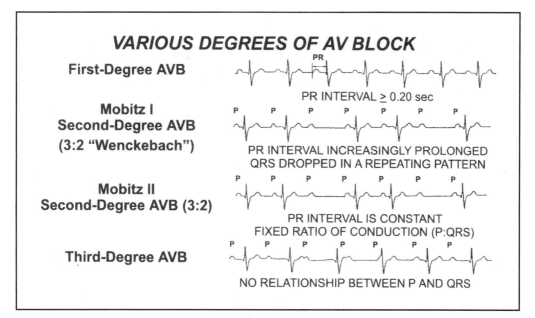

VARIOUS DEGREES OF AV BLOCK

First-Degree AVB

PR INTERVAL ≥ 0.20 sec

Mobitz I
Second-Degree AVB
(3:2 "Wenckebach")

PR INTERVAL INCREASINGLY PROLONGED
QRS DROPPED IN A REPEATING PATTERN

Mobitz II
Second-Degree AVB (3:2)

PR INTERVAL IS CONSTANT
FIXED RATIO OF CONDUCTION (P:QRS)

Third-Degree AVB

NO RELATIONSHIP BETWEEN P AND QRS

Note: When evaluating the various degrees of AV block, keep in mind the following mnemonic: IF the "R" is far from "P", then you have FIRST DEGREE; If longer, longer, longer, DROP! – then you have WENCKEBACH; If some "Ps" don't get through, then you have MOBITZ II; If "Ps" and "Qs" just don't agree, then you have THIRD DEGREE (from the Heart Block Poem by the Princeton Surgical Group).

Figure 3-51

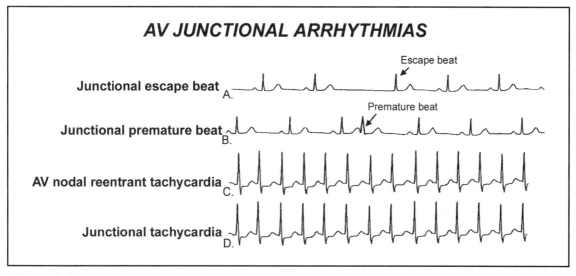

AV JUNCTIONAL ARRHYTHMIAS

Junctional escape beat A.

Escape beat

Junctional premature beat B.

Premature beat

AV nodal reentrant tachycardia C.

Junctional tachycardia D.

Figure 3-52

very rapid ventricular rate and bizarre looking wide QRS complexes (so-called "wacky"-cardia) that can mimic polymorphic ventricular tachycardia ("torsades de pointes") (**bottom**) as seen in patients with long QT syndrome. Keep in mind the possibility of preexcited atrial fibrillation in any young patient who presents to the emergency department with a rapid, irregular wide complex tachycardia. Rapid atrial fibrillation in such a patient can result in ventricular fibrillation if AV nodal blocking agents (e.g., digitalis, beta blocker, verapamil) are administered (which increase the refractory period in the AV node and paradoxically allow even more atrial impulses to get through the accessory pathway to the ventricle). These patients require careful evaluation and electrophysiologic study.

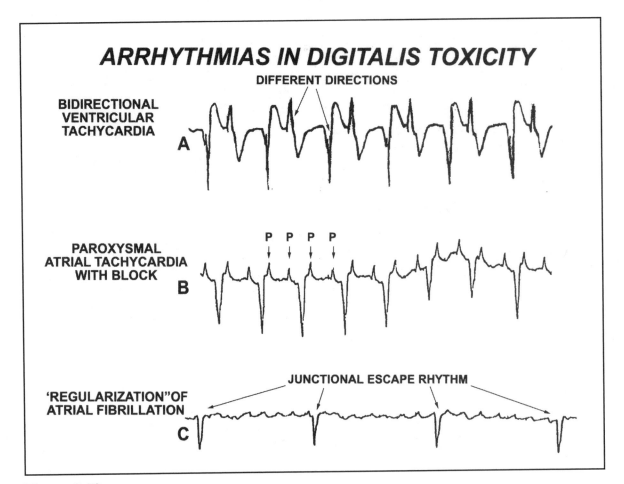

Figure 3-53

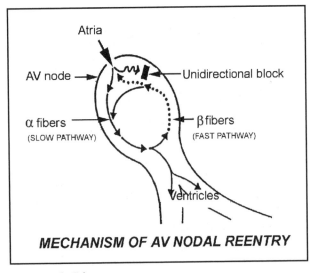

Figure 3-54

Figure 3-58. 12 lead ECG in a patient with a history of palpitations and WPW. Note the short PR interval (e.g., lead II) and delta wave.

Although the presence of an accessory pathway may be detected on an ECG, not everyone with WPW will develop tachycardia or require special treatment.

Figure 3-59. *Lown-Ganong-Levine (LGL) syndrome.* Atrial impulses may bypass the AV node using a fast conducting accessory pathway, but rejoin the bundle of His, thereby producing a short PR interval, but normal QRS complex (no delta wave). A tachyarrhythmia may result if impulses spread backward along the rapidly conducting accessory pathway to stimulate the atria at a rapid rate. Patients with a short PR interval on the ECG are prone to atrial tachyarrhythmias.

Bundle Branch Block
The characteristics of right and left bundle branch block were presented above in the discussion on analysis of the QRS complex.

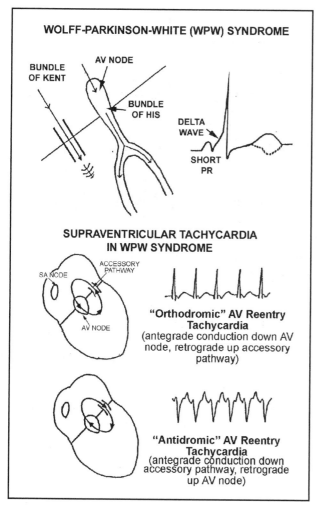

Figure 3-55

Figure 3-60. 12 lead ECG tracing demonstrating the characteristic features of *right bundle branch block*. Note the QRS is wide (>0.12 sec), an rSR′ pattern (so-called "rabbit ears") is present in leads V1 and V2, and a wide S wave is seen in leads I, aVL and V6.

Figure 3-61. 12 lead ECG tracing demonstrating the characteristic features of *left bundle branch block*. Note the QRS is wide (>0.12 sec), monophasic (or notched, not shown) R waves are present in leads I, aVL and V6, the QRS is mostly negative in V1–V3, the ST segment is in the opposite direction of the QRS, and is elevated in leads V1–V3. These ST-T changes are secondary to the conduction defect.

An ECG abnormality should always be interpreted in the context of the "company it keeps". For example, right bundle branch block, although it may be seen in congenital heart disease (e.g., atrial septal defect), and conditions affect-

ing the conduction system (e.g., sclerodegenerative disease), may not have a serious import if it appears as an isolated finding (congenital abnormality) in a young, otherwise healthy individual. It is not unusual to detect RBBB in patients with no other clinical evidence of heart disease. On the other hand, if RBBB develops in the setting of an acute MI, it often has significant prognostic importance. (**Note:** A specific entity known as *Brugada syndrome* has been described in which RBBB with persistent ST segment elevation (coved or saddleback) in precordial leads V1–V2 is associated with the susceptibility to VT/VF and sudden cardiac death.)

In contrast, the new appearance of LBBB is decidedly more ominous. LBBB is usually associated with organic heart disease and is only occasionally seen in normal subjects. It is associated with significantly reduced long-term survival, with 10-year survival rates as low as 50%. It is commonly associated with long-standing hypertension, CAD, dilated cardiomyopathy, calcific aortic valvular disease, and degenerative conduction system disease. LBBB may be the first clue to underlying heart muscle disease (e.g., cardiomyopathy). In the setting of symptoms highly consistent with myocardial ischemia, the presence of a new (or presumably new) LBBB on the ECG should raise the suspicion of acute MI with proximal occlusion of the LAD. In general, patients with CAD and LBBB often have a higher incidence of multivessel disease, LV systolic dysfunction and a poorer prognosis.

Fascicular blocks (also known as *hemiblocks*) represent disturbed conduction in either the anterior or posterior division, or fascicle, of the left bundle branch. The anterior fascicle is long and thin and has a single blood supply (LAD), which makes it more vulnerable to block than the posterior fascicle, which is short and thick and has a dual blood supply (LAD and right coronary artery).

Figure 3-62 illustrates the *hemiblock* patterns in the limb leads. The "anterior" papillary muscle of the left ventricle is above (rather than inferior) and lateral to the "posterior" papillary muscle, and the two divisions of the left bundle branch course towards their respective papillary muscles. If the anterior division is blocked (*left anterior hemiblock*), initial forces are directed downwards and to the right (toward the posterior papillary muscle), inscribing a Q wave in lead I and an R wave in lead II. The subsequent forces are directed mainly upwards and to the left (toward the anterior papillary muscle), inscribing an R wave in lead I and an S wave in lead II, producing a left axis deviation. In *left posterior hemiblock,* the opposite holds true. The initial forces spread upwards and to the left, inscribing an R in lead I and a Q in lead II. Subsequent forces are directed downwards and to the right, producing a right axis deviation. Although hemiblock can occur by itself, left anterior hemiblock is often, and left posterior

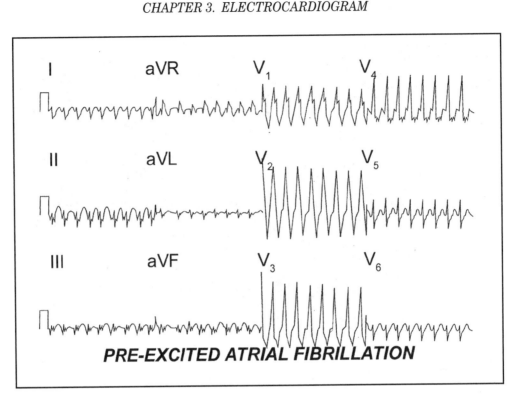

Figure 3-56

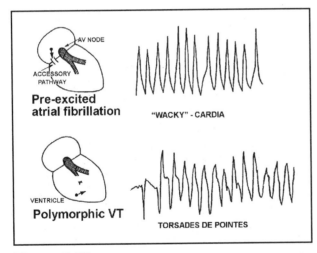

Figure 3-57

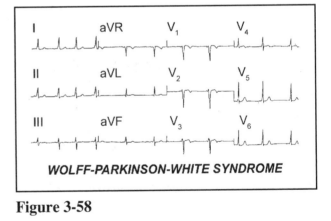

Figure 3-58

hemiblock almost always, associated with RBBB. Hemiblock, like bundle branch block, is commonly caused by CAD. Other causes include cardiomyopathy, sclerodegenerative disease, and aortic valve calcification.

As an aside, remember, "primum non nocere" (i.e., first do no harm). An unkind or thoughtless approach to evaluating or talking to a patient can cause harm before any treatment has had the opportunity to do so. Some heart disease terms should be avoided in the presence of patients or,

if used, explained properly. For example, when the ECG term "block" is used (e.g., heart block, left or right bundle branch block, hemiblock), it is important to tell the patient that this is an electrical term and does not connote blockage of blood in the heart or circulation. Speak in plain English. Keep in mind that many patients do not even know what a coronary artery or a ventricle is. Asking the patient his or her understanding of what was said often provides the opportunity to clarify any potential areas of misunderstanding.

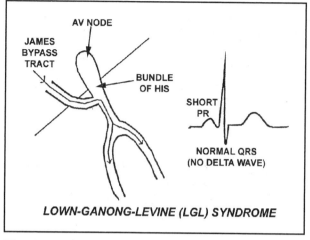

Figure 3-59

* * *

Ten "Take-Home" Points Regarding the ECG:

1. The ECG is the test of first choice for patients presenting with chest pain, syncope, or dizziness.
2. The ECG is useful as a baseline in the initial assessment of patients with known cardiovascular disease and/or dysfunction, and as part of the preoperative evaluation in patients >40 years of age, and in any patient with risk factors for CAD and/or known or suspected heart disease who are undergoing cardiac or noncardiac surgery (especially if a major operation, associated with large fluid shifts, or aortic or peripheral vascular surgery).
3. Serial ECGs may be helpful in certain conditions (e.g., evolving acute MI). Serial ECGs permit evaluation of the response to treatment (e.g., thrombolytic therapy for acute MI) and of progression, remission or persistence of any abnormality noted on the baseline tracing.
4. The ECG is an imprecise tool. A patient may have serious heart disease with little abnormality on the ECG, or no detectable heart disease, but an abnormal tracing.
5. Don't over-interpret the ECG. The range of normal is wide, and there is considerable overlap between normal and abnormal.
6. Before interpreting the ECG, make sure it is taken correctly. Beware of technician errors (e.g., misplaced electrodes, lead reversal). Always check for technical quality of the recording and calibration of the ECG machine. Keep on the lookout for baseline artifact (e.g., from disposable electrodes without proper skin preparation). Beware of patient movement and tremor (e.g., Parkinson's disease).
7. To successfully interpret ECGs, have a systematic and logical approach. (i.e., assess heart rate and rhythm, P wave, QRS complex, ST and T wave, PR interval, QRS and QT intervals, and mean QRS axis; then you won't miss anything.

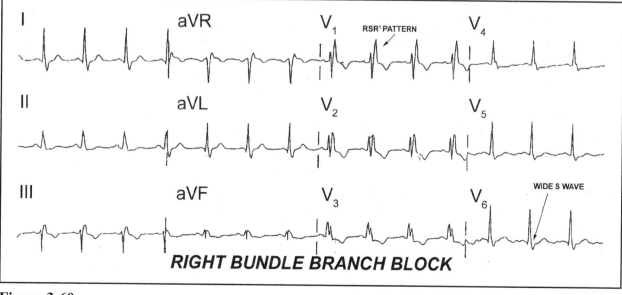

Figure 3-60

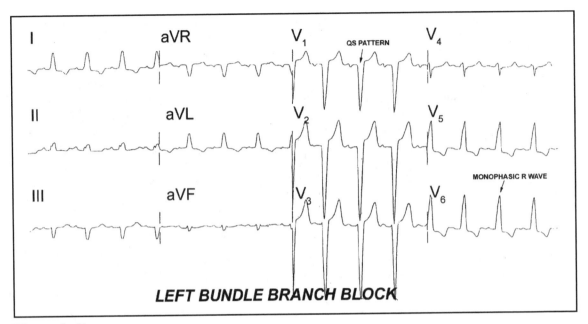

Figure 3-61

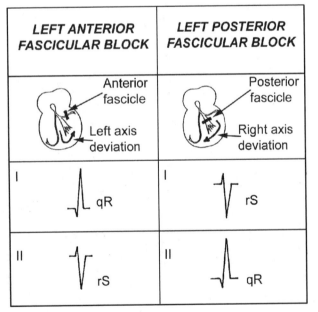

Figure 3-62

8. Beware of the "computer-read" ECG. The ECG interpretation created by the computer is often wrong. In general, computer programs are accurate for measuring heart rate and electrical axes, but do poorly in interpreting intervals, rhythm disturbances, ischemia and infarction. All ECGs require careful over-reading to avert misdiagnosis and possible catastrophic consequences.

9. Don't interpret an ECG without reference to prior tracings. On occasion, a new ECG abnormality can "erase" a previously existing one. A comparison also allows the interpreter to date specific abnormalities and may have important therapeutic implications.

10. All ECG diagnoses must be made in light of the total clinical picture. The accuracy of ECG interpretation is greatly improved when appropriate clinical information (e.g., patient's age, gender, presenting symptoms, and list of pertinent medications) is provided, and any ECG abnormalities detected then are correlated with the other clinical data. For example, diffuse concave ST segment elevation in a young asymptomatic patient is likely to represent early repolarization (a normal variant), whereas the same finding in a patient with chest pain and a friction rub is more likely to represent acute pericarditis. Furthermore, lateral ST segment depression means something different in the setting of acute chest pain, hypertension or digoxin therapy. Keep in mind that, along with the clinical history, the ECG is still the simplest, most readily available, and inexpensive tool in the early diagnosis of acute ST elevation MI.

* * *

Figure 3-63 summarizes a systematic approach to ECG interpretation.

Note: Please refer to attached CD for more information and practice in interpretation of ECGs.

FIGURE 3-63

Systematic Approach to ECG Interpretation

Basic Concepts

- Observe name and date (checking to be sure it is the correct patient's ECG).
- Assess age and gender.
- Check for technical quality of ECG and other factors (e.g., voltage calibration of the ECG machine).
- Compare with patient's previous ECGs.

Determine Cardiac Rhythm

- Is the rhythm regular or irregular?
- Identify atrial activity (P waves) and ventricular activity (QRS complexes).
- Determine the P-QRS relationship.

Measure Heart Rate

- Use the following methods.
  - Counting method (300–150–100–75–60–50)
  - Number of beats in 6 seconds × 10
- Is the rate normal (60–100 bpm), bradycardia (<60 bpm), or tachycardia (>100 bpm)?

Evaluate P Wave Morphology

- Inspect P wave in leads II and V1 for right and left atrial enlargement. What are the amplitude, duration and direction?

Assess PR, QRS, and QT Intervals

- PR interval–Is it normal (0.12–0.20 sec.), short or prolonged?
- QRS interval–Is it normal (≤0.10 sec) or abnormal? If ≥ 0.12 sec, check the QRS for bundle branch block.
- QT interval–What is the duration? Normal QT ≤one-half of the R-R interval, (if heart rate is normal).

Determine Mean QRS Axis (in the limb leads)

- Is it normal (+90° to −30°), left axis deviation, or right axis deviation?
- Also assess R wave progression in the precordial leads. Is it normal, poor progression, or early transition?

Evaluate QRS Complex, ST and T Wave Morphologies

- Is a Q wave present or absent? If pathologic Q waves present, check the anatomic distribution: septal leads (V1, V2), anterior leads (V3, V4), lateral leads (I, aVL, V5, V6), and inferior leads (II, III, aVF). Q waves normal width <0.04 seconds; height <25% of QRS complex.
- Is the QRS amplitude normal, increased, or decreased? Check for left or right ventricular hypertrophy.
- Is the ST segment elevated, depressed or isoelectric? Check for ischemia, infarction, pericarditis, metabolic and/or chemical abnormalities.
- Is the T wave upright or inverted?
- Is the amplitude increased or diminished?

Identify Abnormal ECG Patterns

- Myocardial ischemia and infarction
- Cardiac chamber enlargement and hypertrophy
- Arrhythmias and conduction disturbances
- Miscellaneous patterns (e.g., pericarditis, WPW syndrome, electrolyte imbalances, drug effects)
- Is a pacemaker present? If so, is it pacing, capturing, and sensing appropriately?

CHAPTER 4.   CHEST X-RAY

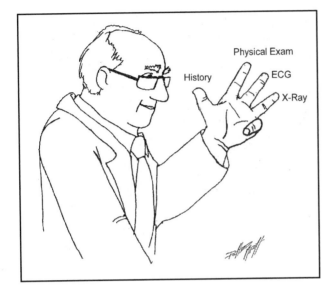

Figure 4-1. The normal cardiac silhouette. SVC = superior vena cava, RA = right atrium, AO = aortic knob, PA = main pulmonary artery, LV = left ventricle, RV = right ventricle, LA = left atrium, IVC = inferior vena cava, PV = pulmonary valve ring, AV = aortic valve ring, MV = mitral valve ring.

Proper analysis of the PA and lateral chest x-ray (CXR) provides much useful information about the status of the heart and lungs. You should (if at all possible) personally view the patient's chest film and correlate the clinical and radiographic findings. In this way, the CXR serves as an extension of the cardiac clinical examination.

When reviewing the chest film, try to resist the natural tendency to focus too quickly on the heart and vasculature. The interpretation of the chest x-ray should proceed in a systematic fashion so that valuable clinical clues in other parts of the film are not overlooked, and technical variations (e.g., rotation, quality, orientation, degree of inspiration) do not lead to incorrect conclusions.

The chest x-ray is an important part of the initial evaluation of a patient with cardiac disease and is a useful noninvasive method for following the progression of disease and/or its response to therapy. The routine chest film includes an upright posteroanterior (PA) projection (taken with the x-ray film placed against the patient's anterior chest) and a left lateral projection (with the left side of the patient's chest adjacent to the film cassette). Chest x-rays may also be taken at the bedside with a portable x-ray machine and the film behind the patient (anteroposterior [AP] view), but interpretation of AP films is significantly limited, particularly in estimating heart size.

THE CARDIOVASCULAR SILHOUETTE, INCLUDING THE CARDIAC CHAMBERS AND THE AORTA

The standard chest x-ray is the simplest and most practical method for determining overall heart size and can provide a rough estimate of the dimensions of individual cardiac chambers and great vessels.

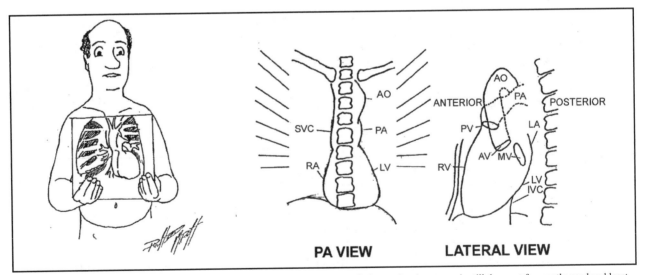

Note: Despite the widespread availability of newer, more sophisticated imageing techniques, the chest x-ray is still the most frequently used and least costly modality for imaging the heart, lungs, and great vessels.

Figure 4-1

Cardiac enlargement, as seen in the PA view, may be present when the cardiothoracic ratio (i.e., the ratio of the transverse diameter of the cardiac silhouette to the transverse diameter of the thorax at the level of the diaphragm is >0.5) (**Figure 4-2**).

Figure 4-2. Measurement of cardiothoracic ratio. A vertical line at the center of the spine serves as a reference. The greatest distance of the right and left cardiac borders from the reference line are measured (A + B). The cardiothoracic ratio is this distance (A + B) divided by the widest transverse diameter of the thoracic cage (C). The normal value of this ratio is 0.5 or less. If it is >0.5, cardiac enlargement is present. It is essential for the CXR to be taken in the posteroanterior (PA) view, since the heart is magnified in the anteroposterior (AP) projection.

Figure 4-3. *LA enlargement* (e.g., due to chronic MR, rheumatic MS, LV failure) is suggested when the left-sided heart border is straightened, the left mainstem bronchus elevated, and a "double density" within the cardiac silhouette is present, representing enlargement of the left atrium over to the right side.

RA enlargement (as may be seen in tricuspid valve disease, right atrial tumor, pulmonary hypertension, and cardiomyopathy) may be present when the right-sided heart border bulges toward the right.

Figure 4-4. *RV enlargement* (e.g., in LV failure, rheumatic MS, pulmonary hypertension), occupying the retrosternal clear space, is best visualized on the lateral view.

LV enlargement shows up as a prominence of the left side of the silhouette, a downward and lateral displacement of the apex. *LV hypertrophy* may present as a rounding of

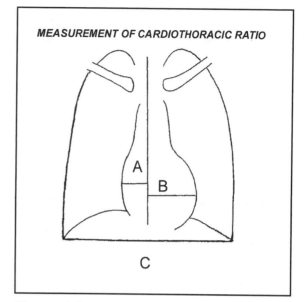

Figure 4-2

the cardiac apex. Hypertrophy alone (as may occur in systemic hypertension, valvular AS, and HOCM), however, may not result in radiographic abnormalities since it generally occurs at the expense of the LV internal volume and produces little or no change in overall heart size. LV hypertrophy is more readily suspected from changes in QRS voltage on the ECG and can be accurately quantitated from measuring wall thickness on echo.

The detection of LV enlargement may provide a clue to the presence of chronic volume overload (e.g., AR, MR) or dilated cardiomyopathy. A previous history of MI or the

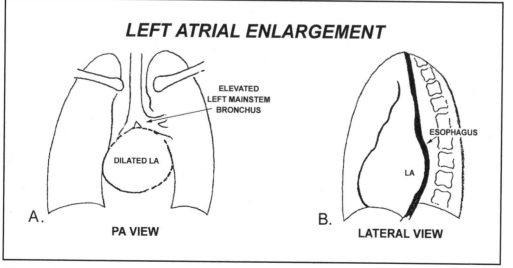

Figure 4-3

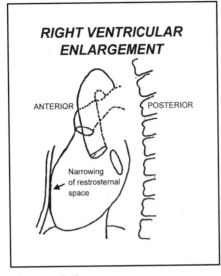

Figure 4-4

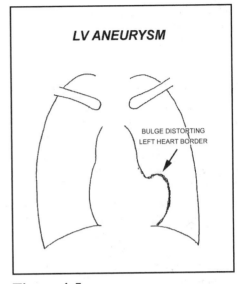

Figure 4-5

presence of pathologic Q waves on the ECG provide clues to an ischemic origin for the enlargement. Occasionally, in such patients, the CXR may reveal an angulated distortion of the left heart border, often with calcification, suggesting the presence of an *LV aneurysm* (**Figure 4-5**). In LV volume overload (e.g., AR) the LV tends to enlarge primarily in its long axis, displacing the apex downward and to the left (**Figure 4-6A**). In dilated cardiomyopathy, on the other hand, LV length and width are generally both increased, causing the heart to appear globular (**Figure 4-6B**). Dilated cardiomyopathy causes not only LV but also generalized car-

diac dilation. The heart may appear falsely enlarged, however, when it is displaced horizontally (e.g., poor inspiration, obesity, pectus excavatum) and if the film is taken in the anteroposterior (AP) projection (which magnifies the heart shadow) or when the patient's body is rotated (which may produce a spurious abnormality of the cardiac silhouette).

The chest x-ray may also help identify:

• Increased pulmonary blood flow or "shunt vascularity", as seen in left-to-right shunts (e.g., *atrial septal defect*)

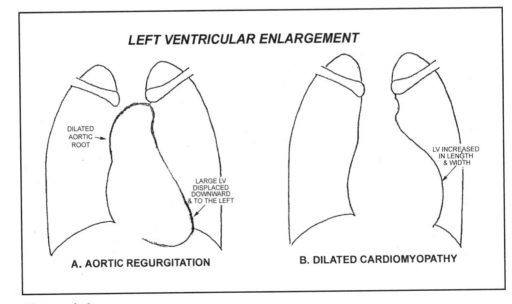

Figure 4-6

- *Pulmonary venous hypertension* (as occurs in CHF and mitral valve disease)
- Mediastinal widening or a dilated ascending aortic shadow (clues to proximal *aortic dissection or aneurysm*)
- *Calcification of the aortic valve*, along with post-stenotic dilatation of the aorta (as occurs in significant valvular aortic stenosis)
- *Calcification of the mitral valve* (rheumatic MS) or its surrounding annulus
- *Calcification of the pericardium* (as may be seen on the lateral view in as many as 50% of patients with long-standing *constrictive pericarditis*)
- *Calcification of the coronary arteries*. Image intensification fluoroscopy and particularly electron

beam CT scanning, though, are much more sensitive than radiography in detecting coronary artery calcification. Such calcifications, although indicative of coronary atherosclerosis, do not necessarily imply clinically significant CAD.

Figure 4-7. Cardiac calcification on CXR:
    A. Aortic dissection showing separation between the calcification in the aortic intima and media (dark shading) and the outer edge of the aorta.
    B. Severe calcific valvular aortic stenosis, with calcification of the aortic valve and post-stenotic dilatation of the ascending aorta (arrow). The presence of LV hypertrophy results in a rounding of the cardiac apex.

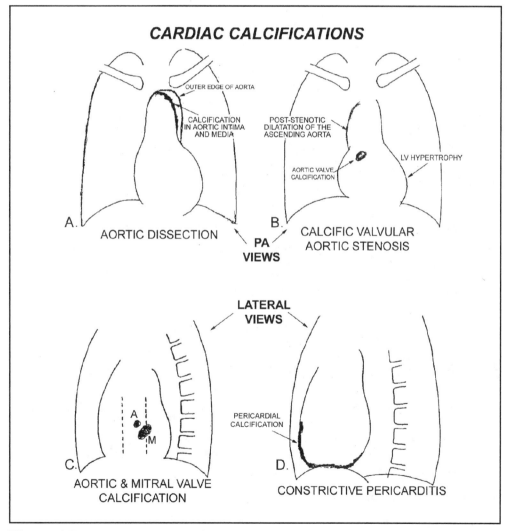

Figure 4-7

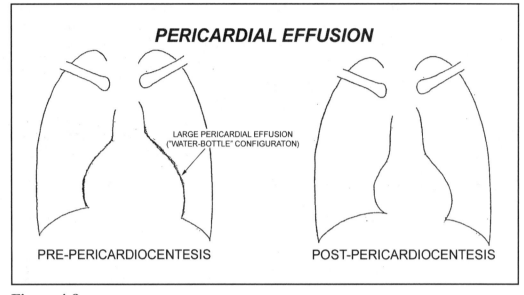

Figure 4-8

C. Calcification in the aortic and mitral valves (lateral view).

D. Constrictive pericarditis (lateral view). Note linear pericardial calcium (dark markings) particularly on the anterior and inferior surfaces.

The plain chest film may also reveal previous cardiac surgery, including stainless steel sternal sutures, metal clips or loops marking saphenous vein coronary bypass grafts, as well as clues to the type of prosthetic heart valves or rings, and the manufacturer and model number of cardiac pacemakers and defibrillators along with the location and condition of the leads. Fluoroscopy may also help in evaluating the function of mechanical prosthetic valves.

With a large pericardial effusion, the cardiac silhouette increases on both sides, without evidence of pulmonary venous congestion. Approximately 200 to 250 cc of pericardial fluid may be needed to produce an enlargement on the chest x-ray. The heart may appear globular (classic "*water-bottle*" configuration), and there is loss of the distinctive borders and outline of the hilar vessels (i.e., no pulmonary distention) despite an enlarged heart on the lateral film. A distinct stripe separating the subepicardial fat from the subxiphoid fat (*epicardial fat pad sign*) is a highly specific (but relatively insensitive) clue to pericardial effusion. The only clue to a relatively small effusion may be a noticeable change in heart size compared with that on previous films (**Figure 4-8**).

THE PULMONARY VASCULATURE

Figure 4-9. The pulmonary vasculature on CXR, showing the pulmonary arteries (clear) and pulmonary veins and left atrium (shaded). Changes in vascular appearance arise from increased or decreased pulmonary blood flow and from pulmonary hypertension.

Elevation of the LA and pulmonary venous pressure (e.g., due to LV failure, MS) are reflected in the radiographic findings of redistribution of pulmonary blood flow to the upper lobes ("cephalization"), increased interstitial markings,

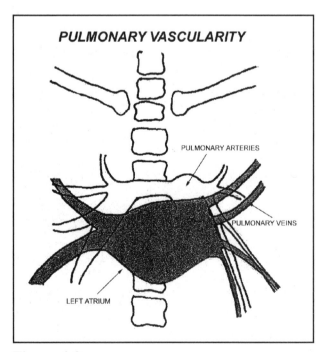

Figure 4-9

and frank alveolar edema. With LA pressures in excess of 15 mmHg, there is dilatation of upper lobe veins ("*antler pattern*"). Higher pulmonary venous pressures (to ~25 mmHg or more) lead to pulmonary edema (**Figure 4-10**).

Figure 4-10. CXR findings in congestive heart failure. Note cardiomegaly, along with cephalization of blood flow (prominent upper lobe pulmonary vessels), interstitial pulmonary edema with Kerley B lines (linear, horizontal markings in the outer and lower lung fields due to edema of the interlobar septa, alveolar edema (bilateral hilar clouding, "butterfly" or "bats wing" appearance), and pleural effusion (right > left). The CXR findings in CHF can be remembered by the mnemonic "**ABCDE**": **A**lveolar edema, Kerley **B** lines, **C**ardiomegaly, **D**ilated prominent upper lobe vessels, and pleural **E**ffusions.

Pleural fluid may also accumulate in the minor fissure, forming an ovoid density simulating a tumor ("pseudotumor"), which when caused by CHF, disappears with effective diuresis.

Chest radiography is particularly valuable when an S3 gallop cannot be heard because of noisy respiration in a patient who is dyspneic. The CXR may provide the first clue to underlying CHF by showing unsuspected increases in pulmonary vasculature (even before pulmonary crackles are heard). Usually the heart is enlarged, unless MS or diastolic dysfunction is present.

Because dilatation takes time to develop, recent lesions (e.g., acute MR/AR) may present without apparent cardiomegaly. The presence of acute pulmonary edema, along with a normal (or nearly normal) size heart, thus, should alert the astute clinician to the presence of an acute event, e.g., acute MI, acute MR/AR, or the acute onset of rapid atrial fibrillation.

Problems in interpretation of the chest x-ray in LV failure include:

- Interpretation is greatly influenced by the technical quality of the film. An under-penetrated film may exaggerate pulmonary vascular markings, heightening the illusion of LV failure.
- The chest x-ray also may not correlate in time with the patient's immediate condition. For example, when CHF begins, there may be as much as a 12 hour diagnostic lag in x-ray appearance, and there may be a *post-therapeutic* lag in x-ray appearance of up to 4 days after the clinical resolution of CHF.
- Although the chest x-ray is an accurate reflection of hemodynamics in patients with *acute* left heart failure, it may not be reliable in *chronic* CHF because increased lymphatic clearance can result in clear lung fields.

Enlarged pulmonary arteries (due to increased pulmonary blood flow) are present in a variety of conditions *including congenital heart disease* (e.g., ASD, VSD, PDA) with a left-to-right shunt ("shunt vascularity") and *pulmonary hypertension* (primary or secondary).

Figure 4-11. CXR findings (PA view) in a patient with pulmonary hypertension. In contrast to both centrally and peripherally dilated pulmonary arteries in left-to-right shunts, in pulmonary hypertension the pulmonary vessels in the outer portion of the lung fields are quite inapparent compared with the enlargement of the main pulmonary artery and its primary branches (which may attain aneurysmal

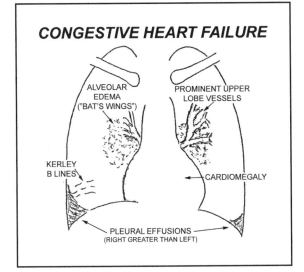

Figure 4-10

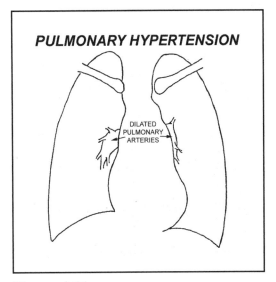

Figure 4-11

proportions, and on occasion even become calcified). Right ventricular enlargement may also be present.

THE LUNG FIELDS

The radiographic appearance of the pulmonary parenchyma may provide important cardiac clues:

- *Pulmonary embolism* may present as chest pain or dyspnea, with findings on the chest x-ray (e.g., atelectasis, blunted costophrenic angle, elevated diaphragm, decreased pulmonary vascular markings).
- The lung fields may show pneumonic infiltrates from septic pulmonary emboli (e.g., IV drug use) and may be a clue to the presence of tricuspid valve endocarditis.
- CXR findings of emphysema or pulmonary fibrosis may provide the explanation for chronic right heart failure (cor pulmonale) or shortness of breath in a patient taking amiodarone.

THORACIC CAGE ABNORMALITIES

Inspection of the chest x-ray for abnormalities of the thoracic cage can also yield valuable diagnostic information. Abnormalities may include *straight back, pectus excavatum* (funnel chest) or *carinatum* (pigeon chest) as seen in mitral valve prolapse, the classic *"bamboo spine"* of ankylosing spondylitis (associated with AR and AV block) and *rib notching* (as in coarctation of the aorta).

Figure 4-12. Coarctation of the aorta. CXR shows dilated ascending aorta and aortic arch, and the "figure of 3" sign produced by dilatation of the descending aorta above and below the site of coarctation, enlarged LV, and rib notching (arrows showing scalloped appearance of the inferior margins of the ribs).

Although the CXR is a routine preadmission and preoperative test, it is of little value for CAD unless complications (e.g., CHF) occur, because cardiovascular structures may appear normal in CAD. As with all diagnostic tests, the findings on CXR are best interpreted when integrated in the context of the other findings on the cardiac clinical examination.

Figure 4-13 summarizes a systematic approach to the chest x-ray.

* * *

Pearls:

- A cardiothoracic ratio >50% on the upright PA chest film indicates an enlarged cardiac silhouette,

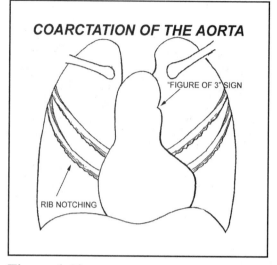

Figure 4-12

suggesting either cardiomegaly or a pericardial effusion.
- Radiographic signs of CHF include cardiomegaly, pulmonary vascular redistribution with prominent upper lobe vessels, "butterfly" pattern of alveolar edema, Kerley B lines, and pleural effusion (right > left).
- Pericardial effusion on the CXR is suggested by a globular ("water bottle") shaped heart.
- When diagnosing cardiomegaly, check the technical quality of the CXR. A supine (AP) film, poor inspiration, or rotation may make the heart look larger, mimicking cardiomegaly. A poor penetration may mimic pulmonary edema; over penetration may give falsely clear lung fields.
- Increased pulmonary blood flow centrally and peripherally ("shunt vascularity") may be visible on the CXR with a significant left to right shunt (e.g., ASD, VSD, PDA).
- Enlargement of the central pulmonary arteries with rapid tapering of the vessels ("pruned tree" appearance) is seen with pulmonary hypertension.
- Aortic abnormalities on the CXR include aneurysm, tortuosity, and calcification. Aortic dissection is suggested if mediastinal widening and a separation between the calcification and the aortic border is present.
- Coarctation of the aorta on the CXR is indicated by the "figure of 3" sign produced by dilatation of the descending aorta above and below the site of

---

FIGURE 4-13

Systematic Approach to CXR Interpretation

Basic Concepts

- Observe name and date (checking to be sure it is the correct patient's film).
- Assess age and gender.
- Check for technical quality of film and other factors.
  - Left or right markers (prevents missing dextrocardia)
  - Type of projection (upright [PA], or supine [AP] view)
  - Size of the patient (obesity may enlarge appearance of the heart)
  - Degree of inspiration (poor inspiration can make heart appear larger)
  - Emphysema (hyperinflation can make heart appear smaller)
  - Chest configuration (straight back, pectus excavatum can make heart appear larger); pectus carinatum, rib notching
  - Position of patient (AP supine or rotated film can make heart appear larger)
  - Exposure (underpenetrated film may exaggerate, and overpenetrated film may obscure, pulmonary vascular markings)

Cardiovascular Silhouette, including Cardiac Chambers and the Aorta

- Position
- Overall heart size
- Specific chamber enlargement
- Calcifications
- Pericardium (effusion)
- Check for pacemakers, prosthetic heart valves, sternal wires

Pulmonary Vasculature

- Pulmonary venous congestion
- Pulmonary arteries (increased blood flow ["shunt vascularity"], pulmonary hypertension)

Lung Fields

- Interstitial and alveolar edema
- Infiltrates
- Atelectasis
- Emphysema, pulmonary fibrosis
- Pleural effusions

---

coarctation, along with rib notching (due to enlargement of the intercostal arteries).

- Calcifications on the CXR may be seen in severe valvular AS (with post-stenotic dilatation of the ascending aorta), the mitral valve (rheumatic MS), the mitral annulus (ring-shaped), the coronary arteries, an apical LV aneurysm, and the pericardium (constrictive pericarditis).
- The CXR may reveal metal sutures, clips, or loops from previous CABG surgery, as well as clues to the presence and type of prosthetic heart valve. Fluoroscopy may help in evaluating the function of me-

chanical valves, by assessing for "rocking" (caused by dehiscence) and prosthetic leaflet motion. Keep in mind that a single lead in the RV apex indicates the presence of an electronic ventricular pacemaker (or ICD), 2 leads indicate a dual chamber (AV sequential) pacemaker, and 3 leads a biventricular pacemaker.

* * *

Note: Please see attached CD for more detailed coverage of the CXR in heart disease.

CHAPTER 5.   CARDIAC DIAGNOSTIC LABORATORY TESTS

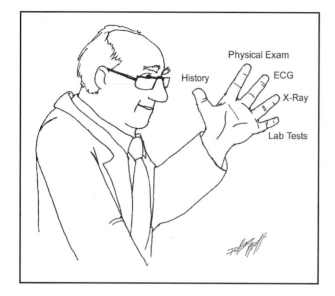

When considering ordering a laboratory test, several questions should be addressed. Specifically, will the results of the test or procedure arrive at a more precise diagnosis? Will the test alter the therapy and/or the patient's prognosis? Do the benefits justify the potential risk and/or cost (not only financial, but physical and mental as well)? Too much testing can be detrimental to patient care. These tests are often expensive, time-consuming, and potentially hazardous. They may delay treatment, heighten the patient's (and practitioner's) anxiety, and may at times lead to additional and unnecessary laboratory tests (the "cascade effect"). Furthermore, obtaining too many tests reflects a basic insecurity on the part of the practitioner, and, on occasion, may be motivated by medicolegal (fear of malpractice suit) and/or economic considerations (**Figure 5-1**).

The best clinicians order the fewest tests. They select diagnostic tests only as needed, based upon the clues derived from the history and physical examination. Experienced clinicians use the cardiac laboratory to confirm their clinical suspicion of heart disease, rather than to establish the diagnosis, or "rule-out" the almost limitless less likely diagnostic possibilities. If laboratory tests are needed to answer a specific question, then cost, convenience, and risk should all be considered, particularly when more than one method can offer similar useful information. Furthermore, the level of expertise of the laboratory providing the service, and the skill and experience of those interpreting the tests should be taken into consideration before a test is ordered. Although very sophisticated tests are available to help diagnose heart disease, no test is perfect. The astute practitioner must appreciate the fallibility and limitations of these tests and procedures. Differences in techniques or thor-

oughness can affect the diagnostic yield markedly. In many laboratories these tests have a high diagnostic accuracy, whereas in others the number of "false positives" and "false negatives" is so great as to render the results virtually worthless.

BLOOD TESTS

Routine Chemistries

Since prevention of heart disease is highly desirable, certain blood tests may be useful in those with a family history of CAD, to evaluate risk and guide therapeutic intervention. These tests include *fasting lipid profile*, including *total cholesterol, LDL* and *HDL cholesterol*, and *triglyceride levels* (which screen for dyslipidemia), *plasma homocysteine* and *lipoprotein (a) levels* (which may be an independent risk factor for CAD), and *fasting serum glucose* and *hemoglobin A_{1C}* levels (which assess for diabetes mellitus and the degree of glycemic control). Biochemical markers of inflammation e.g., *C-reactive protein* (CRP), measured by a high sensitivity assay, have recently been found to be helpful in predicting long-term prognosis and in identifying those patients at risk for ischemic events who might benefit from more aggressive treatment, e.g., with "statins" (which lowers CRP in addition to LDL cholesterol levels).

A *thyroid profile*, including serum TSH and serum thyroxine (T4) level, should be a part of the diagnostic work-up of new onset SVT and/or atrial fibrillation (particularly in patients receiving amiodarone, which can cause hypo- or hyperthyroidism).

Some common blood tests can provide clues to such conditions as:

- Anemia (decreased *hemoglobin* and *hematocrit*), which can exacerbate ischemic chest pain
- Electrolyte imbalance (low *serum potassium* [K^+] and/or *magnesium* [Mg^{++}] which increase risk for ventricular arrhythmias)
- Renal insufficiency (elevated *blood urea nitrogen* [*BUN*] and *serum creatinine*), as may result from decreased cardiac output or damage secondary to contrast media
- Hepatitis and/or myositis (liver and/or skeletal muscle [*creatine phosphokinase, CPK*] enzyme elevations), as may be caused by lipid lowering therapy; and
- Clotting abnormalities and/or function (activated *partial thromboplastin time* [*PTT*], *prothrombin time* [*PT*], and *international normalized ratio* [*INR*]), as may occur in patients receiving anticoagulation therapy.

Abnormalities of renal or hepatic function may be the initial clues to previously unsuspected heart disease. Eleva-

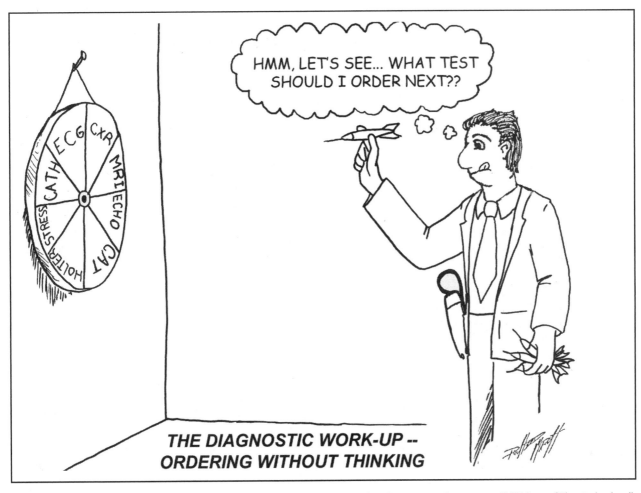

THE DIAGNOSTIC WORK-UP --
ORDERING WITHOUT THINKING

Note: Cardiovascular testing is an essential part of the patient work-up. Not every patient, however, needs every test. Skillful use of "low technology", the history and physical exam, leads to intelligent cost-effective use of "high-technology". Remember, *hands before scans!*

Figure 5-1

tion of the BUN may indicate intrinsic kidney disease. If the elevation is out of proportion to the serum creatinine level (i.e., in prerenal azotemia, due to a low cardiac output to an intrinsically normal kidney), the BUN elevation often provides a clue to decreased renal perfusion secondary to CHF. In patients with right-sided CHF, *liver function tests* (e.g., *aminotransferases, alkaline phosphatase, bilirubin levels*) may be minimally (or even markedly) elevated. Some patients with marked hepatic congestion have evidence of poor synthetic function (i.e., elevated *PT*, reduced *albumin* levels).

Certain blood chemistries can help identify patients with CHF who are at risk for poor outcomes, including hyponatremia, abnormal liver function, renal insufficiency (so-called cardiorenal syndrome), anemia, and elevated BNP and troponin levels (see below).

Rapid measurement of circulating levels of *BNP* (*B-type* or *brain natriuretic peptide*) or *NT-pro BNP* are

newer blood tests that have been found to be helpful in differentiating CHF from lung disease in patients presenting with dyspnea. BNP was first identified in the brains of pigs, and, in humans, is produced by the ventricular (and to a lesser extent atrial) myocardium in response to an increase in volume and pressure. A normal circulating BNP level virtually excludes the diagnosis of CHF. BNP levels are a good indicator of CHF severity and prognosis, and correlate well with treatment efficacy. A declining BNP indicates a good response to therapy and portends a more favorable outcome. A rising BNP indicates a greater risk of adverse outcome, warranting a more aggressive treatment strategy. Keep in mind, however, that factors other than CHF, e.g., older age, women, renal failure, cirrhosis, LV hypertrophy (e.g., in valvular AS, hypertension), acute coronary syndromes, myocarditis, pulmonary embolism, and pulmonary hypertension, can elevate BNP levels. Recent data suggests that measurement of BNP is an important addition to our current tools for risk stratification.

Cardiac Biomarkers

Serum biomarkers of myocardial injury in acute MI, e.g., *cardiac troponins* and *creatine kinase* and the *MB isoenzyme (CK-MB)* reflect ischemic necrosis or cell death. The height and duration of elevation of these biomarkers usually correlate with the size of acute MI if allowed to run its full course untreated.

Figure 5-2. Sequential changes in cardiac serum markers following an acute MI. The total creatine kinase (CK) and CK-MB isoenzyme rise several hours after the acute event and peak at 24 hours. The smaller molecule, myoglobin, is detected in the serum earlier, but is less specific for myocardial necrosis. Cardiac specific troponins are the preferred biomarkers since they are highly sensitive and specific for myocardial injury (troponin isoform I more so than isoform T). They are detectable in the serum 3–6 hours after an acute MI begins, and remain detectable in the serum for 10–14 days after the acute event. LDH serum levels rise more gradually and peak at 3–5 days after the acute event. Since cardiac troponins detect lesser degrees of myocardial necrosis, it is useful to diagnose microinfarcts in CK–MB negative patients with acute coronary syndromes (ACS), or to rule out myocardial injury if a "false positive" CK-MB is suspected. Patients with ACS who "rule out" for acute MI by CK–MB criteria, but have detectable levels of troponin, have a higher risk of adverse cardiac events.

Although troponin elevations are mostly related to ischemic myocyte injury due to ACS ("type 1" MI), other conditions that can result in a supply-demand ischemic mismatch ("type 2" MI), e.g., anemia, tachyarrhythmias, hypo- or hypertension, or that cause myocardial cell damage e.g., perimyocarditis (due to inflammation), pulmonary embolism (due to RV ischemia), severe CHF, cardiotoxic drugs (e.g., anthracyclines), radiofrequency catheter ablation, electrical cardioversion and/or defibrillation, cardiopulmonary resuscitation, PCI and CABG, may release these serum markers. Vigorous exercise, sepsis, critical illness, and severe renal impairment (for unclear reasons) may also increase these serum markers. Detectable increases in these enzymes, therefore, is not synonymous with an acute MI due to coronary atherosclerosis.

Cardiac isoforms of *troponin T and I* (which are more sensitive and specific for myocardial injury than CK-MB measurements) may be released in patients with ACS (who have no MI by CK-MB or ECG criteria), offer earlier warning, and correlate well with a four times greater risk of short-term adverse outcome (i.e., death, MI).

Elevated serum troponin levels in patients with ACS may, in reality, reflect watershed injury or minor degrees of myocardial necrosis (microinfarction) that result from microemboli from an unstable coronary atherosclerotic plaque. It is now clear that these patients should be labeled as non-ST segment elevation MIs and that an elevated troponin level represents a powerful marker of increased risk. These isoforms, which begin to rise 3–6 hours after the onset of an acute MI, reach 95% to 99% sensitivity and specificity by 10 hours. They remain detectable for 10–14 days after the acute event (4 times longer than CK levels), allowing for the diagnosis of acute MI even more than a week after its onset. It is estimated that ~30% of patients with an acute coronary syndrome who present with rest pain without ST segment elevation, and would otherwise be diagnosed as having unstable angina because of a lack of CK-MB elevation, actually have non-ST segment elevation MI when assayed with cardiac-specific troponin levels. These patients may receive a greater treatment benefit from intravenous platelet glycoprotein (GP) IIb/IIIa inhibitors, low molecular weight heparin (LMWH), and an early invasive strategy.

Since troponin levels may not rise for up to 6 hours after the onset of symptoms, the measurement should be repeated if initial troponin levels are negative at <6 hours. Keep in mind that although *myoglobin* is released more rapidly from infarcted myocardium than is CK-MB or the troponins, and may be detected as early as 2 hours after the onset of myocardial necrosis, it is not cardiac specific. However, because of its high sensitivity, a negative myoglobin within the first several hours after the onset of chest pain is useful in "ruling out" an MI.

Worthy of mention, in patients with elevated CK levels from noncardiac sources e.g., skeletal muscle injury (from trauma, surgery, IM injections), myopathy or myositis (due to statins), or hypothyroidism, cardiac troponins are

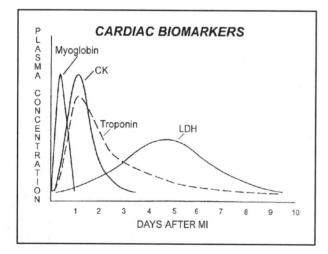

Note: A rise and/or fall of cardiac biomarkers, preferably troponin, in a clinical setting compatible with ischemia, helps to establish the diagnosis of acute MI.

Figure 5-2

more specific for myocardial injury than CK-MB. Although newer troponin assays with higher sensitivity may supplant the current markers, they have diminished specificity for MI since they detect myocardial injury in a variety of clinical settings. The diagnosis of acute MI, therefore, requires a rise and/or fall in cardiac troponin levels above the 99th percentile of the normal range (for the assay used) along with a clinical picture compatible with acute myocardial ischemia.

SPECIALIZED NONINVASIVE TESTS

Cardiac noninvasive and invasive testing is playing an increasingly prominent role in the diagnosis and treatment of patients with known or suspected heart disease. Over the past few decades, new techniques have been developed and old ones improved, providing increased sensitivity and specificity. *When used appropriately,* the following noninvasive laboratory studies can supplement the clinical data.

Transthoracic M-Mode and Two-Dimensional Spectral and Color-Flow Doppler Echocardiography

A complete *M-mode* and *two-dimensional (2-D) transthoracic echocardiographic* (echo) study, including *spectral* (pulsed and continuous wave) and *color flow Doppler,* is one of the most versatile and valuable noninvasive imaging tests in the initial and serial evaluation of the cardiac patient. It is rapid, accurate, readily available, and portable. A transducer is placed on the surface of the patient's chest and sound waves, reflected from blood-tissue interfaces within the heart and great vessels, provide a "picture" of the cardiac

anatomy along with a detailed image of cardiac blood flow. Indeed, cardiac ultrasound has become the most commonly requested cardiac diagnostic imaging modality employed in the office, at the bedside, in the intensive care unit, the operating room, and/or in the emergency department.

In M-mode transthoracic echo (which detects motion along a single beam of ultrasound) the ultrasound image is recorded against time (*time-motion study*), while the echo keeps the angle of the single "ice-pick" ultrasound beam stationary. In 2-D transthoracic echo the angle is rapidly moved within a sector, with multiple ultrasonic beams transmitted through a wide arc, producing a "sector scan", like the appearance of an MRI section. Both M-mode and 2-D echograms are recorded as movies.

Transthoracic Doppler echo is used to evaluate:

- *Cardiac chamber size*
- *LV and RV wall thickness and function,* including ejection fraction (that fraction of end-diastolic blood volume ejected from the ventricle during each systolic contraction)
- *Valve structure and motion,* e.g., bicuspid aortic valve, mitral valve prolapse or stenosis, with superimposed calcification, vegetation, or flail leaflet
- *Intracardiac shunts, pressures* and hemodynamics.

Figure 5-3. *Transthoracic M-mode echocardiogram.* Left. Ultrasound beams are directed across the chest wall to obtain images of the heart. Right. Schematic representation of the heart showing the structures through which the ultrasonic beam passes as it is directed from the left ventricle

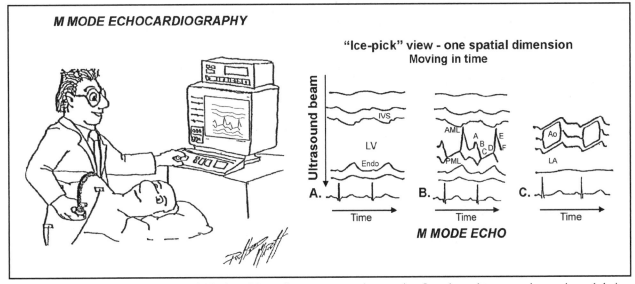

Note: M mode echo can provide a 1D ("ice pick") view of the cardiac structures moving over time. It can be used to assess valve opening and closing, chamber size and thickness, and subtle abnormalities of ventricular wall motion (which are better displayed on M mode than 2D echo).

Figure 5-3

toward the base of the heart. A, B, and C are the three standard "ice pick" views of the heart with M-mode echo. The transducer is placed on the chest wall and angulated to provide a view of:

(**A**) the left ventricle, (**B**) mitral valve, (**C**) the aortic valve, root, and left atrium. IVS = interventricular septum, LV = left ventricle, Endo = endocardium, RV = right ventricle, LA = left atrium, Ao = aortic valve, AML = anterior mitral valve leaflet, PML = posterior mitral leaflet.

Figure 5-4. Schematic diagram of M Mode echocardiogram in various cardiac disease states. The normal anterior and posterior mitral valve has a typical "M or W-shaped" appearance respectively. (**A**) Mitral valve prolapse. Note the late systolic bowing of the mitral valve leaflets (typical "buckle" or "question mark on its side" configuration). (**B**) Mitral stenosis. Note the thickened and calcified mitral valve leaflets with reduced diastolic (EF) slope and paradoxical motion of posterior leaflet. (**C**) Hypertrophic obstructive cardiomyopathy. Note asymmetric septal hypertrophy (ASH) and systolic anterior motion (SAM) of the anterior mitral leaflet. (**D**) Dilated cardiomyopathy. Note dilated and severely hypocontractile LV with "double diamond" mitral valve along

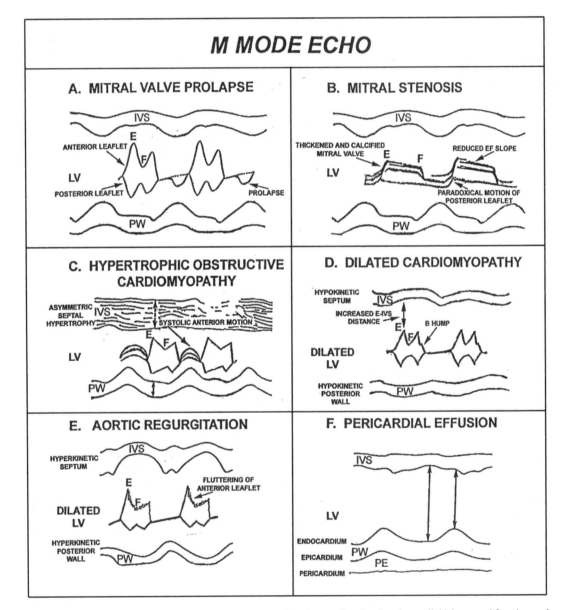

Note: M mode echo can be used to evaluate valve structure and motion, cardiac chamber size, wall thickness and function, and pericardial effusion.

Figure 5-4

with "B hump" due to elevated LV end–diastolic pressure. The distance between the E point of the anterior leaflet of the mitral valve and the interventricular septum (double arrows) is also increased. (**E**) Aortic regurgitation. Note diastolic "fluttering" of the anterior mitral valve leaflet along with dilated LV and exaggerated septal and posterior wall motion. (**F**) Pericardial effusion. Note echo-free space behind the LV posterior wall between the LV epicardium and the pericardium.

Figure 5-5. *Transthoracic two-dimensional echocardiography,* showing the four major views of the heart:

A. Parasternal long axis view. The echo beam creates a "slice" along the long axis of the heart from the aorta to the mid-LV, excellent for studying the aortic and mitral valves, the interventricular septum (IVS), posterior wall of the left ventricle (LV), the left atrium, and the right ventricular (RV) outflow tract.

B. Parasternal short axis view, mid LV level. This view shows both ventricles in cross section. LV wall motion abnormalities can be assessed. When the echo beam is moved cephalad, the mitral and aortic valves can be visualized.

C. Apical four-chamber view. LV wall motion abnormalities, along with mitral and tricuspid valve motion and atrial dimensions can be evaluated.

D. Apical two-chamber view. Allows visualization of the apex, which is usually missing on the parasternal long axis view, along with anterior and inferior LV wall motion.

Transthoracic Doppler echo is far superior to the ECG or CXR for diagnosing hypertrophy or enlargement of any cardiac chamber, and is a powerful noninvasive imaging tool for assessing cardiac systolic and diastolic function. It can also determine the direction and velocity of blood flow in cardiac chambers, across valves, and through the great vessels, thus permitting the detection of regurgitant or stenotic lesions and shunts. Flow moving toward the transducer is color coded in red, and away from the transducer in blue. Very high velocity of flow is assigned a speckled or green color.

Figure 5-6A. Schematic diagram of mitral Doppler inflow (LV filling) patterns in diastolic dysfunction.

Figure 5-6B. Schematic diagram demonstrating 2-D Doppler flow imaging in valvular regurgitation. **Left.** 2-D Doppler echo of aortic regurgitation and mitral regurgitation from parasternal long axis view. **Right.** 2-D Doppler echo of tricuspid regurgitation and mitral regurgitation from apical 4 chamber view.

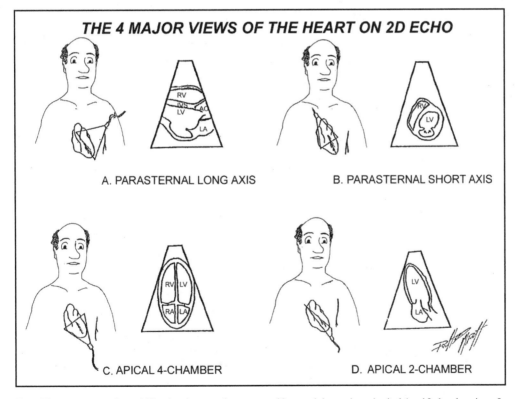

THE 4 MAJOR VIEWS OF THE HEART ON 2D ECHO

A. PARASTERNAL LONG AXIS

B. PARASTERNAL SHORT AXIS

C. APICAL 4-CHAMBER

D. APICAL 2-CHAMBER

Note: The most commonly used 2D echo views are the parasternal long and short axis, and apical 4 and 2 chamber views. In the parasternal long axis view, the septum and posterior wall, as well as mitral and aortic valves, are well visualized. The apical 4 chamber view demonstrates both ventricles and atria, as well as the mitral and tricuspid valves. In some patients, e.g., those with COPD (hyperinflated lungs), the heart can not be adequately visualized. In such patients the subcostal view provides better quality echo images.

Figure 5-5

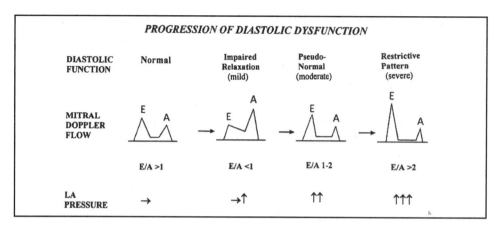

PROGRESSION OF DIASTOLIC DYSFUNCTION

DIASTOLIC FUNCTION	Normal	Impaired Relaxation (mild)	Pseudo-Normal (moderate)	Restrictive Pattern (severe)
MITRAL DOPPLER FLOW	E/A >1	E/A <1	E/A 1-2	E/A >2
LA PRESSURE	→	→↑	↑↑	↑↑↑

Note: Schematic diagram of transmitral Doppler flow patterns in various stages of diastolic dysfunction (DD). In mild DD (impaired relaxation), there is a decrease in early transmitral flow (E wave) with a compensatory increase in late diastolic flow during atrial contraction (A wave). As DD progresses from moderate (pseudonormal) to severe (restrictive pattern), LA pressure rises to compensate, and the E wave becomes more prominent than the A wave.

Figure 5-6A

Transthoracic Doppler echo techniques can be useful in evaluating:

- Global (generalized) and regional (localized) ventricular wall motion and systolic and diastolic function (thereby discriminating between systolic [reduced EF] and diastolic [preserved EF] heart failure)
- LV diastolic function and filling pressures (using mitral Doppler flow [E/A ratio] and tissue Doppler imaging [E/é]) (**Figure 5-6 A**)
- Right heart and pulmonary arterial pressures (RV systolic pressure = 4 × [TR velocity]^2 + RA pressure)
- Transvalvular pressure gradients (Peak gradient = 4 × [peak velocity]^2) and valvular orifice areas in stenotic aortic or mitral valves (**Figure 15-4**)
- Valvular regurgitation (e.g., MR, AR, TR) and estimating its severity (**Figure 5-6B**)
- Prosthetic valve function
- Intracardiac shunts (e.g., ASD, VSD)

- Intracardiac masses, e.g., valvular vegetation, LA or LV thrombus, LA tumor (myxoma)
- Myocardial disease (e.g., dilated cardiomyopathy, HOCM, and restrictive cardiomyopathy) (**Figure 5-4**)
- Pericardial effusion, as in pericarditis. Although an echo is useful in detecting the size and location of a pericardial effusion (often as small as 20–30 cc), it is not a reliable test for diagnosing pericarditis. Patients may have pericarditis without a pericardial effusion, and a pericardial effusion may be present in the absence of pericarditis. (**Figure 5-4**).
- Cardiac tamponade (RA and RV collapse)
- Acute aortic dissection.

Transesophageal Echocardiography

Figure 5-7. Schematic diagram illustrating *transesophageal echo* (TEE). In transthoracic echo, the sound waves are reflected back to the chest surface and recorded. In TEE, an

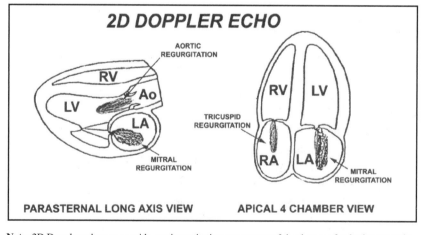

Note: 2D Doppler echo can provide semiquantitative assessment of the degree of valvular regurgitation (mild, moderate, or severe). The presence of mild or trivial ("physiologic") regurgitation, however, should not be construed as pathology, since minor degrees of regurgitant flow occur normally.

Figure 5-6B

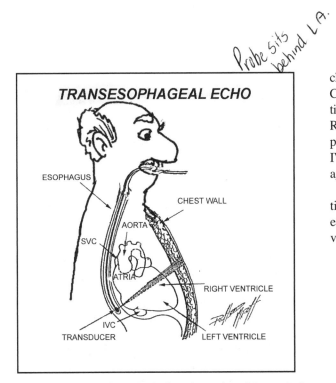

Probe sits behind LA.

TRANSESOPHAGEAL ECHO

ESOPHAGUS

CHEST WALL

AORTA

SVC

ATRIA

RIGHT VENTRICLE

IVC

TRANSDUCER

LEFT VENTRICLE

Note: TEE is used to rule out aortic dissection, endocarditis, prosthetic valve dysfunction, and LA thrombus prior to cardioversion for atrial fibrillation. With TEE, the transducer is posterior to the heart, and the thoracic aorta, mitral valve, and the LA and LA appendage are more easily seen than with transthoracic echo.

Figure 5-7

endoscopic ultrasound transducer is passed through the mouth into the esophagus and two-dimensional images are obtained from the posterior aspect of the heart. Because of the transducer's posterior location and the fact that it is not limited by imaging through adipose tissue, air or rib spaces, TEE can often provide more detailed information than conventional transthoracic echo imaging of posterior cardiac structures (especially the mitral valve, LA, and thoracic aorta). It is particularly suited for the detection of LA thrombi or spontaneous echo contrast (so-called "smoke", which represents stagnant blood) before cardioversion, a patent foramen ovale (PFO), small (<2 mm) mitral valve vegetations, a thoracic aortic dissection, and aortic atheroma with a high degree of accuracy. TEE provides superb visualization of the LA and its appendage, and, when no thrombus is seen, cardioversion may be performed with minimal embolic risk in patients with atrial fibrillation.

In those patients with suspected endocarditis (especially involving a prosthetic valve, particularly mitral) and a negative transthoracic echo, a TEE, which has a high (>90%) sensitivity, should be considered. A negative TEE, however, does not exclude the diagnosis.

TEE, along with real-time *3D echo*, is now being used in the operating room during surgical procedures to monitor LV function and to determine the accuracy of repair of congenital and valve lesions. It can help in the guidance of pericardiocentesis.

Rest or stress echo can assist in the initial diagnosis of patients with chest pain or suspected acute coronary syndromes. It can provide an assessment of myocardial is-

chemia and/or infarct size and location, define the extent of CAD, determine regional wall motion abnormalities, and identify post-MI mechanical complications, e.g., infarct expansion, RV infarction, LV aneurysm, LV thrombus, ischemic MR and papillary muscle rupture, acute VSD, and pericardial effusion. IV echo *contrast agents* can opacify the LV and improve image quality when acoustic windows are poor.

Because of its ability to evaluate structural, functional, and hemodynamic abnormalities of the heart, it is easy to see the potential utility of Doppler-echo in a wide variety of clinical situations:

- To evaluate the patient with a "significant" heart murmur, to confirm the clinical impression of its cause or to characterize the morphologic and hemodynamic abnormalities responsible for its production.
- To determine the cause of unexplained symptoms:
  1. Chest pain (due to CAD, AS, HOCM, MVP, pericarditis, or aortic dissection)
  2. Shortness of breath (e.g., systolic and/or diastolic dysfunction due to CAD, cardiomyopathy, valvular heart disease)
  3. Stroke (cardiac source of an embolus, e.g., MS, LA or LV mural thrombus, vegetation, atrial myxoma) A right to left shunt through a patent foramen ovale (PFO) may also be demonstrated by agitated saline *contrast echocardiography* ("bubble study").
- To evaluate those in an intensive care setting who are critically ill and have hypotension or shock syndrome. The presence of segmental wall motion abnormalities in a patient with a dilated cardiomyopathy, although not specific, favors CAD as an etiology. For patients with mitral and/or aortic regurgitation, echo evidence of progressive LV dilatation despite medical therapy with vasodilators should help lead the clinician to the consideration of surgical intervention (valve repair or replacement) to prevent irreversible LV dysfunction.

Although the Doppler-echo is potentially useful in the evaluation of systolic murmurs, it should not be ordered if, on clinical grounds, the patient is felt to have an "innocent" systolic murmur. The yield of echo is very low for asymptomatic patients with typical flow murmurs detected on physical examination. Doppler-echo is indicated in the evaluation of heart murmurs in symptomatic patients or patients whose murmur has a moderate probability of reflecting structural heart disease.

Doppler-echo will detect even the slightest amount of valvular regurgitation, even in individuals without any clinical evidence of cardiac disease. This raises the possibility that a murmur heard may not truly correlate with what is found by Doppler-echo. For example, if a systolic murmur is detected, which is thought to be due to MR, but in reality is an innocent murmur, and the Doppler-echo reveals trivial or mild MR, the clinician may assume the systolic murmur is indeed due to

MR when, in fact, it is not. Furthermore, color flow Doppler echo is a more accurate reflection of flow velocity than actual flow, and may over-estimate the severity of high velocity small volume regurgitant jets. Care should be taken, therefore, not to overinterpret these Doppler-echo findings.

In addition, an echo has a substantial "false positive" rate for the diagnosis of mitral valve prolapse. A slight alteration of the orientation of the transducer can lead to the appearance of MVP. Despite its versatility, therefore, echo is best applied and integrated in the context of a given clinical presentation.

Another area of innovation has been the miniaturization of echo recorders (i.e., "handheld" devices), to permit easy "point of care" evaluation of cardiac patients. For some clinicians, *handheld echo* has replaced the stethoscope. Echo, however, should be considered an extension of a careful cardiac clinical examination, not a substitute for it. It is best utilized as a definitive test to confirm a clinical suspicion of heart disease, rather than as a screening diagnostic tool. It is the challenge of today's clinician to order echo studies in a cost-effective manner, while providing the best possible care for his or her patients.

Note: Please refer to the attached CD for more in depth information about echocardiography.

Ambulatory Electrocardiography: Holter Monitoring and Transtelephonic ECG/Event Recording

Figure 5-8. Ambulatory ECG (Holter) monitoring is a useful non-invasive technique to detect arrhythmias and other ECG abnormalities during ordinary daily activities in a 24-hour period. Accurate correlation of the ECG recording with a diary of the patient's symptoms is crucial, and can provide valuable clues to proper interpretation. Keep in mind that many patients will not have symptoms during the 24 hour monitoring period; ~20% will have a normal Holter recording during symptoms; and ~10% will have an arrhythmia coinciding with symptoms. Since the majority of patients will not have symptoms during the monitoring period, an *event recorder* that the patient can activate during an episode may offer better results.

Episodes of palpitations, dizziness, near-syncope or syncope, particularly if frequent, may be evaluated by Holter monitoring if a cardiac rhythm (e.g., brady or tachyarrhythmia) and/or conduction disturbance (e.g., heart block) is suspected as a contributing factor. Patients with significant complaints of palpitations that correlate with periods of normal sinus rhythm should be further evaluated for underlying psychologic disorders. Dizziness is a common symptom that may or may not be related to an irregular heart rhythm. It is important to document the time of occurrence of dizziness and correlate this with what is happening on the Holter monitor. If a tachy or bradyarrhythmia is associated with dizziness, appropriate therapy can be instituted. In the absence of symptoms during monitoring, however, finding transient or no arrhythmias does not rule out arrhythmic syncope. Conversely, ambulatory recording often reveals clinically insignificant asymptomatic arrhythmias. Cardiac arrhythmias are common (especially in adults >65

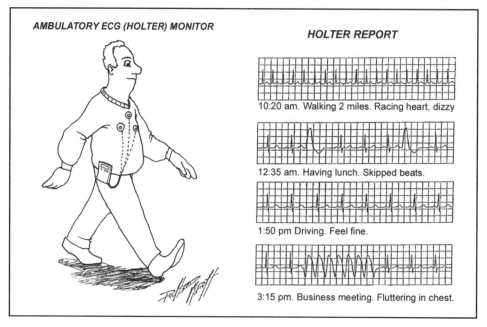

AMBULATORY ECG (HOLTER) MONITOR

HOLTER REPORT

10:20 am. Walking 2 miles. Racing heart, dizzy

12:35 am. Having lunch. Skipped beats.

1:50 pm Driving. Feel fine.

3:15 pm. Business meeting. Fluttering in chest.

Note: Patients with frequent (at least daily) palpitations or dizzy spells are commonly investigated by a 24 hour ambulatory ECG (Holter) monitor. A patient diary allows correlation between symptoms and heart rate and rhythm. Patients with less frequent episodes require longer term (external or implantable) event monitoring.

Figure 5-8

years of age). It is important, therefore, to make sure that symptoms occur with the arrhythmia or conduction abnormality observed during monitoring before assuming that you have identified the cause. The presence of high grade AV block, especially if correlated with symptoms, can provide a clue to the need for permanent pacemaker implantation. In contrast, if nothing abnormal is occurring on the Holter during dizziness, other causes must be entertained.

Holter monitoring is also useful in:

- The evaluation of *episodic chest pain* suspicious for exertional (ST segment depression) or rest-related, variant or Prinzmetal's (ST segment elevation) angina
- The diagnosis of *silent ischemia* (i.e., ischemic ST segment changes on the ECG in the absence of chest pain), although it is of limited specificity
- The assessment of the effectiveness or aggravation (proarrhythmic, i.e., arrhythmia exacerbating effect) of anti-arrhythmic drugs, cardiac ablation, and/or device (e.g., pacemaker, defibrillator) therapy.

Patients with infrequent and unpredictable episodes of cerebral or cardiac symptoms may benefit from the use of portable external (or rarely subcutaneous implantable) *event recorders,* with a memory loop, that can be activated by the patient at the time of onset or after the cardiac event. This device will allow a recording of the ECG from the minutes immediately *preceding* a symptomatic episode which can be transtelephonically transmitted for interpretation. A small, wearable and wireless adhesive device (ZIO patch) is a promising new option for arrhythmia detection. These devices are more cost-effective for occasional symptomatic arrhythmias than 24-hour ambulatory ECG monitoring.

Signal Averaged Electrocardiography and T Wave Alternans

In certain settings (e.g., following an acute MI), a relatively simple, noninvasive, computerized technique known as the *signal-averaged ECG (SAECG)*, averages multiple QRS complexes, eliminates artifactual "noise", and thus may detect low amplitude electrical signals from the heart called "late potentials" in the terminal portion of the QRS complex. These "late potentials" are generated by asynchronous conduction through ischemic/fibrotic myocardium. They serve as a helpful clue in identifying patients at an increased risk for sudden death from sustained ventricular arrhythmias (due to reentrant circuits), especially those with depressed LV function and poor ejection fractions (< 40%).

Figure 5-9. Left. Abnormal signal-averaged ECG demonstrating late potentials. **Right.** Mechanism of reentrant VT in a patient with a previous MI. In the peri-infarction area (dark circle) a critically timed premature electrical impulse is conducted down one of two pathways in the ventricular Purkinje fibers (1) but is blocked down the other (2). This impulse not only depolarizes the ventricle, but may also conduct retrograde through the previously blocked pathway, thereby initiating a reentrant VT. The SAECG may provide clues to the presence of such reentrant circuits.

The predictive value of a *normal* SAECG is quite good (>90%) for identifying post-MI patients unlikely to

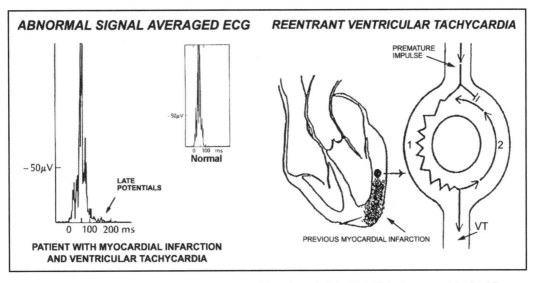

Note: Left. Abnormal signal averaged ECG with late potentials at the end of the QRS. Right. Late potentials after MI are an independent marker of risk for reentrant ventricular tachycardia.

Figure 5-9

have a ventricular tachyarrhythmia, whereas the predictive value of an *abnormal* SAECG is much lower. Patients with normal SAECG have a very low risk for developing potentially malignant ventricular tachyarrhythmias. Those with an abnormal SAECG have an overall arrhythmic risk of ~20% (half of those being fatal events).

Studies have shown that *T wave alternans* (microvolt beat-to-beat variation in T wave morphology and/or amplitude), detectable by computer-averaging techniques during exercise or pacing, is a useful non-invasive tool in identifying patients at increased risk for VT-VF and sudden cardiac death.

Tilt-Table Testing

Head-up tilt-table testing (with or without concurrent administration of isoproterenol, a beta agonist, or nitroglycerin, a vasodilator used to provoke syncope) can be a useful, noninvasive diagnostic tool in evaluating those patients with suspected vasovagal (*neurocardiogenic*) syncope. In the latter, vagal tone increases and sympathetic tone decreases on the upright posture, leading to hypotension (secondary to vasodilation) and/or bradycardia along with syncope or presyncope (a feeling that syncope is imminent). This testing is particularly helpful in patients with no evidence of associated heart disease by history, physical examination, ECG, or other noninvasive testing. The pathophysiologic mechanism involves increased venous blood pooling in the lower extremities, decreased venous return and ventricular filling,

which, in turn, causes vigorous myocardial contraction and activation of ventricular mechanoreceptors, which leads to increased vagal tone and decreased sympathetic tone.

Figure 5-10. Tilt-table testing in a patient with neurocardiogenic syncope. The tilt-table test is designed to provoke a syncopal event while the patient's heart rate, rhythm and blood pressure response is closely monitored. When syncope or presyncope related to hypotension or bradycardia occurs during upright tilt, the test is considered positive and the patient is returned to the supine position. A baseline shows supine heart rate and blood pressure. In this case, after 22 min. of upright tilt, BP falls to 70/25 mmHg, and full syncope occurs (courtesy of Dr. Albert A. Del Negro).

In general, 30–40% of patients who are thought to have neurocardiogenic syncope have a true positive test without a drug challenge, and up to 80% if isoproterenol or nitroglycerin is added. Of note, efficacy of treatment e.g., high salt diet, increased fluid intake, and fludrocortisone (Florinef), to expand intravascular volume; beta blockers and disopyramide, which reduces the force of LV contraction, along with other potential therapies, e.g., selective serotonin reuptake inhibitors (SSRIs), transdermal scopolamine, ephedrine, theophylline, midodrine, and pacemaker therapy remains inconclusive, and repeating the head-up tilt after therapy has been implemented is not recommended due to its poor predictive value. It should be realized that the results of tilt-table testing are not always reproducible. Conversely, 15–20% or more of patients without neurocardiogenic syncope may

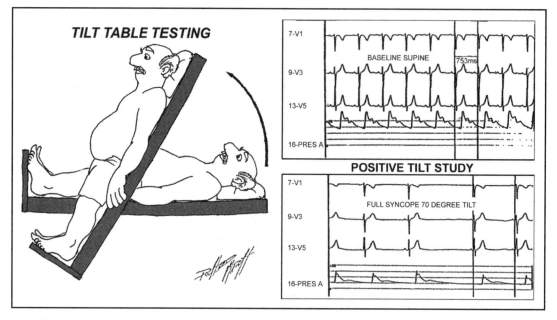

Note: Tilt table testing may be useful in patients with severe or recurrent syncope or in those in whom the diagnosis of neurocardiogenic syncope is suspected, but cannot be confirmed by history and physical exam. Note the mixed vasodepressor (↓BP) and cardioinhibitory (↓HR) vagal response to upright tilt along with the induction of syncope.

Figure 5-10

have a false-positive tilt-table study (particularly if a more extensive protocol is used). For patients with syncope and no structural heart disease, however, the diagnostic yield of tilt-table testing in the initial work-up is much greater than that of electrophysiology studies (EPS — where electrodes introduced into the heart can finely record an "internal ECG").

Exercise and Pharmacologic Stress Testing, including Nuclear and Echocardiographic Imaging

Exercise ECG stress testing is one of the most helpful and widely available noninvasive tools in cardiology. The most common indications for stress testing include establishing a diagnosis of CAD in patients with chest pain, assessing prognosis and functional capacity in patients with stable angina or after an MI, evaluating exercise-induced arrhythmias, and assessing for ischemia after myocardial revascularization (PCI, CABG).

Figure 5-11 summarizes the definite and possible indications for exercise testing.

In the standard ECG stress test (Bruce protocol), the patient exercises for 3-minute intervals at increasing speed and incline on a motorized treadmill while being monitored for symptoms during the test, peak heart rate achieved, BP, and ECG response (specifically ST segment displacement, its magnitude, time of onset, and resolution), arrhythmias and exercise capacity. Contraindications include unstable angina, acute MI, rapid atrial or ventricular arrhythmias, poorly controlled CHF, severe valvular AS, myocarditis, recent illness or an uncooperative patient.

Figure 5-12. Patient undergoing a treadmill exercise stress test. Note, in this case, the downsloping ST segment depression persisting 5 minutes into the recovery period consistent with a markedly positive response for ischemia, as may be seen in patients with left main or triple vessel CAD.

In general, exercise capacity (i.e., duration of exercise) is a very strong prognostic indicator in patients with CAD. Those who are able to exercise >9 minutes on the treadmill (Stage III according to the standard Bruce protocol) and achieve at least 85% of age-predicted maximum heart rate (220 minus age) have a much better prognosis in comparison to those who cannot exercise beyond 6 minutes (Stage II). In the Bruce protocol the work load (i.e., speed, grade) is increased every three minutes from Stage I–1.7 miles per hour [mph], 10% grade elevation to Stage II–2.5 mph, 12% grade; Stage III–3.4 mph, 14% grade; Stage IV–4.2 mph, 16% grade, etc.)

FIGURE 5-11

Clinical Indications for Exercise Testing

Definite indications

- To assist in diagnosis of symptomatic patients with possible CAD (particularly middle aged males with atypical chest pain who have an intermediate likelihood of CAD).
- To assess functional capacity and prognosis of patients with known CAD.
- To evaluate patients with symptoms of exercise-induced arrhythmias (e.g., palpitations during sports).
- To evaluate functional capacity of selected patients with congenital, valvular or hypertensive heart disease or chronic heart failure.
- To evaluate functional status in possible heart transplant candidates (cardiopulmonary exercise testing).

Possible indications

- To evaluate asymptomatic middle aged patients with multiple risk factors for CAD.
- To evaluate females with atypical chest pain and risk factors for CAD.
- To assist in the diagnosis of CAD in patients taking digitalis or with ECG abnormalities which would hinder interpretation.*
- To evaluate response to therapy (medical, interventional, and/or surgical)**
- To evaluate serially (1–2 yr intervals) patients with known CAD.
- To evaluate risk prior to vascular surgery or after an acute MI.
- To evaluate significance of residual CAD post-infarct artery PCI.
- To evaluate asymptomatic men aged 40+ yrs and women aged 50+ yrs who plan to start vigorous exercise program or who are involved in occupations in which impairment might affect public safety (e.g., pilots, police, fire fighters, bus drivers).

---

*Stress testing with nuclear or echo imaging is a reasonable option in these patients. Nuclear imaging is more sensitive, but less specific, than stress echo for detection of ischemia. Exercise testing (without adjunctive imaging) is the initial diagnostic test of choice in most patients with suspected CAD who are able to exercise and who have a normal (or near normal) resting ECG.

Note: Anti-anginal medications should be held if trying to diagnose CAD, but should be continued when assessing the efficacy of current medical therapy.

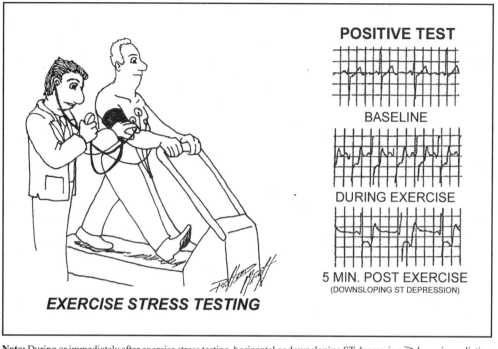

POSITIVE TEST

BASELINE

DURING EXERCISE

5 MIN. POST EXERCISE
(DOWNSLOPING ST DEPRESSION)

EXERCISE STRESS TESTING

Note: During or immediately after exercise stress testing, horizontal or downsloping ST depression ≥ 1 mm is predictive of CAD, but does not localize the ischemic territory involved. ECG stress testing with nuclear (perfusion) or echo (regional wall motion) imaging improves diagnostic accuracy and helps identify areas of ischemic myocardium.

Figure 5-12

Clinical clues to high risk (i.e., severe CAD) on exercise stress testing include:

- Inability to complete 6 minutes (Stage II) on Bruce protocol without ischemia
- Low workload (e.g., ≤ 6.5 METS). One MET (metabolic equivalent) is the unit of energy that is required for basal metabolism, i.e., an individual at complete rest. It approximates 3.5 ml of oxygen per kg of body weight per minute.
- Early positive test, e.g., ischemia in less than 3 minutes, or ischemia at low peak heart rate (e.g., <120 beats/min) without beta-blocker therapy (beta blockers lower the heart rate)
- Systolic blood pressure drop (e.g., >10 mmHg) or flat response (peak <130 mmHg)
- Marked horizontal or downsloping ST segment depression (e.g., >2mm)
- ST segment depression in multiple leads
- Prolonged ST segment depression (e.g., >6 min) after cessation of exercise
- ST segment elevation without pathologic Q wave
- Signs of LV dysfunction (pulsus alternans, pulmonary rales, S3 gallop, murmur of MR)
- Frequent PVCs or VT during or after exercise
- Delayed decrease or delayed recovery in heart rate after exercise
- Severe exercise-induced angina

- Large and/or multiple reversible perfusion defects or regional wall motion abnormalities, along with exercise-induced LV cavity dilatation (and increased lung uptake of radioisotope) on stress nuclear or echo imaging.

With few exceptions, exercise stress testing is the test of choice for initial evaluation of suspected CAD. It should be realized, however, that the predictive value of stress testing for the diagnosis of CAD depends on the pre-test likelihood of CAD. That is, the frequency of "false positives" (finding ECG changes in a patient who does not have CAD) and "false negatives" (missing CAD in a patient who has it) relates to the prevalence of the disease in the population being tested (*Bayes theorem*). Exercise testing is most useful in patients in whom the pretest probability of CAD is in the intermediate range (e.g., a middle-aged male with atypical chest pain and a normal resting ECG). If typical chest pain and ≥1 mm horizontal or downsloping ST depression 0.08 sec after the J point develops during exercise testing, the predictive value is >90%, whereas the likelihood of CAD is only 10% in patients who have a negative exercise test. Exercise testing adds little in detecting CAD in patients with a high pretest probability (i.e., a history of typical angina and risk factors in middle-aged or older males and older females), and may lead to false reassurance that no further evaluation or treatment is necessary if a "false negative" test results. Conversely, testing of young, asymptomatic individuals, especially women with no risk factors (in whom the likelihood

140

of CAD is very low), may be more likely to generate "false positive" than "true positive" results, which may therefore lead to unwarranted disability and unnecessary additional and even invasive testing and/or interventions.

As public awareness of testing modalities for CAD increase, requests among low-risk patients for stress testing are likely to escalate. This should be tempered, however, since such testing will only increase cost without improving diagnostic accuracy. Patients with a moderate or intermediate pre-test likelihood of CAD are the best candidates for exercise testing, since a markedly positive result can essentially establish the diagnosis whereas a clearly negative result can decrease the possibility to a low level.

"False positive" exercise-induced ST segment changes (i.e., not due to myocardial ischemia) are commonly seen with:

- Pre-existing ST segment depression >1 mm at rest
- Pressure overload (e.g., hypertension, valvular aortic stenosis, hypertrophic cardiomyopathy)
- Electrolyte imbalance (e.g., hypokalemia)
- Drugs (e.g., digitalis)
- Women with mitral valve prolapse
- Premenopausal women with ST segment changes (which may, in part, be due to the higher incidence of CAD in younger men)
- LV hypertrophy with "strain" pattern
- Left bundle branch block (LBBB)
- Paced ventricular rhythm
- Preexcitation (WPW) syndrome
- Hyperventilation

For patients who are unable to undergo adequate exercise on the treadmill or bicycle (due to severe peripheral vascular disease, orthopedic disability, or pulmonary disease) pharmacologic stress testing may be performed using:

- Potent *vasodilators,* e.g., dipyridamole (Persantine), regadenoson (Lexiscan), or adenosine (particularly for those with LBBB or paced ventricular rhythm), combined with thallium or sestamibi "cold spot" scanning that create a "steal" of coronary blood flow from constricted vessels and demonstrate relative hypoperfusion and decreased tracer uptake, or
- *Inotropic agents* (e.g., dobutamine) that increase heart rate and blood pressure (particularly for those with severe lung disease or asthma). The dobutamine echo stress test is said to be positive for myocardial ischemia when new LV hypokinesis or akinesis is observed during dobutamine infusion. *Improvement* of abnormal resting wall motion with low doses of dobutamine suggests the presence of stunned or hibernating but viable myocardium.

Figure 5-13 summarizes the indications for pharmacologic stress testing.

The diagnostic accuracy of exercise testing in the detection of significant CAD improves from a mean sensitivity of ~65% (lowest in single vessel disease, highest in multivessel disease) to the 85–90% range, by combining exercise testing with:

- *Radionuclide* e.g., thallium-201 or technetium-99m sestamibi (Cardiolite) or tetrofosmin (Myoview) rest and stress myocardial perfusion imaging using single-photon emission computed tomography (SPECT). This may demonstrate a reversible decrease in tracer uptake (ischemia) and/or fixed (infarction) perfusion defects ("cold spots").
- *Echo studies,* which may reveal diminished or absent systolic wall thickening and/or new or worsening wall motion abnormalities e.g., *hypokinesis* (decreased wall motion), *akinesis* (no wall motion), *dyskinesis* (paradoxical wall motion). These valuable imaging techniques increase the sensitivity (and especially the specificity) in identifying a "false positive" stress ECG result.

FIGURE 5-13

Candidates for Pharmacologic Stress Nuclear Perfusion Scan or Echo*

- **Patients unable to exercise**
  a) Orthopedic problems of the lower extremities
  b) Rheumatologic illnesses
  c) Neurologic illness
   (1) Paralysis secondary to cerebrovascular accidents
   (2) Severe neuropathy involving the lower extremities
   (3) Primary skeletal muscle disorders
  d) Severe lung disease or asthma
- **Peripheral vascular disease**
  a) Claudication of the lower extremities
  b) Large abdominal aortic aneurysms
  c) Venous insufficiency with severe edema of the lower extremities
- **Severe cardiovascular deconditioning**
- **General debility**
- **Drug therapy** with beta blockers or calcium channel blockers which may prevent heart rate increases above 85% of maximum predicted for age.

---

*Note: Pharmacologic stress imaging is indicated for those patients who cannot exercise and do not have contraindications to the agent used (e.g., acute bronchospasm [adenosine], or severe hypertension [dobutamine]). Aminophylline or caffeine can reverse the effects of adenosine.

Figure 5-14. Patient undergoing nuclear myocardial perfusion imaging. Myocardial perfusion is assessed using thallium-201 or technetium sestamibi (Cardiolite) injected prior to treadmill exercise. The test compares the myocardial radionuclide distribution right after exercise as compared with rest. In one case, where there is stress induced ischemia, the schematic illustration shows a radionuclide defect that disappears with rest. In the other, where there is an old myocardial infarction, the defect persists. If the patient is unable to exercise, intravenous dipyridamole (or adenosine) in combination with thallium or sestamibi imaging, or a dobutamine stress echo study can be performed.

Figure 5-15. Schematic diagram of stress echo study. The test compares the systolic wall motion immediately after exercise with the systolic wall motion at rest. **Left.** Normal systolic wall motion is present at rest. **Right.** Immediately after exercise there is transient hypokinesis of the anteroseptal and apical walls (arrows) indicating the presence of a high grade stenosis of the LAD coronary artery.

Stress echo compares favorably in cost-effectiveness and provides similar levels of accuracy (slightly less sensitive but more specific) for detecting CAD to that of nuclear stress testing. (**Figure 5-16**) Stress echo may be of particular value in patients who have a questionable defect on perfusion imaging. Both stress echo and radionuclide stress testing are noninvasive imaging modalities that help in situations in which clarification of the presence, distribution, or threshold of inducible myocardial ischemia is required.

These situations include high clinical suspicion of CAD but negative exercise stress test, low clinical suspicion but positive exercise stress test, non-diagnostic exercise stress test, "culprit" vessel identification in multivessel CAD, assessment post-CABG surgery or after PCI.

Nuclear or dobutamine echo stress is useful in helping decision-making when considering revascularization and risk stratification prior to major noncardiac surgery (e.g., vascular surgery). Multiple areas of reversible ischemia (myocardial perfusion defects and/or echo wall motion abnormalities) at low workload, transient LV cavity dilatation, along with an increase in lung uptake of radioisotope on nuclear stress testing (evidence of LV dysfunction), are clues to patients with CAD at high risk. These patients should be considered for coronary angiography and potential revascularization prior to elective noncardiac surgery.

"*False positive*" nuclear studies may result from soft tissue attenuation artifacts, as can be seen in women with large breasts (breast attenuation artifacts of the anterior wall) and patients with elevated diaphragms (diaphragmatic attenuation artifacts of the inferior wall) or LBBB (septal perfusion defects). In addition, abnormal septal wall motion may be seen in patients with RV volume overload, LBBB, WPW syndrome, and after cardiac surgery.

"*False negative*" nuclear studies can occur when collateral circulation masks single vessel CAD, or "balanced" hypoperfusion disguises multivessel disease. For example, global ("balanced") ischemia from triple-vessel disease may

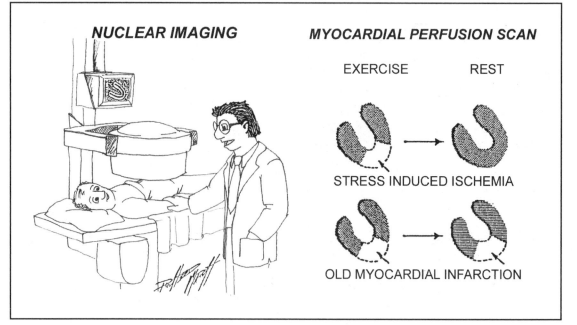

Note: With nuclear imaging, perfusion defects that appear only with stress suggest reversible myocardial ischemia; whereas perfusion defects that appear on both stress and rest images suggest irreversible scar (infarcted myocardium).

Figure 5-14

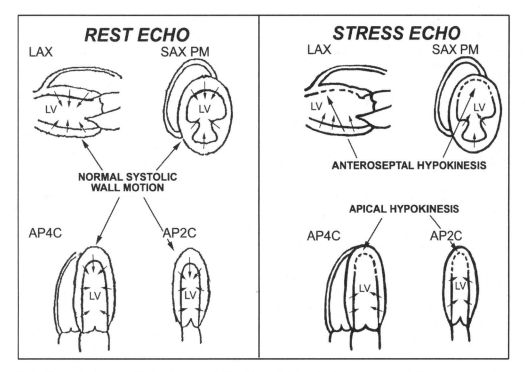

Note: Stress echo images of the heart prior to (left) and immediately following exercise (right). Note the decreased anteroseptal and apical LV wall motion (hypokinesis) post-treadmill stress (arrows) in a patient with ischemia in the LAD distribution. Dobutamine pharmacologic stress echo can be substituted for patients who cannot exercise.

Figure 5-15

on occasion be overlooked because of a uniform decrease in tracer uptake on nuclear scanning. The overall sensitivities for detecting significant stenoses in the LAD, RCA and left circumflex artery are ~ 85%, 80% and 65% respectively. Likewise, difficulty in obtaining a good ultrasound image (due to body habitus, chronic lung disease, or technician inexperience) and the need to image as close to peak exercise as possible may result in a non-diagnostic echo study. Under these circumstances, coronary arteriography may need to be performed to evaluate a "false positive" or "false negative" result. In general, the choice between stress echo and nuclear imaging modalities is determined by patient factors, e.g., ultrasound imaging windows (ability to adequately visualize cardiac structures by echo), and breast tissue and/or

FIGURE 5-16

Stress Echocardiography

LV Wall Motion at rest	LV Wall Motion at peak stress	Clinical Significance
Normal wall motion and endocardial thickening	Hyperdynamic and symmetric wall thickening	Normal or very low likelihood of CAD
Normal wall motion and endocardial thickening	Hypokinetic, akinetic or dyskinetic	CAD (ischemia) without MI
Hypokinesis or akinesis with partial or full endocardial thickening	Augmented (increased wall motion), hypokinetic, akinetic or dyskinetic	Nontransmural MI with viable stunned (if augmented), ischemic (if worsens), or hibernating myocardium (if a biphasic response noted).
Akinetic and thinned wall	Akinetic or dyskinetic	Transmural MI, no viability

diaphragmatic attenuation artifacts on nuclear scan, or by local expertise, availability and cost.

Whenever possible, exercise testing (as opposed to pharmacologic) is the preferred mode of stress testing in patients with suspected or even known CAD. This is because certain exercise variables, such as those used in the Duke treadmill score (*exercise time* in minutes on the Bruce protocol −5 × mm *ST deviation* −4 × *exercise angina* [0 = none, 1 = non-limiting, 2 = limiting]), can provide valuable prognostic information for separating patients into high risk (score < −10), moderate risk (score −10 to +4), and low risk (score ≥ +5) subsets.

Clues to advanced triple vessel or left main CAD include early onset of limiting angina accompanied by marked (≥2 mm) downsloping ST segment depression, occurring in multiple leads, at low workload, lasting for >6 minutes into the recovery period, along with exercise-induced hypotension, chronotropic incompetence (inability of the SA node to pick up speed), and high grade ventricular arrhythmias. When exercise testing is combined with nuclear and/or echo imaging studies, large reversible myocardial perfusion defects or multiple echo wall motion abnormalities, as well as increased lung uptake of radionuclide (leakage, as with CHF fluid), and transient LV cavity dilatation provide additional clues to LV systolic dysfunction caused by severe ischemia.

The diagnostic and predictive accuracy of the exercise ECG is dependent on the population of patients studied, and "false positive" tests results are relatively common in women, especially in those with a low probability of CAD. Keep in mind that the exercise ECG is not diagnostically useful in the presence of LV hypertrophy, LBBB, WPW syndrome, or digitalis therapy (which may confuse the ECG appearance). In these instances, adjunctive nuclear or echo imaging may be useful in detecting signs of ischemia.

Figure 5-17. Pre and post thallium-201 stress scintigrams and ECGs obtained before (left) and after (right) percutaneous transluminal angioplasty (PTCA) to the left anterior descending (LAD) coronary artery. **Left.** Note presence of angina pectoris and marked downsloping ST segment depression at 5.5 min of exercise along with anterior wall perfusion abnormality **Right.** Post-PTCA ECG tracing and perfusion scan is normal, and the patient was symptom-free at 12.5 min of exercise.

Radionuclide Ventriculography and Positron Emission Tomography

The ECG-gated cardiac blood pool scan, also known as the multi-unit gated acquisition (*MUGA*) nuclear scan or radionuclide ventriculogram, is another valuable tool. This scan uses a tracer dose of radioactivity (technetium 99M labeled red blood cells) to "look" directly at LV and RV chamber size, configuration, regional and global wall motion and function (ejection fraction).

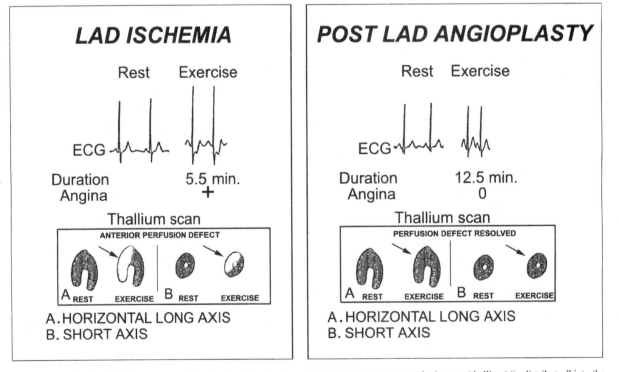

Note: LAD ischemia (left). The anterior wall perfusion defect during exercise disappears at rest as the isotope (thallium) "redistributes" into the ischemic area. Post-LAD angioplasty (right). The perfusion scan is normal during exercise and at rest.

Figure 5-17

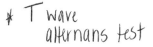
CHAPTER 5. CARDIAC DIAGNOSTIC LABORATORY TESTS

Figure 5-18. Radioisotope ECG gated cardiac blood pool (MUGA) scan which is essentially a radionuclide ventriculogram (LAO view). Using radionuclide-labeled red blood cells, images are triggered or "gated" by the R wave on the ECG and acquired over many cardiac cycles. The amount of radiation in the LV and RV can be measured at end diastole and end systole and their ejection fractions calculated. In this case, end diastolic and end systolic frames depict normal LV and RV wall motion and function.

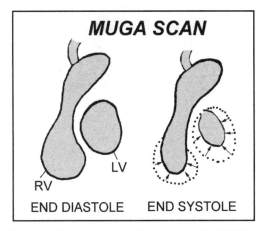

Note: Schematic diagram of multi-unit gated acquistion (MUGA) nuclear scan at end diastole and end systole indicating normal wall motion and function.

Figure 5-18

MUGA scan can be useful in risk assessment or in the serial evaluation of ejection fraction in patients with CHF and MR or AR, and especially in monitoring the effects of chemotherapeutic agents, e.g., doxorubicin (Adriamycin) on LV performance, where accurate LV EF measurement is critical. Echo is the study of choice among many practicing cardiologists, since it is generally less expensive, simpler (i.e., does not involve radioactivity and its attendant problems) and provides additional important detailed anatomical information regarding cardiac structure and valvular function (e.g., assessment of valvular disease, LV hypertrophy and LA size, pericardial effusion, LV thrombus). The MUGA scan requires venipuncture and radiation exposure.

In patients with CAD, regional and global LV dysfunction leading to a reduced ejection fraction on MUGA scan or echo can be the result of irreversible myocardial necrosis (scar), or severely ischemic, but viable (hibernating), myocardium which is likely to regain function after coronary revascularization. Myocardial viability can be assessed non-invasively by *positron emission tomography* (PET), a specialized nuclear imaging technique that uses the metabolic agent 18-Fluorodeoxyglucose (FDG), a glucose analogue taken up by myocardial cells, and a blood flow tracer, e.g., 13-N ammonia or Rubidium-82, to assess both myocardial metabolism and perfusion simultaneously. The presence of increased FDG uptake in regions of reduced blood flow (metabolism-blood flow "mismatch") is characteristic of viable (hibernating) myocardium. Although PET imaging is considered the "gold standard" for the assessment of myocardial viability, its use is limited by its high cost and lack of widespread availability. Hibernating myocardium can also be identified by demonstrating improved (> 50%) tracer uptake (preserved cellular integrity) in "fixed" perfusion defects on late-delayed (24 hour) redistribution or rest-reinjection SPECT myocardial perfusion imaging with thallium-201 or technetium-99m agents, or by demonstrating improved wall motion (contractile reserve) on stress echo in response to inotropic stimulation with low dose dobutamine.

Computed Tomography and Magnetic Resonance Imaging

Conventional *computed tomography* (CT) uses thin X-ray beams to obtain detailed cross-sectional images of the heart, pericardium, and great vessels. Although non-invasive, CT imaging exposes the patient to ionizing radiation and frequently requires the use of intravenous iodinated contrast agents. Its main application is in the detection of aortic dissection and aneurysm, pulmonary emboli, and the evaluation of pericardial and myocardial diseases.

A more recent imaging modality that has received much attention in the evaluation of the cardiac patient is the electron beam CT (EBCT) or ultrafast CT scan. Largely as a result of widespread marketing, the so-called "heart scan" is growing in popularity, particularly among the "worried well" (i.e., individuals without a previous diagnosis of CAD and/or angina) or in those with atypical chest pain, as a rapid, non-invasive "screening" method for assessing the potential risk for CAD. EBCT is far superior to the plain chest film and fluoroscopy in being able to detect coronary artery calcium.

Figure 5-19A. Patient undergoing EBCT. Note large amounts of calcification (white) in the coronary arteries. The amount of calcium can be quantified using the "Agatston score" (< 100 = mild, 100–400 = moderate, > 400 = severe). The greater the amount of coronary calcification, the greater the atherosclerotic plaque burden, and the greater the risk of coronary events.

Although coronary calcium is a well accepted marker for atherosclerosis, its presence does not necessarily indicate significant luminal narrowing or the precise location of stenosis. The test also cannot detect noncalcified, asymptomatic soft plaque, which if ruptured can lead to significant cardiac events. Plaque rupture, a common cause of acute coronary syndromes, is related to the lipid content and inflammatory nature of a plaque, not to the amount of calcium. In general, however, a low coronary calcium score (although it cannot exclude the presence of coronary atherosclerosis) does suggest a lower likelihood of fixed obstructive CAD.

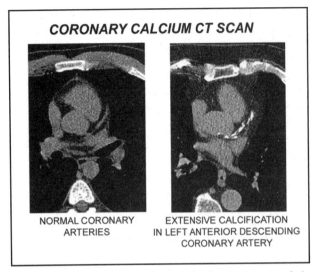

Note: CT coronary calcification correlates closely with the extent of atherosclerotic plaque burden, but does not predict the % of coronary stenosis, nor the presence of a rupture-prone lesion.

Figure 5-19A

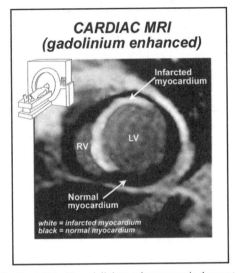

Note: Cardiac MRI with gadolinium enhancement is the most sensitive imaging technique to detect and quantitate the extent of infarcted myocardium.

Figure 5-19B

Conversely, although a high coronary calcium score is associated with advanced plaque burden (often with an obstructive lesion), many atherosclerotic plaques contain calcium but are not flow-limiting. Indeed, coronary calcification may even be found in patients whose coronary angiograms are considered "normal". Since the EBCT scan cannot directly determine coronary blockage (nor the physiologic effect of such blockage) or identify unstable ("rupture-prone") atherosclerotic plaques, it should not be considered a substitute for nuclear and/or echo stress testing, or for coronary angiography in the delineation of coronary anatomy.

The current role of the EBCT coronary calcium score in the diagnosis and management of patients with suspected CAD is uncertain. The extent to which coronary calcium scores predict future coronary events independently of the traditional risk factors remains to be determined. Therefore, the use of EBCT for risk assessment must be weighed against the costs (financial as well as emotional) and the risk that the results of the test may create enough concern for the patient and practitioner to lead to inappropriate, invasive, and expensive coronary evaluation. The general screening of asymptomatic adults is currently not recommended by professional societies. Selective use of coronary calcium scores, however, may be helpful in the screening of individuals at apparently intermediate risk to help guide aggressive lifestyle and risk factor modification, as well as for the evaluation of patients at low risk for CAD who have atypical chest pain.

Thin slice multidetector row CT (MDCT) is another noninvasive imaging technique that correlates well with EBCT in the detection and quantification of coronary calcium. Unlike EBCT, which uses a rapidly oscillating electron beam to sequentially acquire individual CT slices in a

"stop and shoot" fashion as the patient's table is advanced into the CT scanner, MDCT uses the simultaneous rotation of the X-ray tube and continuous movement of the patient's table to acquire the data rapidly in a spiral or helical fashion. The newer MDCT scanners rotate around the patient faster and can acquire up to 64 slices (or higher) per rotation. Contrast-enhanced CT angiography is now being used to noninvasively visualize coronary artery stenoses, and assess the patency of coronary stents and bypass grafts. Limitations include poor visualization of distal vessels and smaller stents (diameter < 3mm), and artifact from metal clips, stent struts, and calcified plaques. The high negative predictive value of MDCT makes it a particularly useful tool in excluding significant coronary stenoses in symptomatic patients with a low to intermediate pre-test likelihood of CAD. With the availability of novel technologies (e.g., fractional flow reserve) that provide physiological assessment of coronary stenosis, coronary CT angiography may evolve from a useful compliment, to a viable alternative, to invasive coronary angiography in selected patients (**Figure 5-33**).

Cardiac *magnetic resonance imaging* (MRI) is yet another noninvasive imaging technique that uses a strong magnetic field and radiofrequency waves to generate high resolution images of the heart, pericardium, and great vessels, without exposure to ionizing radiation or the use of iodinated contrast agents. Like CT, MRI provides detailed anatomic information and is useful in the assessment of aortic aneurysm and dissection, pericardial disease, myocardial abnormalities, cardiac masses, RV dysplasia, and many congenital heart defects. Rapid acquisition sequences can produce high quality cine-mode images demonstrating LV function and wall motion. Dobutamine stress MRI is thus a useful alternative to dobutamine stress echo when acoustic windows are suboptimal. Recent advances have been made in imaging the proximal coronary arteries, congenital coronary anomalies, and bypass grafts, and in assessing myocardial perfusion with the use of intravenous gadolinium, a paramagnetic contrast agent. The vasodilator adenosine can be used with MRI to provoke myocardial ischemia as a type of pharmacologic stress perfusion imaging study. Delayed contrast enhanced MRI imaging, using intravenous gadolinium, has been shown to reliably identify infarcted tissue (scar) which retains contrast and appears "hyperenhanced" relative to viable, reversibily ischemic, myocardium.

Figure 5-19B. Contrast enhanced cardiac MRI (short axis view) in a patient with an anteroseptal MI. Note infarcted, nonviable myocardium appears hyperenhanced (white), compared with normal, viable myocardium (black).

MRI is relatively contraindicated in patients with pacemakers and ICDs. With the exception of older ball-cage valves, MRI can be performed safely in patients with mechanical valves and coronary stents. Patients with claustrophobia, however, may have difficulty in the confined space of the "tunnel-like" MRI scanner. Of note, the use of gadolinium has been linked to a rapidly progressive form of systemic sclerosis called nephrogenic systemic fibrosis and should be avoided, if possible, in patients with impaired renal function.

SPECIALIZED INVASIVE TECHNIQUES

The modern cardiac catheterization and electrophysiology laboratories are a complex environment in which various types of diagnostic and therapeutic procedures are often performed on critically ill patients. This section discusses the appropriate clinical indications and practical applications of these elaborate and expensive catheter-based techniques in this cost-driven era of aggressive cardiac intervention and managed care.

Cardiac Catheterization: Coronary Angiography and Left Ventriculography

Nowadays, cardiac catheterization, including *coronary angiography* and *left ventriculography,* is the "gold standard" for the diagnosis and quantification of the location, extent and severity (% stenosis) of CAD, and for making treatment decisions regarding whether medical therapy, percutaneous coronary intervention (PCI), or bypass surgery should be considered. By means of a cardiac catheter, pressures in the heart can be measured, oxygen saturation can be assessed, and by injecting radio-opaque contrast medium, coronary and great vessel anatomy along with left ventricular wall motion and function can be determined.

Figure 5-20. Cardiac catheterization. A guiding catheter is inserted into the femoral (brachial or radial) artery in the groin (arm or wrist) via a sheath and advanced through the aorta to the coronary arteries. X-ray contrast medium is injected to detect any narrowing. The schematic diagram illustrates significant narrowing of the proximal portion of the left anterior descending coronary artery. Note varying degrees of segmental wall motion abnormalities that can be detected: *hypokinesis* (decreased wall motion), *akinesis* (no wall motion), *dyskinesis* (paradoxical wall motion) as may be seen on left ventriculography.

Clinical symptoms which favor referral for cardiac cath include:

- Unstable or worsening angina
- CHF and valve dysfunction

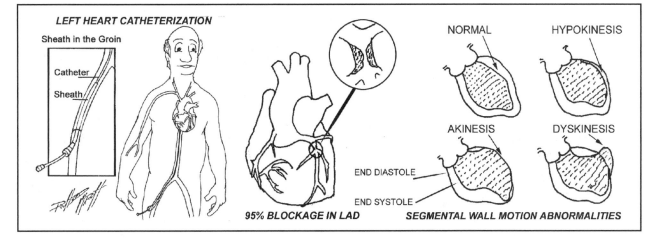

Note: The femoral artery is the most common access site in the U.S. The radial artery approach, although technically more challenging, is gaining in popularity (earlier ambulation, decreased access site bleeding complications, improved patient comfort), particularly in patients with severe PAD or morbid obesity.

Figure 5-20

- Suspected acute MI or cardiogenic shock
- An obscure or confusing problem that appears to be cardiac in origin

Coronary angiography should also be considered in patients with severe angina refractory to optimal medical therapy, strongly positive stress tests with evidence of extensive myocardial ischemia, those with angina who have survived sudden cardiac death, or those who have had PCI or CABG with subsequent recurrence of symptoms. It can be used to determine whether bypass grafts or native vessels are occluded (or restenosed), if CAD is present in patients with cardiomyopathy of unknown cause, and, in patients with valvular heart disease undergoing valve surgery, to determine whether concomitant CABG should be performed if the anatomy is compelling.

There are some patients who suffer from recurrent chest pain along with repeated and costly hospitalizations ("frequent flyers"), in whom noninvasive testing has yielded negative or equivocal results. These patients may be severely disabled by these symptoms and may also benefit from coronary arteriography to exclude CAD, and thereby remove uncertainty, provide reassurance and expedite the patient's return to a normal active life.

In patients with suspected variant angina and normal coronary arteries, ergonovine maleate (a drug that causes coronary vasospasm producing focal spasm in ~90% of patients) can be used as a provocative agent during the procedure. Since life-threatening arrhythmias and/or profound spasm unresponsive to nitrates may develop, however, ergonovine provocation should not be used outside a closely-monitored setting.

Less common indications for cardiac catheterization include patients with a strong family history of premature CAD and/or death, and a "need to know" situation (e.g., airline pilots). Not every patient with "possible" angina pectoris, however, needs coronary angiography, particularly if the pre-test likelihood of significant CAD is extremely low and the patient has no evidence of myocardial ischemia on adequate (85% of age-predicted maximal heart rate) noninvasive stress testing.

Cardiac cath will answer such questions as, "Does the patient have significant CAD?" (defined as $\geq$ 50% narrowing of the left main and $\geq$ 70% narrowing of the other coronary arteries); "Is the patient a suitable candidate for coronary intervention, and if so, which intervention (PCI/CABG) is most appropriate?" *Intravascular ultrasound* (IVUS) and *optical coherence tomography* (OCT) imaging, which allows direct visualization of the vessel wall, and coronary pressure wire derived *fractional flow reserve* (FFR), which provides physiologic determination of the pressure difference across a coronary blockage, are adjunctive techniques used to assess the anatomic and functional severity of "intermediate" (40-70%) coronary stenoses, and help guide angioplasty and stent procedures.

In general, the most common indications for percutaneous transluminal coronary angioplasty (PTCA) and stenting include:

- Significant anatomic ($\geq$70%) or physiologic (FFR < 0.80) stenosis in one or more coronary arteries with evidence of refractory or unstable angina, severe ischemia, "high risk" stress test
- Acute MI with plaque rupture/thrombus of the infarct-related coronary artery.

PCI has progressed in the past several years and can now be performed in patients with multivessel CAD, left main stenosis, chronic total occlusions, and diseased vein grafts. Efforts to solve coronary artery restenosis have centered on limiting neointimal hyperplasia through intravascular radiation (*brachytherapy*), which has fallen out of favor, and more recently, *drug-eluting stents*.

In addition to defining the anatomy and providing a "road map" of the coronary arteries, cardiac catheterization, specifically *left ventriculography* and *supravalvular aortography,* can be helpful in assessing LV chamber size, regional wall motion abnormalities, global LV function (ejection fraction), structural abnormalities (e.g., LV aneurysm, thrombi) and the presence and severity of mitral and/or aortic valve disease in patients being considered for mechanical (PCI, valvuloplasty) and/or surgical intervention. Left ventriculography in patients with CAD may demonstrate reversible wall motion abnormalities after an extrasystolic beat (PVC) or nitroglycerin administration. Such reversible hypokinetic or akinetic wall motion often shows improvement after CABG or PCI.

Figure 5-21. Schematic diagram of coronary arteriogram (Left coronary artery in the right anterior oblique [RAO] view and the Right coronary artery in the left anterior oblique [LAO] view).

Figure 5-22. Schematic diagram of left ventriculogram.

The degree of mitral and/or aortic valvular regurgitation can be roughly estimated from contrast injections in the LV and aorta, respectively, and is expressed as mild to severe based on a grading scale of 1+ to 4+ (**Figure 5-23**).

Figure 5-23. Schematic diagram of contrast angiography showing the severity of valvular regurgitation:

Top. LV angiogram in mitral regurgitation. **Left.** "Whiff" of MR that is rapidly cleared. **Middle.** Moderate MR with complete opacification of the left atrium. **Right.** Severe MR with rapid and complete opacification of the entire left atrium and pulmonary veins.

Bottom. Supravalvular aortogram in aortic regurgitation. **Left.** Mild AR with incomplete LV opacification that is cleared with each beat. **Middle.** Moderate AR with complete LV opacification. **Right.** Severe AR with rapid LV opacification with slow clearing. Enlargement of the chamber receiving the regurgitant volume may occur in patients with chronic valvular regurgitation.

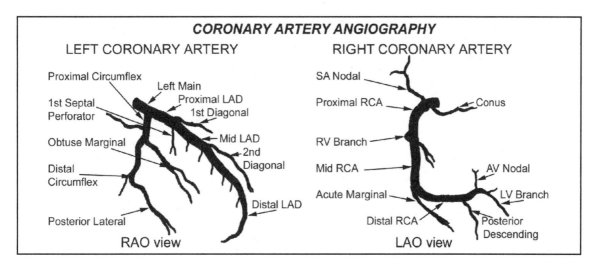

Note: Normal angiographic coronary anatomy. The major arteries are the left main, left anterior descending, left circumflex, and right coronary arteries. In the majority of patients, the posterior descending artery arises from the right coronary artery (right dominant), and from the left circumflex (left dominant) or both arteries (co-dominant) in the remainder. The coronary arteries and their branches should be viewed in two or more projections for adequate visualization.

Figure 5-21

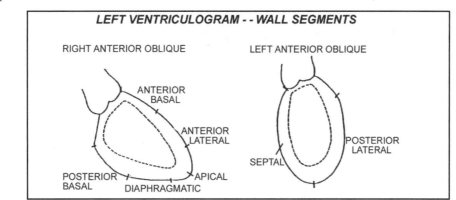

Note: Schematic diagram of left ventriculogram in diastole (solid line) and systole (dotted line) in the RAO and LAO projections, which enables assessment of LV wall motion and function (normal ejection fraction ≥ 55%).

Figure 5-22

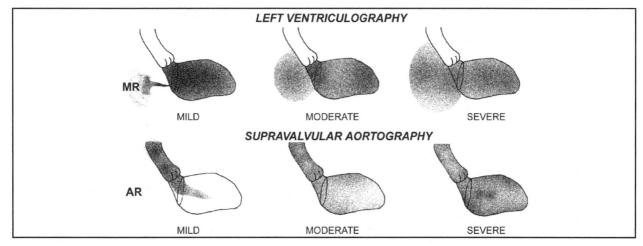

Note: Schematic diagram of left ventriculogram (top) and supravalvular aortogram (bottom), which enables assessment of the degree of mitral and aortic regurgitation respectively.

Figure 5-23

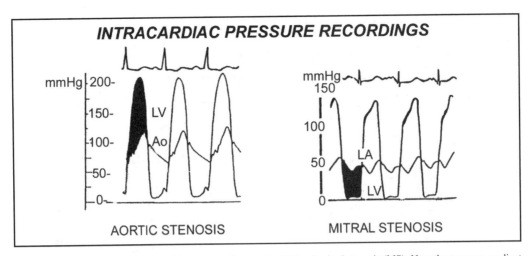

INTRACARDIAC PRESSURE RECORDINGS

AORTIC STENOSIS

MITRAL STENOSIS

Note: Pressure tracings in a patient with severe aortic stenosis (AS) and mitral stenosis (MS). Note the pressure gradient (shaded area) between the left ventricle (LV) and aorta (Ao) during systole in AS (left) and between the left atrium (LA) and LV during diastole in MS (right). The magnitute of the gradient is determined by the severity of the stenosis and the flow across the valve. When the cardiac output is normal, the higher the pressure gradient, the greater the degree of stenosis.

Figure 5-24

Additional information that can be obtained at the time of cardiac catheterization includes measuring the intracardiac pressures, gradients across stenotic valves, and waveform recordings. From these pressure recordings and hemodynamic measurements, the effective valve area can be calculated (*Gorlin formula*) (**Figure 5-24**).

Figure 5-24. Pressure wave forms in aortic stenosis (left) and mitral stenosis (right). **Left.** Note significant systolic pressure gradient between the left ventricle (LV) and the ascending aorta (Ao) in a patient with severe valvular aortic stenosis. The aortic pulse tracing demonstrates an anacrotic notch and a delayed peak typical of a fixed obstruction in the LV outflow tract. An estimation of the stenotic aortic valve area may be made by using a simplified version of the *Gorlin formula:* Aortic valve area equals the cardiac output divided by the square root of the LV–AO pressure gradient (**Figure 15-5**). Thus, for the patient with aortic stenosis with a cardiac output of 5 liters per min. and an LV–AO systolic gradient of 100 mmHg, the aortic valve area = $5 \div \sqrt{100} = 5/10 = 0.5$ cm^2. Note, for the Gorlin formula, that a patient with CHF and severe aortic valve stenosis may have only a relatively low pressure gradient if the cardiac output is also low. **Right.** Note the large diastolic pressure gradient between the left atrium (LA) and left ventricle (LV) in a patient with severe mitral stenosis. The left atrial pressure is elevated due to obstruction to blood flow across the mitral valve in diastole ("mitral block").

By combining both a right and left heart catheterization, and measuring oxygen saturation in the cardiac chambers and vessels, it can be determined whether there is a "step-up" in oxygen saturation and an intracardiac shunt (e.g., ASD, VSD, or PDA) (**Figure 5-25**).

Intracardiac pressure recordings (**Figure 5-26**) can help in evaluating the severity of HOCM (**Figure 16-5**), dilated cardiomyopathies and constrictive pericarditis. (**Figure 19-9**). Right heart catheterization can also be used to determine the presence and severity of pulmonary hypertension, test pulmonary vasoreactivity, and guide therapy (**Figure 20-3**).

Figure 5-26. Normal intracardiac pressure recordings during right heart catheterization. Keep in mind the "rule of 6's" i.e., right atrial (RA) pressure ≤ 6 mmHg, right ventricular (RV) pressure $\leq 30/6$ mmHg, pulmonary artery (PA) pressure $\leq 30/12$ mmHg, pulmonary capillary wedge pressure (PCWP) ≤ 12 mmHg.

Figure 5-27. Left. Schematic representation of flow-directed balloon-tipped (Swan-Ganz) catheter being floated into the pulmonary artery. Note the pulmonary artery (PA) catheter tip wedged into a branch of the pulmonary artery sensing pressure reflected back from the left atrium. **Right.** Pulmonary capillary wedge (PCW) pressure in a patient with an acute inferior MI with papillary muscle rupture and acute severe mitral regurgitation. Note the characteristic tall V waves that reflect marked regurgitation into a normally small, nondistendible left atrium.

Although the risk of catheterization is relatively small, a definite morbidity is involved, along with a certain degree of patient discomfort. The most common complications of cardiac catheterization and interventional procedures include:

- Myocardial perforation by the catheter
- Coronary artery dissection, air or thromboembolism
- Abrupt closure
- Acute MI
- No reflow syndrome (i.e., failure to restore normal blood flow despite removal of coronary obstruction)
- Occlusion of side branch vessels (*"stent jail"*)
- Vascular injury (pseudoaneurysm, AV fistula)
- Dislodgement of atherosclerotic plaque
- Infection
- Precipitation of arrhythmias and conduction blocks
- Hematoma/retroperitoneal bleeding
- Stent thrombosis, and most frequently native coronary and in-stent restenosis
- Allergic reaction to contrast; renal failure

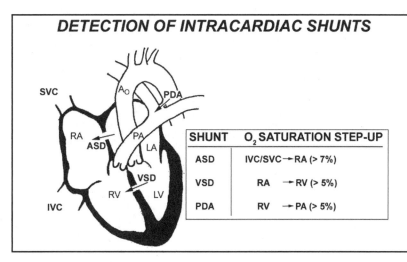

Note: Detection of an intracardiac shunt can be accomplished by measuring oxygen (O_2) saturation in the right heart chambers and vena cava. A "step-up" in O_2 saturation between the proximal chamber and the shunted chamber localizes the site of a left-to-right shunt (e.g., ASD, VSD, or PDA).

Figure 5-25

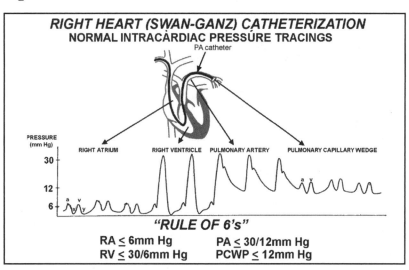

Note: Passage of a balloon-tipped catheter, permits recording of pressures in the right side of the heart. Keep in mind the "rule of 6's" when considering the range of normal intracardiac pressures.

Figure 5-26

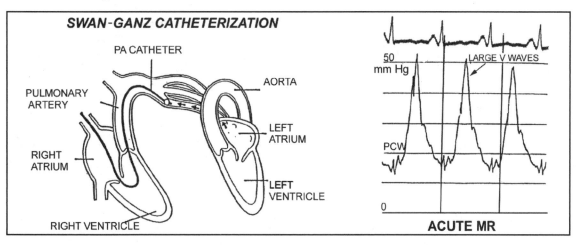

Note: Left. Diagram of PA flotation catheter with the balloon inflated in the pulmonary capillary wedge position (PCWP reflects left atrial pressure). Right. In acute severe MR, tall V waves are present on the PCWP tracing.

Figure 5-27

Furthermore, catheterization is relatively costly compared to other diagnostic evaluations. It should not be employed, therefore, as a "screening" procedure in patients without suspected significant underlying heart disease. The balance of risk and benefit is not the same for all patients with a positive stress test. Coronary angiography is sensible, for example, in a symptomatic, but otherwise "fit" patient with a markedly positive stress test, because the prognosis and symptoms may be altered by coronary artery bypass surgery. The same is not necessarily true for an older, asymptomatic patient with chronic pulmonary disease, since bypass surgery may not be an option anyway. With the availability of various noninvasive techniques to confirm clinical diagnoses, invasive catheterization studies should generally be reserved for those patients in whom a therapeutic (interventional, surgical) as well as diagnostic decision needs to be made. It is important to keep in mind that certain general medical factors can influence the outcome of an interventional or surgical procedure. These include preexisting infection, severe anemia, active bleeding, metabolic derangements, severe peripheral vascular disease, cerebrovascular disease, renal insufficiency, hypersensitivity to radiographic contrast agents, and certain medications, e.g., metformin (Glucophage, an oral hypoglycemic agent, which should be held in diabetics around the time of iodinated contrast since both the contrast and the metformin predispose to lactic acidosis).

Electrophysiologic Studies (EPS)

Cardiac arrhythmias are often difficult to identify since they may occur intermittently. In many patients a precise diagno-

sis may be difficult to obtain with noninvasive techniques. For such an individual, intracardiac electrophysiologic studies (EPS) using multipolar electrode catheters introduced into either the venous or arterial circulation and advanced to various positions in the heart, allow for the detection and recording of the timing and conduction of electrical impulses (like an "internal ECG"), and/or the induction of an arrhythmia and the elucidation of its mechanism and characteristics. These tests are expensive, invasive and generally not useful in patients without heart disease or an abnormal ECG since the yield is then very low (~10%). EPS should be used only when the information cannot be obtained in any noninvasive way and if it is likely to alter prognosis or therapy.

Figure 5-28. Left. Schematic representation of the electrophysiological anatomy of the right atrium and ventricle. **Right.** Common catheter positions for recording electrical events in the high right atrium **A)** His bundle **B)** RV apex **C)** RV outflow **D)** and coronary sinus **E)** and **F)** (courtesy of Drs. Ross D. Fletcher and Albert A. Del Negro).

EPS can be a valuable tool in the evaluation of patients with unexplained syncope or in survivors of sudden cardiac death to help determine the underlying cause, decide on the appropriate treatment, or quantify risk in patients with known or suspected VT or SVT, especially if catheter ablation of an abnormal pathway or an implantable cardioverter-defibrillator (ICD) is being considered. It may help to evaluate sinus node function and uncover an AV conduction abnormality (block in the AV node, His bundle, or bundle branches), and the need for a pacemaker that cannot be determined by clinical means alone. EPS may also be useful in revealing reentry circuits at the AV node, and in the evaluation of preexcitation

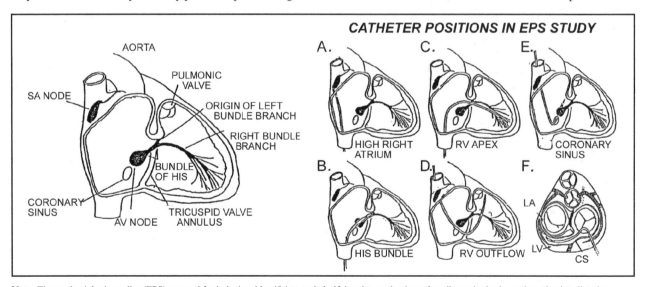

Note: Electrophysiologic studies (EPS) are used for inducing, identifying, and clarifying the mechanism of cardiac arrhythmias and conduction disturbances as well as for potential treatment (e.g., catheter ablation). Electroanatomical mapping is commonly used to localize sites for ablation and to follow catheter position.

Figure 5-28

(WPW) syndromes to map bypass tracts and therapeutically terminate tachyarrhythmias (radiofrequency ablation of an AV nodal or accessory pathway).

Additionally, through programmed electrical stimulation of the ventricle, it can be determined whether VT can be induced in the laboratory under controlled circumstances, and if the implantation of a cardioverter defibrillator is warranted, with or without antiarrhythmic therapy (e.g., amiodarone), or ablation of arrhythmic foci.

The most common arrhythmia detected by EPS is VT, and the most powerful predictor of a positive EPS is an EF of <40%. In patients with underlying heart disease (e.g., previous MI), for example, particularly if the SAECG shows late potentials, a ventricular tachyarrhythmia is likely to be the cause of syncope, and EPS testing is generally a better initial diagnostic test than tilt-table testing. In patients without structural heart disease, invasive EPS testing may be useful if recurrent syncope remains unexplained in the face of negative tilt-table test results. It must be understood, however, that failure to elicit an arrhythmia during EPS does not provide absolute assurance that the patient will not suffer from the rhythm disturbance in another setting. In addition, false-positive EPSs do occur.

Figure 5-29 summarizes the clinical indications for EPS testing.

SUMMARY: NON-INVASIVE AND INVASIVE TEST INDICATIONS AND APPLICATIONS

Figure 5-30 and **5-31** summarize the overall clinical indications and practical applications for cardiac noninvasive and invasive laboratory tests.

Keep in mind that no test is "fool-proof". False positives and negatives occur, even in the best of hands. Visual estimates used to define coronary narrowing, for example, may vary from one catheterization laboratory to the next, depending on the operator. Before ordering a diagnostic test, you should ask, "What additional information will the test provide"?, and "what will be done with the results"? If the treatment plan is the same regardless of the test results, then the test may be unnecessary.

Whenever possible, select those tests that are safe, convenient, and cost-effective (**Figure 5-32**). Redundancy must be avoided to achieve a favorable cost/benefit ratio. For example, a MUGA scan will often yield information regarding LV function that can be obtained from an echo, and both methods may be superfluous if the patient is destined to undergo left ventriculography as part of a cardiac catheterization procedure. While cardiac catheterization has long been considered the "gold standard" for detecting coronary stenoses, 64-and higher-slice CT angiography

---

FIGURE 5-29

Clinical Indications for Electrophysiologic Testing

Syncopal Indications

- Suspected structural heart disease and syncope that remains unexplained after appropriate evaluation.
- Recurrent unexplained syncope without structural heart disease and a negative head-up tilt test.
- Sinus node dysfunction or His-Purkinje block (high-grade AV block) is suspected as the cause of symptoms (but a causal relation has not been established).
- Nonspecific intraventricular conduction delay where the cause of symptoms is not known.
- Syncope plus presence of ventricular preexcitation (WPW) syndrome.
- Palpitations preceding syncope.

Major Nonsyncopal Indications

- Frequent or poorly tolerated episodes of supraventricular tachycardia that do not adequately respond to drug therapy.
- Wide QRS complex tachycardia where the correct diagnosis is unclear.
- Evaluation for catheter ablation of an accessory pathway.
- Other risk factors for future arrhythmic events, (e.g., low ejection fraction, positive signal-averaged ECG, and nonsustained VT on ambulatory ECG recordings) where electrophysiologic studies will be used for further risk assessment and for guiding therapy in patients with inducible VT.
- Cardiac arrest without evidence of an acute STEMI or occurring more than 48 hrs after the acute phase of MI in the absence of a recurrent ischemic event.

test Review Summary

FIGURE 5-30

Cardiac Noninvasive Laboratory Tests

TEST	CLINICAL INDICATIONS	PRACTICAL APPLICATIONS
2D color-flow Doppler transthoracic echo (TTE)	Assesses valve function and pathology, detects myocardial and pericardial disease, measures chamber dimensions and ventricular function, right heart and pulmonary pressures, intracardiac shunts, and identifies cardiac masses and tumors.	Assists in the evaluation of "significant" (not "innocent") heart murmurs, symptoms of chest pain, dyspnea, or stroke; assesses LV and RV systolic and diastolic function (ejection fraction, ventricular filling patterns) and resting wall motion abnormalities in patients with CAD, CHF, cardiomyopathy or valve disease, (especially if worsening symptoms), and identifies mechanical complications in patients post-MI.
Transesophageal echo (TEE)	Provides unimpeded view of LA, mitral valve apparatus and descending aorta.	Higher sensitivity and specificity than transthoracic echo in identifying source of emboli (LA thrombus, PFO, atrial myxoma), native and prosthetic valve disease, small vegetations in infective endocarditis and thoracic aortic dissection. Helps direct mitral and aortic valve repair and guidance of pericardiocentesis.
Ambulatory (Holter) ECG monitoring	Documents frequent tachy and/or bradyarrhythmias and conduction disturbances.	Correlation of symptoms (e.g., patients with unexplained palpitations, dizziness, syncope) possibly related to rhythm or conduction disturbance. Helps assess therapeutic response (e.g., antiarrhythmic drugs, pacemaker and ICD function, catheter ablation).
Event recording	Detects episodic paroxysmal arrhythmias.	Correlation of symptoms and rhythm abnormalities that are infrequent or unexpected.
Signal averaged ECG	Detects late potentials in the terminal portion of the QRS complex.	Identifies patients at increased risk for VT or sudden death after MI.
T wave alternans testing	Detects microvolt beat-to-beat variation in T wave morphology and/or amplitude during exercise or pacing.	Identifies patients at increased risk of VT/VF and sudden cardiac death.
Tilt table testing	Elicits vasodepressor response (↓ BP, ↓ HR).	Confirms neurocardiogenic (vasovagal) syncope as mechanism in patients without structural heart disease.
Stress test Exercise or Pharmacologic (dipyridamole, adenosine, dobutamine), if unable to exercise (e.g., severe peripheral vascular disease, orthopedic disability)	Detects obstructive CAD, identifies location and extent of ischemia, assesses the need for or adequacy of revascularization.	Helpful in diagnosing the presence and severity of CAD, risk stratification, functional class assessment and prognosis, especially in patients with intermediate probability chest pain, and in patients after MI and before noncardiac surgery. Cardiopulmonary exercise testing (stress ECG combined with ventilatory gas exchange analysis) helps in differentiating a cardiac from a pulmonary cause of impaired exercise capacity, and in assessing the need for cardiac transplantation in select patients with advanced CHF.

FIGURE 5-30

Cardiac Noninvasive Laboratory Tests (*continued*)

TEST	CLINICAL INDICATIONS	PRACTICAL APPLICATIONS
Adjunctive imaging • **nuclear** (Thallium, sestamibi) • **echo**	Especially useful in patients with abnormal baseline ECG (e.g., resting ST-T abnormalities, digoxin therapy, LV hypertrophy, preexcitation (WPW) syndrome, LBBB, electronically paced ventricular rhythm) or to evaluate functional significance of a known coronary lesion.	Early, marked (>2 mm) and persistent ST segment depression in multiple leads accompanied by angina, exercise-induced hypotension or VT, along with large, multiple, fixed (infarction or scar) and/or reversible (ischemia) nuclear perfusion defects, or echo wall motion abnormalities, transient LV dilatation, ↑ lung tracer uptake is associated with a poor prognosis and/or more severe CAD. Helps assess myocardial viability.
MUGA scan (Radionuclide ventriculogram)	Measures LV (and RV) function (ejection fraction) and wall motion.	Helps in assessing global LV (and RV) function, especially in patients receiving cancer chemotherapy (e.g., anthracycline-induced [doxorubicin] cardiomyopathy).
Positron emission tomography (PET)	Assesses myocardial perfusion and metabolism.	Distinguishes viable myocardium from scar tissue.
Conventional computed tomography (CT)	Provides detailed anatomic images of the heart, pericardium, and great vessels.	Helps in the detection of aortic dissection and aneurysm, pulmonary emboli, and the evaluation of pericardial and myocardial diseases.
EBCT scan	Detects coronary artery calcification.	Indicator of atherosclerotic plaque burden (does not identify "vulnerable" plaque or precisely determine degree of coronary blockage). May assist in risk stratification.
MDCT scan	Visualizes coronary stenoses, anomalous coronary arteries, and atherosclerotic plaque.	Helps in the detection of CAD (high negative predictive value), and the assessment of coronary stent and bypass graft patency.
MRI	Provides high resolution images of heart, pericardium, and great vessels.	Helps in the assessment of aortic and pericardial disease, myocardial abnormalities, cardiac masses, RV dysplasia, congenital heart defects, anomalous and proximal coronary arteries, myocardial perfusion and viability.

FIGURE 5-31

Cardiac Invasive Laboratory Tests

TEST	CLINICAL INDICATIONS	PRACTICAL APPLICATIONS
Cardiac catheterization	Delineates coronary anatomy and severity of stenoses in chronic stable and acute unstable coronary syndromes, assesses LV contractile function, quantitates stenotic valve gradient, area, and regurgitation, and detects shunt lesions.	The "gold standard" in the diagnosis and treatment of CAD; valvular, myocardial, and congenital abnormalities and for making treatment decisions (e.g., medical, interventional, or surgical).
EPS	Defines conduction system disease, elicits SVT and VT.	Helps in the diagnosis and treatment of patients with severe, life threatening or hemodynamically important arrhythmias (e.g., RF catheter ablation, ICD). Measures response to pharmacologic and/or pacing/device intervention.

FIGURE 5-32

Cost of Selective Diagnostic Methods

- Electrocardiogram — $
- Chest x-ray (PA and lateral) — $
- Exercise stress test — $$
- Ambulatory (Holter) monitor — $$+
- Color-flow Doppler echocardiogram — $$$
- Transesophageal echocardiogram — $$$+
- Exercise radio-isotope scanning, — $$$$
  e.g., Thallium, Cardiolite
- Cardiac catheterization — $$$$$
  with angiography
- Cardiac clinical examination — *Priceless!*

---

may be a viable alternative in symptomatic patients with a low to intermediate probability of CAD or in those with an equivocal stress test. Both procedures require iodinated contrast and expose the patient to radiation. A normal coronary CT angiogram (CCTA) has a very high negative predictive value (99%) for significant CAD. The quality of images in CCTA, however, is limited by calcification and the presence of cardiac motion, which can be reduced by slowing the heart rate with β-blocker therapy. Current CT technology can also be used as a powerful "triple rule-out"

in the diagnosis of CAD, aortic dissection, and pulmonary embolism, in patients presenting with chest pain in the emergency department (**Figure 5-33**).

Figure 5-33. MDCT: the "triple rule-out". **Left.** 64-slice CT coronary angiography, 3 dimensional volume rendered image, demonstrating high grade stenosis of the left anterior descending (LAD) coronary artery. **Middle.** Contrast-enhanced CT scan demonstrating aortic dissection. **Right.** Spiral CT pulmonary angiography demonstrating bilateral pulmonary thromboembolism.

In general, the more complicated and expensive tests should be reserved for patients who have a higher chance of having significant heart disease and for those in whom the results of simpler clinical and/or noninvasive methods do not elicit a clear-cut or logical answer. Furthermore, it is not always necessary to perform invasive or noninvasive testing to assess the results of therapeutic intervention. Symptomatic improvement and changes in functional class can often be assessed on clinical grounds alone. In patients with CHF, for example, a reduction in heart rate, peripheral edema, and jugular venous pulse, resolution of rales and pulsus alternans, a decrease in severity of secondary MR (due to papillary muscle dysfunction), and disappearance of the S3 gallop are all important indicators of improvement in cardiac performance. As more elaborate and higher risk procedures are being used, you must be certain that the risks to which the patient is exposed are justified by the benefits to be gained.

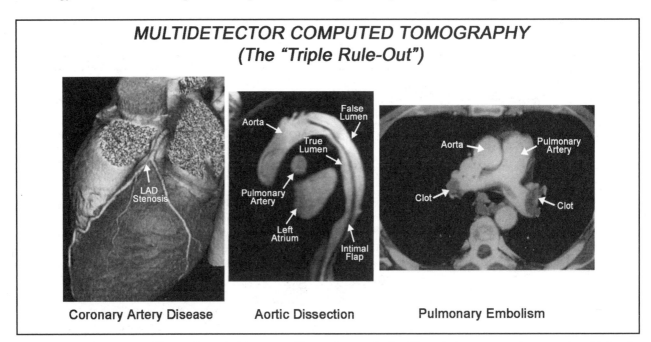

MULTIDETECTOR COMPUTED TOMOGRAPHY (The "Triple Rule-Out")

Coronary Artery Disease   Aortic Dissection   Pulmonary Embolism

Note: For patients who present with acute chest pain, it is now possible to perform an ultrafast CT scan in the emergency department that will allow for the simultaneous evaluation of CAD, aortic dissection, and pulmonary thromboembolic disease – the so-called "triple rule-out". The procedure requires higher doses of radiation and iodinated contrast, however, for simultaneous opacification of the coronary arteries, aorta, and pulmonary arteries.

Figure 5-33

PART II.   CARDIOVASCULAR THERAPEUTICS

The following chapters provide a practical overview of cardiovascular therapy. Major emphasis will be placed on the various therapeutic modalities used to treat the myriad cardiac problems encountered in clinical practice. It is important to understand the natural history of the cardiac disease, both untreated and treated, before recommending drug, device or surgical interventions. Keep in mind that a disease encountered during an earlier stage may require less aggressive intervention than at a later stage in the natural history. Decisions regarding the appropriate treatment of the cardiac patient are based on the best scientific evidence available and guided by sound clinical judgment. This can be acquired only through clinical experience gleaned by caring for many patients over a long period of time. Remember, *good judgment comes from experience…which often comes from bad judgment.*

CHAPTER 6.
CARDIOVASCULAR THERAPY:
AN OVERVIEW

GENERAL CONSIDERATIONS AND TREATMENT GOALS

Before considering what may be life-long treatment for the patient, you should consider the long-term efficacy of the drug and/or procedure, and what negative effects can be expected (i.e., is the treatment worse than the disease?). The risk of treatment should be outweighed by its benefit to the patient. It is surprising how uncritical today's practitioners can be in embracing new therapies without asking critical questions regarding proof of efficacy. With new treatments being advertised to the lay public (through the Internet, television commercials, and other print media), and patients often requesting them before they can be properly evaluated, you should develop a healthy skepticism about claims regarding a new drug's efficacy and/or safety, and seek out objective sources before prescribing them. The history of cardiovascular therapeutics includes many examples of new treatments initially recommended enthusiastically, but later abandoned as useless or worse, even harmful. Some of these new therapies were actually tested by well-designed clinical trials with results seemingly indicative of effectiveness, yet later disproved, and even taken off the market after discovery of serious side effects. You would do well to follow a conservative strategy of "watchful waiting" whenever pos-

sible, before pushing your patient too rapidly into new treatments. There are times, however, when a major "breakthrough" in management is demonstrated to be safe and effective and therefore should be utilized sooner.

The haphazard administration of a large number of drugs is more likely to create harm than benefit. Always keep in mind factors such as side effects, ease of administration, desires and/or compliance of the patient, and cost considerations when determining the appropriate therapy for the individual patient. Remember to take a "good look" at your patient. After all, you are not treating a disease, you are treating a patient who has the disease. Two patients with the same cardiac condition may respond differently to the same medication. What may be an effective medication for one patient may be toxic for another. Most drug side effects can be prevented by a careful review of the patient's clinical database (i.e., age, liver and kidney function, presence of associated diseases, and other medications). Adverse drug reactions are often dose-dependent, and correct dosing minimizes patient's risk.

In addition to compiling a list of medications and their side effects, specifically inquire about whether your patient is allergic to iodine, which is present in the contrast medium used during cardiac catheterization and CT scanning. Keep in mind that patients, who claim to have an aspirin allergy, but instead have had GI upset, are usually able to tolerate aspirin after undergoing stent implantation.

Figure 6-1. Ask your patients (or their spouses) to describe how they take their medication. Safe and appropriate medication use requires close adherence to the five "*rights*": *right* patient, *right* drug, *right* dose, *right* route, *right* time.

It is important to find out what medicines, prescription or nonprescription (i.e., over-the-counter, including herbal remedies) the patient is taking and how they are being administered. Are they being swallowed, inhaled (e.g., bronchodilators, steroids) or applied topically (e.g., timolol eye drops)? Some cardiac medications may actually harm patients, and even increase their chances of dying. Sometimes cardiac medications can mimic the very signs and symptoms for which they were given! For example: class IA and III antiarrhythmic agents used in the treatment VT can prolong the QT interval, and cause the VT called "*torsades de pointes*" and recurrent syncope, and thus, ironically produce the same fatal ventricular arrhythmia that one is trying to prevent.

Other causes of this potentially lethal ventricular arrhythmia include diuretics (due to hypokalemia, hypomagnesemia), phenothiazines, tricyclic antidepressants, liquid protein diets, and the use of certain non-sedating antihistamines, e.g., terfenadine (Seldane), astemizole (Hismanal) in combination with cytochrome P-450 inhibitors (e.g., erythromycin, and other macrolide antibiotics) and grapefruit juice. This is not merely "pulp fiction"! You should instruct your patients to refrain from drinking grapefruit juice when they are taking drugs that are known to be susceptible to this interaction.

A dry, nonproductive cough is a particularly annoying side effect of long-term ACE inhibitor therapy. It occurs in ~5-20% of patients, and is thought to be caused by increased bradykinin levels. There is no relationship between the dose of the ACE inhibitor and the development of cough. Although cough most often occurs within the first few weeks of therapy, it may occur 6 months after the initiation of an ACE inhibitor. In patients with known CHF, the presence of chronic cough may also be a manifestation of suboptimal treatment. Keep in mind that a patient who has developed a cough from an ACE inhibitor in the past will not be pleased to find out that his or her "new" medication is another form of the offending agent. Switching to a different ACE inhibitor is rarely effective in reducing this bothersome side effect. ARBs are a better alternative for most patients with intractable cough.

Worthy of mention, antiarrhythmic drugs are not recommended for PVCs in asymptomatic patients without cardiac disease. Instead, you should encourage your patient to avoid stimulants (e.g., nicotine, caffeine, alcohol). Keep in mind that hypokalemia and hypomagnesemia, which may occur in patients taking diuretics, can also precipitate PVCs, and should be corrected.

Figure 6-2 summarizes potential side effects (both cardiovascular and non-cardiovascular) that can arise from drugs currently utilized for the treatment of various heart conditions.

Cardiac patients should be counseled regarding the risks of using drugs e.g., sildenafil (Viagra) to treat erectile dysfunction. Sildenafil is potentially hazardous in patients with acute coronary syndromes, CHF, borderline hypotension and low volume status, and complicated antihypertensive therapy since this agent is also a systemic vasodilator and it may exacerbate hypotension. Recent nitrate use is an absolute contraindication to use of Viagra-like agents (due to the potential for severe hypotension). In the management of acute coronary syndromes developing after sildenafil use, no nitrates should be administered within the first 24 hours (but other routine therapy should not be withheld). Viagra is now allowing older men who have previously not been able to have sex to resume sexual activity. What these patients may not realize is that the sexual environment has changed. Often, they do not use condoms and incorrectly believe that they are not at risk for acquiring HIV infection or other sexually trans-

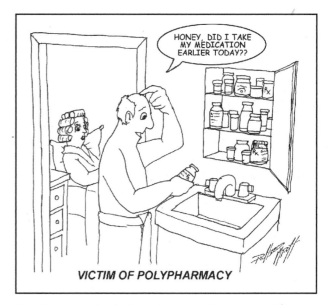

Note: Patients are frequently victims of polypharmacy, and despite the best of intentions, often make inadvertent medication errors (especially the elderly).

Figure 6-1

mitted diseases. Patients should be informed about safer sex practices in conjunction with the use of sildenafil. Also keep in mind that erectile dysfunction may be one of the side effects seen in patients taking certain cardiac medications (e.g., beta blockers and antihypertensive agents).

The goals of treatment in cardiology are to relieve symptoms, improve quality of life, slow disease progression, and prolong survival. Examples include:

- Restoration of normal sinus rhythm by chemical or electrical cardioversion
- Control of rapid ventricular response of atrial fibrillation and other SVTs by beta blockers, rate-slowing calcium channel blockers, digoxin, or catheter ablation
- Control of blood pressure by antihypertensive medication
- Reducing elevated blood cholesterol levels by "statins" and other lipid-reducing agents
- Prevent stroke and TIA in atrial fibrillation with warfarin or novel oral anticoagulants (NOACs)
- Restoration of coronary blood flow by thrombolytic therapy or direct PCI
- Cure of infective endocarditis by antibiotics
- Correction of valvular stenosis and/or regurgitation by valve repair or replacement
- Treatment of CHF by ACE inhibitors, ARBs, ARNI, beta blockers, diuretics, and digoxin

FIGURE 6-2

Symptoms Attributable to Cardiovascular Drugs*

SYMPTOM	CARDIOVASCULAR DRUG/MECHANISM
CNS	
Headache	Nitroglycerin
Syncope	Class IA and III antiarrhythmic agents (torsades de pointes)
	Beta blockers } bradycardia
	Diuretics, vasodilators (e.g., nitrates, calcium channel blockers, α-blockers), ACE inhibitors, hydralazine } hypotension
	Warfarin—blood loss
Tremor, ataxia	Amiodarone
Tremor, confusion, stupor, coma, seizures	Lidocaine
Confusion, delirium, disorientation	Digitalis
Gastrointestinal	
Xerostomia	Disopyramide
Anorexia	Digitalis
Nausea, vomiting	Quinidine, digitalis
Diarrhea	Quinidine
Constipation	Verapamil, cholestyramine
Peptic disease	Nicotinic acid
Pulmonary	
Cough	ACE inhibitors
Pulmonary fibrosis	Amiodarone
Genitourinary	
Nocturia	Diuretics
Hesitancy	Disopyramide
Impotence	Beta blockers
Renal insufficiency	ACE inhibitors, contrast medium
Endocrine	
Hyper/hypothyroid	Amiodarone
Diabetes aggravated	Nicotinic acid
Hypoglycemia masked	Beta blockers
Musculoskeletal	
Arthritis, lupus	Procainamide, hydralazine
Muscle weakness, cramps	Diuretics/electrolyte depletion
Muscle aches and pains (Myositis syndrome)	"Statins"
Cutaneous	
Sunlight sensitivity	Amiodarone
Flushing	Nicotinic acid
Fatigue/lethargy	Beta blockers
Gynecomastia	Digitalis, spironolactone

*Note: Most of the drugs used in cardiology have unwanted, and sometimes serious, side effects on the heart and other organs. These adverse effects must be carefully sought in all patients taking cardiac drugs.

FIGURE 6-3

Drug-Drug Interactions

Common Drug Interactions	Clinical Effect
• Digoxin ± beta blocker ± non dihydropyridine calcium channel blocker (diltiazem, verapamil) ± amiodarone	Sinus bradycardia
• Nitrates ± diuretic ± vasodilator ± α -blocker ± calcium channel blocker	Postural hypotension
• ACE inhibitor ± spironolactone ± NSAID	Hyperkalemia
• Terfenadine, astemizole ± class I or III antiarrhythmic agent ± macrolide antibiotic ± grapefruit juice	Prolongation of QT interval and torsades de pointes
• Aspirin ± clopidogrel ± warfarin ± ginkgo biloba ± vitamin E	Increased bleeding
• ACE inhibitor ± diuretic ± NSAID	Azotemia
• Insulin ± oral hypoglycemic agent ± beta blocker	Hypoglycemic episode—prolonged or unrecognized (masking of hypoglycemic symptoms)
• Beta agonist ± theophylline ± anticholinergic agent	Aggravation of angina and/or arrhythmias
• Digoxin ± amiodarone ± quinidine ± verapamil ± propafenone	Increased serum digoxin levels and/or signs of digitalis toxicity
• Clopidogrel ± proton pump inhibitor (PPI)	PPI may decrease antiplatelet effect of clopidogrel

---

- Relief of angina pectoris by nitrates, beta blockers, calcium channel blockers, PCI or CABG surgery
- Treatment of acute MI by reperfusion therapy
- Treatment of syncope due to potentially life-threatening pauses or ventricular tachyarrhythmias by implantable pacemaker or ICD

It is not possible to manage heart disease as an isolated entity. Many patients with heart disease have other medical problems that may influence their condition adversely, and treatment of their cardiac problem may worsen other coexistent conditions. Furthermore, several cardiac drugs may manifest some form of interaction with each other or with noncardiac drugs. (**Figure 6-3**). For example, studies have implicated certain proton pump inhibitors (PPIs), particularly omeprazole (Prilosec), used concomitantly to decrease the risk of GI bleeding, as drugs that can interfere with hepatic cytochrome P450 2C19 enzymatic activation of clopidogrel (Plavix), and decrease its antiplatelet effect. Although some PPIs may interfere with platelet inhibition, there is no convincing evidence to date of an impact on clinical outcome. Nevertheless, it is vital for the practitioner to be aware of these interactions, which may be potentially harmful to patients.

EVIDENCE-BASED MEDICINE AND CLINICAL PRACTICE GUIDELINES

Over the past few decades, randomized clinical trial data, so-called "*evidence-based medicine*," has emerged as an important tool to improve the quality of patient care. A large number of practice guidelines in cardiology are now available to assist the practitioner in clinical decision making. Good clinical judgment, however, is required to determine whether the guidance applies to the individual patient or if exceptions exist ("no one size fits all").

As in all of medicine, the goals of cardiovascular therapy, whether pharmacological, interventional, or surgical, must be clear in the practitioner's mind, and the patient should be educated as to the potential benefits and risks. If there is no anticipated mortality benefit, and the patient is not feeling ill, potentially risky treatment is not advisable. Keep in mind the dictum, "*primum non nocere*", i.e., first, do no harm. In many cases, patient education and promotion of preventative measures, including a "heart healthy" diet; exercise; smoking cessation; BP, lipid, and glucose control; and weight reduction (if appropriate), ultimately may be the more effective therapy than treating the immediate problem. Remember, "an ounce of prevention is worth a pound of cure."

CHAPTER 7. CARDIAC DRUGS

The introduction of new cardiac drugs and the new applications of standard drugs has resulted in significant changes in the clinical management of the patient with cardiovascular disease. This chapter discusses the common cardiac drugs and their mechanisms. These drugs may have multiple uses for various cardiac conditions. The "putting it all together" section of the book in Part III will focus on the common (and not so common) cardiac conditions encountered in clinical practice, and show how the drugs discussed in this chapter are used in those situations.

The different kinds of problems in cardiology require different pharmacologic treatment strategies:

- Acute and chronic coronary ischemic syndromes: Try to improve coronary artery blood flow through dilation of coronary arteries. Decrease myocardial oxygen demand through dilation of peripheral veins (preload reduction) and arteries (afterload reduction) and decreased myocardial contractility. Deal with acute and chronic thrombosis with thrombolytics, antiplatelet and antithrombotic agents and anticoagulants.
- Congestive heart failure with problems of systolic or diastolic dysfunction: When there is systolic dysfunction, it may help to increase cardiac contractility and/or decrease peripheral resistance (e.g., lowering blood pressure) to make it easier to pump out the blood and increase cardiac output. With diastolic dysfunction, slowing the heart to allow more time for diastolic filling may be beneficial.
- Hypertension: Lower the blood pressure. Raise BP in significant hypotension.
- Dyslipidemia: Correct the lipid abnormality.
- Cardiac arrhythmias: Speed up a pathological bradycardia; slow a tachycardia; reduce the excitability of an ectopic focus in the atria, His-bundle system, or ventricles; decrease conduction along an aberrant pathway.

Advances in pharmacology, including combination medications (so-called "polypills"), have provided the practitioner with a wide array of effective cardiac drugs. Certain agents have become the "cornerstones" of modern cardiac therapy. These include:

- Beta blockers
- Calcium channel blockers
- Nitrates
- Angiotensin-converting enzyme (ACE) inhibitors
- Angiotensin receptor blockers (ARBs)
- Digitalis and other inotropic agents
- Diuretics
- Aspirin and other antiplatelet agents

- Thrombolytic agents and anticoagulants
- Lipid controlling drugs
- Antiarrhythmic agents

BETA BLOCKERS

Drugs that act on the adrenergic receptors of the sympathetic nervous system have particular value in cardiology.

Figure 7-1. Location and effects of stimulation of adrenergic receptors. Beta-1 receptors are found on cardiac muscle cells, including the modified muscle cells of the SA and AV nodes, which are part of the pacemaker and conduction system of the heart. Stimulation of beta-1 receptors increases heart rate (by stimulating the SA node), increases conduction velocity through the AV node, cardiac muscle contractility, and automaticity of the pacemakers, with a net increase in cardiac output. Stimulating these receptors (beta-1 agonists) may be of value to increase cardiac output, but blocking (beta-1 antagonists) may be of value when there is need to:

- Decrease the oxygen demand of the heart by decreasing heart rate and contractility
- Decrease a tachyarrhythmia by slowing conduction through the AV node and decreasing the automaticity of an abnormal ectopic pacemaker.

Beta-1 receptors are also found on granular cells in the kidney, where stimulation increases renin secretion. Renin initiates a chain reaction that results in the production of angiotensin II and aldosterone. Angiotensin II has powerful vasoconstrictive effects and aldosterone stimulates the renal tubules to reabsorb sodium (and, passively, water), thereby increasing blood pressure and blood volume (**Figure 7-3**). Increasing blood pressure may be useful in hypotensive states, but decreasing BP through beta-1 blockers may also be important, e.g. to reduce the stress (afterload) on cardiac contraction, or to treat hypertension.

Beta-2 receptors are found in the trachea and bronchioles and arterioles (but not in the skin or brain arterioles). Stimulating them will cause *vasodilation* and also dilation of the trachea and bronchioles. Thus, beta-2 blockers may aggravate coronary vasospasm, Raynaud's phenomenon, and intermittent claudication by inhibiting arteriolar vasodilation and leaving α-mediated vasoconstriction unopposed. They may also induce bronchospasm. It is therefore very important, when using a beta-blocker to understand whether it nonspecifically blocks both beta-1 and beta-2 receptors (and/or alpha receptors) or acts more specifically. In general, beta-1 specific blockers are preferred in cardiology.

[handwritten margin note: ← lungs]

[handwritten margin note: Spasm of arteries cause episodes of ↓ BF.]

LOCATION AND EFFECTS OF STIMULATION OF ADRENERGIC RECEPTORS	

ALPHA-1 RECEPTORS
 	
Arterioles and Veins:
  constriction (epinephrine and norepinephrine)
 	
Glands:
  ↓ secretions
 	
Eye:
  constriction of radial muscle
 	
Intestine:
  ↓ motility
	ALPHA-2 RECEPTORS
	
	CNS Postsynaptic Terminals:
	  ↓ sympathetic outflow from brain
	
	CNS Presynaptic Terminals:
	  ↓ norepinephrine release
	
	Beta Islet Cells of Pancreas:
	  ↓ secretion

BETA-1 RECEPTORS
 	
Heart:
  ↑ heart rate (SA node)
  ↑ contractility
  ↑ conduction velocity
  ↑ automaticity
 	
Kidney:
  ↑ renin secretion
	BETA-2 RECEPTORS
	
	Trachea and Bronchioles:
	  dilation
	
	Pregnant/nonpregnant Uterus:
	  relaxation
	
	Arterioles (no beta-2 receptors in skin or brain):
	  dilation (epinephrine)

Figure 7-1

Alpha-1 receptors reside on arterioles and veins. Stimulating them will cause *vasoconstriction*. Stimulating alpha-1 receptors thus will *increase* blood pressure, while alpha-1 blockers tend to *decrease* blood pressure. Parasympathetic nerves do not significantly innervate peripheral blood vessels.

Alpha-2 receptors are found in the central nervous system. Stimulating them increases their normal function of inhibiting sympathetic outflow from the brain. Thus, alpha-2 agonists reduce blood pressure.

Beta blockers, both *non-cardioselective* (β-1 and β-2), e.g., *propranolol* (Inderal), *timolol* (Blocadren), *nadolol* (Corgard), and β-1 *cardioselective*, e.g., *atenolol* (Tenormin), *metoprolol* (Lopressor, Toprol-XL), *acebutolol* (Sectral), *bisoprolol* (Zebeta), IV *esmolol* (Brevibloc) block the beta-division of the adrenergic (sympathetic) nervous system, reducing heart rate, blood pressure, and the strength of cardiac contraction. These drugs have thus assumed an important role in the management of patients with:

- CAD (by decreasing myocardial oxygen demand), including stable angina pectoris, unstable angina, acute MI (reduce infarct size) and post-MI (reduce recurrent MI and death)
- Hypertension (through decreased cardiac output and decreased renin secretion)
- CHF (blunts cardiotoxic effects of excess circulating catecholamines and improves LV size and shape [reverse-remodeling])

- Supraventricular and ventricular tachyarrhythmias (increasing refractory period and conduction time of AV node, decreasing automaticity of Purkinje fibers, inhibition of cardiac sympathetic activity)
- HOCM (reducing ventricular contraction force and allowing time for diastolic filling of contracted ventricle thereby reducing LV outflow tract obstruction)
- MVP (inhibits cardiac sympathetic activity)
- Marfan's syndrome and aortic dissection (reduces shear force, blood pressure, and ventricular contractility, and thus slows the rate of aortic dilatation and reduces the risk of rupture)
- Neurocardiogenic syncope (blocks sympathetic increase and intense LV contraction that may precipitate paradoxical vagal reflex)
- Prolonged QT syndrome (beta blockers do not prolong QT interval as do many other drugs)

Drugs that nonselectively antagonize both β-1 and β-2 receptors run the risk of inducing bronchospasm and vasospasm, because β-2 stimulation is important in maintaining broncho- and vasodilation. Agents that are "cardioselective" have a greater effect on β-1 (cardiac) adrenoreceptors than on β-2 adrenergic receptors of the bronchi and blood vessels. You should avoid using nonselective beta blockers and use agents with β-1 selectivity cautiously (if at all) in patients with asthma and COPD, since β-1 selectivity is dose dependent, and these drugs become less selective as the dosage is increased. As primary preventive therapy, beta blockers are less effective than other antihypertensive agents at reducing the risk of stroke in older patients with isolated hypertension. In the post-MI setting, beta blockers limit infarct size; suppress ventricular arrhythmias; reduce the incidence of angina, reinfarction, and sudden cardiac death; and improve survival. These agents are effective in slowing the ventricular response in patients with atrial fibrillation or flutter, converting paroxysmal SVT to normal sinus rhythm, and preventing atrial tachyarrhythmias following cardiac surgery.

Beta blockers (e.g. *long-acting metoprolol succinate, carvedilol, bisoprolol*) have been shown to be helpful in prolonging life in carefully treated patients with CHF as well (as do ACE inhibitors/ARBs and the aldosterone antagonists, spironolactone and eplerenone). *Labetalol* (Trandate, Normodyne), either orally or IV, also has α -adrenoreceptor blocking (vasodilating) properties, which makes it particularly useful in patients with hypertensive emergencies or aortic dissection. *Carvedilol* (Coreg), another combined α and nonselective β blocker, is effective in the patient with compensated CHF due to systolic dysfunction. *Nebivolol* (Bystolic), a highly selective β-1 receptor blocker with nitric oxide mediated vasodilating properties, has recently been approved for use in hypertension. Since beta blockers can transiently worsen CHF, these agents should be started at the lowest dose and titrated upward gradually. IV *esmolol* (Brevibloc) is useful in the treatment of SVT and hypertensive emergencies. It has an ultra-short half life of 9 minutes, and therefore is particularly useful in the patient at risk for the common complications of beta blockade.

Potential side effects of beta blockers include:

- Symptomatic bradycardia and heart block
- Exacerbation of Prinzmetal's (vasospastic) angina and cocaine-induced chest pain and/or MI (by inhibiting the vasodilatory β -2 receptor and causing unopposed α-mediated vasoconstriction)
- Peripheral vascular disease (claudication)
- Bronchospasm (asthma)
- Raynaud's phenomenon (by inhibiting β -2 receptors and causing vasoconstriction)
- Lethargy, fatigue, and weight gain
- Decreased libido, impotence
- Disordered sleep patterns, vivid dreams
- Cold hands and feet
- Acute mental disorders, and worsened depression
- Beta blockers may raise triglyceride levels and lower HDL ("good") cholesterol levels.

Highly *lipid soluble* compounds (e.g., *propranolol*) have a high brain penetration, whereas *hydrophilic* compounds (e.g., *atenolol, nadolol*) have a low brain penetration, and theoretically may influence the presence of some of the central nervous system effects. Furthermore, beta blockers with intrinsic sympathomimetic activity (e.g., *pindolol* [Visken]) have partial agonist activity, and therefore, cause less reduction in cardiac output and heart rate, and negligible peripheral vasoconstriction. Keep in mind that beta blocker therapy should be discontinued by tapering slowly, since sudden withdrawal may lead to a distinct worsening of angina or even an MI (due to excessive catecholamine response). Beta blockers may also potentially mask or exacerbate diabetic hypoglycemia (by increasing beta islet cell insulin secretion), and blunt the catecholamine surge associated with hypoglycemia.

CALCIUM CHANNEL BLOCKERS

Calcium channel blockers block the inward movement of calcium ions across cell membranes, thereby decreasing contractility of vascular smooth muscle cells and cardiac muscle cells, resulting in vasodilatation and decreased cardiac cell contractility (negative inotropic effect). These agents are useful in treating patients with hypertension as well as classic effort and vasospastic angina, by reducing myocardial oxygen demand and increasing myocardial oxygen supply. They include the *dihydropyridines* (*nifedipine* [Procardia, Adalat], *amlodipine* [Norvasc], *felodipine* [Plendil], *isradipine* [DynaCirc], *nicardipine* [Cardene], *nisoldipine* [Sular]), and *clevidipine* [Cleviprex]), which are the more potent vasodilators, and the *nondihydropyridines* (*verapamil* [Isoptin, Calan, Verelan], and *diltiazem* [Cardizem, Tiazac, Dilacor]), which are the less potent vasodilators. Verapamil and diltiazem, in particular, are also useful in treating supraventricular arrhythmias since they also decrease conduction velocity and increase the refractory period of the AV node (by blocking slow inward calcium current).

Controversies regarding the safety of calcium channel blockers emerged during the early 1990s. Administration of the short acting rapid release agents (particularly nifedipine) has been curtailed due to increased cardiovascular mortality witnessed in certain categories of patients. Extended release formulations of the calcium channel blockers (including nifedipine), when indicated, are generally considered effective and safe. Their ability to block calcium-mediated electromechanical coupling in contractile tissue enables these agents to increase blood flow to the heart by dilating the coronary arteries and decreasing oxygen demand by lowering BP, heart rate (e.g., verapamil, diltiazem), and contractility.

Certain calcium channel blockers can be used if anginal symptoms or hypertension are not controlled with beta blockers and ACE inhibitors, or if patients cannot tolerate beta blockers. They do not, however, appear to be universally effective in patients with previous MI, and are not equivalent to beta blockers in post-MI patients. Exception: *Diltiazem* has been demonstrated to be helpful in preventing recurrent MI, but only after non ST segment elevation MI in those with good LV function. Furthermore, short-acting first generation calcium channel blockers (e.g., *nifedipine*) have been implicated in increased morbidity and mortality (in the setting of acute MI) and should not be used. Rate-slowing agents (e.g., diltiazem, verapamil) can be useful in patients with supraventricular tachyarrhythmias (e.g., SVT, atrial fibrillation or flutter).

Aggressive BP reduction can cause myocardial and cerebral ischemia and/or infarction. Short-acting preparations (particularly SL or oral nifedipine) may worsen ischemia (by lowering blood pressure and reflexly increasing heart rate), cause excessive hypotension and stroke, and should be avoided. Long-acting agents should be used. An exception is intravenous clevidipine, an ultra short acting dihydropyridine with little to no reflex tachycardia, approved for use in severe hypertension. In general, calcium channel blockers should not be used alone to treat stable angina pectoris unless there is a clear contraindication for beta blockers or nitrates. However, patients with variant (Prinzmetal's) angina (where vasoconstriction is the predominant mechanism of myocardial ischemia) are best treated with nitrates and calcium channel blockers, since *beta blockers may worsen coronary spasm (due to unopposed alpha vasoconstriction) in Prinzmetal's angina.* Calcium channel blockers are useful as first line agents in these patients.

Since verapamil and diltiazem can induce significant bradycardia, they should be used with caution if a beta blocker is part of the regimen.

Verapamil (by depressing myocardial contractility) can be helpful in selected patients with HOCM.

Calcium channel blockers may be preferred in patients with COPD, pulmonary hypertension, peripheral vascular disease, Raynaud's phenomenon, or SVT.

The afterload-reducing effect of extended release nifedipine may delay the need for aortic valve replacement in patients with AR. Frequent or adverse side effects of calcium channel blockers include dizziness, headache, gingival hyperplasia, bradycardia and AV block (verapamil, diltiazem), flushing, constipation (verapamil) and precipitation of CHF in patients with marginal LV function. In otherwise well-treated patients with CHF, *amlodipine* is more "vascular selective" and may be cautiously added if essential (e.g., for control of hypertension). Currently amlodipine and felodipine have the safest "track-record" in patients with LV systolic dysfunction.

Verapamil can raise digoxin levels and precipitate digitalis toxicity.

Keep in mind that peripheral edema can occur as a side effect of calcium channel blockers (and therefore should not be confused with a sign of CHF).

In patients with diabetic hypertension, ACE inhibitors and ARBs, along with calcium channel blocker therapy (particularly dihydropyridines) have been shown to be effective.

NITRATES

Sublingual, oral, cutaneous, and parenteral nitrates have been the mainstay of treatment for patients with stable and unstable angina pectoris due to atherosclerotic CAD, coronary artery spasm (Prinzmetal's angina), and acute MI. By conversion to nitric oxide (NO), also known as endothelium-derived relaxing factor, organic nitrates stimulate formation of cyclic guanosine monophosphate (GMP) which mediates vascular smooth muscle cell relaxation. (**Figure 7-2**)

Figure 7-2. Mechanism of action of organic nitrates.

These agents induce coronary vasodilation (including dilation at sites of coronary artery stenoses) and dilate peripheral veins, thereby reducing venous return to the heart, and thus decrease heart size, which lowers myocardial oxygen demand. Nitrates lessen symptoms of CHF and, in combination with hydralazine (a peripheral vasodilator), improve survival and delay progression of LV dysfunction (although not as well as ACE inhibitors). Despite their extensive "track-record" in relieving symptoms and improving exercise tolerance and the quality of life for patients with CAD, there is no evidence that nitrates reduce mortality. Nitroglycerin is available as a *SL tablet* (e.g., Nitrostat) or *spray* (Nitrolingual) to shorten or prevent an anticipated angina attack, *long-acting oral tablets* (e.g., *isosorbide dinitrate* [Isordil], *mononitrate* [Ismo, Imdur,

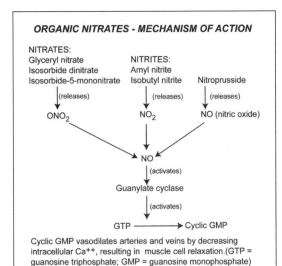

Figure 7-2

Monoket], *topical ointment* (e.g., Nitro-Bid 2%) or *patch* (e.g., Nitro-Dur, Transderm-Nitro, Minitran), as well as an *IV preparation* (e.g., Tridil). If angina occurs under predictable circumstances (e.g., taking a walk, climbing a flight of stairs), nitroglycerin can be used prophylactically before the activity to prevent it from occurring. Nitrates decrease the heart's demand for oxygen by reducing preload and increase blood supply by relaxing the coronary arteries.

Keep in mind that all nitrates are subject to "tolerance", i.e., with continuous use their effects may wane or even disappear. Eccentric dosage schedules with a "nitrate-free interval" of 8–10 hours is generally recommended to preserve efficacy in long-term treatment. Transdermal nitroglycerin preparations, although initially greeted with enthusiasm, are being replaced, for the most part, by extended-release oral preparations. Use nitroglycerin with caution in patients with acute inferior MI with RV involvement. (Patients with RV infarction have a stiff, noncompliant ventricle that depends on high filling pressures; thus, these patients may not tolerate the reduction in preload or venodilation induced by these medications.) Do not administer nitroglycerin to patients who present with an ACS, including unstable angina, who have used phosphodiesterase 5 (PDE-5) inhibitors for erectile dysfunction e.g., *sildenafil* (Viagra), *vardenafil* (Levitra), or *tadalafil* (Cialis) within the previous 24-48 hours. These agents are also vasodilators and marked and potentially dangerous hypotension may result with resultant myocardial ischemia. Other problems with nitroglycerin include the fact that 10% of patients do not respond and another 10% have associated intolerable headaches that may necessitate discontinuation. Patients who have frequent angina, or angina at night (during the nitrate-free period) should be treated with a second drug (e.g., beta blocker, calcium channel blocker).

ANGIOTENSIN CONVERTING ENZYME (ACE) INHIBITORS

The renin-angiotensin-aldosterone system plays an important role in regulating blood pressure and maintaining cardiovascular homeostasis (balance). Drugs that act on this system (e.g., ACE inhibitors, ARBs) are of great value in cardiology (**Figure 7-3**).

The enzyme renin is secreted into the bloodstream by the juxtaglomerular cells of the kidney in response to decreased renal blood flow and increased sympathetic nervous system (beta-1 adrenergic) activity (as may occur in CHF). Renin then acts to convert angiotensinogen (from the liver) to the inactive precursor, angiotensin I. Angiotensin converting enzyme (ACE) in the pulmonary capillaries facilitates the conversion of angiotensin I to active angiotensin II, a potent vasoconstrictor and stimulator of aldosterone secretion by the adrenal cortex (aldosterone promotes absorption

of sodium from the distal nephron), which raises arterial blood pressure and improves cardiac output and renal blood flow, thus turning off the renin-activated system.

These "compensatory" mechanisms, however, can have deleterious effects in the failing heart. Excessive vasoconstriction increases peripheral vascular resistance (increases afterload) which can decrease LV function and cardiac output, and salt and water retention by the kidney can worsen the already elevated ventricular filling pressure (increases preload).

Figure 7-3. The renin-angiotensin-aldosterone system and sites of drug intervention. Blockade of the renin-angiotensin-aldosterone system can take place at five pivotal sites: (1) Inhibiting the release of renin from the juxtaglomerular cells of the kidney with beta-adrenergic blockers; (2) Blocking the activity of renin with direct renin inhibitors; (3) Blocking the conversion of angiotensin I to angiotensin II with ACE inhibitors; (4) Blocking the AT type I receptor with ARBs; and (5) Antagonizing the effects of aldosterone at the distal renal tubule with aldosterone antagonists. **Note:** Unlike ACE inhibitors, the ARBs do not affect serum bradykinin levels and, therefore, cough is not a common side effect.

ACE inhibitors, by preventing the conversion of angiotensin I to angiotensin II, reduce systemic blood pressure by promoting vasodilation, and reduce sodium reabsorption from the distal nephron. These agents also increase levels of bradykinin and vasodilatory prostaglandins. By reducing peripheral vascular resistance (decreasing afterload) ACE inhibitors reduce the stress (impedance) to the heart and increase cardiac output in heart failure. They are also useful as antihypertensive agents.

ACE inhibitors include *captopril* (Capoten), *enalapril* (Vasotec), *lisinopril* (Zestril, Prinivil), *ramipril* (Altace), *fosinopril* (Monopril), *quinapril* (Accupril), *benazepril* (Lotensin), and *trandolapril* (Mavik). These vasodilators are the mainstay of therapy for patients with CHF due to LV systolic dysfunction (reduces mortality and hospitalization in patients with symptomatic CHF and in those who are asymptomatic with poor LV function). While treating hypertension, they help provide renoprotection in patients with diabetes and proteinuria.

They are useful in decreasing morbidity and mortality in patients with acute MI (with EF < 40%). Therapy should be started early in stable, high-risk patients, e.g., anterior MI, previous MI, Killip class II (S3 gallop, rales, radiographic CHF). Afterload reduction with an ACE inhibitor is of value in the management of chronic AR. Side effects may include

- Hypotension
- Worsening of renal function with volume or salt-depletion or concomitant use of diuretics
- Hyperkalemia in patients with renal dysfunction (particularly diabetics) and in those receiving

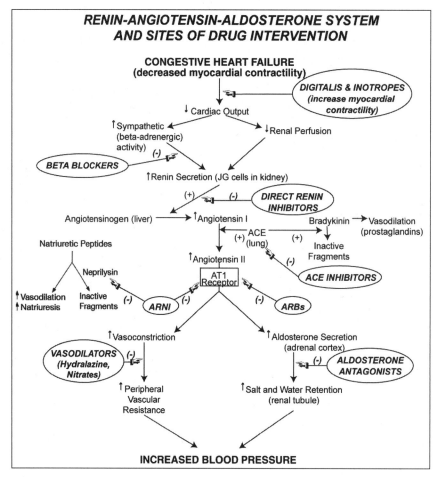

RENIN-ANGIOTENSIN-ALDOSTERONE SYSTEM AND SITES OF DRUG INTERVENTION

Figure 7-3

potassium supplements or potassium-sparing diuretics

- Acute renal failure in patients with bilateral renal artery stenosis (or stenosis in the artery to a solitary kidney).
- Cough, loss of taste, rash, or rarely angioneurotic edema.

To minimize the hypotension risk in diuretic treated patients, diuretics should either be held or reduced in dose (if possible) before starting ACE inhibitor therapy. You should exercise caution in volume depleted or hyponatremic patients. Keep in mind that a bothersome dry *cough* (which may relate to increased bradykinin levels) may result, which at times can be mistaken for the symptoms of CHF. Since ACE inhibitors can impair renal function, the BUN, creatinine and serum potassium levels should be monitored. Hyperkalemia may occur especially if ACE inhibitors are used with other drugs that increase potassium (e.g., potassium-sparing diuretics), and if renal insufficiency is present. Mild increases in potassium may be tolerated; however, significant increases are indications to discontinue the drug. These agents should not be used by pregnant women.

ANGIOTENSIN RECEPTOR BLOCKERS (ARBs)

Angiotensin receptor blockers (ARBs), e.g., *losartan* (Cozaar), *candesartan* (Atacand), *irbesartan* (Avapro), and *valsartan* (Diovan), *olmesartan* (Benicar), *telmisartan* (Micardis), *eprosartan* (Teveten), and *azilsartan* (Edarbi) specifically block the angiotensin II receptor AT$_1$ which causes effective blockade of the renin-angiotensin system. These agents act at a different site from ACE inhibitors to block the effects of angiotensin II and theoretically have the benefits of ACE inhibition, except formation of bradykinin, and without adverse side effects, particularly cough (**Figure 7-3**). ARBs represent a major breakthrough in the management of hypertension and CHF and are now being used more often (at least in ACE-intolerant patients). **Note:** although ARBs are clearly better tolerated than ACE inhibitors, producing a far smaller incidence of cough or angioneurotic edema, it should not be expected that renal insufficiency, hypotension, or hyperkalemia will occur less frequently with ARBs compared with ACE inhibitors. As with ACE inhibitors, to minimize the hypotensive risk in diuretic treated patients, diuretics should be held or reduced (if possible) before using ARBs. These agents should not be taken by pregnant women. Caution is advised when considering these agents if a history of ACE inhibitor angioedema is present.

ANGIOTENSIN RECEPTOR NEPRILYSIN INHIBITORS

A new class of drug called angiotensin receptor neprilysin inhibitor (ARNI), which combines an ARB (valsartan) with a neprilysin inhibitor (sacubitril), marketed as Entresto, has been shown to be superior to an ACE inhibitor (enalapril) in reducing cardiovascular mortality and hospitalization in patients with CHF. The drugs ability to block the renin-angiotensin system and inhibit the enzymatic breakdown of endogenous natriuretic and vasodilatory peptides provides a novel approach to the treatment of CHF. Of note, symptomatic hypotension is more common with an ARNI than with an ACE inhibitor or ARB. (**Figure 7-3**)

DIRECT RENIN INHIBITORS

Aliskiren (Tekturna) is the first direct renin inhibitor approved by the FDA for treatment of hypertension, either alone or in combination with other antihypertensive agents. Unlike ACE inhibitors and ARBs, which target the renin angiotensin aldosterone system at later stages, direct renin inhibitors, e.g., aliskiren, target the renin angiotensin aldosterone system at the first and rate-limiting step. By blocking the action of renin, this agent decreases the production of angiotensin and aldosterone, and thus reduces systemic blood pressure by promoting vasodilation and reducing sodium retention from the distal renal tubule. (**Figure 7-3**) Direct inhibition of renin does not increase

bradykinin levels thought to be responsible for the angioedema and cough seen with ACE inhibitors. These agents should not be used by pregnant women. Results of long-term clinical outcome studies are needed to establish the precise role of this novel class of antihypertensive medication.

INOTROPIC AGENTS

Digitalis Glycosides

The digitalis glycosides inhibit the Na^+-K^+ ATPase pump in myocardial cell membranes. This increases intracellular sodium (and extracellular potassium) which, in turn, increases intracellular calcium (by sodium-calcium exchanger) which increases the force of myocardial contraction.

Figure 7-4. Digitalis—Mechanism of action.

By its unique combination of increasing the force of ventricular contractions (positive inotropic effect) and decreasing the ventricular rate in SVTs (vagally-induced inhibition of AV nodal conduction and sympatholytic effects), *digoxin* (Lanoxin) is particularly useful in the treatment of patients with CHF due to impaired LV systolic function, especially when atrial fibrillation, flutter, and other atrial tachyarrhythmias are also present. In patients with stable mild to moderate heart failure and substantial LV systolic dysfunction (ejection fraction $\leq 35\%$) the withdrawal of digoxin from triple therapy (i.e., ACE inhibitor, diuretic, digitalis) results in clinical deterioration. Although long-term prospective data show that digoxin decreases hospitalization, it does not confer added mortality benefit as do beta blockers, ACE inhibitors and spironolactone; therefore its use in normal sinus rhythm remains optional. For patients with significant symptomatic LV systolic dysfunction, digoxin provides benefit when digoxin levels are 0.5 to 1.0 ng/ml. The therapeutic-toxic window is narrow. Data suggests that patients

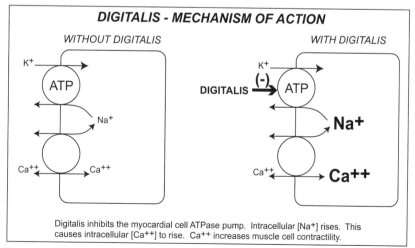

DIGITALIS - MECHANISM OF ACTION

WITHOUT DIGITALIS   *WITH DIGITALIS*

Digitalis inhibits the myocardial cell ATPase pump. Intracellular [Na++] rises. This causes intracellular [Ca++] to rise. Ca++ increases muscle cell contractility.

Note: Acute digitalis toxicity can cause *hyper*kalemia (digoxin blocks the Na^+ - K^+ ATPase pump, so more K^+ remains outside the cells), but *hypo*kalemia can predispose to chronic digitals toxicity (digoxin competes with K^+ for the same ATPase binding site, so more digoxin is available to exert its effects).

Figure 7-4

with serum digoxin levels of 1.0–2.0 ng/ml (previously regarded at "therapeutic") and women (who tend to have higher serum levels on fixed doses of digoxin than men) have an increased mortality risk. Serum digoxin levels are particularly valuable in assessing patients suspected of having digitalis toxicity. However, the serum digoxin level is not a substitute for a complete clinical assessment of the patient. Patients with hypoxemia, hypokalemia, and hypomagnesemia, for example, may have toxic manifestations of digitalis excess even in the absence of an elevated serum digoxin concentration.

Digitalis toxicity: Despite the best of intentions, patients often make inadvertent medication errors (especially the elderly). For example, a patient may take a certain medication, e.g., digoxin, several times a day, thinking that it was a different medication and wonders why he or she is becoming nauseated! Common early clues to digitalis intoxication include GI complaints (e.g., nausea, vomiting, anorexia), along with visual disturbances (e.g., blurred, yellow-green and/or halo vision), electrolyte abnormalities (e.g., hyperkalemia), and neurologic symptoms and/or signs (e.g., headache; fatigue, disorientation, delirium, and confusion). Cardiac arrhythmias are additional clues to digitalis toxicity (**Figure 3-53**). These include PVCs, paroxysmal atrial tachycardia with AV block, bidirectional VT (QRS complexes from two different ectopic foci alternate in morphology), "regularization" of atrial fibrillation (regular R-R intervals). Gynecomastia is a rare sequela. Digitalis toxicity is frequently seen in advancing age, renal insufficiency, diuretic use, hypothyroidism or accidental/deliberate overdose. Therapy for digoxin toxicity generally requires simply withholding the drug and monitoring the patient. Tachyarrhythmias can be treated with antiarrhythmic agents e.g., lidocaine (Xylocaine), phenytoin (Dilantin), and beta blockers. Hypokalemia can precipitate this condition and therefore should be corrected. Keep in mind that amiodarone, verapamil, and quinidine can raise digoxin levels and increase the risk of digitalis toxicity. Life-threatening digitalis intoxication requires immediate attention and can be treated with digoxin-specific antibodies, e.g., Digibind.

Sympathomimetic Amines (e.g. Dopamine, Dobutamine)

When additional inotropic support is needed in the treatment of CHF, intravenous sympathomimetic amines (e.g., *dopamine* [Intropin], *dobutamine* [Dobutrex]) and phosphodiesterase inhibitors (e.g., *milrinone* [Primacor]) may be administered, usually as a short-term continuous infusion. Their hemodynamic effect is to shift a depressed ventricular performance (Frank-Starling) curve in an upward direction, so that for a given ventricular filling pressure, stroke volume and cardiac output are increased (**Figure 12-1**).

Intravenous dopamine and dobutamine are commonly used sympathomimetic amines in the treatment of acute CHF. At low doses (2–5 ug/kg/min), dopamine has primarily a renal vasodilating action (dopaminergic effect), and may selectively improve renal blood flow and promote diuresis in oliguric patients. At moderate doses (5–10 ug/kg/min), the inotropic (β-1 agonist) effect of dopamine predominates, and at high doses, its primary action is vasoconstriction (α agonist effect). Dopamine may increase pulmonary capillary wedge pressure and should be reserved, therefore, for the patient with significant hypotension. If the patient is normotensive or only mildly hypotensive, dobutamine is the preferred inotropic agent.

Dobutamine primarily stimulates cardiac β-1 receptors with little α or β-2 adrenergic activity and has the advantage of having less chronotropic effect than dopamine. Doses of 2.5–15 ug/kg/min lead to an increase in cardiac output without a marked increase in peripheral vascular resistance or heart rate. Dobutamine should not be used alone, however, if the patient is markedly hypotensive since it has minimal vasoconstrictive activity. As a result, it causes a fall in systemic arterial and pulmonary capillary wedge pressure. The combination of low dose dopamine with dobutamine improves myocardial contractility, maintains systemic blood pressure, enhances renal blood flow and reduces pulmonary capillary wedge pressure and thus may be an extremely effective regimen.

Phosphodiesterase Inhibitors (e.g., Amrinone, Milrinone)

Tachyphylaxis (rapidly decreasing response after a few doses) to the hemodynamic effects of dobutamine can occur after 2 to 3 days of continuous therapy and may require either increasing the drug dose or switching to another intravenous inotrope, i.e., a phosphodiesterase -3 inhibitor e.g., *milrinone* (Primacor), *amrinone* (Inocor). Inhibiting phosphodiesterase in cardiac muscle and smooth muscle of peripheral vessels with milrinone preserves intracellular cyclic adenosine monophosphate (cAMP) which results in enhanced myocardial contraction (positive inotropic effect) and peripheral vasodilation (vasodilator effect), the so-called "inodilator" effect. Cardiac output and stroke volume increase while pulmonary capillary wedge pressure and peripheral vascular resistance decrease due to mixed cardiac and vascular effects. Milrinone appears to be more potent than amrinone and has less major adverse side effects (e.g., thrombocytopenia). Since these drugs cause vasodilation, hypotension may be aggravated and can be a limiting factor. As with sympathomimetics, these drugs can cause mild tachycardia and aggravation of ventricular arrhythmias.

There can be surprisingly different hemodynamic responses to dobutamine and milrinone in individual patients, with much greater increase of cardiac output when switching from one to the other. Although intermittent intravenous inotropic therapy in advanced CHF patients has been shown to increase physical capacity, there is concern for aggravated arrhythmias and sudden death. Since quality of life is often the issue more than quantity of life in these patients, intermittent inotropic treatment may be a reasonable option.

DIURETICS

Diuretics are a mainstay in the treatment of hypertension and CHF. In CHF, they help to eliminate excess sodium and water through renal excretion and can ease shortness of breath (due to pulmonary congestion) and swelling (due to peripheral edema) within hours or days, whereas other agents (e.g., digitalis, vasodilators) may take weeks or even months. In hypertension, diuretics act, in part, by elimination of intravascular volume. Because the compensatory response to most other classes of antihypertensive medications involves sodium retention, diuretics can lead to improved blood pressure control. The three most commonly used groups of diuretics are the thiazide diuretics, loop diuretics, and potassium-sparing diuretics. A new class of diuretics currently under evaluation are the aquaretics ("vaptans"). (**Figure 7-5**) These classes can be distinguished by their site of action in the kidney tubule, their mechanism, and form of diuresis that they elicit (solute vs. water diuresis [i.e., aquaresis]).

    Figure 7-5. Sites of action of diuretics. Thiazide diuretics inhibit sodium and chloride reabsorption in the distal convoluted tubule. Loop diuretics inhibit sodium, potassium, and chloride reabsorption in the thick ascending limb of the loop of Henle. Potassium sparing diuretics inhibit potassium secretion and influence sodium excretion in the cortical collecting tubule. Aquaretics, also known as vasopressin antagonists ("vaptans"),

are now being used in the treatment of euvolemic or hypervolemic hyponatremia. These agents block the antidiuretic (water retaining) effects of vasopressin on the renal collecting duct, resulting in an increase in solute-free water excretion, along with an increase in serum sodium concentration.

Thiazides

Thiazides, e.g., *hydrochlorothiazide* (HydroDIURIL), *chlorothiazide* (Diuril), *chlorthalidone* (Hygroton), and *indapamide* (Lozol), act on the distal renal tubule and collecting segment and are standard therapy for chronic CHF when edema is mild to modest, either alone or in combination with loop diuretics. These agents are less potent than loop diuretics, but because of their longer duration of action, are beneficial in chronic conditions, e.g., mild to moderate CHF (except in patients with renal dysfunction, i.e., serum creatinine level > 2 mg/dL). Thiazides are also useful in treating hypertension. Chlorthalidone is stronger and longer acting than hydrochlorothiazide, and due to its superior clinical outcome data, may be the preferred agent in controlling hypertension.

Loop Diuretics

With more advanced degrees of CHF the stronger loop diuretics, which impair absorption in the thick ascending limb of the loop of Henle, and/or combinations of diuretics, e.g., thiazide or a thiazide-like agent *metolazone* (Zaroxolyn, Diulo) and a loop diuretic e.g., *furosemide* (Lasix), *bumetanide* (Bumex), *torsemide* (Demadex) may be needed. Both these agents administered together tend to be effective even in the setting of

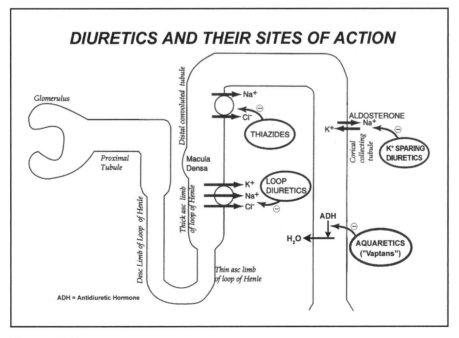

Figure 7-5

impaired renal function. A more prominent natriuretic effect results than with either agent alone since they act on different segments of the renal tubule ("sequential nephron block"). Thiazide diuretics alone are ineffective in the setting of diminished renal function (when the serum creatinine is >2.5 mg/dL). Loop diuretics e.g., furosemide (Lasix), bumetanide (Bumex), torsemide (Demadex), all sulfonamide derivatives, are effective in patients with renal insufficiency and CHF and/or hypertension. *Ethacrynic acid* (Edecrin), a non-sulfonamide derivative, is useful in patients allergic to sulfa drugs (but is more ototoxic). Intravenous loop diuretics are of great value in the acute management of pulmonary edema. In addition to its diuretic effect, and even preceding it, these drugs may induce venodilation (by promoting prostaglandin and nitric oxide release from endothelial cells which act to relax vascular smooth muscle), and thereby decrease venous return and reduce pulmonary congestion.

Potassium Sparing Diuretics

Potassium sparing diuretics, e.g. *spironolactone* (Aldactone), *triamterene* (Dyrenium), and *amiloride* (Midamor), are relatively weak diuretics that are useful when maintenance of serum potassium is crucial. These drugs are rarely used alone and are often combined with thiazide or loop diuretics to offset urinary potassium loss. Spironolactone (Aldactone) is an aldosterone antagonist that acts on the aldosterone-sensitive region of the cortical collecting tubule. When added to an ACE inhibitor and a loop diuretic, with or without digoxin, this agent has been shown to improve CHF symptoms and reduce mortality rates by competitively inhibiting the adverse effects of aldosterone on *myocardial remodeling* (i.e., the process whereby the failing heart undergoes changes in LV size, shape, and thickness to maintain adequate forward flow). The other potassium-sparing agents e.g., dyrenium and amiloride act independently of aldosterone.

Diuretic effects should be monitored carefully since excessive administration may result in a drop in cardiac output, hypotension and prerenal azotemia. The most common side effects of the thiazide and loop diuretics include intravascular volume depletion, hypokalemia and hypomagnesemia (which predisposes to ventricular arrhythmias), metabolic alkalosis, weakness, fatigue, sexual dysfunction, elevated lipid levels (increased LDL cholesterol and triglyceride levels), hyperuricemia (and possible precipitation of gout) due to decreased clearance of uric acid, and hyperglycemia (because of impaired pancreatic insulin release and/or decreased peripheral glucose utilization). The most serious potential adverse effects of the potassium sparing diuretics is the development of hyperkalemia, resulting from impaired excretion of potassium. Spironolactone also possesses antiandrogenic activity and may produce gynecomastia in men. Newer aldosterone antagonists, e.g., *eplerenone* (Inspra), have been shown to improve survival in post-MI patients with LV systolic dysfunction and CHF. These agents may reduce some of the side effects associated with aldosterone (e.g., gynecomastia) while providing a diuretic and potassium conserving activity similar to that of spironolactone.

ANTIPLATELET AGENTS

Aspirin

Aspirin (acetylsalicylic acid) is the most widely used antiplatelet agent in cardiology. This simple, over-the-counter pill, has proved to be a cornerstone of therapy for patients with atherosclerotic vascular disease. If an individual has already had a heart attack or stroke, a daily dose of aspirin will substantially reduce the odds of another event or even death from cardiovascular disease. Furthermore, aspirin dramatically improves survival for patients in the throes of an MI. *The use of just one aspirin tablet chewed (or swallowed) at the onset of symptoms of a heart attack can cause a 25% reduction in the incidence of MI or death. Keep in mind that nitroglycerin, although it may relieve anginal pain, does not prevent a heart attack or save lives.* Moreover, in patients with stable angina pectoris without a history of acute MI, aspirin lessens the occurrence of subsequent MI and mortality. As with all medications, however, any benefit must be weighed against risk. In the case of aspirin, these risks include bleeding into the brain or GI tract (especially in older patients). Those who have active peptic ulcer disease, consume > 2 alcoholic beverages a day, have severe uncontrolled hypertension, or are taking blood thinners, e.g., warfarin (Coumadin) are at high risk for bleeding. Although aspirin plays an important role in secondary prevention, i.e., in patients with known ischemic vascular disease, it is not clear that otherwise healthy individuals who are not at high risk should routinely take aspirin for cardiovascular protection. The decision to use aspirin, particularly for primary prevention (i.e., in individuals without a history of CAD), should be made on a case-by-case basis, weighing the patient's risk of bleeding against potential benefit.

Platelets play a key pathophysiologic role in the development of the atherosclerotic plaque and the acute phase of coronary thrombosis. By irreversible inhibition of the cyclooxygenase enzyme, aspirin prevents platelet production of thromboxane A2, a vasoconstrictor and an important substance for induction of platelet aggregation. (**Figure 7-6**)

Figure 7-6. Pathways to thrombosis and sites of drug intervention. After disruption of a vulnerable atherosclerotic plaque, tissue factor and subendothelial collagen are exposed, which initiates platelet activation and aggregation (white clot pathway) and the coagulation cascade (red clot pathway), ultimately resulting in a fibrin clot. Antiplatelet drugs interfere with platelet function at various sites along the platelet activation and aggregation pathway. Aspirin irreversibly inhibits cyclooxygenase and thus decreases platelet production of thromboxane A2, an important activator of platelets. Thienopyridines (e.g., clopidogrel, ticlopidine, prasugrel) and nonthienopyridines (e.g. ticagrelor) inhibit the binding of adenosine diphosphate (ADP) to the P2Y12 platelet receptor, which also blocks platelet activation. Thrombin receptor antagonists (e.g., vorapaxar) inhibit the binding of thrombin to the protease-activated receptor, PAR-1, on the platelet surface, which blocks platelet aggregation. Glycoprotein (GP) IIb/IIIa inhibitors (abciximab, eptifibatide, tirofiban) block fibrinogen binding to the platelet GP IIb/IIIa receptor and thus block the critical and final common pathway to platelet aggregation. Anticoagulant drugs interfere with the coagulation factors at various sites along the clotting cascade. Unfractionated heparin and low molecular weight heparin (LMWH), combined with their cofactor antithrombin III (AT III), both inhibit

thrombin activation from prothrombin. Unfractionated heparin inhibits factor Xa and thrombin to a similar degree, whereas LMWH inhibits factor Xa more potently than it inhibits thrombin. Factor Xa inhibitors, both indirect (e.g., fondaparinux) which binds with AT III, and direct (e.g., rivaroxaban, apixaban, edoxaban), selectively inactivate factor Xa, and indirectly inhibit thrombin generation. Direct thrombin inhibitors (bivalirudin, lepirudin, argatroban) predominantly inhibit thrombin itself. Warfarin inhibits the formation of reduced vitamin K and thus decreases production of functional prothrombin. Thrombolytic agents (e.g., tPA, rPA, TNK-tPA) convert plasminogen to plasmin, thereby activating the endogenous fibrinolytic system. These agents lyse fibrin and dissolve occlusive clots that have already formed.

The clinical benefits for aspirin have been shown in patients with acute and chronic CAD, post-CABG (lowers the likelihood of graft occlusion), PCI (prevents thrombotic complications following coronary stenting), nonvalvular atrial

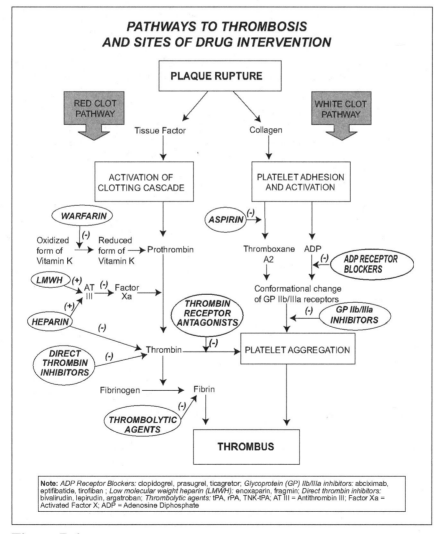

Figure 7-6

fibrillation, prosthetic valves, and TIAs (reduces the risk of stroke). In ACS, aspirin alone has been shown to be effective in reducing acute MI in patients with unstable angina as well as augmenting the benefit of heparin (by reducing the incidence for post-heparin rebound thrombosis). Similarly, in acute ST elevation MI, aspirin alone reduces the risk for adverse events when combined with thrombolytic therapy. Of note, dipyridamole, a relatively weak platelet inhibitor, in combination with low dose aspirin (marketed as Aggrenox) has been shown to be superior to aspirin monotherapy, but not more effective than clopidogrel alone, in preventing recurrent stroke.

Despite its widespread use, the optimal dose of aspirin has not been established. According to previous practice guidelines, higher doses (162–325 mg) of aspirin are recommended immediately in patients with ACS (preferably non-enteric coated and chewed for rapid absorption), and for at least 1 month, and up to 3–6 months, in patients undergoing PCI with a bare metal or drug eluting stent respectively, followed by a lower dose (75–162 mg) of aspirin daily thereafter. More recent studies, however, have shown that lower doses of aspirin are safer and as effective as higher doses for reducing the risk of cardiovascular events. Accordingly, updated guidelines recommend a low dose (81 mg) of aspirin indefinitely in most patients with acute or chronic ischemic vascular disease, including those who have undergone PCI, unless specifically contraindicated. In special circumstances, e.g., post-CABG, a higher maintenance dose (325 mg) of aspirin may be preferable (at least for the first year) to help maintain graft patency.

Adenosine Diphosphate (ADP) Receptor Antagonists (e.g., Clopidogrel, Ticlopidine, Prasugrel, Ticagrelor, Cangretor)

If aspirin use is contraindicated (because of hypersensitivity or intolerance), *clopidogrel* (Plavix), a thienopyridine that irreversibly inhibits the binding of adenosine diphosphate (ADP) to the P2Y12 receptor on platelets, should be considered (**Figure 7-6**). Clopidogrel inhibits ADP-induced platelet aggregation and has been shown to have favorable effects on cardiovascular events (particularly in combination with aspirin, on reducing the incidence of stent thrombosis) and does not present the hematologic complications (e.g., neutropenia, thrombotic thrombocytopenic purpura) associated with *ticlopidine* (Ticlid), an older thienopyridine. The combination of clopidogrel, the most widely used agent in this class, plus aspirin (indefinitely) provides benefit in patients with unstable angina, non ST elevation MI, ST elevation MI (when combined with fibrinolytic therapy), and in those with stable CAD or ACS who undergo coronary stent implantation. The optimal loading dose, timing, and duration of clopidogrel therapy, however, remains unresolved. To achieve effective levels of platelet inhibition more rapidly, a standard loading dose of 300 mg of clopidogrel, followed by a daily maintenance dose of 75 mg is recommended. Compared to the conventional loading dose of 300 mg, a loading dose of 600 mg provides even faster

and higher degrees of platelet inhibition, without a significant increase in bleeding, and is currently being used in many centers. In addition to aspirin, in patients with stable CAD, updated guidelines recommend a minimum of 1 month of clopidogrel therapy after bare metal stenting (BMS). and at least 6 months after newer generation drug eluting stent (DES) implantation. In patients with ACS, at least 12 months of clopidogrel therapy is recommecded, with or without a coronary stent (BMS or DES), to reduce the risk of future MI and stent thrombosis in patients who are not at high risk for bleeding. Although clopidogrel has been shown to be of benefit if started prior to PCI, a minority of patients will require CABG, which makes the "upstream" use of clopidogrel (i.e., before catheterization) somewhat problematic (due to concerns it will delay surgery or increase the risk of bleeding). Clopidogrel should be discontinued at least 5 days prior to CABG to allow for its antiplatelet effect to wear off and to minimize the risk of perioperative bleeding. It may be prudent, therefore, to wait until the coronary anatomy is identified and decisions about revascularization (PCI vs. CABG) are made before initiating clopidogrel treatment. Of note, not all patients respond to clopidogrel with similar benefit. Clopidogrel is a prodrug that requires hepatic metabolism to its active form by the cytochrome P 450 (CYP) enzymatic system, particularly CYP2C19. Patients on clopidogrel who carry a reduced-function allele of the CYP2C19 gene, especially those taking a proton pump inhibitor, e.g., omeprazole, that inhibits CYP2C19 activity, metabolize clopidogrel poorly, have lower degrees of platelet inhibition (so-called "clopidogrel resistance"), and may be more likely to develop adverse cardiovascular events, especially stent thrombosis after ACS or PCI.

Newer ADP receptor blockers have been developed to address these shortcomings. *Prasugrel* (Effient) is an irreversible, oral thienopyridine with more rapid, potent, and consistent platelet inhibition than clopidogrel. In high risk ACS patients undergoing PCI (particularly those with diabetes or a drug eluting stent), prasugrel has been shown to further reduce ischemic events and stent thrombosis, but at a cost of increased risk of bleeding, particularly in patients who are older (> 75 years), with low body weight (< 60 kg), and in those with a history of prior TIA or stroke (in whom the drug is contraindicated).

Ticagrelor (Brilinta) is the first reversible, oral non-thienopyridine ADP receptor blocker, in a new class called cyclopentyltriazolopyrimidine. Like prasugrel, it provides faster, greater, and more consistent platelet inhibition than clopidogrel, but with a more rapid "offset" of action. In ACS patients managed medically or with PCI, ticagrelor results in fewer vascular deaths, MIs, and stent thromboses than clopidogrel, without an increase in overall major bleeding, but with an increased rate of non-CABG related bleeding, and other adverse effects (e.g., dyspnea, ventricular pauses). Due to the faster recovery of platelet function, ticagrelor may be stopped 5 days before CABG or other surgery, rather than 7 days recommended for prasugel. Its twice-daily dosing and faster "offset" of antiplatelet effect, however, underscores the importance of patient compliance. Maintenance doses of aspirin above 100 mg daily may decrease the effectiveness of ticagrelor and should be avoided. Of note, *cangrelor* (Kengreal) is a potent, reversible IV nonthienopyridine ADP receptor blocker recently approved to reduce the risk of thrombotic events in ACS patients undergoing PCI who have not been pretreated with an oral P2Y12 platelet inhibitor. With its short half-life (3-6 minutes) and very rapid onset and offset of action, cangrelor may find a niche role for bridging off of other antiplatelet agents or as an alternative to GP IIb/IIIa receptor antagonists.

Thrombin Receptor (PAR-1) Antagonist

Vorapaxar (Zontivity), a first-in-class, selective, reversibly binding, oral thrombin receptor (PAR-1) platelet antagonist, has recently been approved as "add-on" therapy to aspirin and/or clopidogrel to reduce the risk of thrombotic cardiovascular events in select patients with prior MI or PAD. However, the increased risk of bleeding, particularly intracranial, precludes its use in patients with a history of stroke or TIA.

Glycoprotein IIb/IIIa Receptor Inhibitors (e.g., Abciximab, Eptifibatide, Tirofiban)

The most effective antiplatelet agents are the glycoprotein (GP) IIb/IIIa inhibitors. These agents reversibly inhibit the critical and final common pathway of platelet aggregation— the binding of activated GP IIb/IIIa receptors to fibrinogen and von Willebrand factor—and thus prevent platelets from sticking to one another, thereby impairing the formation of a hemostatic plug. (**Figure 7-6**) Intravenous GP IIb/IIIa inhibitors may be used in high-risk ACS patients (i.e., ST depression, elevated troponin levels), especially those with recurrent ischemia, a large thrombus burden, and/or inadequate pre-treatment with dual antiplatelet therapy at the time of PCI. These agents have been shown to reduce adverse cardiac events (e.g., MI, death). The currently approved agents include the small molecules *eptifibatide* (Integrilin) and *tirofiban* (Aggrastat) for use in ACS, as well as the monoclonal antibody *abciximab* (ReoPro) for use in high-risk PCIs (e.g., patients with diabetes, chronic renal insufficiency, ST elevation MI). Recent studies in patients with acute ST elevation MI have demonstrated that intravenous GP IIb/IIIa inhibitors given in combination with a reduced dose of a thrombolytic agent reduces reinfarction, but does not confer a mortality benefit, and is associated with an increased risk of bleeding, particularly in the elderly. Rarely, an immune-mediated thrombocytopenia may also occur. Of note, oral GP IIb/IIIa inhibitors have been developed but have not demonstrated beneficial outcomes in clinical trials.

THROMBOLYTICS AND ANTICOAGULANTS

Thrombolytic Agents (e.g., Streptokinase, Alteplase, Reteplase, Tenecteplase)

With rupture of a coronary artery atherosclerotic plaque, a platelet plug forms. In addition, the biochemical coagulation pathway may also be activated, resulting in a thrombus, containing not only platelets, but red blood cells and the reaction end products of the blood clotting processes, particularly fibrin. Once a thrombus has formed, the only clinically useful pharmacologic strategy involves degrading fibrin with thrombolytic therapy. Thrombolytic agents convert plasminogen to plasmin, thereby activating the endogenous fibrinolytic system and dissolving occlusive fibrin clots (**Figure 7-6**).

In the treatment of acute MI, thrombolytic therapy is aimed at rapid and complete restoration of coronary blood flow through the infarct-related artery; it is indicated for patients who present within 12 hours of the onset of chest pain with either ST segment elevation MI (where there is complete thrombotic coronary artery occlusion) or new (or presumably new) LBBB (suggesting an acute coronary thrombosis has taken place). The goal is to minimize "door-to-needle" time to less than 30 minutes. Early reperfusion reduces infarct size, preserves LV function, reduces the risk of arrhythmias, and improves survival.

Streptokinase (Streptase) is an older non-clot selective agent that stimulates the conversion of circulating plasminogen to plasmin, thus producing a systemic lytic response. *Alteplase* (tPA, Activase), along with the newer fibrin selective agents, *reteplase* (rPA, Retevase), and *tenecteplase* (TNK-tPA, TNKase) activate circulating plasminogen to a lesser extent than surface bound (intracoronary clot) plasminogen. All agents, however, activate circulating plasminogen to varying degrees and, as a result, bleeding is the most important risk of thrombolytic drugs. Since the major risk of thrombolysis is bleeding, contraindications to thrombolytic include patients with a history of a recent stroke, active peptic ulcer disease or an underlying bleeding disorder, severe uncontrolled hypertension (BP ≥ 180/110 mmHg) or those who are recovering from recent major surgery or trauma. Thrombolytic agents have not been proven effective for non-ST segment elevation MI or unstable angina and, in fact, there is evidence that these agents may be harmful.

Recognition of the importance of coronary thrombosis in the pathogenesis of acute MI has led to the intensive development and application of the newer fibrinolytic agents (i.e., double bolus *reteplase* [rPA] and single bolus *tenecteplase* [TNK-tPA] injection). These newer agents, both mutants of tPA with longer half lives, are currently favored over the "gold standard" tPA because of the ease of bolus administration vs. infusion. No thrombolytic agent is ideal for all patients, however, and each has its own advantages and disadvantages. Regardless of which agent is chosen, appropriate and prompt administration is the key to improving survival and quality of life. Specifics of the indications and precautions for the thrombolytic drugs are discussed in the approach to the patient with acute MI in Chapter 11.

Unfractionated and Low Molecular Weight Heparin, Direct Thrombin Inhibitors, and Factor Xa Inhibitors

Heparin anticoagulation (both IV *unfractionated heparin* [UFH] and subcutaneous *low molecular weight heparin* [LMWH] e.g., *enoxaparin* [Lovenox], *dalteparin* [Fragmin]) has also received renewed attention for the treatment of acute coronary syndromes. Heparin enhances the natural anticoagulant properties of antithrombin III, which prevents activation of the coagulation cascade (increases the rate of destruction of activated clotting factors II [thrombin], IX, X, XI, XII), and interferes with the ability of fibrinogen to form fibrin (**Figure 7-6**). Unfractionated heparin is administered parenterally as an intravenous bolus followed by a continuous infusion. Commercial preparations of IV unfractionated heparin are obtained from bovine or porcine sources. The adequacy of anticoagulation with unfractionated heparin can be determined by monitoring the activated partial thromboplastin time (aPTT) or the activated clotting time (ACT). Weight based protocols have become more popular in light of studies that have demonstrated their superiority over non-weight based treatment.

The most common clinical settings in which UFH is being used include unstable angina, non-STEMI, STEMI with PCI or fibrinolytic therapy (i.e., tPA, rPA, TNK-tPA), pulmonary embolism or deep vein thrombosis (DVT). When administering heparin, keep in mind additional drug-drug interactions. IV nitroglycerin may interfere with the anticoagulant effects of heparin. When using both these agents together, patients may require higher doses of IV heparin and should have their PTT levels monitored carefully. Discontinuation of nitroglycerin while heparin treatment is maintained may increase the risk of bleeding and thus require careful monitoring of PTT. Abrupt discontinuation of heparin therapy may result in a rebound effect.

The most important side effect of heparin is bleeding. Another potential adverse effect is immune-mediated, *heparin-induced thrombocytopenia* (HIT) (~3% of cases). HIT can lead to life-threatening bleeding, and has also been associated, paradoxically, with an increased risk of thrombosis (caused by antibodies directed against heparin-platelet complexes, resulting in platelet activation, aggregation, and clot production). The incidence of HIT may be reduced with porcine heparin compared to bovine heparin and with LMWH. Treatment of documented HIT includes discontinuation of all heparin products (SQ, IV, heparin flushes and heparin-coated catheters, as well as LMWH), and institution of alternative anticoagulation i.e., *direct thrombin inhibitors*, that block both circulating and clot-bound thrombin, e.g., lepirudin (Refludan), a recombinant hirudin; argatroban, and bivalirudin (Angiomax), or *factor Xa inhibitors*, e.g., fondaparinux (Arixtra), that indirectly inhibit thrombin generation. Of note, IV bivalirudin is approved for use in patients with ACS undergoing PCI, and has been shown to reduce bleeding events, but at an increased risk (and cost) of acute stent thrombosis, when compared with heparin with or without GP IIb/IIIa inhibitors. Sub Q fondaparinux has been shown to be superior to UFH in patients with STEMI, and superior to LMWH in patients with non-ST elevation ACS, but with less bleeding. In patients undergoing PCI, however, UFH must be added since fondaparinux alone increases the risk of catheter thrombosis.

In addition to a lower risk of HIT, LMWH offers several other advantages over unfractionated heparin. LMWH has a long half life and can be easily administered SQ twice daily. It has greater anti-Xa activity than unfractionated heparin, resulting in a greater inhibition of thrombin generation. Due to its enhanced bioavailability and more reliable anticoagulation effect, there is no need for PTT measurements with LMWH. Furthermore, the use of LMWH is associated with similar or less bleeding than standard IV unfractionated heparin. LMWH is a suitable (may be preferable) alternative to unfractionated heparin in patients with unstable angina, non-ST/ST elevation MI, and in those undergoing PCI. Current clinical indications for LMWH also include prevention and/or treatment of DVT (with or without pulmonary embolism). The use of LMWH, however, has not been adequately studied for thromboprophylaxis in patients with mechanical prosthetic heart valves. Cases of prosthetic heart valve thrombosis (including in pregnant women) have been reported.

Vitamin K Antagonists (e.g., Warfarin) and Novel Oral Anticoagulants (e.g., Dabigatran, Rivaroxaban, Apixaban, Edoxaban)

An increased risk of thromboembolism is associated with many common cardiac disorders, including atrial fibrillation (especially in patients >65 years of age, or those who have hypertension, a history of stroke or TIA, CHF, an LV ejection fraction < 40%, and diabetes mellitus), rheumatic mitral valve disease, acute MI (particularly anterior MI with LV dysfunction, LV aneurysm, and mural thrombus formation), and mechanical prosthetic heart valves. The long-term management, with oral anticoagulation therapy, of selective cardiac conditions associated with an increased risk of thromboembolism has resulted in a significant reduction in morbidity and mortality. The mainstay of oral anticoagulation therapy in patients with cardiovascular disease is *warfarin* (Coumadin), a vitamin K antagonist. Warfarin interferes with the formation of the reduced form of vitamin K, which is necessary in the activation of coagulation factors II (prothrombin), VII, IX, and X (**Figure 7-6**). The dose response differs significantly from patient to patient. Keep in mind that the half-life of factor VII (3–6 hours) is shorter than the half-life of factor II (~72 hours). Warfarin can elevate the prothrombin time (PT) before achieving a true antithrombotic state. Since warfarin's anticoagulation action has a delayed onset (2–7 days), unfractionated heparin or LMWH should be used concurrently at first (so-called "bridging") if an immediate effect is needed. Furthermore, because warfarin also impairs the function of certain vitamin K dependent natural coagulation inhibitors e.g., protein C (which also has a shorter half-life than factor II), theoretical concern exists regarding precipitating a hypercoagulable state before achieving a true antithrombotic state, if heparin-warfarin therapy is not overlapped. Warfarin's effect on coagulation must be monitored closely until individual doses are determined. Over the past several years, the international normalized ratio (INR), obtained by either venipuncture or by simple "finger-stick", has replaced the prothrombin time (PT) as the standard for monitoring oral anticoagulation. The desired therapeutic range for the INR in most cardiac conditions is 2–3. For patients with mechanical heart valves (particularly mitral), or those with higher risk characteristics, the INR should be 2.5–3.5. Of note, many experts recommend the addition of low dose aspirin to warfarin in patients with mechanical heart valves unless there is a contraindication. For select patients at increased risk of bleeding (e.g., those with coronary stents and atrial fibrillation), who require dual antiplatelet therapy and warfarin (so-called "triple therapy"), a low dose (81 mg) of aspirin (for a relatively short duration of time) along with clopidogrel and warfarin (with a target INR of 2.0-2.5), may be reasonable.

If your patient is on warfarin, many different drugs and/or foods can effect the INR levels, so caution should be exercised whenever new medications are administered, or dietary changes take place. (**Figure 7-7**). The safest rule is to tell your patient not to use any new or over the counter drugs (including herbal medicines) without first consulting with you. Commonly used herbal supplements include: Dong quai, Feverfew, Garlic, Ginger, Ginkgo Biloba, Glucosamine sulfate/ chondroitin sulfate (which may increase risk of bleeding when combined with warfarin), Coenzyme Q10, Ginseng, and green tea (which may decrease risk of bleeding in patients on warfarin). Whenever these medications are started or stopped, more frequent monitoring of the PT/INR is necessary. Foods e.g., fish oil, mango, grapefruit juice, and cranberry juice, may raise the PT/INR, whereas high vitamin K containing green salads may lower the PT/INR level. Reduction of warfarin dose is required in the presence of decreased liver blood flow (CHF), liver damage (alcohol, malnutrition), or renal impairment.

FIGURE 7-7

Commonly Used Medications and Foods that Affect Anticoagulation

Increases PT/INR	Decreases PT/INR
Acetaminophen	Barbiturates
Allopurinol	Cholestyramine and
Amiodarone	colestipol
Anabolic steroids	Corticosteroids
Antibiotics (e.g., erythromycin, metronidazole, fluoroquinolones, trimethoprim-sulfa, 2nd and 3rd generation cephalosporins)	Green leafy vegetables (e.g., broccoli, brussel sprouts, lettuce, spinach)—high vitamin K intake
Cimetidine	Herbal medicines (e.g., ginseng, St. John's Wort, Coenzyme Q10)
Fibrates	Rifampin
Heparin	Sucralfate
Herbal medicines (e.g., garlic, ginger, ginkgo, glucosamine)	Vitamin C (high dose)
Isoniazid	
Nonsteroidal anti-inflammatory agents (including celecoxib [Celebrex], rofecoxib [Vioxx])	
Propafenone	
Quinidine	
Thyroxine	
Verapamil	
Vitamin E (high dose)	

Anticoagulation must be reversed for most types of surgery. However, minimally invasive procedures (e.g., dental cleaning) usually can be performed with the patient anticoagulated. Surgery generally can be done once the INR has fallen below 1.5. If the patient needs to remain on anticoagulation therapy as close to the time of surgery as possible, IV unfractionated heparin or SQ low molecular weight heparin, e.g., enoxaparin (Lovenox) can be started while the PT/INR is drifting down toward baseline, discontinued 6 hours prior to surgery, and resumed (usually without a bolus) ≥12 hours after surgery (in the absence of overt bleeding). In cases where the risk of thromboembolism is low (e.g., nonvalvular atrial fibrillation), warfarin may be discontinued several days before surgery and resumed shortly thereafter, without the use of perioperative heparin. The most common adverse effect of warfarin is bleeding.

The risk of bleeding is directly related to the intensity and duration of therapy and may be increased by concomitant treatment with antiplatelet agents, age >65 years, and the use of medications that can elevate the PT/INR. If serious bleeding arises, warfarin's effect can be reversed within hours by the administration of Vitamin K, or even more quickly by transfusing fresh frozen plasma, which directly replenishes functional circulating clotting factors. Warfarin is teratogenic and should not be taken during pregnancy, especially in the first trimester.

Novel (non-vitamin K-dependent) oral anticoagulants (NOACs), e.g., the direct thrombin inhibitor, *dabigatran* (Pradaxa), and factor Xa inhibitors, *rivaroxaban* (Xarelto), *apixaban* (Eliquis) and *edoxaban* (Savaysa), produce reliable anticoagulation without the need for PT/INR monitoring, and are safe and effective alternatives to warfarin for the prevention of stroke and systemic embolism in patients with "nonvalvular" atrial fibrillation (i.e., without a mechanical valve or rheumatic MS), and the treatment of DVT and pulmonary embolism. In contrast to warfarin, NOACs can be given at fixed doses, have a rapid onset of action (that obviates the need for bridging therapy), fewer dietary and drug interactions, and less intracranial bleeding, but are more expensive and, as yet, have no specific antidotes (with the exception of *idarucizumab* [Praxbind], a reversal agent for dabigatran), to reverse their anticoagulation effect. (**Note:** *Andexanet* alfa, a factor Xa inhibitor antidote, is under investigation)

LIPID CONTROLLING AGENTS

Serum lipids play an essential role in the pathogenesis of atherosclerosis. Lipid controlling drugs, particularly statins, can slow the rate of progression, improve clinical outcomes, and reduce mortality rates. Treatment strategies focus first on diet (low in saturated and trans fats, and if the patient is overweight, in total caloric intake) and exercise (which increases serum concentration of HDL). Drug therapy is generally reserved for patients who fail to respond to these lifestyle measures. Lipid controlling agents act on various aspects of lipid absorption and metabolism (**Figure 7-8**). Since these agents work by different mechanisms, they are sometimes combined to achieve a greater effect than possible by monodrug therapy alone.

Figure 7-8. Lipid pathways and sites of drug intervention. (Modified from Goldberg, S. Clinical Physiology Made Ridiculously Simple). Exogenous pathway: Lipids in the diet are taken up by intestinal cells and formed into chylomicrons. Chylomicrons are released into the bloodstream and are hydrolyzed by lipoprotein lipase in fat and muscle cells. The action of lipoprotein lipase liberates triglycerides and releases chylomicron remnants. Chylomicron remnants are taken up by the liver and cleaved, resulting in free cholesterol. Endogenous pathway: The liver synthesizes very low density lipoproteins (VLDLs). VLDLs are released into the bloodstream and cleaved by lipoprotein lipase. This results in the liberation of triglycerides and intermediate density lipoproteins (IDLs). IDLs can either be taken up by low density lipoprotein (LDL)-receptors on the liver or further hydrolyzed to release triglycerides and form LDLs. LDLs bind to their receptors on extrahepatic or hepatic tissues. HDLs are formed by peripheral cells and serve to transport cholesterol to the liver. The effects of drug therapy can be understood from these pathways. *Statins* inhibit the HMG Co-A reductase enzyme and decrease the synthesis of cholesterol and secretion of VLDL, and increase the activity of LDL receptors. *Bile acid binding resins* increase the secretion of bile acids (along with

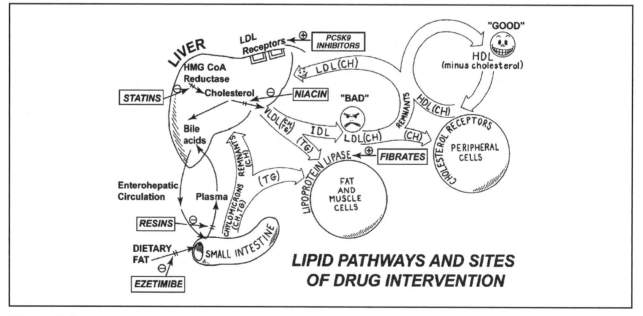

LIPID PATHWAYS AND SITES OF DRUG INTERVENTION

Figure 7-8

cholesterol). *Niacin* increases the secretion of VLDL and the formation of LDL and increases the formation of HDL. *Fibrates* decrease the secretion VLDL and increase the activity of lipoprotein lipase, thereby increasing the removal of triglycerides. *Ezetimibe* inhibits the intestinal absorption of cholesterol (both from the diet and via enterohepatic reabsorption), and lowers LDL cholesterol. *PCSK9 inhibitors* block the degradation of hepatic LDL receptors, which in turn increases the clearance of LDL cholesterol from the blood. Of note, lipoprotein (a) [Lp (a)], a genetic variant of LDL, is synthesized and secreted primarily by the liver, but the receptors that bind and mediate its catabolism are not well understood.

The most commonly used drugs used in the treatment of dyslipidemia include the following:

HMG-CoA Reductase Inhibitors ("Statins")

"Statins" e.g., *lovastatin* (Mevacor), *pravastatin* (Pravachol), *simvastatin* (Zocor), *atorvastatin* (Lipitor), *fluvastatin* (Lescol), *rosuvastatin* (Crestor), and *pitavastatin* (Livalo) inhibit the enzyme HMG CoA reductase, a key rate-limiting component in the biochemical pathway for the synthesis of cholesterol. Inhibition of this pathway results in increased synthesis of LDL receptors, which lowers serum cholesterol. They are highly effective in reducing "bad" LDL cholesterol (↓ 18–55%) and moderately effective in raising "good" HDL cholesterol (↑ 5–15%) and in reducing triglyceride levels (↓ 7–30%). The benefits of statin therapy may extend beyond lipid-lowering. These agents can potentially improve endothelial dysfunction, inhibit platelet aggregation, impair thrombus formation, and reduce inflammation and thus "stabilize" atherosclerotic plaques, which makes them less prone to rupture and consequently reduces clinical CAD events and mortality. They are generally well tolerated but may occasionally raise liver enzymes and blood sugar levels, can cause headache, fatigue, memory loss, constipation, flatulence, dyspepsia, and abdominal pain, and rarely skeletal muscle damage (muscle pain, tenderness or weakness), particularly if used in high doses or when combined with niacin or a fibrate (especially gemfibrozil). Blood tests, e.g., liver function tests (LFTs), creatine kinase (CK), should be obtained initially and when clinically indicated thereafter, to determine whether statins need to be discontinued (**Note:** If LFTs > 3 times and/or CK ≥ 10 times the upper limit of normal, stop statin therapy). Although risk for muscle toxicity exists with all statins, concern has been raised about a potentially greater risk with high dose simvastatin.

Nicotinic Acid (Niacin)

Niacin reduces the production of the triglyceride-containing very low density lipoproteins (VLDLs) in the liver, which in turn, lowers serum LDL cholesterol levels. It is inexpensive and effective in lowering LDL cholesterol (↓ 5–25%), and particularly at raising HDL cholesterol (↑ 15–35%) and lowering Lp(a), an LDL-like lipoprotein that carries an independent risk of ASCVD, by up to 30-40% (but the clinical benefit is uncertain), and triglyceride levels (↓ 20–50%). Compliance can be a problem, however, because of flushing and prominent side effects, e.g., headache, itching, GI upset (do not use in patients with peptic ulcer), liver function abnormalities, increased glucose and uric acid levels. Taking aspirin a half hour before the niacin dose can help ameliorate the flushing reaction. Side effects are better tolerated with extended release preparations. Niaspan is a more recent extended-release form of niacin that has less hepatic toxicity and flushing than former controlled-release forms.

Bile Acid Sequestrants (Resins)

Bile acid sequestrants, e.g., *cholestyramine* (Questran), *colestipol* (Colestid), *colesevelam* (Welchol), are anion exchange resins that bind bile acids in the intestinal lumen, thereby promoting their loss from the GI tract. The resultant interruption of the enterohepatic circulation of bile acids promotes the conversion of cholesterol to bile acids in the liver. Reducing hepatic cholesterol content stimulates the formation of LDL receptors, which reduces serum cholesterol levels. Bile acid sequestrants are used mainly to treat high LDL cholesterol. These agents lower LDL cholesterol (↓ 15–30%) but either do not change or increase triglyceride levels, and have only a minimal effect at raising HDL cholesterol (↑ 3–5%). They are especially useful in combination with "statins". Resins may cause constipation, flatulence, nausea, heartburn, and can decrease the absorption of other medications (e.g., warfarin, digitalis).

Fibric Acid Derivatives

The fibric acid derivatives e.g., *gemfibrozil* (Lopid), *fenofibrate* (Tricor), *fenofibric acid* (Trilipix), increase the activity of the enzyme lipoprotein lipase, which enhances catabolism of triglyceride-rich VLDLs and IDLs, and reduces serum triglyceride levels. These agents lower high triglyceride levels (↓ 20–50%) more effectively than high LDL cholesterol levels (↓ 5–20%) and increase HDL cholesterol (↑ 10–20%). They are generally well tolerated but may cause GI upset (nausea, abdominal pain), cholelithiasis, worsen renal insufficiency, potentiate the effects of warfarin, and can cause myositis or rhabdomyolysis when used alone or in combination with a "statin". Consider fibrates or niacin if HDL cholesterol level is low or triglyceride level is high. Reduction in elevated triglyceride levels can decrease the risk of pancreatitis.

Cholesterol Absorption Inhibitors (e.g., Ezetimibe)

Ezetimibe (Zetia), a *cholesterol absorption inhibitor,* which prevents dietary and biliary cholesterol from crossing the intestinal wall and getting into the blood stream, reduces LDL cholesterol (↓ 18–25%), increases HDL cholesterol (↑ 1–3%) and reduces triglyceride levels (↓ 8–14%). The drug is generally well tolerated, but may raise liver enzymes, particularly

FIGURE 7-9

Antiarrhythmic Drug Therapy

Vaughan-Williams Drug Classification	Clinical Indications	Side Effects
Class I A	Conversion/prevention of atrial fibrillation, atrial flutter, ventricular tachycardia. Prevention of ventricular fibrillation.	
Quinidine (Quinidex)		Diarrhea, proarrhythmia ($\uparrow$ QT, torsades de pointes), thrombocytopenia, 1:1 flutter (vagolytic effect), rash, cinchonism (tinnitus, hearing loss)
Procainamide (Procan)		Nausea, lupus-like syndrome, drug fever, agranulocytosis, proarrhythmia ($\uparrow$ QT, torsades de pointes), 1:1 flutter (vagolytic effect)
Disopyramide (Norpace)		Myocardial depression, proarrhythmia ($\uparrow$ QT, torsades de pointes), 1:1 flutter, anticholinergic effects (urinary retention, dry mouth, blurred vision, constipation)
Class I B	Treatment of ventricular tachyarrhythmias	
Lidocaine (Xylocaine)		Drowsiness, slurred speech, confusion, seizures, respiratory arrest.
Mexiletine (Mexitil)		Nausea, tremor, gait disturbance
Class I C	Conversion/prevention of atrial fibrillation, atrial flutter, ventricular tachycardia. Prevention of ventricular fibrillation.	
Flecainide (Tambocor)		CNS, visual, and GI disturbances, VT (proarrhythmia), 1:1 flutter, CHF
Propafenone (Rythmol)		Metallic taste; CNS, visual, and GI disturbances, VT (proarrhythmia), CHF, increases serum digoxin and INR (warfarin) levels
Class II	Rate control for atrial fibrillation, atrial flutter; prevention of supraventricular tachycardia, with adjunctive ventricular antiarrhythmic therapy.	Marked bradycardia, AV block, bronchospasm, fatigue, depression, cold hands and feet, vivid dreams, memory loss, impotence. May worsen CHF and diabetic control.
β-blockers		
Class III		
Amiodarone (Cordarone)	Conversion/prevention of atrial fibrillation, atrial flutter, ventricular tachycardia.	Thyroid abnormalities, pulmonary fibrosis, hepatitis, corneal microdeposits, bluish-gray skin discoloration, neuropathy, $\uparrow$ QT, increased sensitivity to warfarin.
Sotalol (Betapace)	Prevention of atrial and ventricular fibrillation.	Fatigue, bradycardia, exacerbation of ventricular arrhythmia, $\uparrow$ QT, torsades de pointes
Ibutilide (Corvert)	Conversion of atrial fibrillation/flutter	Torsades de pointes, hypotension, nausea
Dofetilide (Tikosyn)	Conversion/prevention of atrial fibrillation/flutter	$\uparrow$ QT, torsades de pointes, headache, dizziness
Dronedarone (Multaq)	Prevention of atrial fibrillation/flutter	Nausea, vomiting, diarrhea, abdominal pain, asthenia, $\uparrow$ QT

Potassium Channel blockers

FIGURE 7-9

Antiarrhythmic Drug Therapy (*continued*)

Vaughan-Williams Drug Classification	Clinical Indications	Side Effects
Class IV		
Calcium channel blockers Verapamil (Calan, Isoptin), Diltiazem (Cardizem)	Rate control for atrial fibrillation/ flutter, conversion of SVT	Bradycardia, AV block, edema, may worsen CHF, hypotension, constipation (verapamil).
Other Agents		
Digoxin (Lanoxin)	Rate control for atrial fibrillation/flutter	GI and visual disturbances, AV block, ventricular and supraventricular arrhythmias
Adenosine (Adenocard)	Conversion of SVT	Facial flushing, chest pain, dyspnea, transient hypotension and/or atrial standstill (lasting <10 seconds)

---

when combined with a statin, and on rare occasion has been associated with myalgias, rhabdomyolysis, acute pancreatitis, and thrombocytopenia. Ezetimibe may be an additional drug to consider if the LDL cholesterol level remains high despite the maximum recommended and/or tolerated dose of statin. Recent data has shown that the addition of ezetimibe to a statin in high risk ACS patients further reduces cardiovascular events when compared to statin therapy alone.

Proprotein Convertase Subtilisin-Kexin type 9 (PCSK9) Inhibitors

Injectable monoclomal antibodies, e.g., *alirocumab* (Praluent) and *evolocumab* (Repatha) that inhibit the function of proprotein convertase subtilisin-kexin type 9, so-called *PCSK9 inhibitors*, block the degradation of hepatic LDL receptors, which in turn increases LDL cholesterol clearance, and reduces serum LDL cholesterol levels ($\downarrow$40-70%). These agents have been approved as an adjunct to statin therapy for high risk patients with familial hypercholesterolemia or known ASCVD, and may become suitable alternative therapy for patients who are statin-intolerant.

ANTIARRHYTHMIC AGENTS

The pharmacologic treatment of patients with cardiac arrhythmias requires substantial knowledge about the rhythm disorder and antiarrhythmic drugs. It is necessary to choose the effective drug that is least likely to harm the patient. The major factors to be considered include side effects, the presence and severity of LV dysfunction, hepatic and renal insufficiency, and the drug profile. (**Figure 7-9**). The most common classification of drugs used for the treatment of cardiac arrhythmias (based on their electrophysiologic actions) is the modified *Vaughan-Williams classification*. This system includes:

- Classes IA, B and C (*sodium channel blockers*)
- Class II (*beta-receptor blockers*)
- Class III (*potassium channel blockers*) and
- Class IV (*calcium channel blockers*)

An understanding of the mechanism by which action potentials are propagated through conducting cells facilitates learning about the mechanism of antiarrhythmic action (**Figure 7-10**).

Figure 7-10. Left. Relationship of the phases (0–4) of a cardiac action potential from a Purkinje fiber (top) to the cardiac electrical activity on the surface ECG (bottom). Top. Phase 0: Voltage-dependent Na^+ channels open and a rapid movement of sodium ions inward stimulates (depolarizes) the cell. Phase 1: Early phase of repolarization, caused by inactivation of Na^+ influx and the activation of a transient outward K^+ current. Phase 2: Plateau phase, characterized by low membrane conductance and the activation of a slow inward Ca^{++} current (and relatively low K^+ efflux). Phase 3: Rapid repolarization to resting potential results from outward K^+ current. Phase 4 (diastole): Outward K^+ current is deactivated and an inward Na^+ current reduces transmembrane potential. In normal ventricular muscle cells, the resting potential during phase 4 remains in the region of -80 to -90 mV. Bottom. Phase 0 depolarization is reflected in the QRS complex on the ECG. The repolarization period (phases 2 and 3) constitutes the action potential duration that governs the refractory period of heart muscle, and is represented on the surface ECG by the QT interval. **Right.** Sinus node action potential. Not all cells in the cardiac conduction system rely on sodium influx for initial depolarization. In sinus node (shown here) and AV nodal cells, spontaneous diastolic (phase 4) depolarization is mediated primarily by a slow inward movement of calcium ions and, to a lesser extent, sodium ions (I_f "funny" current).

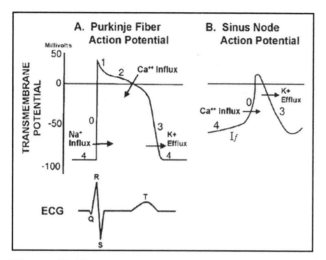

Figure 7-10

Antiarrhythmic drugs influence cardiac conduction properties (usually by modifying ion conductance) and may revert an abnormal rhythm to normal sinus rhythm. They work primarily by reducing ectopic pacemaker activity and/or altering conduction in reentrant circuits. Each class of antiarrhythmic drugs acts on a different phase of the action potential. Class I agents (sodium channel blockers) decrease the upstroke velocity during phase 0 of the action potential. Class II agents (beta blockers) inhibit phase 4 spontaneous depolarization (and indirectly close calcium channels). Class III agents (potassium channel blockers) block the outward potassium channel during phase 3 and prolong the action potential duration and refractoriness (resistance to stimulation). Class IV agents (the rate slowing calcium channel blockers [i.e., verapamil and diltiazem]) inhibit the influx of calcium, which is most responsible for pacemaker automaticity and conduction in the sinus and AV nodes.

Although the electrophysiological effects of most of the antiarrhythmic agents have been defined, their use in controlling arrhythmias remains largely empirical. They must be used carefully since in certain settings they can exacerbate arrhythmias ("proarrhythmic effect"), and most can depress LV function. They should be used with caution, if at all, for patients with life-threatening ventricular arrhythmias and symptomatic SVTs. The following points are of practical use to the clinician and deserve special mention.

Class I Agents

Classes I A, B, and C antiarrhythmic drugs predominately slow the maximum velocity of the upstroke of the Purkinje fiber action potential (phase 0) by blocking the influx of sodium ions into the cell (which decreases the rate of depolarization). (**Figure 7-10**). In clinical trials, these agents have not been shown to decrease mortality in many subsets of patients at risk for sud-

den cardiac death. In fact, they have been shown to increase mortality (proarrhythmic effect) in certain subsets of patients with structural heart disease (particularly those with the most advanced LV dysfunction) and to have no effect on the mortality of others. There is evidence, however, that beta blockers reduce mortality rate, especially in patients with CAD and CHF. In patients who have survived a cardiac arrest or who present with symptomatic VT/VF, guided therapy with group I drugs is inferior to guided therapy with sotalol (Betapace, a Class III antiarrhythmic agent with both Class II beta blocker properties and Class III activity), empiric treatment with amiodarone (Cordarone, a Class III drug), or therapy with an ICD. The use of class I drugs is increasingly being relegated to patients who have symptomatic arrhythmias with no demonstrable structural heart disease. Although proarrhythmic effects may occur in these patients, they are not usually fatal.

Class IA agents (e.g., Quinidine, Procainamide, Disopyramide) (*Figure 7-9*)

Class IA agents moderately slow the rate of rise of the Purkinje fiber action potential and prolong its duration, thus slowing conduction, prolonging repolarization, and increasing refractoriness. These agents particularly affect Purkinje fibers and ectopic pacemakers. These actions can prolong the QRS and QT intervals on the surface ECG. Class IA agents are effective at converting and suppressing a variety of reentrant and ectopic SVTs (e.g., atrial fibrillation and flutter, paroxysmal SVT) as well as suppressing ventricular ectopy (however, they are associated with significantly increased mortality, when used in patients who have structural heart disease). When given to a patient with atrial fibrillation or flutter, class IA agents may increase the ventricular response rate as the atrial rate slows since these agents can also enhance conduction through the AV node by means of their vagolytic effects. A drug with AV nodal blocking properties (e.g., digoxin, beta blockers, verapamil, diltiazem) should be given first. Since *quinidine* (sulfate and gluconate) increases serum digoxin levels, the maintenance dose of digoxin will have to be decreased.

Procainamide (Procan, Pronestyl) is more commonly used in the acute management of arrhythmias. Hypotension may result with rapid IV loading doses. Sixty to seventy percent of patients who receive procainamide develop antinuclear antibodies. Long-term use is associated with a clinical lupus-like syndrome in ∼30% of patients (reversible on stopping the drug).

Disopyramide (Norpace) has prominent anticholinergic effects (especially urinary retention, dry mouth, blurred vision, constipation, aggravation of narrow angle glaucoma) and may worsen established heart failure. Disopyramide has significant negative inotropic properties (i.e., decreases ventricular contractility) and should be used with extreme caution (if at all) in patients with LV systolic dysfunction. Class IA agents present a risk of cardiovascular mortality (proarrhythmic effect—"torsades de pointes"). As a result, use of the entire class IA drugs is gradually shifting to other agents (e.g., class III drugs) or devices for chronic use.

Class IB agents (e.g., Lidocaine, Mexiletine, Tocainide, Phenytoin) (*Figure 7-9*)

Class IB agents mildly slow the rate of rise of the Purkinje fiber action potential and decrease its duration, shorten refractory period and repolarization, and slow conduction velocity through ischemic myocardium (suppresses ventricular automaticity). These agents cause no QRS or QT interval changes, so there is less risk of inducing a proarrhythmia than Class 1A drugs. IV *Lidocaine* (Xylocaine) is recommended for the treatment of symptomatic or life-threatening ventricular arrhythmias. Its primary use is for ischemic-related ventricular arrhythmias in the acute phase of an MI. Prophylactic lidocaine, however, is no longer recommended in the management of acute MI. In fact, it may be detrimental (increased mortality) in this setting. The loading and maintenance dose of lidocaine should be reduced in patients who metabolize the drug slowly (e.g., those with CHF, liver dysfunction, and in those >70 years of age). Toxicity is manifest primarily as central nervous system alterations ranging from tremor and lightheadedness to confusion, stupor, coma, and seizures.

Mexiletine (Mexitil) can be given orally for serious ventricular arrhythmias. As a single agent, potency is low and it is frequently combined with other antiarrhythmics.

Phenytoin (Dilantin), an anticonvulsant drug used extensively for the treatment of epilepsy, is particularly effective in treating atrial and ventricular arrhythmias caused by digitalis toxicity.

Class IC agents (e.g., Propafenone, Flecainide, Encainide) (*Figure 7-9*)

Class IC agents markedly slow the upstroke rate of the Purkinje fiber action potential. They cause such a dramatic slowing of conduction in all cardiac tissues, thereby prolonging the PR and QRS intervals. The QT interval will be affected primarily because of QRS prolongation and not a repolarization effect (because these drugs do not profoundly influence repolarization). Class IC agents are effective in suppressing ventricular arrhythmias, but have a high proarrhythmic potential, particularly in the setting of CAD. Patients at highest risk for proarrhythmia have a history of MI or a low ejection fraction. When administered to post-MI patients with asymptomatic ventricular arrhythmias, flecainide and encainide (and moricizine, a class IA agent) were associated with an increase in mortality (when compared to placebo).

Both *flecainide* (Tambocor) and *propafenone* (Rythmol) have been shown to be effective in preventing recurrent episodes of paroxysmal atrial fibrillation and AV nodal reentrant tachyarrhythmias. Flecainide remains an effective and relatively safe therapy for SVTs (especially paroxysmal atrial fibrillation) in patients with structurally normal hearts and should be used, therefore, only in patients without underlying heart disease. Reports of atrial proarrhythmia include conversion of atrial fibrillation or flutter to flutter with 1:1 conduction. Propafenone is similar to flecainide but with weak beta blocking effects and therefore may exacerbate bradycardia, heart block, CHF, and bronchospasm. Propafenone should be administered with caution, therefore, in patients receiving beta blockers. Propafenone can also increase the serum level of digoxin and the INR with oral anticoagulants (warfarin).

Class II Agents (i.e., Beta Blockers, e.g., Propranolol, Metoprolol, Atenolol)

Class II agents are beta blockers. These drugs inhibit sympathetic nervous system stimulation of cardiac tissue by depressing phase 4 depolarization, thereby decreasing sinoatrial (SA) node automaticity and prolonging atrioventricular (AV) conduction. They prolong the PR interval on the ECG but have little (slightly shorten) or no effect on the QT interval. Beta blockers may be effective in slowing the ventricular response rate in atrial fibrillation or flutter, suppressing episodes of paroxysmal atrial fibrillation, converting paroxysmal reentrant SVTs, suppressing ventricular arrhythmias, preventing post-MI sudden death, suppressing MVP or catecholamine-induced ventricular ectopy, and minimizing QT-related "torsades de pointes" VT (since beta blockers do not prolong the QT interval). They have been shown to reduce the incidence of sudden death in a variety of patient populations and should, therefore, be considered in the therapy of patients with malignant VTs, especially in the setting of LV dysfunction or CAD.

Intravenous *esmolol* (Brevibloc) is useful, in view of its short half-life (∼ 9 minutes) in patients at risk for the common complications of beta blockade (e.g., bradycardia, hypotension) Beta blockers as a class consistently reduce mortality (both total and sudden death). The increased prevalence of hypertension and CAD in patients with recurrent arrhythmias encourages the use of beta blockade for combined antiarrhythmic, antihypertensive, and antiischemic actions. Their long-term proven safety and efficacy makes these agents the best initial choice for primary or adjunctive treatment of patients with supraventricular and ventricular arrhythmias.

Class III Agents (e.g., Sotalol, Amiodarone, Bretylium, Ibutilide, Dofetilide, Dronedarone)

Class III agents exert their antiarrhythmic effects primarily by blocking potassium channels during phase 3 of the action potential. They increase the action potential duration, prolong repolarization and refractoriness, widen the QRS complex, and prolong the QT interval. These agents decrease automaticity and conduction. All Class III antiarrhythmic drugs have proarrhythmic potential.

Sotalol (Betapace) is a non-selective beta blocker that also has Class III properties. It prolongs the QT interval (and therefore may precipitate torsades de pointes). Sotalol has been shown to be effective in the management of ventricular arrhythmias (superior to class I agents) and in the prevention and treatment of atrial fibrillation, but should be used with caution in patients with impaired LV function, as well as reduced renal function. It should not be initiated as an outpatient, if underlying structural heart disease is present.

Amiodarone (Cordarone) is an effective therapy for a wide range of supraventricular and ventricular arrhythmias, including atrial fibrillation and flutter, VT, and SVTs (including those involving bypass tracts). It is recommended as a first line agent for the prevention or treatment of atrial fibrillation in patients with CHF and has been shown to be more effective than class IA agents for the treatment of ventricular arrhythmias. In addition, amiodarone may decrease arrhythmic death after MI, but in patients with moderate to severe ischemic or nonischemic systolic CHF, long term use does not improve survival and may even be detrimental. Amiodarone may be administered IV for the acute treatment of hemodynamically significant and refractory life-threatening ventricular tachyarrhythmias, and is a first line drug for the emergency treatment of VT/VF during cardiac resuscitation. IV use may cause hypotension. When administered orally, it exerts a powerful suppressant effect on PVCs and non-sustained VT, and provides control in 60% to 80% of patients with recurrent VT/VF in whom conventional drugs have failed. However, serious adverse side effects, e.g., pulmonary fibrosis (rarely but occasionally irreversible), thyroid dysfunction, elevated liver enzymes, ataxia, peripheral neuropathy, as well as photosensitivity, blue-gray skin discoloration, corneal microdeposits may occur. Because of the multiple toxicities, patients taking amiodarone should undergo CXR examination and pulmonary function testing (to look for pulmonary fibrosis), liver function tests (to screen for hepatitis), and thyroid function studies (to check for hypo- or hyperthyroidism) every 6 months, along with a slit-lamp ophthalmic examination yearly (to look for corneal microdeposits). Low doses have demonstrated a major decline in the overall incidence of serious adverse reactions, and have been shown to be effective in suppressing SVTs, converting paroxysmal atrial fibrillation, and maintaining normal sinus rhythm after conversion. It has also recently been shown to be effective when administered IV to suppress sustained VT and prevent recurrent VF. QT prolongation is mild with only

rare incidence of proarrhythmic "torsades de pointes". Amiodarone is contraindicated in patients with marked sinus bradycardia and second or third degree heart block in the absence of a functioning pacemaker. During long-term therapy, there is no impairment of LV function. Keep in mind that the drug has a long half-life (averaging 25–60 days) and therefore it takes a long time for the drug to reach therapeutic levels and to be cleared by the body. Amiodarone can increase the serum level of digoxin by 70% and the INR with oral anticoagulants (warfarin) by 100%.

IV *bretylium* has been used mainly in the past in the acute treatment of life-threatening ventricular arrhythmias unresponsive to other agents. Because of limited data to support its use, however, bretylium has been removed from the advanced cardiac life support (ACLS) list of antiarrhythmic agents for patients with pulseless VT or VF.

IV *ibutilide* (Corvert) is a parenteral class III agent approved for the rapid conversion of recent onset atrial fibrillation or flutter. Its role in clinical practice continues to evolve. It restores normal sinus rhythm in ~60–70% of patients with recent-onset atrial flutter and ~35–50% of patients with recent-onset atrial fibrillation and also enhances the success of electrical cardioversion. When effective, acute conversion occurs in the first hour after administration. Prolongation of the QT interval along with torsades de pointes may occur in 5–10% of cases. The reported proarrhythmic effects of IV ibutilide generally occur in the first 4 hours after termination of the IV infusion. Patients treated with ibutilide (and other antiarrhythmic agents that prolong the QT interval) should undergo continuous telemetry monitoring to follow for QT prolongation and the development of torsades de pointes.

Dofetilide (Tikosyn) is a recently approved oral class III antiarrhythmic drug that shows promise as a safe and effective treatment in patients with atrial fibrillation or flutter for inducing a reversion to normal sinus rhythm and maintaining sinus rhythm once it has been achieved. Similar to other class III agents (other than amiodarone), dofetilide's major adverse effect is QT prolongation complicated by torsades de pointes in a small percentage of patients. Therefore, its administration must be performed in the hospital during careful electrocardiographic monitoring.

Another class III agent recently approved is *dronedarone* (Multaq), a deiodinated analog of amiodarone with a much shorter half life (1 to 2 days vs. months) and the potential for less thyroid and pulmonary toxicity. Clinical trial data show a reduced risk of cardiovascular related hospitalization, along with rhythm and rate control, in hemodynamically stable patients treated for atrial fibrillation. Because of an increase in mortality, however, dronedarone is contraindicated in patients with permanent atrial fibrillation and advanced or recently decompensated CHF. Common adverse side effects include nausea, vomiting, diarrhea, and abdominal pain. Similar to amiodarone, dronedarone is rarely associated with torsades de pointes. However, dronedarone is substantially less effective than amiodarone in maintaining sinus rhythm. Patients taking dronedarone should undergo periodic liver function testing, since case reports of rare, but severe liver toxicity have emerged in association with its use.

Class IV Agents (i.e., Calcium Channel Blockers e.g., Verapamil, Diltiazem)

Class IV agents e.g., verapamil and diltiazem, are the slow calcium channel blockers. They are most potent in tissues in which the action potential depends on calcium currents, e.g., the SA and AV node. Within nodal tissue, rate slowing calcium channel blockers decrease SA node automaticity and prolong AV conduction and refractoriness. The ECG may show a prolonged PR interval or slowing of the sinus rate. These agents are useful in the treatment of reentry rhythms involving the AV node, and for slowing the ventricular response to atrial fibrillation and atrial flutter. IV verapamil and diltiazem, therefore, are effective in terminating paroxysmal reentrant SVTs and controlling the rapid ventricular response rate in atrial fibrillation or flutter. IV use can be complicated by hypotension and bradycardia (particularly in patients receiving beta blockers). Chronic oral therapy may be useful in preventing SVTs.

Diltiazem (Cardizem) can be used in conjunction with digoxin for rate control of atrial fibrillation. It is important to note, however, that *verapamil* (Calan, Isoptin) may raise digoxin levels. Beta blockers and rate-slowing calcium channel blockers, by virtue of their ability to selectively slow conduction in the AV node, may increase conduction down a bypass tract, and therefore, are contraindicated in patients with WPW syndrome. The dihydropyridine calcium channel blockers (e.g., nifedipine and amlodipine) do not cause electrophysiologic changes and are not used as antiarrhythmics. They are used primarily to treat patients with hypertension and CAD, including stable, unstable, or variant angina.

Other Agents

All antiarrhythmic drugs do not fit neatly into the above four classifications. As previously mentioned, sotalol possesses characteristics of both Class II and Class III drugs. Some drugs used to treat arrhythmias (e.g., digitalis, adenosine) do not fit into the classification system at all.

Digitalis

Digitalis, a cardiac glycoside, inhibits the Na^+/K^+-ATPase pump that maintains the sodium/potassium transmembrane gradients. It increases cardiac contractility and prolongs the refractory period of the AV node. Digitalis has visible effects on the ECG, i.e. coving or valley-like ST segment depression. Digitalis holds a firm place in the treatment of rapid atrial fib-

rillation and flutter by slowing conduction in the AV node. It is useful for controlling the ventricular response to an SVT and may also be effective in treating AV nodal and AV reentrant tachyarrhythmia. *Digoxin* (Lanoxin) is the drug of choice for rate control in the setting of CHF. Effects of IV digoxin are delayed for 6 to 12 hours; therefore, IV calcium channel blockers or beta blockers are preferred for immediate rate control. Digoxin has minimal efficacy in the presence of high circulating catecholamines (e.g., during exercise or acute illness). Cardiac effects of digitalis toxicity include SA and AV blocks and junctional and ventricular arrhythmias.

Adenosine

Adenosine (Adenocard), a naturally occurring nucleoside that activates potassium channels, has substantial electrophysiologic effects on the sinus and AV nodes. This agent acts on the AV node to slow conduction and inhibit reentry pathways. It can be administered rapid IV bolus to terminate AV nodal or AV reentrant tachycardia (but is not effective in atrial fibrillation or flutter) in ~95% of cases. Transient side effects are common, including sinus bradycardia, AV block, flushing, chest pain, and dyspnea. Metabolism is very rapid with a half-life of 2 to 6 seconds, and adverse effects wear off within 1 minute. The drug should be used cautiously in patients with asthma or those receiving dipyridamole (Persantine). Higher doses may be needed if the patient is on theophylline or caffeine (since these methylxanthines competitively antagonize the adenosine receptor), and lower doses if the patient is on dipyridamole (since dipyridamole inhibits the breakdown of adenosine and enhances its effect).

Ivabradine

Ivabradine (Corlanor), is a novel agent that acts by selectively blocking the hyperpolarization-activated cyclic nucleotide-gated (HCN) channel, thereby inhibiting the inward Na^+/K^+ "funny current" (I_f) in the sinoatrial node, resulting in a dose dependent reduction in heart rate. The drug is approved for use as add-on therapy to reduce the risk of hospitalization (but not mortality) for worsening heart failure in patients with stable, symptomatic chronic heart failure with a reduced ejection fraction $\leq 35\%$, who are in sinus rhythm with a resting heart rate ≥ 70 beats per minute, and who are on maximum tolerated doses of beta blockers or have a contraindication to their use. Unlike beta blockers, ivabradine has no effect on myocardial contractility (no negative inotropic effect). Side effects include bradycardia, atrial fibrillation, and visual disturbances, called phosphenes (flashes of light), which are generally mild and resolve spontaneously. Ivabradine should not be used in combination with agents that prolong the QT interval and must be used cautiously with inhibitors (including grapefruit juice) or inducers of CYP3A4.

CHAPTER 8.   CARDIAC NONPHARMACOLOGIC AND INTERVENTIONAL TECHNIQUES

The inability of certain drugs to control a number of cardiac conditions, along with their potential side effects and cost, make non-pharmacologic treatment an appealing option in selected patients. The field of *interventional cardiology* has greatly increased the options for treatment of coronary and structural heart disease. These non-surgical techniques offer the advantages of reduce discomfort, avoidance of general anesthesia, shorter hospital stays, and substantial cost savings. The next few chapters discuss the catheter-based techniques, devices, and surgical procedures used in cardiology.

PERCUTANEOUS CORONARY INTERVENTION (PCI): PERCUTANEOUS TRANSLUMINAL CORONARY ANGIOPLASTY (PTCA) AND STENTING

In percutaneous coronary intervention (PCI) a catheter is maneuvered from a peripheral artery (femoral, brachial or radial) into a stenotic coronary artery where an attempt is made to widen the stenotic area through local balloon dilatation (angioplasty) or insertion of a stent.

PCI was initially employed mainly in the treatment of single-vessel CAD and select cases of double-vessel CAD, but has been expanded in recent years to patients with multivessel CAD, left main stenosis, chronic total occlusions, acute MI (direct or primary PCI, rescue PCI after failed thrombolysis, cardiogenic shock, routine early PCI following pharmacologic reperfusion), and post-CABG.

Figure 8-1. Left. Significant narrowing of the proximal right coronary artery. **Right.** Plain old balloon angioplasty (POBA) procedure. A small inflatable balloon is passed through the guiding catheter and positioned within

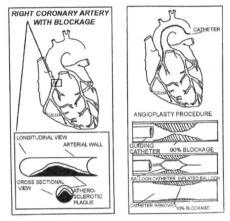

Figure 8-1

the narrowed section of the artery. Inflation of the balloon reduces the blockage. The balloon is then deflated and removed from the artery. Note significant improvement in luminal diameter after angioplasty.

Figure 8-2. Left. Significant narrowing of the proximal portion of the left anterior descending (LAD) coronary artery. **Right.** Angioplasty and stenting. Note that the balloon compresses the plaque against the blood vessel wall. The stent is a small metallic scaffold that expands until it fits the inner wall of the vessel. It stays in place permanently, holding the vessel open and improving the flow of blood. Stents have revolutionized treatment, improving acute results ($\downarrow$ emergency CABG and MI) and long-term results (restenosis) when compared with angioplasty alone. Intravascular radiotherapy (brachytherapy), which has fallen out of favor, and more recently, drug-eluting stents (DES), are advancements that have been developed to address the occurrence of restenosis (see below).

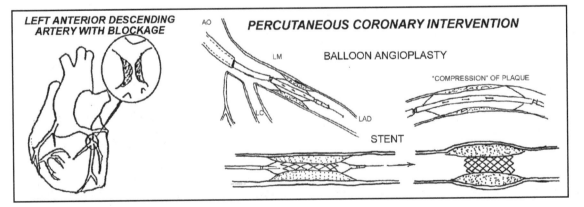

Note: Percutaneous coronary intervention (PCI) includes balloon angioplasty and stenting. Compared with conventional balloon angioplasty, coronary stents, particularly DES, decrease restenosis rates, and reduce the need for repeat target vessel revascularization. Because stents are thrombogenic, dual antiplatelet therapy (lifelong aspirin plus a P2Y12 receptor antagonist, e.g., clopidogrel) is crucial after stent implantation.

Figure 8-2

Optimal lesions for PCI are relatively proximal, non-eccentric, free of significant calcification or plaque dissection, and removed from the origin of large branches. PCI may improve symptom status in some medically refractory patients with stable CAD, but does not decrease the future risk of MI or death (as it does in patients with ACS). Direct PCI for acute ST segment elevation MI is superior to thrombolytic therapy, however, logistics limit its general use. The major advantages compared to CABG include: shortened hospital lengths of stay, decreased initial cost, and decreased recovery time (**Figure 8-3**). Relief of ischemia and objective improvement in heart function occur in the great majority of patients. Disadvantages include renarrowing of the vessel, i.e., *"restenosis"* (the "Achilles heel" of angioplasty) and is often heralded by the recurrence of symptoms.

Over the past few decades, use of a small, metallic device (*stent*) as a scaffold to maintain vessel patency has been shown to reduce restenosis rates by as much as 50 to 75%. Antiplatelet agents e.g., aspirin, ADP receptor blockers (clopidogrel, prasugrel, ticagrelor), GP IIb/IIIa inhibitors (abciximab, eptifibatide, tirofiban), and antithrombotic therapy (IV unfractionated and SQ low molecular weight heparin), along with adjunctive plaque modification devices that debulk fibrocalcific lesions (atherectomy), evacuate clots (thrombectomy), and remove atherosclerotic debris in SVGs (embolic protection), have significantly reduced the atherothrombotic complication rates with PCI.

PCI (angioplasty/stenting) can now be achieved with high success rates (~95%) and at a relatively low risk (coronary artery dissection and acute thrombosis, resulting in acute MI and emergency CABG, occur in ~3% of cases). Restenosis (due to elastic recoil, vascular remodeling, and neointimal hyperplasia) usually occurs within 6 months after the procedure. It occurs angiographically in up to 30 to 40% of patients treated with PTCA alone. Coronary stents are now being used in >90% of PCIs. Coronary stents can be used to treat procedure-related dissection resulting in a decreased need for emergent CABG to <1%. Bare metal stents (BMS) significantly reduce the rate of symptomatic restenosis to 15 to 20%. Although restenosis resulting from vessel elastic recoil is greatly diminished by bare metal stents, neointimal hyperplasia caused by smooth muscle cell proliferation and extracellular matrix production, remains an important cause of in-stent restenosis and recurrent ischemic symptoms (**Figure 8-4**). To address this problem, adjunctive techniques, e.g., intravascular radiation therapy (*brachytherapy*), and more recently, *drug eluting stents* (DES) were developed. Although brachytherapy initially appeared promising in reducing in-stent restenosis, high rates of stent-edge restenosis, i.e., smooth muscle cell proliferation at the edges of the stent have been reported. Furthermore, angiographic studies performed one year after brachytherapy have shown ongoing intrastent luminal loss, suggesting that irradiation may be delaying, but not preventing, long term in-stent restenosis.

A more promising method to prevent in-stent restenosis has been the introduction of coated stents that elute antiproliferative agents (e.g., sirolimus, paclitaxel) into the vessel wall (*"drug-eluting" stents*). *Sirolimus (rapamycin)*, a naturally occurring

---

FIGURE 8-3

Advantages and Disadvantages of Mechanical Revascularization*

	Percutaneous Coronary Intervention	Coronary Artery Bypass Graft Surgery
Advantages	Less invasive than CABG	Effective in relieving symptoms in medically refractory cases
	Decreased hospital stay and easier recuperation	More effective for long term relief of symptoms than PCI
	Lower initial cost	Increased survival in specific anatomic subsets (e.g., left main, severe triple vessel CAD with LV systolic dysfunction, two vessel disease with severe LAD stenosis, especially in diabetics)
	Effective in relieving symptoms (? role of placebo effect)	
	Newer generation DES have lower rates of stent thrombosis, restenosis, and repeat target vessel revascularization than older generation DES and BMS	More complete revascularization
		Less subsequent hospitalization and revascularization
Disadvantages	Incomplete revascularization (limited to suitable anatomic lesions)	Higher initial cost
	"Restenosis" (usually within 6 months)	Increased risk of a repeat procedure due to late graft closure (90% patency rate of internal mammary artery grafts vs 50% patency of saphenous vein grafts at 10 years)
	More subsequent hospitalization, and revascularization	
	PCI does not reduce risk of MI or death in stable CAD.	Increased morbidity and mortality risk of surgery.
		Higher risk of stroke than PCI.
	Poor outcome in diabetics with multivessel CAD.	Longer initial hospital stay and recovery

*Note: Optimal medical therapy is the first line approach for most patients with chronic stable CAD and mild to moderate symptoms. Patients with persistent and/or disabling anginal symptoms, an ACS, and severe (left main or multivessel) CAD, poor LV function, or diabetes may be candidates for PCI/CABG.

macrocyclic antibiotic, is a potent immunosuppressive agent that virtually eliminates neo- intimal proliferation. *Paclitaxel*, a taxane derivative, is a microtubule stabilizing agent that inhibits vascular smooth muscle cell proliferation and migration. Initially, indications for the use of drug-eluting stents (DES) were limited to symptomatic patients with single de novo lesions in a native coronary artery. Current data suggests that treatment of de novo coronary lesions with a DES is safe and is capable of reducing in-stent restenosis to less than 10%. DES have also been shown to be effective in a wide range of subsets, e.g., patients with diabetes, small vessels, long lesions, left main disease, chronic total occlusions, and focal lesions in saphenous vein grafts. Prolonged and uninterruped antiplatelet therapy with aspirin indefinitely and clopidogrel, prasugrel, or ticagrelor for at least 6-12 months is recommended following DES implantation since DES delay endothelialization and late stent thrombosis has been reported after premature withdrawal of these agents. Data for DES using 1st generation sirolimus (Cypher stent) and paclitaxel (Taxus stent), and more recently, 2nd generation everolimus (Xience V/Promus stent) and zotarolimus (Endeavor/Resolute stent), is evolving rapidly. Recent data suggests that PCI with newer generation DES are associated with lower rates of stent thrombosis, restenosis, and repeat target vessel revascularization than older generation DES and BMS. Novel bioresorbable DES have been developed and are under investigation. Early trial data, however, suggests an increased risk of stent thrombosis compared with commonly used DES.

Figure 8.4. Mechanisms of restenosis. PTCA compresses the atherosclerotic plaque and creates a larger immediate lumen in the coronary artery. Restenosis occurs in 30–40% of cases and results from 3 mechanisms: early elastic recoil, late constrictive arterial remodeling, and scar tissue formation due to vessel injury, i.e., neointimal hyperplasia. Bare metal stents reduce restenosis by controlling elastic recoil and arterial remodeling, but do not reduce (and may even promote) neointimal hyperplasis. Drug eluting stents deliver antiproliferative agents (over several weeks) into the vessel wall that inhibit neointimal hyperplasia and result in lower incidence of restenosis (5–10%) than bare metal stents (15–20%).

Patients with CAD may have different prognoses depending on their coronary anatomy, LV function, and comorbidities. When evaluating your patient for PCI or CABG, keep in mind the following:

1. Significant (≥50%) narrowing of the left main coronary artery is the most ominous (the "widow-maker") and usually mandates CABG. (PCI may be considered if not a candidate for CABG.)
2. Triple-vessel disease has a worse prognosis than double-vessel disease. PCI is comparable to CABG in double-vessel and select triple-vessel disease (normal LV function, no diabetes, limited number of discrete lesions [low SYNTAX score]).

3. Single-vessel disease, in most cases, has a good prognosis and can be treated with optimal medical therapy or PCI (if large area of ischemia). Surgery is rarely indicated (unless restenosis occurs after failed PCI, especially for proximal LAD lesions)
4. Significant (≥70%) narrowing of the proximal portion of the coronary arteries has a worse prognosis, especially disease of the proximal LAD, and usually requires intervention (PCI or CABG).
5. In most patients either the RCA or left circumflex is large (dominant) and supplies the inferior wall of the left ventricle. The nondominant vessel (most often the left circumflex) does not supply much heart muscle, and rarely requires interventional treatment.
6. Prognosis is better in those who have a normal LV and worse in those who suffer one or more MIs and whose LV function is below normal. Patients with complex and diffuse triple-vessel disease (high SYNTAX score) and sub-normal LV function (diminished EF) have a particularly poor prognosis, and as a rule benefit from CABG (especially if diabetic).

PERCUTANEOUS BALLOON VALVULOPLASTY, VALVE REPLACEMENT AND/OR REPAIR

Percutaneous balloon valvotomy may be attempted in cases of symptomatic valvular aortic stenosis where surgery is contraindicated because of other concomitant illnesses.

Figure 8-5. Left. Technique of percutaneous aortic balloon valvuloplasty. The balloon is advanced from the femoral artery over a guide wire positioned across the stenotic aortic valve. **Right.** Simultaneous aortic (AO) and left ventricular (LV) pressures before and after aortic valvuloplasty in a patient with severe valvular aortic stenosis. Note marked reduction in aortic valve gradient. This procedure, however, is associated with a high rate of restenosis (50% restenose within 6 months), which limits long term benefit. It is generally reserved for high risk patients with symptomatic severe aortic stenosis who have severe comorbidities (e.g., cardiogenic shock) that preclude aortic valve replacement, or as a "bridge" to definitive surgical correction. In the absence of these indications, the procedure of choice, even in elderly patients, is aortic valve replacement.

Because of its marginal improvement in hemodynamic state and short duration of effect, valvulotomy for adults with calcific valvular AS should be considered a palliative procedure only. On the other hand, balloon valvotomy produces excellent, long-lasting results in selective patients with rheumatic mitral stenosis.

New approaches to percutaneous valve therapy are being investigated. Percutaneous stent mounted valve prostheses have been successfully implanted in the aortic position in

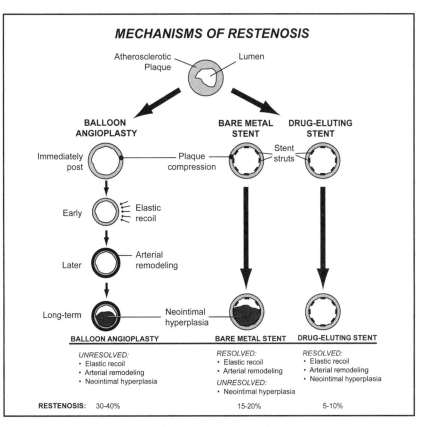

Note: Coronary stents are now being used in > 90% of percutaneous coronary interventions. Compared with balloon angioplasty, coronary stenting provides a larger luminal diameter, maintains arterial patency, and reduces restenosis. Drug eluting stents inhibit cell proliferation and are generally favored over bare metal stents in patients who can take dual antiplatelet therapy for at least 6-12 months, have no upcoming procedures that necessitate premature discontinuation of antiplatelet therapy, are at low risk of bleeding, and/or at high risk for restenosis (e.g., those with diabetes, small vessels, and long lesions). Balloon angioplasty is usually reserved for patients with very small arteries, or when a stent cannot be delivered.

Figure 8-4

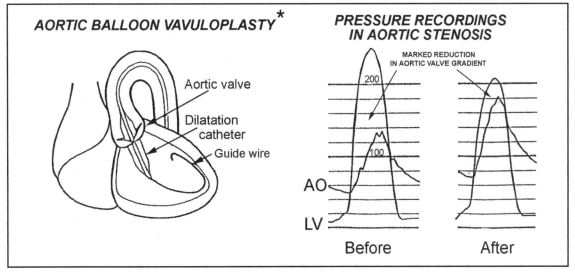

*Note: Transcatheter aortic valve replacement (TAVR), with a balloon-expandable Edwards SAPIEN valve or a self-expanding Medtronic CoreValve, is a viable treatment option for patients with severe symptomatic aortic stenosis who are deemed inoperable or at intermediate to high risk for surgery.

Figure 8-5

symptomatic patients with severe AS who are at intermediate, high, or prohibitive surgical risk. Percutaneous mitral valvuloplasty and repair is also being developed for MR.

Figure 8-6. Left. Mitral balloon valvuloplasty via the transseptal approach. The balloon(s) are advanced up the inferior vena cava into the heart across the atrial septum to the left atrium and across the stenotic mitral valve. This procedure is appropriate for symptomatic patients with severe MS who have mobile, minimally calcified valves, with little or no MR, and no LA clot. In certain cases, open mitral commissurotomy can result in excellent relief of mitral obstruction when balloon valvotomy cannot. If the valve is too severely damaged and calcified, however, mitral valve replacement should be performed.

CATHETER ABLATION

Apart from drugs, which have many side effects, the treatment armamentarium for cardiac arrhythmias now includes radiofrequency (RF) energy (heat) and cryothermal (cold) catheter ablation techniques. RF catheter ablation has become the primary treatment modality for many cardiac tachyarrhythmias. The appeal of a safe, highly effective therapy for symptomatic tachyarrhythmias that avoids the need for long-term medication and its potential attendant problems and that can be performed at the time of an initial diagnostic EPS is evident. Problems with long-term medication include adverse medication side effects, multiple daily doses (non-compliance), and failure to cure. RF ablation is successful in well over 95% of patients with the common forms of paroxysmal SVT. It is effective in eliminating AV reciprocating tachycardias caused by accessory pathways (e.g., WPW syndrome) or AV nodal

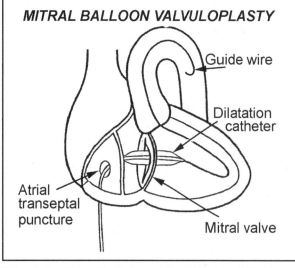

MITRAL BALLOON VALVULOPLASTY

Guide wire

Dilatation catheter

Atrial transeptal puncture

Mitral valve

Note: Grading (1-4 each) of leaflet mobility, thickening, calcification, and subvalvular fibrosis (Wilkins echo score) can predict outcome of mitral balloon valvuloplasty (A total valve score ≤ 8 is favorable).

Figure 8-6

reentrant tachycardias due to dual pathways in the AV node. RF ablation is also used in certain atrial tachycardias, flutter and fibrillation, and in VT, especially the idiopathic variety when there is no underlying structural heart disease. The success rate of ablation for atrial flutter is ~90%. In patients with atrial fibrillation refractory to attempts at cardioversion or pharmacologic rate control, AV nodal ablation and pacing offers a definitive method of controlling the ventricular rate.

Ablation techniques are currently being developed to treat and potentially cure atrial fibrillation as well, delivering wide circumferential lesions outside the ostia of the pulmonary veins (which decreases the risk of pulmonary vein stenosis) with additional linear ablation in the LA. Success rates are ~ 70% (but more than one procedure may be required), with the best results in patients with paroxysmal atrial fibrillation and no structural heart disease. These procedures are generally safe, although there is a low incidence of stroke, perforation of the atria (atrio-esophageal fistula) or RV that may result in pericardial tamponade and sufficient damage to the AV node to require permanent pacing in < 5% of patients.

ELECTRICAL CARDIOVERSION AND DEFIBRILLATION

Tachyarrhythmias (supraventricular or ventricular) that produce chest pain, shortness of breath, decreased level of consciousness, hypotension, shock, CHF, or acute myocardial ischemia, may require emergency cardioversion. External cardioversion rapidly establishes normal sinus rhythm. In elective circumstances, cardioversion should always be performed after the patient has fasted for 8 hours, and in the synchronized mode (*synchronized to the QRS complex and not on the T wave, which may precipitate VF*).

Figure 8-7. The anteroapical position for cardioversion or defibrillation. Proper electrode position is key.

Figure 8-8. Left parasternal anterior-posterior electrode placement for synchronized direct current (DC) cardioversion. Provides optimal current flow through atria and is more effective for cardioversion of atrial fibrillation (courtesy of Dr. Gordon A. Ewy).

Electrical *cardioversion* (shock delivered synchronously with the QRS complex, thus avoiding the vulnerable phase of the cardiac cycle) and *defibrillation* (shock delivered on an emergency basis during cardiac arrest without synchronization to the QRS complex (to terminate VF) appear to terminate most effectively those tachycardias presumed to be due to reentry. Reentry tachycardias include atrial flutter and fibrillation, AV nodal reentry, reciprocating tachycardias associated with WPW syndrome, most forms of VT, ventricular flutter and VF. Generally, any tachycardia that produces hypotension, CHF, or angina, and that does not respond quickly and appropriately to

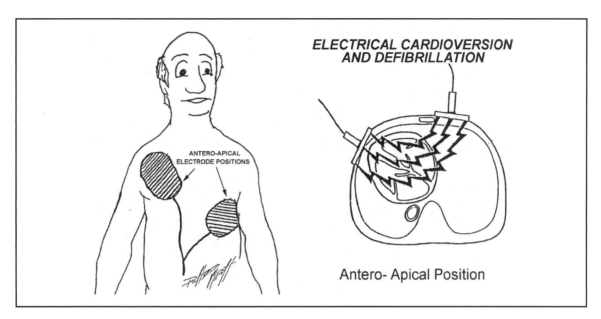

Figure 8-7

medical management should be terminated electrically. Electrical cardioversion restores normal sinus rhythm in 70% to 95% of patients (depending on the type of tachyarrhythmia).

Electrical cardioversion is frequently performed to restore sinus rhythm and relieve symptoms of atrial fibrillation. There are a number of predictors of successful sustained cardioversion. These include duration of atrial fibrillation, LA size (success is less with a large atrium, where there may be disruption of the normal electrical pathways), the presence and etiology of heart disease, and precipitating factors. Most studies indicate that duration of atrial fibrillation is the most important predictor. Cardioversion should be performed as soon as it is safe for the patient. In patients in whom the duration of atrial fibrillation is unknown or is believed to be > 48 hours,

therapeutic oral warfarin anticoagulation (to an INR of 2 to 3) or NOAC is recommended for ≥3 weeks before cardioversion. Pre-cardioversion TEE has been used to evaluate the presence of atrial thrombi in non-anticoagulated patients. Because mechanical atrial function may not return for several weeks after cardioversion *("atrial stunning")*, all patients should receive anticoagulation therapy for at least 4 weeks after the procedure, even if the TEE detected no atrial thrombi. In patients with prior risk factors for stroke (e.g., age > 65 years, hypertension, diabetes, CHF, history of TIA or stroke), chronic anticoagulation should be considered even if NSR is thought to be maintained (since recurrent episodes of atrial fibrillation may be asymptomatic and go undetected [i.e., "silent" atrial fibrillation]).

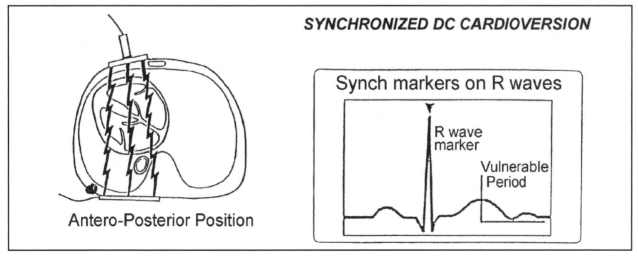

Figure 8-8

CHAPTER 9.   CARDIAC DEVICE THERAPY

CARDIAC PACEMAKERS AND RESYNCHRONIZATION THERAPY

Pacemakers are described by a 4-letter code:

- The first letter refers to the chamber(s) *paced,* i.e., Atrial (A), Ventricular (V), or Dual (D).
- The second letter refers to the chamber(s) *sensed* (A, V, or D).
- The third letter refers to the pacemaker *mode,* i.e., Inhibited (I), Triggered (T), or Dual (D).
- The fourth letter refers to *programmable functions.* The letter R = rate responsiveness, which denotes that the device has a sensor that increases the pacing rate in response to a perceived physiologic requirement.

A typical *single-chamber* demand (back-up) pacemaker is a VVI, which paces in the right ventricle, senses in the ventricle, and inhibits ventricular pacing if there is a sensed QRS. A typical *dual-chamber* pacemaker is the DDDR (paces and senses both the right atrium and right ventricle), and inhibits and triggers a paced response. Both pacemaker types are rate-responsive to exercise (by sensing body motion or respiratory rate). (**Figure 9-1**). A pacemaker that senses and paces in both chambers is the most physiologic approach to pacing patients who remain in sinus rhythm. Dual chamber pacing is most useful for individuals with LV systolic or, perhaps more importantly, diastolic dysfunction (since they preserve "atrial kick").

For many years, most cardiac pacing was ventricular in either the fixed-rate or demand (stand-by) mode. Present pacemaker technology has made early fixed-rate pacemakers obsolete. Only demand-type pacemakers are in current use. VVI or VVIR (ventricular leads only) pacing is particularly appropriate when there is chronic atrial fibrillation (i.e., no "atrial kick") and when there is a short life expectancy and low risk for *pacemaker syndrome* (fatigue, weakness, dyspnea, diminished exercise tolerance, even to the point of CHF, lightheadedness). Patients with VVI pacemakers, however, may develop pacemaker syndrome, due to loss of AV synchrony, resulting in a drop in cardiac output of up to 20 to 40%, especially in stiff, noncompliant ventricles (e.g., CAD, hypertension, valvular AS, HOCM).

Figure 9-2. Left. A patient with a single chamber ventricular demand (VVI) pacemaker. The pacemaker generator is placed beneath the skin below the clavicle in the pectoral region, while the tip of the transvenous pacing electrode is lodged in the apex of the right ventricle. **Right.** Pacemaker syndrome. Note that normal sinus rhythm with a blood pressure of

150/95 mmHg is initially present. A ventricular demand pacemaker captures the ventricle with resultant AV dissociation and loss of atrial contribution ("atrial kick") to stroke volume in beats 4–9 (arrow). Note the prompt drop in BP to levels as low as 110/75 mmHg. In the upright position or during physical activity, such a rapid fall in BP may cause symptoms of low cardiac output (e.g., lightheadedness, near-syncope, or even syncope), clinically manifest as the pacemaker syndrome. This syndrome can be treated by restoring AV sequential contraction. Pacemaker syndrome has been resolved with dual-chamber (DDDR) AV sequential pacing (preserves AV synchrony).

Figure 9-3. Left. A patient with a dual chamber (atrial and ventricular) pacemaker. **Right.** ECG tracing demonstrating AV sequential pacing (DDD, DVI) with mode switching. The atrium, ventricle, or both can be paced or sensed electronically. In the last complex, the atrial electrode paces the atrium, and after a programmed delay, signals the ventricular electrode to pace the ventricle (AV sequential pacing). If the patient's intrinsic sinus rate is faster than the programmed atrial pacing rate, the pacemaker switches to a P triggered mode (6–8th complexes). If the patient's AV conduction resumes and the sinus rate is fast enough, both the atrial and ventricular pacing will be inhibited (1st and 2nd complexes). If the AV conduction becomes normal, but the sinus rate is not fast enough, the pacemaker switches to an atrial pacing mode (3rd–5th complexes). Patients with DDD pacemakers may develop *pacemaker mediated tachycardia,* whereby a ventricular premature or paced beat is conducted to the atrium and is sensed by the atrial lead as a retrograde P wave, which triggers ventricular stimulation in a rapid repeating cycle (so-called "endless loop" reentrant tachycardia.)

For patients with chronotropic incompetence, rate adaptive pacing is important to provide adequate heart rate response to exercise or stress. Recent devices can automatically switch the pacing mode (*"mode switching"*) from DDDR to VVIR if the patient goes into atrial fibrillation. For patients with paroxysmal atrial fibrillation, during sinus rhythm, the pacemaker would be in DDD, and during atrial fibrillation it would convert to VVI to avoid ventricular tracking of atrial fibrillation.

Permanent pacing is recommended for patients with symptomatic (or potentially significant) heart block, sinus bradycardia, and atrial fibrillation with symptomatic bradycardia off medications (*sick sinus syndrome*). Permanent pacing also assists with the treatment of the sick sinus syndrome since any antiarrhythmic therapy (used for tachyarrhythmia) will exacerbate the bradycardic aspects of this entity. Reversible and self-limited causes (e.g., drug toxicity, acute MI) of these arrhythmias must first be excluded. After MI, a permanent pacemaker is indicated for patients with

---

FIGURE 9-1

Common Pacing Modes

VVI–Ventricular demand pacemaker

Does not preserve AV synchrony (single lead in right ventricle)

Not rate responsive

Used for backup when bradycardia is infrequent and brief

Used in chronic atrial fibrillation with symptomatic pauses; after AV nodal ablation for rate control; or in old, debilitated patient.

May cause pacemaker syndrome (syncope/presyncope, orthopnea, PND, CHF) due to loss of AV synchrony.

AAI–Atrial demand pacemaker

Preserves AV synchrony

Not rate responsive.

Requires intact AV condition.

Used for symptomatic sinus pauses with otherwise normal sinus node function and AV conduction.

DVI–AV sequential pacemaker

Does not sense in atrium.

Not rate responsive.

Preserves AV synchrony with atrial rate ≤ pacemaker rate.

DDD–Dual chamber pacing and sensing

Atrial sensing allows atrial tracking with rate responsiveness.

Requires intact SA node function for rate increase.

Preserves AV synchrony (leads in both right atrium and right ventricle).

May cause pacemaker mediated tachycardia (so-called "endless loop" reentrant tachycardia).

VDD–Atrial tracking pacemaker

Preserves AV synchrony and rate responsiveness.

Does not pace atrium at time of atrial slowing.

Pacemaker code: The first letter represents chamber paced; the second letter, chamber sensed; and the third letter, response to sensed beat. (**A** = atrial, **V** = ventricular, **I** = inhibited.) A rate responsive feature (**R**) can be added to either a single or dual chamber system if the patient does not have the ability to increase his or her rate appropriately with exercise. If rate responsiveness is incorporated, the pacing code would be changed from VVI to VVIR or DDD to DDDR, etc. A mode switching feature can also be used if any paroxysmal atrial arrhythmias occur.

Note: In patients with LV systolic dysfunction, RV pacing alone can lead to LV dyssynchrony, precipitate CHF, and worsen outcomes. In such patients, consideration should be given to biventricular pacing (cardiac resynchronization therapy).

---

persistent second and third degree AV block with associated BBB (typically in the setting of anterior MI). Recurrent syncope after carotid sinus stimulation (hypersensitive carotid sinus syndrome) and documented > 3 second pauses are indications for permanent pacing. (**Figure 9-4**).

Other special pacing modes and/or indications include *antitachycardia pacing,* to terminate VT, *"rate drop response" pacing* for vasovagal (neurocardiogenic) syncope, pacing to reduce LV outflow tract obstruction in HOCM, *biventricular pacing* (cardiac resynchronization therapy [CRT]), for CHF, and *leadless pacing,* to reduce the risk of device complications.

Biventricular pacing, using leads that stimulate the RV from the apex and the LV from the lateral wall via the coronary sinus, appears to be a promising therapeutic approach in patients with CHF due to LV systolic dysfunction who remain symptomatic despite aggressive medical therapy. Patients with wide QRS complexes, reduced ejection fractions, and NYHA Class III–IV CHF who received multisite pacing have demonstrated an increase in ejection fraction and improvement in symptoms and exercise tolerance. Definitive data on morbidity or mortality shows that CRT offers a beneficial effect. Devices that combine biventricular pacing and intracardiac cardioverter-defibrillator (ICD) capabilities are also now available (see below). For select Class I–II CHF patients, particularly women with nonischemic cardiomyopathy and LBBB, the use of a combined CRT-ICD device may improve quality of life and functional status, reduce hospitalizations, and improve survival.

Early permanent pacemakers were powered by mercury zinc batteries. These have been replaced by lithium

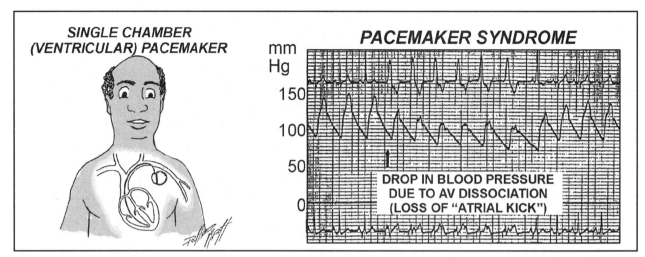

Note: In a single chamber ventricular demand (VVI) pacemaker, 1 pacing lead is implanted in the apex of the right ventricle. Of note, a recently approved, entirely leadless RV pacemaker is a promising treatment option for select bradycardic patients.

Figure 9-2

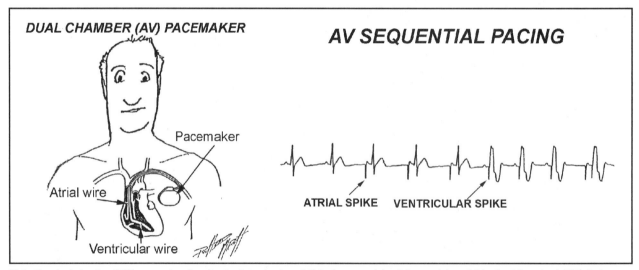

Note: In a dual chamber (AV) pacemaker, 2 pacing leads are implanted (1 in the apex of the right ventricle and 1 in the right atrium). This is the most common type of implanted pacemaker.

Figure 9-3

batteries, which have improved longevity (4–10 years). The insertion of a permanent pacemaker is frequently lifesaving and improves the quality of life. Several potential issues, e.g., keeping cautery distant from pacemaker during surgery, keeping hand-held cellular phones 6 or more inches from the pulse generator, avoiding magnets (including MRI) close to the pulse generator, should be discussed with the patient to ensure his or her safety and device longevity. Airport metal detectors are safe, however, and most electrical equipment found in the home (e.g., microwave ovens, electric shaver) will not cause damage, particularly to the newer devices. Although complications of permanent pacing are uncommon, they may occur. These include pneumothorax, myocardial perforation, hematoma, venous thrombosis, infection,

impulse generator migration, and malfunction due to lead displacement or fracture.

IMPLANTABLE CARDIOVERTER DEFIBRILLATOR

The implantable cardioverter defibrillator (ICD) is an important therapeutic modality whose indications are noted in **Figure 9-5.** The ICD can detect malignant ventricular arrhythmias and deliver appropriate electrical treatment for the rhythm disturbance. In addition, they are programmable for various modes of antitachycardia pacing, low energy as well as higher energy shocks, antibradycardia pacing, and telemetry function, and can perform some electrophysiologic testing noninvasively.

FIGURE 9-4

Clinical Indications for Permanent Pacemakers

- Sinus node dysfunction with symptoms of cerebral hypoperfusion.
- Acquired complete or high grade AV block with wide QRS complex and symptomatic bradycardia, asystolic pauses > 3 sec., or escape rates < 40/min.
- Second degree AV block with symptomatic bradycardia.
- Atrial fibrillation with 5 second pauses.
- Neurocardiogenic syncope with bradycardia during head-up tilt table testing.
- Carotid sinus hypersensitivity with symptomatic bradycardia or asystolic pauses > 3 sec., provoked by carotid sinus massage.
- Post catheter ablation of the AV junction.
- Resynchronization therapy with biventricular pacing for severe systolic heart failure and widened QRS complex.

Note: In general, the patient should be free of any drug, electrolyte abnormality, or condition (e.g., ischemia) which when reversed would eliminate the need for a pacemaker. On occasion, a pacemaker may be placed for symptomatic bradycardia caused by some medications for which there is no acceptable alternative.

FIGURE 9-5

Clinical Indications for ICD Implantation*

Secondary Prevention
- Survivors of cardiac arrest due to VF or VT not due to a reversible cause.
- Spontaneous sustained VT in the presence of structural heart disease.
- Syncope and inducible sustained VT/VF on EP study.

Primary Prevention
- Prior MI (≥ 40 days) with EF ≤ 30%
- Ischemic and noniachemic cardiomyopathy (for ≥ 3 months) with an EF ≤ 35%
- Familial or inherited conditions e.g., Brugada syndrome (with syncope or VT), long QT syndrome (with syncope or VT despite β-blocker therapy), arrhythmogenic RV dysplasia/cardiomyopathy (with extensive RV disease, family history of sudden death, syncope, or VT), and hypertrophic cardiomyopathy with one or more risk factors for sudden cardiac death (e.g., family history of sudden death, unexplained syncope, LV thickness ≥ 30 mm, hypotensive BP response to exercise, or VT).

---

* **Note:** Patients must have an anticipated life expectancy of ≥ 1 year.

Figure 9-6. Left. Implantable cardioverter defibrillator (ICD); early (left) and contemporary (right) models. Note that the early ICD system used epicardial patch electrodes for defibrillation and epicardial leads for rate sensing. This system required thoracotomy for implantation. **Right.** The current model has leads with both sensing and defibrillating function and can sense VT, with antitachycardia pacing and/or shocks. The modern ICD is of sufficiently small size allowing for nonthoracotomy pectoral implant.

The progression through antitachycardia pacing (ATP), low energy, then high energy shocks, is referred to as "tiered" therapy. ICDs are not indicated for patients with arrhythmias caused by reversible and otherwise treatable conditions (e.g., ischemia/infarction, drug effects, electrolyte disturbances).

ICDs have been shown to decrease mortality compared with antiarrhythmic therapy in survivors of VF or hemodynamically unstable VT. Additional antiarrhythmic therapy is often necessary after ICD implantation to decrease the frequency of ventricular tachyarrhythmic events or to control the rate of SVTs so that the number of shocks a patient receives from the device is limited. The initiation of antiarrhythmic drugs, however, must be undertaken with caution. These agents may slow VTs to below the programmed ICD detection rate (i.e., the arrhythmia is not identified) and/or increase the defibrillation threshold (i.e., renders defibrillation ineffective). Patients who have sustained monomorphic VT that is demonstrated to be pace-terminable in the EP laboratory, and who are not good surgical candidates, can receive devices that will pace-terminate tachycardias, which is a much less traumatic experience than shock.

There are currently insufficient data on which to base firm recommendations for the management of patients with asymptomatic nonsustained ventricular arrhythmias. Beta blockers are the first line of therapy, but there is no evidence that antiarrhythmic drugs (with the exception of amiodarone) are beneficial, and they carry substantial risk ("proarrhythmic effect"). Recent data has demonstrated that for patients at least 40 days post-MI, or those with nonischemic cardiomyopathy, who have significant LV systolic dysfunction (EF < 30–35%), with or without spontaneous or inducible ventricular arrhythmias, an ICD provides a much better clinical outcome than does conventional drug therapy. Of note, a wearable cardioverter-defibrillator (LifeVest) may provide some protection against

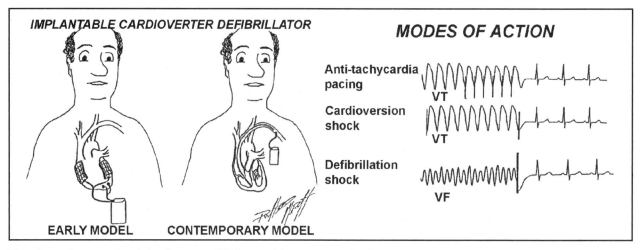

Note: A recently approved, entirely subcutaneous ICD is a promising treatment option for select patients that do not require antibradycardia, antitachycardia, or cardiac resynchronization pacing.

Figure 9-6

sudden cardiac death in select high risk patients, e.g., those < 40 days post-MI, or with newly diagnosed nonischemic cardiomyopathy, who may not qualify for an ICD. Due to the economic implications and potential complications of ICD therapy (e.g., inappropriate shocks and their effects on quality of life), new and improved methods of risk stratification beyond depressed LV function (e.g., T wave alternans analysis) that can more accurately guide patient selection are needed. Worthy of mention, an ICD device combined with biventricular pacing, i.e., cardiac resynchronization therapy (CRT), may be a better option as the initial implant in patients with advanced CHF and significant LV systolic dysfunction (EF ≤ 35%), particularly those with LBBB and wide QRS complexes (≥ 150 msec) (**Figure 9-7**). Recent studies have shown that CRT can improve exercise

capacity, functional status, quality of life, and survival (especially when combined with an ICD) in many of these patients.

A 6-month restriction on private driving should be enforced if the ICD is placed for secondary prevention. It takes between 5 and 15 seconds for the ICD to detect, charge, and deliver a shock. Activities (e.g., driving) place everyone at risk if VF recurs. Patients who experience long periods (e.g., ≥ 6 months) without a shock and/or demonstrate an absence of fainting, even if an event occurs, are generally allowed to return to driving. Patients with ICDs should not have an MRI, and their device should be turned off before (and then on again after) a surgical procedure, since cautery may interfere with the ICD's sensing function, resulting in an inappropriate delivery of antitachycardia pacing and/or shock.

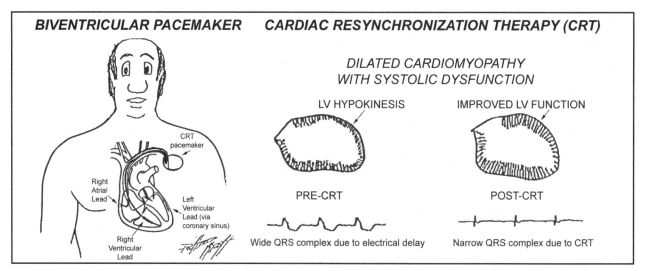

Note: In a biventricular pacemaker (cardiac resynchronization therapy), in addition to pacing leads in the right atrium and right ventricles, a third pacing lead is advanced from the coronary sinus to the lateral wall of the left ventricle (allows pacing of the LV simultaneously with the RV and helps resynchronize cardiac activation thereby improving LV function).

Figure 9-7

CHAPTER 10. CARDIAC SURGERY

CORONARY ARTERY BYPASS GRAFTING

Coronary artery bypass grafting (CABG) remains the most common cardiac surgical procedure performed in the United States. Coronary revascularization can provide significant relief of symptoms in > 80% of patients with angina pectoris refractory to drug therapy. It has a low operative mortality rate (1–2%) in otherwise healthy patients with preserved LV function and carries a low incidence (1–4%) of perioperative MI and stroke. Of these, most have complete relief of angina, while the remainder report that their angina occurs less frequently and is more difficult to induce.

In general, CABG should be limited to those patients whose symptoms can not be managed medically (with lifestyle and risk factor modification, nitrates, beta blockers, calcium channel blockers), patients who have failed PCI, or patients with significant left main or multivessel CAD. CABG is a particular consideration for patients with angiographically complex and diffuse CAD (high SYNTAX score) and for those with diminished LV function (ejection fraction < 50%), especially if diabetic.

Graft closure and recurrence of symptoms continues to be a problem. Since the patency rates for the left internal mammary artery are > 90% at 10 years after surgery (compared to ~50% for saphenous vein grafts) the use of arterial conduits has markedly increased.

Figure 10-1. Schematic diagram demonstrates the left internal mammary artery (LIMA) graft to the left anterior descending (LAD) coronary artery and an aortocoronary saphenous vein graft (SVG) to the right coronary artery (RCA), "bypassing" the blockages in the coronary arteries.

Aggressive lipid lowering (statins) and the daily use of aspirin have been shown to reduce the incidence of SVG occlusion. Minimally invasive approaches to CABG, along with "hybrid" procedures (e.g., LIMA-LAD graft with PCI of other vessels), are gaining in popularity. These approaches include limited sternotomy, lateral thoracotomy, *minimally invasive direct coronary artery bypass* (MIDCAB) or thoracoscopy (Port-access), using robotics technology in selected cases, along with "off pump" procedures utilizing a mechanical coronary stabilizer, that enables CABG to be performed on the beating heart without the assistance of cardiopulmonary bypass (which may lessen the risk of cerebral complications). Although these techniques allow for smaller incisions, along with shorter hospital lengths of stay and the potential for less morbidity and earlier return to normal activity, there is concern that long-term patency rates will not be as good as those performed with the heart arrested. Of note, recent trial data have shown a worse 5 year mortality rate with "off-pump" compared with "on-pump" CABG.

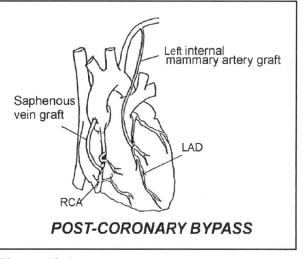

Figure 10-1

Patients with greater degrees of symptoms, greater ischemic burden and more severe angiographic CAD demonstrate the greatest benefit from CABG. Compared with medical therapy, surgery decreases mortality in patients with significant left main disease and in patients with triple-vessel CAD or double-vessel CAD involving the proximal portion of the LAD associated with depressed LV systolic function, especially if they are diabetic. Surgery is more invasive than PCI and has a slightly higher periprocedure mortality rate, but it is also more effective for symptom control, and requires fewer repeated procedures than does PCI. The expected marked decrease in restenosis with drug-eluting stents may favor the use of PCI over CABG in carefully selected patients in the future. Patient risk factors for surgery include LV systolic dysfunction, advanced age, female gender (due to smaller body habitus and target vessel size and later referral for testing—possibly due to atypical symptoms), and the extent and severity of CAD. Overall, patients undergoing CABG surgery within the last 10–15 years tend to be older, with more chronic disease (e.g., diabetes mellitus, renal insufficiency), and have greater severity of CHF and CAD, coexistent valve dysfunction requiring repair or replacement and/or have had a prior CABG. Of note, the mortality rate increases to 4–8% in this high risk population.

VALVE REPAIR AND/OR REPLACEMENT

Repair or replacement of diseased cardiac valves has had a major impact on improving the natural history and the prognosis of patients with valvular heart disease. However, heart surgery continues to carry a certain unavoidable risk of morbidity and mortality, and complications of prosthetic valves (e.g., thromboembolism, infection, malfunction, hemolytic anemia) are so protean and common that the presence of an artificial heart valve should itself be considered a "disease". The practitioner's dilemma about when to recommend valve surgery is compounded by the fact that minimally diseased native valves may serve the patient better and longer than the best prosthetic valve. Conversely, the earlier the surgery, the lower the operative risk. Intervention too early may deny the patient many years of active life without a valve prosthesis, while waiting too long may result in irreversible damage to the myocardium or pulmonary vasculature. In addition to the appropriate timing of surgery, the choice between repair (e.g., for MR), percutaneous balloon valvulotomy (e.g., for MS), or replacement with a bioprosthetic valve (limited durability with the need for eventual reoperation) or mechanical valve (risk of chronic anticoagulation and thromboembolism) are the major issues confronting today's clinician.

Repair of a valve is always preferred because the patient's own native valve may function effectively for many years without risk from anticoagulant therapy or other adverse effects associated with a prosthesis. Cryopreserved aortic homografts are particularly applicable for patients with native or prosthetic valve endocarditis, and offer durability for younger patients without the need for anticoagulation. Malfunction of mechanical prosthetic valves is unusual but may result from thrombus formation, tissue ingrowth leading to obstruction, mechanical disruption of the valve struts and/or disc, or leaks around the suture lines (paravalvular leak) or dehiscence of the prosthesis. Bioprosthesis may develop thickening, calcification, and ultimately obstruction or retraction of the leaflets. Malfunction may be sudden (presenting as acute pulmonary edema) or gradual. It should be suspected when a patient presents with the development of a new regurgitant murmur (e.g., AR, MR), alterations of the timing or quality of opening or closing sounds, embolization in the presence of adequate anticoagulation, increasing severity of intravascular hemolysis, development of CHF, angina, or syncope after a period of improvement. Doppler-echo may help confirm the diagnosis. Repeat surgery is usually indicated.

Mechanical (e.g., bileaflet, tilting disc, caged ball) and bioprosthetic valves (e.g., bovine pericardial or porcine heterograft, human homograft) differ with regard to hemodynamic performance, durability, thromboembolic complications, and the need for anticoagulation.

Figure 10-2. Types of prosthetic heart valves. **A)** Starr-Edwards ball and cage valve; **B)** Medtronic-Hall and Omniscience tilting (single) disc valve; **C)** Hancock and Carpentier-Edwards porcine valve; **D)** St. Jude and Carbomedics bileaflet valve prosthesis.

Mechanical valves have excellent durability, lasting 20 years or longer. The major liability is their inherent thrombogenicity, necessitating long-term anticoagulation with warfarin to avoid thrombosis and embolism. The advantage of bioprosthetic valves is their low risk of thromboembolism. Chronic anticoagulation with warfarin is not required. The major limitation of the bioprosthetic valves (e.g., porcine, bovine), however, is their durability. Valve failure begins to appear 4 to 5 years post-implant and increases progressively thereafter (20% at 10 years, 50% at 15 years); thus these valves generally are not utilized in younger patients. Indications for bioprosthetic valves include patients with contraindications to chronic anticoagulation (e.g., those with risk of falls or injury, travelers, noncompliant patients), the elderly, women of childbearing age who wish to become pregnant (high fetal complication rate from warfarin), and prosthetic replacement of the tricuspid valve (since the incidence of thromboembolism is extremely high with mechanical valves). Frequently, older patients receive a bioprosthesis because these valves deteriorate more slowly in this age group, the need for long-term durability of the valve is less, and the risk of anticoagulation may increase with advancing age. Hemodialysis patients, however, should not receive tissue valves because they have a high failure rate. The prosthesis of choice (in the aortic or mitral position) in patients < 50 years of age who are reasonable candidates for chronic anticoagulation is the artificial mechanical valve. Emboli usually occur because the patient has not maintained an adequate level of anticoagulation (INR of 2-3 for aortic, 2.5-3.5 for mitral). Occasionally, when embolism occurs despite adequate anticoagulation levels, antiplatelet agents (e.g., aspirin, clopidogrel) may need to be added. Clopidogrel is recommended for the first 3-6 months after TAVR in addition to lifelong aspirin. Anticoagulation with warfarin (or NOAC), alone or in combination with antiplatelet agents, may be considered in select TAVR patients at high risk for thromboembolism (e.g., atrial fibrillation, larger valves).

Because prosthetic heart valves are associated with a number of complications (including thrombosis, endocarditis, and hemolysis), the decision to proceed with valve surgery should be made only after the risks of valve replacement are weighed against the potential benefit of symptom relief and/or improved survival. Furthermore, since no "ideal" prosthetic valve has been developed, advantages and disadvantages must be weighed when choosing the appropriate valve for each patient (**Figure 10-3**). The current indications and timing of surgical intervention in patients with valvular heart disease are discussed in Chapter 15. In general, in valvular AS the development of symptoms, e.g., angina, fatigue, shortness of breath, and syncope, is an indi-

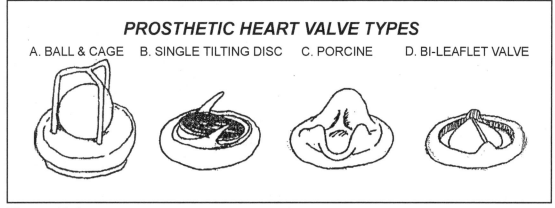

Figure 10-2

FIGURE 10-3

Advantages and Disadvantages of Prosthetic Heart Valves

Mechanical Valves	Bioprosthetic Valves
Good long-term durability, lasting 20 yrs. or longer	Poor long-term durability, limited to 10–15 yrs. (tissue valves degenerate and calcify)
Good flow characteristics in small sizes	Relatively stenotic
Increased risk of thromboembolism	Decreased incidence of thromboembolism (particularly uncommon in aortic position)
Long-term anticoagulation with warfarin (not NOACs) required	Long-term anticoagulation not usually required (some recommend long term therapy for valves in the mitral and tricuspid position)
Increased risk of hemolysis (especially with caged-ball valves or paravalvular leak) and bleeding complications	No hemolysis and fewer bleeding complications

---

cation for rapidly scheduled elective surgery. The Ross procedure (switching the patient's pulmonary valve to the aortic position and placing a bioprosthesis in the pulmonary position, since they do not deteriorate as fast on the right side of the heart) offers another option in younger patients with AS.

Patients with chronic AR should be followed for clinical signs of CHF, e.g., shortness of breath, weakness and fatigue. When LV dysfunction and dilation develop, the clinical course quickly deteriorates. Surgery is indicated as soon as the patient becomes symptomatic or echo evidence of LV systolic dysfunction (EF < 50%) and dilation (end-systolic dimension > 50 mm or end-diastolic dimension > 65 mm) occurs.

Surgery is recommended in patients with chronic MR who are symptomatic despite adequate medical therapy, or who develop signs of increasing heart size (end-systolic dimension ≥ 40 mm) or decreasing LV function (ejection fraction ≤ 60%) on echo.

In patients with rheumatic MS, the indications for surgery include a mitral valve area ≤ 1.5 cm² with symptoms of CHF, evidence of pulmonary hypertension, or systematic embolization.

CARDIAC TRANSPLANTATION

Cardiac transplantation has become a life-saving treatment choice in patients with end-stage CHF of almost any cause. Dilated cardiomyopathy is the most frequent indication. With advances in surgical techniques, the advent of cyclosporine immunosuppressive therapy, and more careful screening of donor hearts, 1 and 5 year survival rates are ~85–90% and 75–80%, respectively. This compares favorably to the 1 year survival in patients with advanced CHF, which can be only about as high as 50% without transplantation. More widespread application for heart transplantation is limited by the scarce donor supply. As a result, implantable left ventricular assist devices (LVADs) are increasingly being used as a "bridge" to transplantation (or heart recovery) and as permanent or "destination" therapy for patients with end-stage CHF. The latest generation devices are externally powered and small enough to allow patients to have unrestricted mobility. Device-related complications (e.g., bleeding, thromboembolism, infection) are frequent, however, and the mortality rate at 2 years remains high. (**Figure 10-4**).

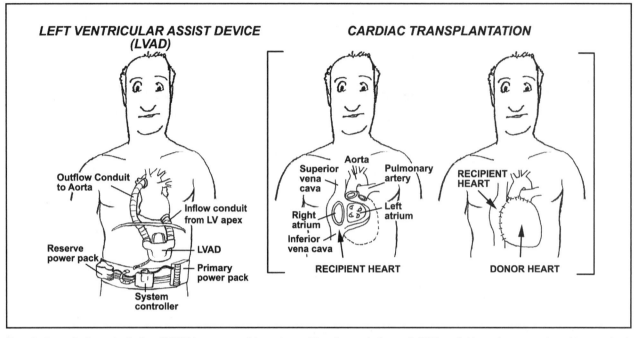

Note: Left ventricular assist devices (LVADs) are reserved for patients with end-stage (refractory) CHF as a bridge to heart transplantation or as destination therapy in selected patients who are not candidates for transplantation.

Figure 10-4

Figure 10-4. Left. Schematic diagram of an implantable LVAD. The LVAD is a mechanical pump type device surgically implanted in the upper part of the abdomen. It receives blood from the heart via an inflow conduit connected to the LV apex, and pumps blood through an outflow conduit into the ascending aorta to the rest of the body. A tube attached to the LVAD is brought out of the abdominal wall and is connected to the battery-operated power source and control system. **Right.** Schematic diagram of cardiac transplantation. During cardiac transplantation, the patient is placed on cardiopulmonary bypass support. The bypass machine receives deoxygenated blood from the superior and inferior vena cava and returns oxygenated blood to the ascending aorta to the rest of the body. Most of the old recipient heart (left) is removed and the new donor heart (right) is attached to the incoming and outgoing blood vessels.

Contraindications to transplant include irreversible pulmonary hypertension, malignancy, active infection, insulin-dependent diabetes mellitus with end-organ damage, and advanced liver or kidney disease. Although advanced age is associated with a higher surgical and 1 year mortality, an age limit for cardiac transplantation is no longer enforced at most centers.

Frequent complications during the first year include systemic infection and rejection of the donor heart. Hypertension and renal dysfunction caused by cyclosporine and immunosuppressant-related cancers have also occurred. Yearly endomyocardial biopsies help to monitor for rejection. The major long-term complication is the development of coronary vasculopathy in the transplanted heart. It occurs in up to 30–40% of recipients within the first 3 years after transplantation.

The diagnosis of transplant CAD may be problematic, since angina is often absent due to cardiac denervation. Because of the unreliability of symptoms in monitoring for new CAD, a reasonable strategy consists of periodic nuclear stress testing to assess functional capacity and discern the physiologic significance of potential coronary stenosis. Since noninvasive testing has proven to be insensitive in definitively detecting transplant CAD, however, coronary angiography (potentially accompanied by intravascular ultrasonography [IVUS]) is currently the "gold standard" in screening for graft atherosclerosis and should be performed yearly after transplantation and periodically thereafter to monitor for significant coronary artery narrowing. This type of atherosclerosis differs from native disease in that it is more diffuse, distally located, and cellular, with less lipid accumulation. In selected patients, discrete lesions appear to respond to PCI. For most patients who develop this complication, however, retransplantation is the only definitive therapy.

PART III.   PUTTING IT ALL TOGETHER

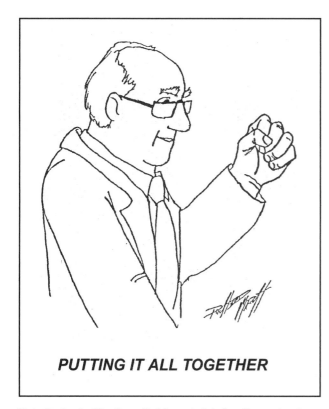

PUTTING IT ALL TOGETHER

Note: Putting the "five fingers" of the total clinical cardiovascular picture together to form a fist, enables one to have a firm grasp on the diagnosis, and is an excellent and efficient way to evaluate and treat patients with known or suspected heart disease.

The previous chapters presented the individual elements of the "five-finger" approach to cardiac diagnosis, as well as pharmacologic and non-pharmacologic therapy in cardiology. The following chapters put these elements together in an integrated whole, presenting the overall diagnostic and therapeutic approaches to patients with a broad spectrum of cardiac conditions. *Reminder:* Despite the current emphasis on technology, the cardiac history and physical examination still remain the most important and cost-effective components of the total clinical cardiovascular evaluation. Often, by the time a careful detailed history and physical examination have been completed, an accurate clinical diagnosis can be made, enabling prompt and appropriate treatment, and in some cases, prevention of heart disease.

Note: Please refer to the attached CD for further discussion of the cardiac conditions presented in this section.

CHAPTER 11.   APPROACH TO THE PATIENT WITH CORONARY ARTERY DISEASE

CAD represents, by far, the most common cardiac problem encountered in clinical practice today. It affects about 16 million Americans and remains the single leading cause of death in the United States. Annually, there are more than 5 million emergency department visits for evaluation of chest discomfort suggestive of an *acute coronary syndrome* (unstable angina, myocardial infarction). Over 1 million Americans experience a new or recurrent *myocardial infarction* (MI) each year. Many more are hospitalized for *unstable angina* and the evaluation and treatment of stable chest pain syndromes. In many cases of acute MI, death occurs early due to VF even before the patient has the opportunity to benefit from current catheter-based PCI and/or thrombolytic reperfusion therapy.

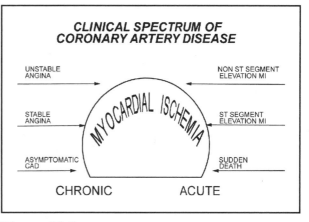

Figure 11-1

Figure 11-1. The clinical manifestations of CAD comprise a spectrum ranging from asymptomatic to sudden death.

In *stable angina,* the symptoms may arise from increased oxygen demand (*exertional angina,* resulting from flow-limiting coronary stenosis), or may follow coronary artery spasm (*variant angina,* also called *Prinzmetal's angina*), or a combination of stenosis and spasm. In *unstable angina,* the pathology is more ominous, involving plaque rupture or erosion with superimposed thrombus formation, which, if persistent, may result in a *myocardial infarction.* Patients with these *acute coronary syndromes* are at risk for *sudden death.*

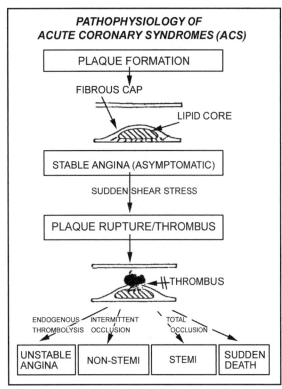

PATHOPHYSIOLOGY OF ACUTE CORONARY SYNDROMES (ACS)

PLAQUE FORMATION

FIBROUS CAP

LIPID CORE

STABLE ANGINA (ASYMPTOMATIC)

SUDDEN SHEAR STRESS

PLAQUE RUPTURE/THROMBUS

THROMBUS

ENDOGENOUS — INTERMITTENT   TOTAL
THROMBOLYSIS   OCCLUSION   OCCLUSION

| UNSTABLE ANGINA | NON-STEMI | STEMI | SUDDEN DEATH |

Figure 11-2

Figure 11-2. Pathophysiology of *acute coronary syndromes (ACS):* Endothelial dysfunction, inflammation, and formation of fatty streaks contribute to the development of an atherosclerotic plaque. Most ACS result from coronary thrombus formation at the site of rupture of a nonobstructive lipid-rich atherosclerotic plaque that is surrounded by inflammation and a thin fibrous cap. Most of these "vulnerable" plaques are not hemodynamically significant before rupture. A partially occluding (platelet-rich) thrombus that impairs coronary blood flow may lead to *unstable angina.* Therapy with antiplatelet agents (e.g., aspirin, clopidogrel, GP IIB/IIIA receptor inhibitor) is most effective at this time. An intermittently occlusive thrombus may cause myocardial necrosis, producing a *non-ST elevation (non-Q-wave) MI* (non-STEMI). If the thrombus totally occludes the coronary artery for a prolonged period, an *ST elevation (Q-wave) MI* (STEMI) results. The clot is rich in thrombin. Early reperfusion therapy by means of prompt fibrinolysis (along with unfractionated or low molecular weight heparin) or direct PCI may limit infarct size and prevent *sudden cardiac death.*

Figure 11-3. The spectrum of stable CAD and the acute coronary syndromes.

Figure 11-4. The CCS classification of disability from angina pectoris. The degree of disability, though, depends not only on the degree of CAD, but also on the patient's normal activities. The patient may consciously or unconsciously scale back his or her activities to avoid precipitating discomfort. Patients with CAD and peripheral vascular disease may not develop chest pain if they are unable to walk more than a short distance due to tiredness or cramps in their calves (*intermittent claudication*). Angina tends to be more readily provoked by early morning activities (e.g., shaving, brushing teeth, drying oneself after a shower). It may occur early in the course of a given activity, e.g., during the first hole of golf, while walking to the bus stop on the way to work ("first-effort" or "warm-up" angina), and then subside as the individual continues on and "walks through" the discomfort. Some patients may be able to tolerate the same or even more strenuous activity after a period of rest ("second-wind" phenomenon). These phenomena have been attributed to the opening of functioning coronary arterial collaterals during the initial episode of ischemia.

The treatment of patients with CAD should be directed toward both the alleviation of symptoms and an improvement in prognosis. In general, this involves several approaches to modify lifestyle and risk factors (e.g., diet, exercise, hypertension, hypercholesterolemia, cigarette smoking, diabetes), along with pharmacologic therapy and coronary revascularization if needed.

* * *

The ABCs of secondary (preventing a recurrent coronary event in patients with known CAD) prevention:

A: **Antiplatelet therapy.** Aspirin indefinitely (or clopidogrel, if aspirin contraindicated)
ACE inhibitor or ARB (especially if post-MI with LV ejection fraction <40%, CHF, hypertension, diabetes mellitus, or proteinuric chronic kidney disease)

B: **Beta blockers** (for up to 3 years post-MI or if LV ejection fraction <40%)
Blood Pressure control (to achieve a goal BP <130/80 mmHg if tolerated)

C: **Cholesterol-lowering therapy** with high intensity "statins" (e.g., atorvastatin 80 mg), if tolerated (to achieve a >50% reduction in LDL cholesterol)
Cardiac rehabilitation (for patients with a recent cardiac event or procedure)
Cigarette smoking cessation (including counseling, nicotine replacement therapy, bupropion, varenicline, and formal cessation program)

D: **Diet.** In general, no more than 25–35% of total calories should come from fat, 15% from protein, and 50–60% from carbohydrates, preferably complex. In addition, less than 7% of the calories should come from saturated fats (including *trans*-fatty acids in products, e.g., margarine and commercial baked goods). The latest dietary

---

FIGURE 11-3

Chronic Coronary Artery Disease and the Acute Coronary Syndromes

Asymptomatic (sub-clinical) Phase

- **Silent Myocardial Ischemia**

Symptomatic Phase

- **Chronic Coronary Artery Disease**

  ■ **Stable (exertional) angina pectoris**—"Fixed threshold" angina secondary to flow-limiting coronary stenoses (demand ischemia)

  ■ **Variant or Prinzmetal's angina**—"Spontaneous" angina at rest secondary to dynamic coronary narrowing (vasospasm) superimposed on obstructive CAD or normal coronary arteries (supply ischemia), often associated with heavy smoking, migraine headaches, and Raynaud's phenomenon. Patient may have angina on initial low level exertion but not with higher activity levels.

STABLE SUBSETS

(Stable "fixed" atherosclerotic plaque)

  ■ **Mixed angina**—"Variable threshold" angina secondary to vasoconstriction superimposed on fixed atherosclerotic plaque (demand and supply ischemia). Patient may have "good" days and "bad" days.

- **Acute Coronary Syndromes (in order of increasing severity)**

  ■ **Unstable angina** (occurs without serologic evidence of myocardial necrosis)
    ❑ *New-onset angina* (severe and <2 months duration)
    ❑ *Increasing (crescendo) angina* (more severe, prolonged, or frequent)
    ❑ *Angina pectoris at rest* (usually prolonged >20 minutes and within a week of presentation)

UNSTABLE SUBSETS

(Unstable "vulnerable" plaque rupture/erosion with superimposed thrombus)

    ❑ *Post-infarction angina* (within 2 weeks of acute MI).

  ■ **Acute myocardial infarction** (confirmed by a rise in serum biomarkers [troponin, CK-MB])*
    ❑ *Non-ST elevation (Non-Q-wave) MI* (transient thrombotic occlusion with early spontaneous reperfusion)
    Smaller infarct size with high risk for recurrent ischemia, re-infarction and sudden death.
    ❑ *ST elevation (Q-wave) MI* (total thrombotic occlusion)
    Larger infarct size with higher in-hospital mortality and complication rate
    Early reperfusion therapy (PCI, thrombolysis) may limit infarct size and prevent sudden death

---

* **Note:** Myocardial infarction can be further classified clinically into 5 types: 1) *spontaneous* MI (i.e., ACS), induced by plaque rupture/thrombus: 2) MI secondary to *supply-demand mismatch*, e.g., from ↑↑ or ↓↓ HR or BP, profound anemia or hypoxemia; 3) MI resulting in *sudden cardiac death* (biomarkers not available); 4) MI related to PCI (4a), stent thrombosis (4b), or restenosis (4c) (↑ troponin > 5 x URL); or 5) MI associated with CABG (↑ troponin > 10 x URL)

---

recommendations from the American Heart Association emphasize the intake of fruits, vegetables, and whole grains, reduction of sweets and salt (if hypertensive), maintenance of normal body weight, and the intake of monounsaturated and polyunsaturated fats, especially oily fish rich in omega-3 fatty acids, and fiber.

Diabetes management (to achieve a hemoglobin [Hb] A1c <7%). Avoid thioglitazones if CHF is present.

E: **Exercise and Education.** Exercise can help to lower elevated BP, LDL cholesterol, and triglyceride levels, raise low HDL cholesterol, improve glucose control, and reduce weight (the major abnormalities comprising the *metabolic syndrome*), along with stress, anxiety and depression. When you counsel a patient with heart disease about physical activity, remember to advise him or her to avoid extremes of exertion and extremes of weather (e.g., bitter-cold, hot-humid). Sexual activity, including the potential dangers involved in treating erectile dysfunction with drugs e.g., sildenafil (Viagra) should be discussed openly with a patient (and significant other) who has heart disease. Most patients can resume sexual activity shortly after returning home from an acute MI or after treatment for other cardiac problems, including cardiac surgery.

F: **Flu and Pneumococcal vaccine** (recommended for all patients with cardiovascular disease).

FIGURE 11-4

The Canadian Cardiovascular Society (CCS) Classification of Angina Pectoris

Class I   Ordinary physical activity, e.g., walking or climbing stairs, does not cause angina. Angina may occur with strenuous, rapid, or prolonged exertion at work or recreation.

Class II   Slight limitation of ordinary activity. Angina may occur with walking or climbing stairs rapidly; walking uphill; in the cold or into the wind; walking or climbing stairs after meals; while under emotional stress; or only during the first few hours after awakening. Walking more than two blocks on a level surface and climbing more than one flight of ordinary stairs at a normal pace and in normal conditions may bring on angina.

Class III   Marked limitation of ordinary physical activity. Angina may occur when walking one or two blocks on the level or climbing one flight of stairs in normal conditions and at a normal pace.

Class IV   Inability to carry out any physical activity without discomfort. Angina may be present at rest.

Adapted from Campeau L: Grading of angina pectoris (Letter). *Circulation* 1976; 54:522–3.

Note: Hormone replacement therapy in older postmenopausal women, antioxidant vitamins C, E, and beta carotene, folic acid with or without vitamins B6 and B12 (aimed at lowering homocysteine), antibiotic treatment (directed against chlamydia pneumoniae), and chelation therapy are not recommended for the secondary prevention of CAD.

*   *   *

ANGINA PECTORIS

Clinical Recognition of Stable Angina Pectoris

Angina pectoris is most commonly caused by the inability of narrowed atherosclerotic coronary arteries to supply oxygen to the heart muscle under conditions of increased myocardial oxygen demand. It is the initial manifestation of CAD in close to 50% of patients. It is diagnosed primarily on the patient's description of his or her symptoms.

Figure 11-5 summarizes the clinical manifestations of angina pectoris in the patient's history.

FIGURE 11-5

Clinical Clues to Classic Angina Pectoris

TIME AND PLACE

- **Location**
  —Retrosternal or slightly to the left of midline
  —Occasionally limited to extrathoracic sites
- **Radiation**
  —To neck, throat ("choking" sensation), lower jaw, teeth ("toothache"), left shoulder, arm (ulnar distribution), occasionally to right arm, interscapular area, epigastrium ("heartburn") or infrascapular (back).
- **Mode of onset, offset and duration**
  —Gradual increase in intensity followed by gradual fading away
  —Usually lasts 2 to 15 minutes
  —New onset, increase in intensity, frequency, duration (> 20 minutes) or occurs at rest ("rest angina"), favors unstable angina or evolving acute MI.

QUALITY AND QUANTITY

- Quality of chest pain or discomfort
  —Tightness, pressure, squeezing, heaviness, burning, aching, fullness (a "heavy weight" or a "band across my chest").
  —Dull and deep (not sharp and superficial).

PROVOCATIVE AND PALLIATIVE

- **Aggravating Factors**
  —Physical exertion (particularly one that involves use of arms, e.g. lifting or carrying heavy objects, emotional stress, sexual activity, after eating heavy meals ("post-prandial angina"), cold or hot-humid environment. Reproducible discomfort with repeated exertion; lying supine ("angina decubitus"—due to increased venous return and extra demand on the heart).
- **Relieving Factors**
  —Relieved with rest, cessation of activity, withdrawal of stress or promptly after taking SL or oral spray NTG.

ASSOCIATED SYMPTOMS
  —Shortness of breath, sweating
  —Dizziness, lightheadedness, syncope, fatigue

Chest pain is considered definite (*typical*) angina if it is:

1. Substernal in location (with characteristic quality and duration)
2. Provoked by exertion or emotional stress, and
3. Relieved by rest or nitroglycerin. Chest pain that fulfills only two of the preceding criteria is considered probable (*atypical*) angina. Chest pain that meets one or none of the criteria is considered noncardiac chest pain (*not angina*).

Although prompt response to nitroglycerin is characteristic of stable angina and is a useful diagnostic consideration in the history, it is important to keep in mind that esophageal spasm and gastroesophageal reflux disease, and even some psychogenic causes of chest pain, may also respond to nitroglycerin. Also, old nitroglycerin can lose its potency over time. Remember to tell your patients to keep the nitroglycerin tablets in the original, dark glass bottle that they came in, and that they should be replaced every 3–6 months. There is much less chance of deterioration of their potency if they are kept in glass, stored in a cool, dry place, and the cotton plug is removed and left out. Avoid fancy or expensive pill containers (occasionally referred to as "gizmos"), often embroidered with jewels, and made of silver or gold. Nitroglycerin tablets are very sensitive and lose their potency when exposed to light, heat, or moisture (**Note:** nitroglycerin spray may retain potency for up to 3 years.) Keep in mind that if the patient no longer obtains relief of ischemic chest discomfort, and/or doesn't experience the usual "sting", "flushing", "fullness of the head", or "headache", it could be a clue that the medication is too old rather than a sign of unstable angina, which often doesn't respond to NTG, or some other non-coronary condition. A surprising number of patients who have seen a practitioner in the past for typical angina pectoris have never been given a prescription for sublingual or oral spray nitroglycerin!

Carotid sinus massage (by increasing vagal tone and decreasing heart rate and BP) may bring about relief of angina in some patients, and, if effective, is a useful diagnostic maneuver. However, it should be applied cautiously, if at all, in older patients, who may have underlying carotid artery disease.

Sublingual nitroglycerin is the drug of choice for the treatment of acute angina episodes. It is also very effective when taken prophylactically to prevent anticipated attacks.

Figure 11-6. Spasm of the left anterior descending coronary artery in a young woman with variant (Prinzmetal's) angina. Both the typical ST segment elevation and chest pain resolve after relief of coronary vasospasm by nitroglycerin.

Angina may also occur with angiographically normal coronary arteries ("*syndrome X*"). The underlying pathophysiology is thought to be due to microvascular and

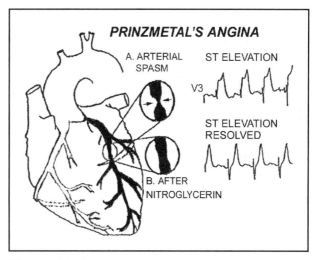

Figure 11-6

endothelial dysfunction. As previously mentioned, ischemia may also be "silent" in some patients (e.g., diabetics, women, the elderly, cardiac transplant recipients) with advanced obstructive CAD because of differences in their perception of pain. Silent ischemic episodes in CAD occur more frequently than symptomatic episodes, and the patient may have substantial ST-T wave changes on their ECGs along with radionuclide perfusion and/or echo wall motion evidence of myocardial ischemia on noninvasive testing. Most authorities favor treating such asymptomatic episodes in the same way that symptomatic angina pectoris is managed.

Women statistically differ from men in the presentation of anginal symptoms. Women:

• Are more likely than men to present with angina than with an acute MI as either the first or subsequent manifestations of CAD.
• Are, on average, 5–10 years older at the time of presentation.
• With an acute MI are more likely to have a history of hypertension, diabetes, hyperlipidemia, and CHF.
• Are more likely than men to have atypical symptoms, e.g., neck and shoulder pain, abdominal pain, nausea, vomiting, fatigue, and dyspnea, in addition to (or instead of) chest pain.
• Have a higher incidence of vasospastic angina and microvascular angina, as well as noncoronary chest pain syndromes, further complicating their clinical assessment.
• Are more likely than men to have an ACS caused by plaque erosion (rather than rupture), especially those who are premenopausal and who smoke.
• Have a higher treadmill exercise "false positive" rate than men, in part because of a lower pretest

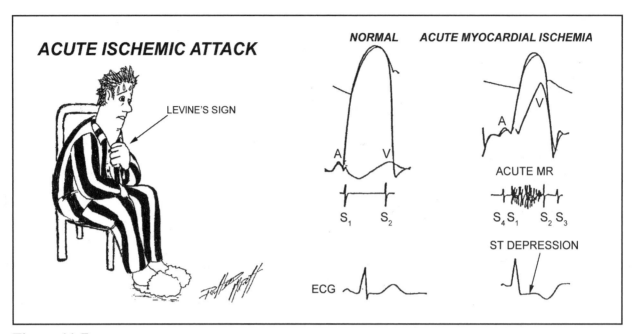

Figure 11-7

likelihood of the disease (along with a higher incidence of MVP) as well as breast attenuation artifact on nuclear perfusion imaging studies.

It is important to differentiate those types of chest discomfort that are not ischemic in nature. Fleeting (lasting only a few seconds), or constant (lasting for days), "sharp", "stabbing", "knife-like" pain, localized to the left infra-mammary area; accentuated with inspiration (pleuritic); produced by change in position or movement of the body; or resulting from palpation over certain areas of the chest wall, are usually musculoskeletal or neurological in etiology and not ischemic in nature. The patient should be reassured that these symptoms are generally not signs of underlying CAD. Keep in mind that in its pre-eruptive stage, herpes zoster (shingles) may cause a band-like chest pain over one or more dermatomes. Clues to the shingles include advanced age of the patient, along with the presence of fever, malaise, hyperesthesia of the involved area, and the subsequent appearance of typical lesions several days after the onset of symptoms.

Don't always assume that palpable chest pain excludes angina. Make sure to ask the patient if the pain produced on palpation is the same type of pain that brought him or her in for evaluation; it might not be.

On the physical exam, the findings of hypertension, carotid or peripheral vascular bruits and/or pulse deficits, or xanthomas, xanthelasmas, and/or corneal arcus senilis (signs of hyperlipidemia), and nicotine-stained fingers or teeth (from cigarette smoking) may provide clues to the presence of underlying CAD.

Although the cardiac examination may be entirely normal between episodes of angina, close evaluation *during* an acute ischemic attack may reveal supportive evidence. Such evidence may include tachycardia, bradycardia, hypertension or marked hypotension (when ischemia is extensive), a transient audible or palpable S4 and S3 gallop, palpable ischemic systolic bulges on the precordium at or medial and superior ("ectopic area") to the cardiac apex (indicative of LV dyskinesia), an apical systolic murmur of MR (due to papillary muscle dysfunction from the ischemia), or rarely a paradoxically split S2 (delay of aortic valve closure due to slow, inefficient LV function) that disappears when the pain subsides (along with disappearance of ST segment depression on the ECG). (**Figure 11-7**). These abnormal physical findings may be caused by failure of the involved LV myocardium to contract and relax normally as a result of ischemia. Relief of chest pain by sublingual nitroglycerin may also be a helpful clue to angina pectoris. Failure of nitroglycerin tablets to relieve chest pain indicates that either the pain is not anginal or, if it is ischemic, that it may represent unstable angina or an acute MI.

Figure 11-7. Clinical findings during an episode of acute myocardial ischemia. Note middle aged male clutching his chest (Levine's sign) with beads of perspiration on his forehead. Note appearance of the systolic murmur of acute mitral regurgitation (due to papillary muscle dysfunction). The murmur decreases in the latter part of systole due to high left atrial pressure (tall V wave). An S4 gallop (due to decreased LV compliance) and an S3 gallop (secondary to decreased systolic function) are also present.

The ECG (below) taken during the ischemic episode reveals transient ST segment depression.

Between attacks of angina pectoris, the ECG may be normal or may show evidence of a prior (possibly "silent") MI. *During* episodes of angina, reversible horizontal or downsloping depression of the ST segment (or transient ST segment elevation, if during Prinzmetal's angina) may occur, or the ECG may be unaffected. Both the choice and timing of noninvasive and invasive tests depend on the pretest likelihood of angina and the perceived urgency or instability of the clinical scenario: ·

- Exercise ECG stress testing may be useful for patients with stable symptoms and/or several risk factors, and a moderate pretest probability of CAD (e.g., a 50 year old male with atypical angina or a 45 year old female with typical angina).
- Among patients with known or suspected CAD, cardiac catheterization and coronary angiography may be beneficial for diagnosis, risk stratification, and the assessment of the appropriateness and feasibility of myocardial revascularization with percutaneous coronary intervention (PCI) (angioplasty/ stenting) or coronary artery bypass graft (CABG) surgery. Cardiac catheterization with coronary angiography is indicated in patients classified at high risk by noninvasive testing, in patients with symptoms refractory to medical therapy, and in those in whom noninvasive tests are unable to establish the diagnosis reliably. Of note, coronary CT angiography can detect coronary stenoses with a high negative predictive accuracy, and may be a viable alternative in symptomatic patients with a low to intermediate probability of CAD or an equivocal stress test.

Clinical Recognition of Unstable Angina

Unstable angina is part of the spectrum of acute coronary syndromes (ACS). It can present as new onset angina, crescendo angina, or rest angina and may be differentiated from non-STEMI, a closely related form of ACS, by the absence of serologic evidence of myocardial necrosis. Symptoms may also be more difficult to relieve with nitroglycerin than those in patients with stable angina. A change in the pattern of onset of previously stable angina must be taken very seriously. This change should alert the clinician to possible progression of CAD, plaque rupture with superimposed thrombus formation, coronary vasospasm, or the reduction of myocardial oxygen supply and/or increase in myocardial oxygen demand (e.g., caused by anemia, tachyarrhythmia, hyperthyroidism, hypoxemia) along with the need for a more aggressive management strategy.

In patients who have had coronary intervention or bypass surgery, the timing of recurrence of chest discomfort suggestive of angina pectoris may be a clinical clue to the pathogenesis. Restenosis is generally the cause of symptoms within 6 months of the angioplasty procedure, whereas recurrence of symptoms after 6 months could indicate either restenosis or progression of disease in another vessel. Recurrence of angina during the first few months after bypass surgery usually denotes graft occlusion.

On physical examination, the patient with unstable angina may have no visible, palpable, or audible cardiac abnormalities at a time when he or she is pain-free. During an episode of chest pain, however, the patient may become anxious, diaphoretic, tachypneic and tachycardic. The cardiac examination may reveal an S4 and S3 gallop and a systolic murmur of MR due to papillary muscle dysfunction. If an ECG is obtained during an episode of chest pain, it often demonstrates transient ST segment depression (or elevation) with or without T-wave inversions.

Patients with ACS and a high ($\geq$ 3) TIMI risk score (age $\geq$ 65 years, $\geq$ 3 CAD risk factors, prior coronary stenosis $\geq$ 50%, ST segment deviation, $\geq$ 2 anginal events in prior 24 hours, aspirin use in past 7 days, and elevated cardiac markers), or those with the high risk features listed in **Figure 11-8** usually have severe underlying CAD with more extensive areas of ischemic myocardium in jeopardy and are at a higher risk for an adverse cardiac outcome. ACS patients with elevated serum creatinine levels (included in the GRACE risk score) are also at higher risk.

FIGURE 11-8

High-Risk Features of ACS

- Accelerating tempo of ischemic symptoms (within 48 hours)
- Prolonged ongoing rest pain
- New ST-segment depression (or transient elevation)
- Elevated troponin levels (indicates cardiac necrosis)
- Recurrent angina or ischemia at rest or with low-level activity despite intensive anti-ischemic therapy
- Recurrent angina or ischemia with symptoms of congestive heart failure, an S3 gallop, pulmonary edema, worsening rales, or new or worsening mitral regurgitation
- High-risk findings on noninvasive stress testing
- Ejection fraction <40%
- Hemodynamic instability (e.g., hypotension, tachycardia)
- Sustained ventricular tachycardia
- Percutaneous coronary intervention within 6 months
- Previous coronary artery bypass graft surgery
- Post-MI angina

Transient hypokinesis, akinesis, or occasionally dyskinetic wall motion abnormalities may be observed in the areas of ischemia during echo examination. Occasionally, patients have normal LV systolic function and ejection fractions but abnormal diastolic function (decreased LV compliance) with impairment of LV filling detectable on echo-Doppler. Compared with men, women with unstable angina are generally older, and are more likely to have diabetes mellitus, hypertension, and prior CHF.

A number of commonly encountered medical conditions can provoke or intensify myocardial ischemia and should be considered when unstable angina occurs. These include severe anemia, fever, infection, uncontrolled hypertension, hypotension, sustained tachyarrhythmias, hyperthyroidism or hypoxemia, and certain medications (e.g., thyroid supplements, vasoconstrictors). However, such secondary causes are absent in most patients with primary unstable angina (caused by rupture or erosion of an atherosclerotic plaque with platelet-thrombus formation and subsequent obstruction to coronary artery blood flow). When cardiac catheterization is performed, most patients with unstable angina are found to have luminal narrowing of one or more of the coronary arteries, often with an eccentric stenosis and a narrow neck, irregular borders and indistinct edges, suggestive of platelet aggregation and/or thrombus formation. Fifteen to thirty percent of patients have multivessel disease or serious obstructive narrowing of the left main coronary artery. An occasional patient has no obstructive CAD and is shown to have coronary spasm (Prinzmetal's variant, cocaine-induced), coronary embolism, ectasia, or spontaneous coronary artery dissection.

Management of Stable Angina Pectoris

The goals of treatment are to provide symptomatic relief of angina and decreased cardiovascular events and mortality, if possible. All patients with angina pectoris should initially be evaluated for a contributing reversible cause. These may include hypertension, CHF, anemia, hypoxemia, sympathomimetic drugs (e.g., vasoconstrictors, inhaled beta agonists, theophylline), and thyrotoxicosis. Medical therapy focuses on increasing coronary blood supply, reducing myocardial oxygen demand, along with stabilization of the atherosclerotic plaque.

Sublingual or oral spray nitroglycerin (for immediate relief) should be prescribed. Patients should be instructed to take one tablet or spray every 5 minutes up to a total of 3 doses, in the sitting or reclining position (to avoid symptomatic postural hypotension), when an anginal attack occurs. Nitroglycerin may also be used prophylactically before an anticipated episode of angina. If the pain lasts longer, they should chew an aspirin (if not contraindicated) and be transported immediately to an emergency department for evaluation. Nitroglycerin tablets should be kept fresh (i.e., the prescription should be renewed every 3–6 months). Beta blockers (to reduce cardiac oxygen demand) are effective as initial therapy, in the absence of contraindications, to reduce anginal symptoms. Since beta blockers have been shown to reduce reinfarction and prolong life in patients with a prior MI or CHF, these agents are a reasonable first choice. The most commonly used beta blockers are atenolol (Tenormin) and metoprolol (Lopressor, Toprol XL). In patients unable to tolerate beta blockers (e.g., due to severe reactive airway disease), a calcium channel blocker (e.g., diltiazem, verapamil), for coronary vasodilation, is a reasonable alternative therapy. In patients with continued angina, combination therapy should be considered. Such therapy includes a beta blocker and a vasodilating calcium channel blocker (e.g., amlodipine, long-acting nifedipine) or an oral long-acting nitrate preparation (e.g., Imdur, Ismo, Isordil). These agents improve the myocardial oxygen supply/demand balance and therefore reduce symptoms and improve exercise tolerance. The most important factor in using oral (or transdermal) nitrates is to allow for a nitrate-free interval of 8–10 hours to avoid nitrate tolerance.

The type of anginal syndrome the patient has determines the kind of anti-ischemic therapy. For example, *beta blockers* (by decreasing heart rate, BP, and contractility, and thus, myocardial oxygen demand) are more likely to be effective in patients with "*fixed threshold*" angina (where the fixed, narrowed coronary artery results in an angina that increases with increased oxygen demand), whereas *calcium channel blockers and nitrates* (by dilating the coronary arteries) are very effective in preventing the spasms of *variant (Prinzmetal's) angina* (where unexpected spasms of the coronary artery result in ischemia). Beta blockers, on the other hand, by leaving the α receptors that mediate vasoconstriction unopposed, may worsen Prinzmetal's angina and increase the duration of the attacks. A careful clinical history, therefore, may not only indicate the cause of chest pain (i.e., ischemia) but may also provide a clue as to the potential underlying mechanism and advisable treatment.

In addition to controlling the patient's symptoms, consider secondary prevention interventions that stabilize the atherosclerotic plaque and decrease the risk of CAD progression and future cardiac events. These include aspirin (or clopidogrel if aspirin-allergic), a "heart healthy" diet, cholesterol-reduction therapy with high intensity "statins", if tolerated, along with exercise (30-60 minutes 5–7 days per week), smoking cessation, and control of hypertension (BP goal <130/80 mmHg if tolerated) and hyperglycemia (HbA1c <7%).

During your initial or subsequent evaluation of a patient with angina, stress testing aids in risk stratification. Patients with symptoms that significantly interfere with their quality of life despite medical treatment, and those with a markedly positive stress test that suggests they are at high risk for future cardiac events, should undergo cardiac catheterization with plans for myocardial revascularization (e.g., PCI, CABG) if anatomically-suitable lesions are found. Survival after the onset of angina pectoris depends on several factors, including the location, severity, and extent of coronary arteries involved by the atherosclerotic process, and the state of LV function. PCI may provide symptomatic relief in some patients with stable angina who are refractory to, or unable to tolerate, medical therapy, but does not decrease the future risk of MI or death (as it does in patients with ACS). Although PCI (angioplasty/stenting) has ~95% immediate success rate, the treated artery may narrow again (restenosis), usually within 6 months. If this happens, repeat PCI or bypass surgery may be recommended. The use of bare metal stents has, in general, been successful in reducing the restenosis rate to ~15–20% (approximately half of that experienced with PTCA alone). More recent developments (e.g., drug-eluting stents) have substantially reduced the restenosis rate even further to less than 10%.

CABG provides excellent relief from symptoms (partial relief in >90% of patients and complete relief in >70%) in patients unresponsive to medical management. CABG also increases survival in those at high risk, i.e., with left main, triple vessel disease or double vessel disease involving the proximal portion of the left anterior descending coronary artery associated with depressed LV function, especially if diabetic.

Occasionally, a patient has severe angina despite medical therapy and/or PCI/CABG. Such a patient may derive symptom improvement with *ranolazine* (Ranexa), a novel antianginal agent that inhibits late sodium entry into ischemic myocardial cells, which reduces calcium overload and LV wall tension, and improves myocardial relaxation and perfusion. In appropriately selected patients, *enhanced external counterpulsation* (EECP), whereby cuffs wrapped around the patient's legs are inflated sequentially (from the lower legs to the upper thighs) in early diastole, may reduce anginal frequency (reducing afterload during systole when the cuffs are deflated and increasing coronary perfusion during diastole when the cuffs are inflated) and extend the time to exercise-induced ischemia. Patients with refractory angina, not amenable to conventional therapy, may also be considered for surgical laser *transmyocardial revascularization* (TMR). The mechanism of benefit is unclear, but may be related to formation of new blood channels, promotion of angiogenesis, myocardial denervation, and/or a placebo effect.

Ongoing medical treatment for stable angina pectoris includes risk factor modification, including statins (which may stabilize plaques and make them less prone to rupture), aspirin, nitrates, beta blockers, and calcium channel blockers. The goal of therapy is to abolish or reduce anginal attacks of myocardial ischemia and to promote a normal life style. *Remember, however, that nitrates and calcium chan-nel blockers can relieve, but beta blockers may worsen, chest pain in patients with variant or Prinzmetal's angina caused by coronary artery spasm (beta blockers prevent vasodilation due to unopposed alpha-vasoconstriction).* Percutaneous transluminal coronary angioplasty with or without stenting (which reduces the restenosis rate) should be considered in patients with anatomically suitable stenoses who remain symptomatic on medical therapy and/or in those with significant ischemic changes on noninvasive (e.g., nuclear and/or echo) stress testing.

Figure 11-9 summarizes the pharmacologic therapy of stable angina pectoris.

Management of Unstable Angina

Individuals with unstable angina have a greater risk of developing MI or dying suddenly than do patients with stable angina. If untreated, unstable angina progresses to nonfatal MI in 10–20% and death in 5–10% of patients. Most of these events occur within days to weeks after symptom onset. Because unstable angina is a potentially serious development, hospitalization for stabilization, assessment, and more aggressive invasive management strategies than for chronic stable angina is often necessary. Acute treatment includes measures to restore balance between myocardial oxygen supply and demand (e.g., beta blockers, nitrates, and/or calcium channel blockers) and stabilization of the intracoronary thrombus (e.g., aspirin and/or clopidogrel, IV unfractionated or SQ low molecular weight heparin).

- All patients with unstable angina should be treated promptly with aspirin and/or clopidogrel, if aspirin is contraindicated due to hypersensitivity or intolerance, as well as an antithrombin agent, e.g., IV unfractionated heparin or SQ low molecular weight heparin. A direct thrombin inhibitor, e.g., IV bivalirudin, or a Factor Xa inhibitor, e.g., SQ fondaparinux, may be acceptable alternatives for patients undergoing an invasive or more conservative medical strategy, respectively.

- In higher risk ACS patients (e.g., ST depression, increased troponin levels), a more rapid and potent antiplatelet agent than clopidogrel, e.g., prasugrel (at the time of PCI only) or ticagrelor, and/or GP IIb/IIIa inhibitors (GPIs) should be considered. IV cangrelor may be considered as an adjunct to PCI in patients not receiving oral P2Y12 inhibitors or planned GPIs. When used appropriately, these agents have been shown to reduce adverse events (e.g., death, MI, recurrent ischemia). The GPIs currently approved for use "upstream", with or without PCI, include eptifibatide and tirofiban. Abciximab is reserved for use only with PCI. Optimal timing of therapy has not yet been estab-

---

FIGURE 11-9

Pharmacologic Therapy of Angina Pectoris

Drug Class	Antianginal Effect	Side Effects

Organic Nitrates (SL, topical, oral)	↓ Myocardial oxygen demand
	  ↓ Preload > afterload
	↑ Oxygen supply
	  Coronary vasodilation
		Headache, hypotension, reflex tachycardia, flushing, tolerance develops with continued use.

β-blockers (e.g., atenolol, metoprolol, nadolol, propranolol)	↓ Myocardial oxygen demand
	  ↓ Heart rate
	  ↓ BP
	  ↓ Contractility
		May aggravate bradycardia, heart block, and CHF, provoke bronchospasm, fatigue, depression, cold hands and feet, vivid dreams, and impotence, may worsen dyslipidemia and mask the symptoms of hypoglycemia. Avoid in Prinzmetal's (vasospastic) angina–can provoke coronary artery spasm and aggravate peripheral vascular disease.

Calcium channel blockers
Dihydropyridines (e.g., nifedipine, amlodipine)
Nondihydropyridines (e.g., verapamil, diltiazem)
	↓ Myocardial oxygen demand
	  ↓ Preload
	  ↓ Heart rate (verapamil, diltiazem)
	  ↓ BP
	  ↓ Contractility (verapamil, diltiazem)
	↑ Oxygen supply
	  Coronary vasodilation
		Headache, flushing, peripheral edema. May worsen CHF, and aggravate bradycardia (verapamil, diltiazem), AV block and hypotension. Constipation (verapamil).
		Short acting formulations (nifedipine) may provoke reflex tachycardia and aggravate angina.

Late sodium current inhibitor
(e.g., ranolazine)
	↓ Myocardial oxygen demand
	  ↓ LV diastolic wall tension
	  No effect on heart rate or BP
	↑ Oxygen supply
	  ↓ Compression of the small
	    intramural blood vessels
		Prolongs the QT interval. Avoid in patients with long QT interval, on QT prolonging drugs, or with liver disease. Approved for use with nitrates, β-blockers, or amlodipine, limit dose with diltiazem or verapamil (which increases the plasma level of ranolazine).

---

lished. Although a theoretical advantage of starting therapy "upstream" is that it allows patients with recurrent ischemia who are awaiting intervention to benefit from the drug, it may well be appropriate perform diagnostic angiography as expeditiously as possible, and administer therapy in the cath lab (especially if large thrombus burden is present) since no clear benefit of routinely starting GPIs prior to PCI has been demonstrated, and there is an increased risk of bleeding. Contraindications to the use of GP IIb/IIIa inhibitors generally include those factors that predispose patients to increased bleeding risks (e.g., active bleeding, prior intracranial hemorrhage, a his-

tory of recent stroke, recent major surgery or trauma, low platelet count).

• Sublingual (tablet or spray), IV and/or oral nitrates should be administered for recurrent episodes of angina. IV and/or oral beta blocker therapy should be considered (if no contraindications exist). When beta-blockers are not tolerated and/or contraindicated, a nondihydropyridine (rate-slowing) calcium channel blocker (e.g., diltiazem or verapamil) may be considered, in the absence of severe LV dysfunction (due to their myocardial depressant effects) or other contraindications. For patients who have recurrent angina despite adequate beta blocker and nitrate therapy, consider a vasodilating calcium channel blocker, e.g., amlodipine (Norvasc).

- *High risk* ACS patients (**Figure 11-8**) should undergo an early invasive strategy (cardiac catheterization within 24 hours with plans for revascularization, if the anatomy is suitable). Patients who are at a *lower risk* and who are clinically stable can be treated more conservatively. They may undergo noninvasive exercise or pharmacologic stress testing (along with nuclear or echo imaging) or coronary CT angiography to screen for provocable ischemia or CAD. In many cases, those patients who have not experienced recurrent chest pain and have no ECG changes, no cardiac enzyme elevations, and/or no evidence of ischemia on exercise testing or imaging procedures, may be discharged directly from the ED (or chest pain observation unit).

- After stabilizing the patient by medication or revascularization, the subsequent long-term treatment should aim at preventing recurrence of episodes of angina and/or MI, and at halting the progression of CAD. An ACE inhibitor should be considered when hypertension, LV systolic dysfunction, or diabetes mellitus is present, along with lipid lowering therapy with high intensity "statins", if tolerated. Specific instructions should be given to the patient regarding smoking cessation, diet, exercise, achievement of optimal weight, hypertension control (to a BP goal of <130/80 mmHg, if tolerated), and control of hyperglycemia if diabetic (HbA1c <7%).

Since in unstable angina, the vessel usually remains patent and the thrombi are undergoing continuous spontaneous formation and thrombolysis, *thrombolytic therapy has not been shown to be effective in improving the outcome* and is not recommended. In general, PCI can be undertaken if there are high grade coronary lesions amenable to the procedure. CABG is a consideration if there is left main or proximal triple vessel disease or two vessel disease involving the proximal portion of the left anterior descending coronary artery, which supplies a large portion of the myocardium, especially when associated with moderate depression in LV function. An occasional high risk patient with unstable angina (particularly those with significant left main coronary artery stenosis) will benefit from intraaortic balloon pump (IABP) counterpulsation in the immediate preoperative and postoperative period. The IABP increases coronary arterial pressure and decreases ventricular afterload, thus reducing myocardial oxygen demand. IABPs have not been associated with increased survival. Early insertion, however, may be of benefit as a "bridge" to emergent PCI.

Figure 11-10. The intraaortic balloon pump (IABP). It is inserted through the common femoral artery and positioned in the descending thoracic aorta just distal to the left subclavian artery. The balloon is inflated during diastole, thereby increasing coronary artery blood flow and perfusion pressure. LV afterload is decreased as the balloon is deflated during cardiac systole, thereby reducing the workload of the heart. Indications for IABP include cardiogenic shock, mechanical complications of MI (e.g., acute MR, VSD), intractable VT, and refractory angina. Contraindications include AR, aortic dissection, and severe peripheral vascular disease.

"To medicate, to dilate, or to operate?"—That is the question: Opinions vary concerning the indications for pharmacologic, interventional, and/or surgical solutions to CAD. However, most would agree that the following patients should be considered for CABG: those with debilitating angina pectoris on medical therapy; those with significant left main, triple vessel, and double vessel CAD involving the proximal portion of the left anterior descending coronary artery, accompanied by decreased LV function (especially if diabetic); and those with ongoing unstable angina or ischemia and/or hemodynamic instability following a failed PCI. Whenever possible, arterial conduits (e.g., internal mammary, radial) should be utilized since their long-term patency rate is far better than for saphenous vein grafts. The availability of drug-eluting stents (DES) (which greatly reduce restenosis) has shifted the paradigm to more PCIs. Concerns over the risk of late stent thrombosis (which is less with newer generation DES) and data demonstrating that PCI, with newer generation DES, in addition to relieving symptoms, offers an advantage over older generation DES and BMS in reducing the risk of stent thrombosis, restenosis, and repeat target vessel revascularization, has added fuel to the debate.

Figure 11-11 summarizes the treatment of ACS. The main aims of treatment are to alleviate symptoms, prolong life, reduce myocardial damage, and prevent recurrences.

ACUTE MYOCARDIAL INFARCTION

Acute myocardial infarction (MI) is a common, often dramatic and potentially fatal form of ACS characterized by a rise and/or fall in cardiac biomarkers (preferably troponin) together with clinical, ECG, and/or imaging evidence suggestive of ischemic myocardial necrosis. MIs may be classified into five types based on whether they are: 1) caused by a primary coronary event (i.e., ACS), 2) secondary to a supply-demand ischemic imbalance, with or without underlying CAD, 3) resulting in sudden cardiac death, 4) related to a PCI procedure, or 5) associated with CABG surgery. Acute MI related to ACS (so-called "type 1" MI) typically results from rupture of a "vulnerable" atherosclerotic plaque (characterized by a lipid-rich core, surrounding inflammation, and a thin overlying fibrous cap) with superimposed occlusive (ST elevation MI) or non-occlusive (non-ST elevation MI) intracoronary thrombus formation. Slowly

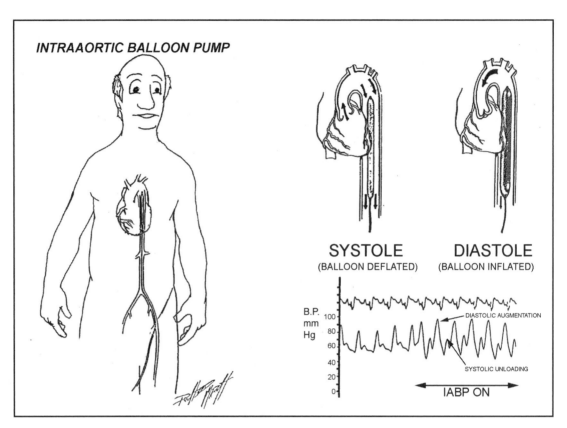

Note: Deflation (systole) of the intraaortic balloon pump (IABP) causes a significant drop in afterload and decrease in cardiac work and myocardial oxygen consumption. Inflation (diastole) of the IABP augments diastolic pressure and coronary perfusion.

Figure 11-10

developing high-grade coronary artery stenoses usually do not precipitate acute MI because of the development of adequate collateral circulation over time. Instead, plaques prone to rupture often are only mild to moderately stenotic (i.e., not flow-limiting) and, therefore, generally do not cause clinical angina. Of note, acute MI can also occur secondary to a supply-demand ischemic mismatch (so-called "type-2" MI), e.g., from anemia, tachyarrhythmias, hypo- or hypertension. Since the extent of myocardial necrosis (with its resultant heart failure, myocardial rupture, and associated ventricular tachyarrhythmias) plays a crucial role in the prognosis and can be successfully treated if diagnosed early, it is essential that the clinician rapidly and accurately establish the diagnosis of acute MI. Then, acute interventions, i.e., PCI/thrombolysis (for "type 1" MI) or therapy directed at the underlying cause (for "type 2" MI) may be initiated to suitable patients as soon as possible.

Clinical Recognition of Acute MI

The patient with acute MI can present in a typical manner or with a variety of atypical symptoms that may obscure the correct diagnosis. (**Figure 11-12**) An accurate and focused clinical history should be obtained as quickly as possible, including investigation as to the indications and potential contraindications to thrombolytic therapy (**Figure 11-13**).

Noting the time of onset of chest pain is important since it predicts the likelihood of myocardial salvage with reperfusion therapy. In the classic clinical presentation, the pain of acute MI, although similar to stable angina in character, location and radiation, is usually (but not always) more intense, longer lasting (>30 minutes) and as likely to occur unexpectedly during inactivity as during effort, not infrequently in the early morning hours (due to a circadian variation in coronary vascular tone, catecholamine stimulation, platelet activation and hypercoagulability). It typically builds in intensity, often becomes severe and unrelenting, although it can be deceptively mild or even "silent" (particularly in diabetics, the elderly, and women). It may be associated with profuse diaphoresis, dyspnea, nausea and vomiting (particularly in inferior MI), lightheadedness, syncope, or a feeling of impending doom and lasts for up to several hours if not relieved by narcotic analgesics or aggressive pharmacological and/or catheter-based intervention (i.e., thrombolysis, PCI).

FIGURE 11-11

Therapy in Acute Coronary Syndromes (ACS)

I. ANTIPLATELET AGENTS
Aspirin (chewed, swallowed) – a cyclooxygenase (COX) inhibitor
—Reduces mortality alone or in conjunction with thrombolysis (for ST segment elevation MI)
—Reduces recurrent ischemia, reocclusion, and reinfarction.

Clopidogrel (Plavix) – an irreversible thienopyridine ADP (P2Y12) receptor antagonist
—If aspirin contraindicated (e.g., intolerance, allergy)
—Reduces mortality and MI in combination with aspirin in non ST elevation MI, and improves infarct-related artery patency and reduces ischemic complications when combined with aspirin and fibrinolytic therapy in ST elevation MI
—Prevents thrombotic complications following PCI (stenting). Recent data suggests decreased antiplatelet effect when clopidogrel is combined with proton pump inhibitors, particularly omeprazole and esomeprazole.

Prasugrel (Effient) – an irreversible thienopyridine ADP (P2Y12) receptor antagonist
—More rapid, potent, and consistent platelet inhibition than clopidogrel.
—Fewer atherothrombotic events when compared with clopidogrel in high risk ACS patients undergoing PCI, albeit at an increased risk of significant bleeding. Use with caution in patients > 75 years of age and those with low body weight (< 60 kg). Contraindicated in patients with history of prior TIA or stroke.

Ticagrelor (Brilinta) – a reversible cyclopentyltriazolopyrimidine ADP (P2Y12) receptor antagonist
—More potent and consistent platelet inhibition than clopidogrel with more rapid "onset" and "offset" of action
—Fewer vascular deaths, MIs, and stent thromboses than clopidogrel in ACS patients with or without ST elevation, without an increase in overall major bleeding, but with an increase in non-CABG related bleeding. Unique side effects include dyspnea and ventricular pauses (thought to be adenosine mediated). Maintenance dose of aspirin above 100 mg daily may decrease the effectiveness of ticagrelor and should be avoided.

Glycoprotein IIb/IIIa receptor antagonist – e.g., abciximab (ReoPro), eptifibatide (Integrilin), tirofiban (Aggrastat)
—Reduces mortality, MI, and recurrent ischemia in high risk ACS patients, especially those undergoing PCI. Eptifibatide and tirofiban are approved for use with or without PCI, whereas abciximab is indicated only with PCI. Abciximab remains the agent of choice in patients at highest risk (e.g., diabetes, renal insufficiency, ST elevation MI), especially those with large clot burden at the time of PCI. Thrombocytopenia can occur, and may require discontinuation of the drug +/– platelet transfusion.
—Use of these agents in combination with reduced dose fibrinolytic therapy in acute ST elevation MI does not confer a mortality benefit, and is associated with an increased risk of bleeding. Decreased dose adjustments for eptifibatide and tirofiban (not abciximab) are required in patients with reduced renal function.

II. ANTICOAGULANTS
Heparin (unfractionated)—IV bolus and drip
—Maintains vessel patency and reduces reocclusion, particularly in conjunction with fibrin-specific thrombolytic agents (e.g., tPA, reteplase, tenecteplase (probably not necessary after SK) and for all patients undergoing direct or adjunctive PCI.
—Reduces mortality and MI (in pre-fibrinolytic era)
—Requires monitoring of PTT levels.
—Sensitivity to heparin may be decreased when it is used concomitantly with IV nitroglycerin (higher doses may be needed to achieve anticoagulation effect).

Low Molecular Weight Heparin–SQ – e.g., enoxaparin (Lovenox), dalteparin (Fragmin).
—Does not usually require laboratory monitoring of activity.
—Enoxaparin approved for prevention of ischemic complications in unstable angina and non ST segment elevation MI when used with aspirin (can be "advantageously" substituted for IV unfractionated heparin (UFH) in the absence of renal failure, unless CABG is planned within 24 hours). Recent evidence favors use of enoxaparin with full dose TNK-tPA in ST elevation MI (in patients < 75 years of age without significant renal dysfunction). Enoxaparin may be a reasonable alternative to UFH for PCI anticoagulation, but has not been shown to be superior to UFH during PCI for preventing ischemic complications.

Direct Thrombin Inhibitors, e.g., IV bivalirudin (Angiomax) and **Factor Xa Inhibitors**, e.g., SQ fondaparinux (Arixtra), a synthetic heparin analog, may be acceptable alternatives to UFH or enoxaparin in patients with ACS. Bivalirudin is also approved for use in patients with, or at risk of, HIT undergoing PCI. Before PCI, UFH must be added to fondaparinux to lessen risk of catheter thrombosis. Fondaparinux does not require laboratory monitoring of its anticoagulant effect. Thrombocytopenia can occur, but HIT has not yet been reported.

Warfarin (Coumadin)
—Prevents thromboembolism, particularly useful in larger anterior MI, with LV mural thrombus, congestive heart failure, apical dyskinesis or aneurysm formation, and atrial fibrillation.
—Evidence suggests warfarin reduces reinfarction and late mortality.

III. ANTI-ISCHEMIC THERAPY
Nitroglycerin (IV, oral)
—acute phase: No effect on survival. (The value of routine administration of IV nitroglycerin to patients also receiving fibrinolytic therapy is indeterminate).
—reduces myocardial oxygen demand: dilates systemic arteries (reduces afterload) and veins (reduces preload).
—increases myocardial oxygen supply: dilates infarct-related coronary vessels, improves collateral blood flow, relieves coronary spasm (spontaneous or cocaine-induced).
—useful for ischemic chest pain, hypertension, CHF, attenuation of LV expansion and remodeling (large anterior MI).
—may be hazardous if hypotension (BP < 90 mmHg) develops, especially in inferior MI complicated by RV infarction (reduced coronary perfusion pressure → worsens myocardial ischemia).
—tolerance may develop after 24 hours of continuous IV therapy.
—avoid use of nitroglycerin in patients who have taken sildenafil (Viagra), vardenafil (Levitra), or tadalafil (Cialis) within 24–48 hours (refractory hypotension and death have been reported).

FIGURE 11-11

Therapy in Acute Coronary Syndromes (ACS) (*continued*)

Beta-blockers (IV, oral)
—acute phase: proven mortality benefit with or without thrombolysis.
—decreases myocardial oxygen demand (↓ HR, ↓ BP, ↓ contractility).
—decreases infarct size, recurrent ischemia, reinfarction, incidence of cardiac rupture, ventricular tachycardia and fibrillation, and mortality.
—useful if hyperdynamic state (tachycardia, hypertension) and ongoing chest pain.
—contraindications include severe hypotension, bradycardia, decompensated LV failure, reactive airway disease, recent cocaine use (controversial).

Calcium Channel Blockers
—acute phase: no proven mortality benefit (or actual harm) for all calcium channel blockers.
—limited role post-MI
—diltiazem: may be beneficial in preventing reinfarction and recurrent angina in subset of patients with non-Q wave MI and intact LV function–detrimental effect noted, however, in subset of patients with LV dysfunction (pulmonary congestion or ejection fraction <40%).
—verapamil: use in late phase (2nd week after acute MI) shown to reduce reinfarction and mortality in patients without heart failure—neither benefit observed, however, in patients with heart failure.
—calcium channel blockers may be considered for post-infarction angina and hypertension (after the acute phase) in beta blocker intolerant patient without congestive heart failure and/or LV dysfunction (since they reduce ventricular contractility), and for ACS precipitated by cocaine use.

IV. OTHER

Angiotensin Converting Enzyme (ACE) Inhibitors (oral)
—acute phase: confers mortality benefit particularly in high-risk groups (e.g., large anterior MI).
—attenuates LV dilation, myocardial remodeling, and aneurysm formation.
—reduces incidence of CHF and recurrent MI in patients with ejection fraction ≤40%.

HMG CoA reductase Inhibitors ("statins")
—e.g., rosuvastatin (Crestor), atorvastatin (Lipitor), simvastatin (Zocor), pravastatin (Pravachol), lovastatin (Mevacor), and others should be administered to reduce LDL cholesterol by at least 50%, if tolerated. Statins have also been shown to be beneficial in reducing vascular inflammation, improving endothelial dysfunction, stabilizing impending plaque rupture, and reducing CAD events and mortality (so-called "pleiotropic effects").

Cardiac catheterization and **coronary intervention**
—includes angioplasty/stenting (for patients with anatomically suitable stenoses), or bypass surgery for patients with significant left main, triple-vessel or double-vessel disease (involving the proximal portion of the LAD) with depressed LV function, especially if diabetic.

Figure 11-14. Left. Direct (primary) percutaneous transluminal coronary angioplasty (PTCA) and stenting of totally occluded proximal left anterior descending coronary artery in a patient with an acute anterior wall MI. **Right.** Left ventriculogram showing marked anteroapical akinesis before PCI, with recovery from myocardial "stunning" and marked improvement in anterior wall motion six months after successful PTCA/stenting of LAD.

Chest pain associated with acute MI generally subsides within 12 to 24 hours. Some patients with persistent pain for more than 12 hours have "*stuttering infarction*" and may be considered candidates for reperfusion therapy. Recurrent or persistent pain beyond 24 hours is an adverse prognostic sign, reflecting the presence of viable, but ischemic myocardium. Post-infarction ischemia and early reinfarction are more common with non ST segment elevation (non Q wave) MIs, as this represents an incomplete thrombotic occlusion of the infarct-related coronary artery. More than 90% of these patients have multivessel CAD.

Keep in mind there are many reasons why patients with acute MI may delay seeking medical attention. When questioned, they often provide such answers as "I didn't think it was anything serious", "I thought the pain would go away", "I didn't think it was my heart", "I didn't want to inconvenience anyone", or even "I would feel foolish if I went to the hospital and they found nothing wrong!" At times, the only clues that such an event even occurred are changes that show up later on a routine ECG or an echo. All too often, individuals have died of an MI because they didn't want to believe (or didn't understand) their symptoms. For example, a patient who thinks he or she has "indigestion" but who is really experiencing an MI may die suddenly while waiting for antacids to relieve the symptoms (**Figure 1-4**). Remember to advise the patient that he or she should seek immediate medical attention if prolonged and unusual discomfort in the chest, neck, arms, or upper abdomen, or unexplained episodes of shortness of breath, profuse diaphoresis, nausea, vomiting, or heartburn should occur and not to worry that it may turn out to be "nothing"! Whether the symptoms are "classic" or atypical, they deserve prompt attention and effective therapy—the keys to a better outcome.

Figure 11-15 reviews the findings in the cardiac physical examination in acute myocardial infarction. The spectrum of clinical findings varies greatly.

Figures 11-16, 11-17, 11-18, and **11-19,** summarize the clinical features of anterior MI, inferior-posterior MI, RV MI, and non-ST segment elevation MI vs. ST segment elevation MI.

- The BP and/or pulse rate may be increased in anterior MI (in ~25% of patients) due to sympathetic nervous system overactivity related to fever, pain, fear or anxiety, and decreased in inferior MI (in ~50% of patients) due to excess vagal tone and/or ischemia of the sinus and AV nodes, especially when associated with an RV infarction.

- Persistent sinus tachycardia may signify significant LV systolic dysfunction and is therefore a poor prognostic sign.

- Fast or irregular pulses due to PVCs and/or VT are common. Atrial fibrillation may be detected, especially when CHF, pericarditis, atrial and/or RV infarction is present.

- On cardiac auscultation, S1 may be faint if LV contractility is diminished, or if the PR interval is prolonged, as may occur in first degree AV block in the setting of inferior wall MI. Variation in the intensity of S1 can be appreciated when the PR interval varies, as in Mobitz Type I (Wenckebach) second degree AV block and complete heart block.

- AV block associated with inferior MI is due to ischemia of the AV node and is commonly transient. AV block associated with anterior MI, on the other

---

FIGURE 11-12

**Clinical Presentations
of Acute Myocardial Infarction**

- **Typical Presentation**
  - Middle-aged, older male; older postmenopausal female.
  - Severe, prolonged (>30 minutes) chest pain (discomfort)—pressure, tightness, heaviness, squeezing, crushing, vise-like, burning.
  - Location—retrosternal, radiating to precordium, neck, jaw, epigastrium, interscapular area, shoulders, arms (left side common).
  - Associated symptoms—nausea, vomiting, diaphoresis, shortness of breath, weakness, anxiety, feeling of impending doom.
  - Not relieved by NTG (requires narcotics and/or thrombolysis or PCI).

- **Atypical Presentation**
  - Pain localized to extrathoracic sites—arms, shoulders, back, jaw, teeth, epigastrium ("arthritis", "bursitis", "toothache", "indigestion").
  - "Gastrointestinal" symptoms alone—nausea, vomiting, heartburn, gas.
  - Profound fatigue, weakness, anxiety, nervousness.
  - Palpitations, dizziness, syncope.
  - Sudden onset of congestive heart failure, pulmonary edema or shock.
  - Cerebral or peripheral embolism (stroke, cold extremity).
  - Acute confusional state, psychosis.
  - Shortness of breath alone.
  - "Silent"—especially elderly, diabetic, female, perioperative state.

---

hand, is generally due to sclerosis of the bundle of His and its fascicles, and may be permanent.

- In the setting of an anteroseptal MI, wide or paradoxical splitting of S2 due to the development of a new right or left bundle branch block, respectively, is generally associated with a poor prognosis, since this usually reflects an extensive amount of damage to the LV. In addition to LBBB, paradoxical splitting of S2 may also be heard when there is LV systolic dysfunction.

- An S4 gallop, indicative of atrial contraction into a noncompliant LV (diastolic dysfunction), can be heard (or felt) in almost all patients (who are in normal

FIGURE 11-13

Thrombolytic Therapy for Acute ST Segment Elevation MI

Patient Selection

A. Indications
- Clinical history of chest pain (or its equivalent) compatible with acute MI and unresponsive to nitroglycerin.
- ST segment elevation $\geq$1 mm in 2 or more contiguous ECG leads, or new (or presumably new) LBBB.*
- <6 hours after symptoms onset (<3 hours most beneficial).
- 6–12 hours (still beneficial), especially if ongoing ischemic chest pain, high-risk patient with large amount of myocardium in jeopardy (extensive anterior MI, inferior MI with precordial ST depression and/or RV infarction).
- Controversial: 12–24 hours after pain onset. Non ST segment elevation MI does not appear to benefit; however, anterior ST depression MI with prominent R wave in leads V2–V3 (left circumflex or true posterior MI) may benefit.

B. Major Contraindications
- Active or recent (within 2–4 weeks) internal bleeding (excluding menses)
- Suspected aortic dissection, or acute pericarditis.
- Recent (<6 weeks) surgical procedure; head trauma; prolonged (>10 minutes) or traumatic CPR.
- History of cerebrovascular accident–hemorrhagic stroke (ever), thrombotic stroke (<12 months), seizures or intracranial mass, neoplasm, AV malformation or aneurysm.
- Known bleeding diathesis or current use of anticoagulants (INR > 2–3).
- Severe uncontrolled hypertension (systolic BP >180, diastolic BP >110 mmHg).
- Previous allergic reaction to the chosen thrombolytic agent, e.g., streptokinase (SK)—infrequently used in current practice.

Note: Time is muscle! All available thrombolytic agents restore coronary blood flow, limit infarct size, preserve LV function and reduce attendant morbidity and mortality. The choice of agent is much less important to survival than is the wider use of reperfusion therapy (PCI/thrombolysis) and the delay time to initiation of treatment. When thrombolytic therapy is chosen as the primary reperfusion strategy, it should be administered within 30 minutes of hospital arrival ("door-to-needle" time). Direct PCI is the preferred reperfusion strategy when available within 90 minutes of presentation ("door-to-balloon" time), or within 120 minutes if transfer to a PCI-capable hospital is required.

*In patients who present with chest pain and a presumed new anterior STEMI, ST elevation in V2-V3 $\geq$ 2 mm in men or $\geq$ 1.5 mm in women improves the diagnostic accuracy. In patients with LBBB, highly specific, but poorly sensitive, ECG criteria can be used to more accurately diagnose a STEMI: (1) ST elevation $\geq$1 mm and *concordant* (in the same direction) with the QRS (strongest predictor); (2) ST depression $\geq$1 mm and *concordant* in leads V1, V2, or V3; and (3) ST elevation $\geq$5 mm and *excessively discordant* (in the opposite direction) with the QRS (weakest predictor) – "Sgarbossa's criteria".

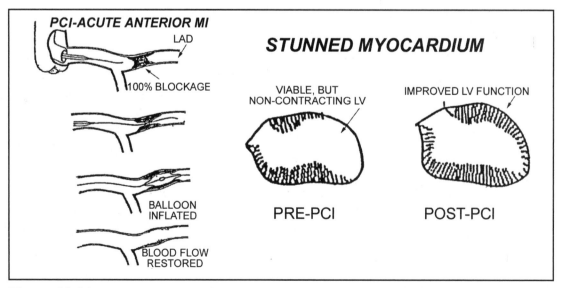

Figure 11-14

FIGURE 11-15

Cardiac Physical Examination in Acute Myocardial Infarction

General
— Anxious, agitated, anguished facies, clenched fist ("Levine's sign")—classic hand gesture.

Skin
— Cool, clammy, pale, ashen.

Low grade fever
— Nonspecific response to tissue necrosis.

Hypertension, tachycardia
— High sympathetic tone (anterior MI).

Hypotension, bradycardia
— High vagal tone (inferior-posterior MI).

Small volume pulses
— Low cardiac output.

Fast, slow or irregular pulse
— Atrial or ventricular arrhythmias, heart block.

Paradoxical "ectopic" systolic impulse
— LV dyskinesis, ventricular aneurysm (anterior MI).

Faint S1
— Decreased LV contractility; first degree AV block (inferior MI).

Paradoxically split S2 (rare)
— Severe LV dysfunction, LBBB.

S4 gallop
— Decreased LV compliance.

S3 gallop, pulmonary rales, pulsus alternans
— LV systolic dysfunction (signs of CHF: > 25% of myocardium infarcted).

Hypotension
— Skin—Cold, clammy, cyanotic; CNS—altered mental status; kidneys—oliguria (signs of cardiogenic shock: > 40% of myocardium infarcted).

Jugular venous distention
— Kussmaul's sign, hypotension, RV S4 and S3 gallops, clear lungs
— RV infarction.

Systolic murmur of mitral regurgitation
— Papillary muscle dysfunction or rupture (apex; palpable thrill rare).

Systolic murmur of ventricular septal defect
— Ventricular septal rupture (left sternal border; palpable thrill common).

Pericardial friction rub
— Early contiguous pericarditis (accompanies transmural MI)–Late post-MI (Dressler's) syndrome.

Signs of cardiac tamponade, electrical mechanical dissociation, pulseless electrical activity
— Cardiac rupture.

---

sinus rhythm) during or shortly after the acute ischemic event. Although the presence of an S4 gallop may not be specific enough to be diagnostic, its absence argues strongly against an acute MI.

- An S3 gallop (along with pulsus alternans) may also be present in as many as 25% of post-MI patients, but only if significant LV systolic dysfunction (along with an elevated LV filling pressure) has developed, and, as such, portends an adverse prognosis.
- Signs of pulmonary edema may appear suddenly (e.g., rales in all lung fields, generalized wheezing) as the first manifestation of acute MI (which may be painful or silent).

Figure 11-20 and 11-21 summarize the complications of acute myocardial infarction and clinical clues to an adverse prognosis. Factors associated with a high risk include advanced age, hypotension, tachycardia, CHF, and anterior MI.

Figure 11-22. The mechanical complications of acute myocardial infarction: VSD, papillary muscle rupture, and LV aneurysm.

- A systolic murmur of MR from papillary muscle dysfunction may occur at least transiently in 30–50% or more of patients within the first 24 hours.
- Approximately 10% of patients with ST segment elevation (transmural) MI have a pericardial friction rub, generally appearing after 48–72 hours. In patients who receive reperfusion therapy, however, the incidence of pericardial friction rubs has diminished dramatically to ≤5%, presumably as a result of limiting transmural extension of the infarction. Although pericarditis itself is usually benign and self-limiting, it may be a clue to a relatively large transmural MI. Overall, patients with pericarditis have lower ejection fractions and a higher incidence

FIGURE 11-16

Clinical Features of Anterior MI

I. **History**
    Symptoms of MI

II. **Physical Examination**
    Tachycardia, hypertension (high sympathetic tone)
    Sign of LV systolic dysfunction–CHF, pulmonary
        edema, cardiogenic shock (Killip class II-IV).
    Higher incidence of:
    • LV free wall rupture
    • Ventricular septal rupture
    • Ventricular aneurysm
    • LV mural thrombus and systemic arterial
        embolism
    • Pericarditis

III. **ECG**
    Sinus tachycardia and atrial tachyarrhythmia
        (associated with LV failure).
    Sudden onset distal heart block (Mobitz type II
        2nd degree, complete heart block) and bundle
        branch block (associated with extensive necrosis).

IV. **Cardiac Cath**
    Left anterior descending coronary artery occlusion
    Larger infarct size, lower ejection fraction.

V. **Prognosis**
    Higher mortality

---

of CHF. Rubs occurring more than 1 week after the onset of acute MI suggest *post-MI (Dressler's) syndrome,* an autoimmune phenomenon very rarely seen in the reperfusion era.

The 12 lead ECG remains the most important initial diagnostic tool in patients with acute MI. An ECG should be obtained immediately (within 10 min) in every patient with chest pain presenting to the emergency department. The rapid diagnosis of ST segment elevation facilitates the triage of patients who would benefit the most from acute reperfusion therapy. (**Figure 3-34**). Typical ECG changes are most commonly seen in patients experiencing their first acute MI, particularly those with occlusion of the left anterior descending (LAD) coronary artery (90% of cases), followed by the right coronary artery (70–80% of cases), and the left circumflex coronary artery (50% of cases), respectively. A pattern "diagnostic" of acute MI, however, is recorded in only

~50% of patients at initial presentation. In approximately 10–20% of cases, the initial ECG may be entirely normal. If the initial ECG does not reveal ST segment elevation, it should be repeated, especially if ongoing ischemic chest pain is present. Episodic ST segment elevations are common in the first few hours of acute MI and may be present on a follow-up ECG, even if absent initially. (**Figure 3-35**).

Anterior *ST segment elevation (Q wave) MIs* (due to occlusion of the LAD) are usually more extensive than inferior or posterior MIs (caused by occlusion of the right or left circumflex coronary arteries), with increased morbidity and long-term mortality (**Figure 11-16** and **11–17**). Patients with a *non ST segment elevation (non Q wave) MI* have a low mortality initially, but a prolonged high risk period of 1 to 2 years, since post-infarction ischemia and early re-infarction are more common. After this interval, the mortality rate is similar to that of an ST segment elevation (Q wave) MI. (**Figure 11-19**).

The resting ECG may be normal in one-half of patients with an MI, and the clinical-pathologic correlation between the anatomic depth of myocardial necrosis (transmural, nontransmural) and changes on the ECG (ST elevation, and non-ST elevation) is imprecise. Nonetheless, the localization of acute MI (using abnormal new Q waves and ST segment and T wave ECG changes) is useful, since the clinical features, course, and prognosis vary with the site and type of infarction. (**Figures 11-16, 11-17, and 11-19**).

The ECG findings generally are limited to the leads that reflect a certain anatomic region of the heart (e.g., anterior, inferior, posterior, or lateral). (**Figures 3-26 to 3-33**). Reciprocal changes may occur elsewhere in the ECG. The ECG diagnosis of MI may be difficult, however, in patients with LBBB or previous MI with residual Q waves, because the development of new Q waves may be masked. Although the ECG diagnosis of acute ST elevation MI may be fraught with difficulty in the presence of a presumed new LBBB, evidence supports the use of reperfusion therapy in this setting when the clinical picture is compatible, particularly if the ST segments are ≥1 mm and concordant or ≥5 mm and excessively discordant with the QRS.

When there is evidence of an inferior wall MI, right-sided ECG chest leads (e.g., V4R) may demonstrate ST segment elevation, indicating the presence of concomitant RV infarction. (**Figure 3-33**).

Serum biomarkers of myocardial necrosis, particularly troponin, play an important role in confirming the diagnosis of acute MI and identifying high risk ACS patients without ST elevation who may benefit from an early invasive strategy. (**Figure 5-2**). Nevertheless, since levels of these biomarkers rise several hours after the onset of infarction, they have no role in the initial decision making process in patients presenting with ST elevation, and may lead to unnecessary delays in administering lifesaving reperfusion therapy.

Echocardiography may help to confirm the diagnosis of acute MI in patients with chest pain and a nondiagnostic ECG and localize the territory at risk. Although the echo often does not detect small non Q wave infarctions and cannot always distinguish new (acute MI) from old (previous MI) injury, the absence of regional or global wall motion abnormalities argue strongly against an acute transmural coronary event. Two-dimensional color flow Doppler-echo may be particularly useful in assessing infarct size (ejection fraction), and, along with TEE, in determining the etiology of cardiogenic shock and detecting the mechanical complications of acute MI. These mechanical complications include RV infarction, perforation of the ventricular septum with resultant left to right shunt, papillary muscle rupture with acute MR, LV aneurysm, pseudoaneurysm (incomplete rupture of the ventricular wall, held up barely by a thrombus plug), infarct extension, mural thrombus formation, and pericardial effusion.

Much valuable diagnostic and prognostic information may be learned from cardiac catheterization and coronary angiography after an acute MI, including delineation of infarct vessel patency, the coronary anatomy (severity, location and extent of obstructive disease), evaluation of residual LV systolic function, and overall hemodynamic status. The proper place of cardiac catheterization and coronary angiography, however, following an acute MI remains controversial. Clinical practice patterns regarding risk stratification using a conservative noninvasive approach vs. a more aggressive invasive strategy vary widely. "Routine" cardiac catheterization and coronary angiography in patients who have received thrombolytic therapy is currently being performed in many centers to identify suitable candidates for PCI or CABG, whereas others reserve it for "selected" high-risk patients only, e.g., those with recurrent ischemia, hemodynamic instability, CHF, or serious ventricular arrhythmias. (**Figure 11-23**). It should be realized, however, that a routine early invasive strategy for all patients with acute MI has not been shown to confer benefit in terms of preventing death or future MI. Nevertheless, with the dramatic advances in interventional cardiology that have taken place in recent years, almost 80% of patients in the United States with uncomplicated MI who have received thrombolytic therapy now undergo coronary angiography before hospital discharge. In suitable post-MI survivors, however, pre-discharge low level or symptom-limited exercise or pharmacologic stress testing, using adjunctive radioisotope imaging or echocardiography, is an effective noninvasive strategy to help identify high risk and low risk patient subgroups. If significant underlying ischemia is detected, coronary angiography should be performed with a view toward revascularization (i.e., PCI, CABG) if the anatomy permits. Because CABG improves mortality for patients with left main and three vessel disease with depressed LV systolic func-

---

FIGURE 11-17

Clinical Features of Inferior-Posterior MI

- **History**
  Symptoms of MI–especially "gastrointestinal" and vasovagal (epigastric or right upper quadrant discomfort, nausea, vomiting, "gas", "indigestion", lightheadedness).

- **Physical Examination**
  Bradycardia, hypotension (high vagal tone). Signs of RV infarction, and papillary muscle rupture and/or dysfunction.

- **ECG**
  Sinus bradycardia
  Proximal heart block (first degree, Mobitz type I 2nd degree [Wenckebach] progressing to complete AV block)–gradual onset, transient AV nodal ischemia

- **Cardiac Cath**
  Occluded right coronary artery (80% of cases) or left circumflex coronary artery (20% of cases). Smaller infarct size, better ejection fraction.

- **Prognosis**
  Lower mortality (Exception: Poorer prognosis associated with ST segment depression in the anterior precordial leads, concomitant RV infarction and complete AV block).

---

tion, current guidelines suggest that coronary angiography be performed in all patients who have a depressed ejection fraction (<40%) to look for severe triple vessel disease or left main CAD. Cardiac MRI has emerged as a powerful imaging modality that can be used to assess myocardial viability after MI, and help identify those patients likely to recover LV function following revascularization. However, since the assessment of viability does not identify patients with a differential survival benefit from CABG vs. medical therapy, the precise role of myocardial viability testing remains controversial.

Management of Acute MI

In patients who present with an ST elevation MI, the importance of immediate patient evaluation and prompt initiation of reperfusion therapies (i.e., thrombolytic agents, PCI) cannot be over-emphasized. Overall, mortality is decreased ~25–30% when reperfusion therapy is given early. The sooner the reperfusion is administered, the better. If treatment is initiated within the first 3 hours, a 50% or greater reduction in mortality can be achieved. The greater the amount of time that lapses

---

FIGURE 11-18

Clinical Features of Right Ventricular Infarction

I. History
Symptoms of inferior-posterior MI ("indigestion", nausea, vomiting, diaphoresis, lightheadedness)

II. Physical Examination
Hypotension
Elevated jugular venous pressure
Kussmaul's sign (inspiratory increase in JVP)
Abnormal jugular venous pulse (prominent A or V waves, steep Y descent)
Clear lungs
RV S4 and S3 gallops
Systolic murmur of tricuspid regurgitation
Pulsus paradoxus
Pericardial friction rub

III. ECG
Inferior-posterior MI
ST segment elevation in V1-V2 and right-sided precordial leads (V4R most sensitive)
Bradycardia, AV block

IV. Chest X-Ray
Clear lung fields

V. Lab

Color Doppler	Tricuspid regurgitation
2-D Echocardiogram and Radionuclide Ventriculography	Regional RV wall abnormalities
Cardiac Catheterization and Hemodynamics	Dilated RV, decreased ejection fraction
	Proximal right coronary artery occlusion
	Elevated right atrial pressure (>10 mmHg)
	Low pulmonary systolic pressure
	Low or normal wedge pressure
	Right atrial pressure/pulmonary capillary wedge pressure >0.8
	RA waveform–large V wave, Prominent Y descent (tricuspid regurgitation).

---

from the onset of chest pain to reperfusion, the greater the loss of viable, functional myocardium which, in turn, results in an increase in morbidity and mortality. Although the magnitude of benefit declines rapidly over time, a 10% relative mortality reduction can still be achieved up to 12 hours after the onset of chest pain. The ultimate goal in patients with acute ST segment elevation MI (or new LBBB) who are within 6 to 12 hours of the onset of symptoms is initiation of fibrinolytic therapy within 30 minutes of hospital arrival ("door-to-needle" time), or even sooner during transport, or direct PCI within 90 minutes of first medical contact ("door to balloon time"), or 120 minutes if transfer to a PCI-capable hospital is required. Direct PCI should be considered the preferred approach, particularly when the patient presents >3 hours after symptom onset, in cardiogenic shock or severe heart failure, or when thrombolytic therapy is contraindicated or the diagnosis is in doubt. Although direct PCI may be preferable, only a minority of hospitals in the U.S. have this capability on an emergency basis, and as a result, thrombolytic therapy is the most commonly used method (when indicated) for attempting reperfusion of a totally occluded infarct-related artery (**Figure 11-24**).

At present, a conservative management strategy (including noninvasive evaluation of LV function and a modified exercise stress test with or without nuclear or echo imaging) is

---

FIGURE 11-19

Clinical Characteristics of ST Segment Elevation MI vs. Non-ST Segment Elevation MI

ST segment elevation MI	Non-ST segment elevation MI
• Presents with ST segment elevation	• Presents with ST segment depression
• Thrombolysis beneficial	• Thrombolysis not recommended
• Total occlusion of infarct-related artery	• Subtotal occlusion of (patent) infarct-related artery (spontaneous reperfusion)
• More myocardial necrosis	• Less myocardial necrosis
• Large infarct size	• Smaller infarct size
• Higher, later time to peak enzyme elevation	• Lower, earlier time to peak enzyme elevation
• Less prominent coronary collaterals	• More prominent coronary collaterals
• Lower ejection fraction	• Higher ejection fraction
• Higher incidence of: —Congestive heart failure —Pulmonary edema —Cardiogenic shock —Cardiac rupture —Ventricular septal rupture —Infarct expansion and LV aneurysm —Mural thrombus and systemic embolism —Pericarditis	• Higher incidence of: —Residual ischemia —Post-infarct ischemia —Infarct extension and re-infarction (more viable ischemic, jeopardized myocardium)
• Higher in-hospital mortality rate	• Lower in-hospital mortality rate
• Equivalent long-term prognosis to non-ST segment elevation MI (reflects extent of myocardium damaged)	• Equivalent long-term prognosis to ST segment elevation MI (reflects greater ischemic instability and potential for re-infarction and death)

being used for most patients after successful thrombolysis for ST elevation MI, and for many patients with non ST elevation MI. After thrombolytic therapy has been administered, emergency PCI is currently reserved for high risk patients with ongoing pain, spontaneous or inducible ischemia, significantly reduced LV function (with "viable" myocardium), or electrical and/or hemodynamic instability. Of note, recent data has demonstrated a beneficial effect of routine early PCI after successful fibrinolysis for patients with ST elevation MI.

It is important to keep in mind that the patient with unstable angina and the one with non ST segment elevation MI may be indistinguishable by history, physical examination, and ECG. The distinction between them is often made only after the results of serum cardiac marker analyses are available. These two entities, therefore, are often collectively termed "non-ST elevation" ACS. The diagnosis of acute MI should be confirmed by an increase in the plasma concentration of troponin T or I (preferred), or the myocardial (MB) fraction of the creatine kinase (CK). Although myoglobin rises early and is a highly sensitive marker of necrosis, it is not specific ("false positive" levels may occur in patients with renal disease or skeletal muscle disease or injury). Troponin is a more sensitive and specific indicator of damage than CK-MB (troponin may be elevated in patients with ACS even if CK-MB levels are normal). Since troponin may be normal in patients who present within the first 6 hours of onset of the acute event, the practitioner must not exclude the diagnoses of a MI on the basis of a normal initial enzyme level (or normal ECG for that matter) alone. Since confirmatory serum enzyme elevations generally take time to evolve (up to 4–6 hours or more), therapeutic interventions should not be delayed pending assay results.

All patients with chest pain and/or symptoms compatible with acute MI ≤12 hours in duration, with ST elevation or new (or presumably new) LBBB, should promptly receive 162-325 mg non-enteric coated aspirin (chewed initially to quicken absorption), and/or clopidogrel (if aspirin contraindicated), ticagrelor, or prasugrel (if PCI planned).

FIGURE 11-20

**Complications of Acute
Myocardial Infarction**

- **Electrical**
  —Arrhythmias, supraventricular and ventricular
  —Conduction disturbances
- **Pump Failure**
  —Congestive heart failure (LV and/or RV dysfunction)
  —Pulmonary edema
  —Cardiogenic shock
- **Mechanical Complications**
  —LV free-wall rupture (cardiac tamponade)
  —Ventricular septal rupture (acute VSD)
  —Papillary muscle dysfunction/rupture (acute mitral regurgitation)
- **Right Ventricular Infarction**
- **Residual Ischemia (Particularly Non-ST Segment Elevation MI)**
  —Post-infarction angina
  —Infarct extension/reinfarction
- **Pericarditis**
  —Early: contiguous pericarditis
  —Late: post myocardial infarction (Dressler's syndrome)
- **Ventricular Aneurysm**
  —True (congestive heart failure, ventricular arrhythmia, thromboemboli)
  —Pseudoaneurysm—blood filling a necrotic area of myocardium (prone to rupture)
- **Arterial and Venous Thrombosis and Embolism**
  —LV mural and systemic
  —Venous and pulmonary

They should also receive an anti-thrombin agent, e.g., IV unfractionated heparin or SQ LMWH (enoxaparin [Lovenox]) to prevent rethrombosis, particularly if a clot-specific agent (e.g., accelerated alteplase [tPA], reteplase [rPA], tenecteplase [TNK-tPA]) is used for thrombolytic therapy. Patients at high risk for systemic emboli (e.g., large anterior MI, atrial fibrillation, LV thrombus) are also candidates for antithrombin therapy. Primary PCI, in conjunction with IV unfractionated heparin (with or without GP IIb/IIIa inhibitors [GPIs]), or bivalirudin (if bleeding risk is high), and the selective (no benefit of routine) use of manual aspiration thrombectomy (if large thrombus burden), is the preferred reperfusion strategy in patients with acute ST elevation MI, as it is associated with lower rates of reinfarction, mortality, and intracranial bleeding when compared to thrombolytic therapy.

After primary PCI, low dose aspirin is continued indefinitely, along with a prolonged course of P2Y12 inhibitor (ticagrelor or prasugrel preferred over clopidogrel) to reduce the rick of ischemic complications and stent thrombosis.

Routine use of a GPI is not recommended in patients who have received fibrinolytics or in those receiving bivalirudin because of an increased risk of bleeding.

ACC/AHA guidelines recommend that SQ LMWH (enoxaparin [Lovenox]) can be "advantageously" substituted for IV unfractionated heparin (UFH) in patients with unstable angina and non-ST segment elevation MI, unless CABG is planned within 24 hours, in which case UFH is preferred (since it has a shorter half life than LMWH and can be rapidly reversed with protamine).

When timely PCI is unavailable, the newer fibrinolytics (e.g., double bolus reteplase [rPA], single bolus tenecteplase [TNK-TPA]) are currently favored over the "gold standard" tPA (and the older non-clot selective agent streptokinase) by some experts because of the ease of bolus administration vs. infusion. More recent evidence suggests a therapeutic paradigm shift towards a regimen that combines LMWH (enoxaparin) with full dose tenecteplase. Thrombolytic agents, however, have not been proven effective for non ST segment elevation MI or unstable angina. In fact, there is evidence that these agents may be harmful, and therefore should not be administered in those conditions. Contraindications to thrombolytic therapy include a history of intracranial hemorrhage; active internal bleeding (excluding menses); severe uncontrolled hypertension (BP $\geq$180/110 mmHg); recent stroke, major surgery or trauma; brain neoplasm, aneurysm or AV malformation; unclear mental status; suspected aortic dissection; and acute pericarditis. When using thrombolytic therapy, adjunctive pharmacologic treatment includes aspirin and/or clopidogrel, beta blockers (in the absence of contraindications), heparin (especially if a fibrin-specific thrombolytic agent [e.g., TPA, rPA, TNK-TPA] is administered), IV nitroglycerin, and ACE inhibitors/ARBs (particularly in patients with diminished LV function [ejection fraction < 40%]).

Irrespective of whether the patient receives thrombolytic therapy or primary PCI, or neither, beta blockers (due to their antiischemic as well as antiarrhythmic influence) should be administered, when hemodynamically stable, unless contraindicated. IV nitroglycerin should be administered to patients with large anterior MI, CHF, hypertension, and/or persistent or recurrent ischemic chest pain. It should be avoided, however, in patients with hypotension and/or RV infarction (where decreasing preload may decrease cardiac output and lead to more hypotension). IV morphine sulfate should be administered if pain is not relieved with nitroglycerin. (Keep in mind the *memory aid:* **"MONA"**— **M**orphine, **O**xygen [if O₂ sat < 90%], **N**itroglycerin, **A**spirin.)

Definitive treatment is to open the infarct-related artery as soon as possible. For patients with acute MI, the greater the amount of time that lapses from the onset of chest pain to initiation of reperfusion therapies, the greater the loss

FIGURE 11-21

Clinical Clues to an Adverse Prognosis in Acute Myocardial Infarction

I. HISTORY

❑ **Patient Characteristics**
- Advanced age (>70 years) (reflects multivessel CAD and previous MI).
- Female gender (may in part reflect older age and associated hypertension, diabetes).
- Hypertension, diabetes mellitus, cigarette smoking.

❑ **Prior History**
- Angina pectoris
- Myocardial infarction (reflects greater extent of CAD and aggregate amount of LV dysfunction—past and present necrosis).

❑ **Hospital Course**
- Delayed time to treatment (> 4 hours) after symptom onset.
- Congestive heart failure (reflects LV dysfunction).
- Recurrent chest pain–especially non-ST segment elevation MI (reflects residual myocardial ischemia— post-infarction angina, infarct extension, reinfarction).

II. PHYSICAL EXAMINATION

❑ **Signs of LV systolic dysfunction (Killip class II to IV)**
- Congestive heart failure
- Pulmonary edema
- Cardiogenic shock

❑ **Signs of complications**
- Systolic murmur of acute VSD (ventricular septal rupture)
- Systolic murmur of acute mitral regurgitation (papillary muscle rupture)
- "Ectopic" systolic impulse—ventricular aneurysm
- Elevated JVP, Kussmaul's sign, RV S4 and S3 gallops, TR murmur (RV infarction)

III. ECG

❑ **Infarct location**
- Anterior MI (reflects greater LV dysfunction, more complicated course)
- ST segment elevation MI (higher in-hospital mortality reflects greater myocardial necrosis)
- Non-ST segment elevation MI—especially ST segment depression (higher late mortality, reflects residual myocardial ischemia and reinfarction)

❑ **Arrhythmias**
- Supraventricular—Sinus tachycardia, atrial flutter-fibrillation (reflects LV failure)
- Ventricular—Symptomatic, complex ventricular tachyarrhythmias.

❑ **Conduction Defects**
- High grade AV block (Mobitz Type II 2nd degree or complete heart block)
- New bundle branch block (reflects greater extent of necrosis)

IV. CHEST X-RAY
- Pulmonary vascular redistribution, interstitial and alveolar edema
- Cardiomegaly

V. LAB

❑ **Enzymes and Chemistries**
- High peak troponin (I or T) and creatine kinase (CK-MB) levels (rough indicator of extent of myocardial damage)
- Elevated leukocyte count (reflects greater myocardial necrosis)
- Elevated BUN and creatinine (decreased renal perfusion due to decreased cardiac output)

FIGURE 11-21

Clinical Clues to an Adverse Prognosis in Acute Myocardial Infarction (*continued*)

❏ **Stress Test, Nuclear Imaging Techniques, 2-D Echocardiography**
- Exercise-induced ischemia (angina, ST segment depression)
- New perfusion (thallium, technetium—Cardiolite) defects and/or echo wall motion abnormalities
- Low ejection fraction (<40%)

❏ **Doppler**
- Visualize site and detect severity of mechanical complications (e.g., ventricular septal defect (VSD), papillary muscle rupture)

❏ **24-Hour Holter Monitor**
- Frequent +/− complex (multiform, repetitive) PVCs, ventricular tachyarrhythmias
- Decreased heart rate variability (an index of abnormal autonomic function)

❏ **Signal-averaged ECG**
- Positive—detects "late potentials" generated by asynchronous conduction through ischemic/fibrotic myocardium (substrate for malignant reentrant ventricular tachycardia [VT])
- Negative—low probability of inducible VT during EPS testing

❏ **EPS Testing**
- Inducible sustained ventricular tachycardia

❏ **Cardiac Catheterization and Hemodynamics**
- Persistent occlusion or suboptimal flow in infarct-related artery
- Increased severity and extent of CAD (left main, advanced triple vessel disease, proximal stenosis of left anterior descending coronary artery)
- Diminished LV function (ejection fraction <40%)
- LV hypokinesis remote from index infarction
- Visualize and quantitate mechanical complications, (e.g., VSD, acute MR, LV aneurysm)
  High LV filling pressure, low cardiac output and index

---

of viable functional heart muscle. Thrombolysis produces the greatest benefit when given within 3 hours of the onset of symptoms, although the patient may still benefit if the drug is given within 12 hours. Since "time is muscle", patients who are eligible should expeditiously receive either thrombolytic therapy ("door-to-needle" time ≤ 30 minutes) or be taken directly to the cath lab for primary PCI, which has been demonstrated to be superior to thrombolytic therapy in expert hands when performed early without prolonged delay (i.e., "door-to-balloon" time ≤ 90 minutes, or ≤ 120 minutes if transfer to a PCI-capable hospital is required). Direct PCI is to be considered when thrombolytic therapy is absolutely contraindicated. "Facilitated" PCI (upstream thrombolysis "on the way to" immediate PCI) offers no advantage over direct PCI, and increases the risk of bleeding, and therefore, is not recommended. "Rescue" PCI is associated with improved outcomes and may be considered after failed thrombolysis. Routine early PCI (within 3-24 hrs) has recently been shown to improve outcomes in ST elevation MI patients following successful fibrinolysis.

Noninfarct artery PCI may be considered at the time of primary culprit PCI, or as a staged procedure, in select patients with ST elevation MI and multivessel CAD.

Patients treated after 12 hours should receive appropriate medical therapy, e.g., nitrates, beta blockers, ACE inhibitors (particularly if large anterior MI with decreased LV function and if patient is diabetic [slows progression of nephropathy]). Patients may be considered candidates for reperfusion therapy on an individual basis. ACE inhibitors have been shown to attenuate LV remodeling (i.e., reduce LV dysfunction and dilatation) and slow the progression of CHF and decrease mortality. Oral anticoagulation with warfarin (preferred) or NOAC is recommended if a large anterior MI with extensive dyskinesis and/or LV thrombus (on echo), or atrial fibrillation is present. Prophylactic lidocaine (or other antiarrhythmic agent) and calcium channel blockers have failed to demonstrate benefit and in fact may even be harmful, and therefore should be avoided (see below).

Calcium channel blockers (particularly the dihydropyridines, e.g., nifedipine) have not been shown to be

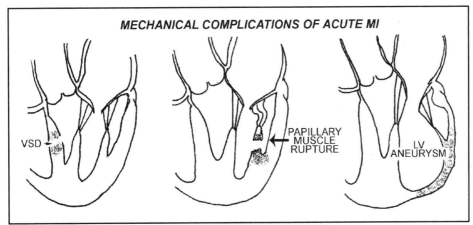

MECHANICAL COMPLICATIONS OF ACUTE MI

VSD

PAPILLARY
MUSCLE
RUPTURE

LV
ANEURYSM

Note: Acute VSD (due to ventricular septal rupture) or acute MR (due to papillary muscle rupture) should be suspected in post-MI patients who abruptly develop CHF/pulmonary edema or cardiogenic shock and a new systolic murmur (parasternal-VSD vs apical-MR). An LV aneurysm should be considered if CHF, ventricular arrhythmias, and arterial thromboemboli occur in the presence of persistent ST segment elevation on the ECG. Unlike pseudoaneurysms, LV aneurysms rarely rupture.

Figure 11-22

FIGURE 11-23

Cardiac Catheterization and Coronary Arteriography After Acute Myocardial Infarction

PHASE	INDICATIONS
Early	• Recurrent or persistent myocardial ischemia. • Congestive heart failure "refractory" to (intensive) medical therapy. • Cardiogenic shock. • Mechanical complications (ventricular septal rupture, acute mitral regurgitation). • Emergency angiography and primary ("direct") PCI, if technically feasible, contraindications to thrombolytic therapy exist, or cardiogenic shock is present. "Rescue" PCI should be considered in high-risk patients with large infarcts who clinically appear to have failed thrombolysis. Routine early PCI (within 3-24 hrs) may also be considered in ST elevation MI patients after successful fibrinolysis. If lysed at a non-PCI capable hospital, consider transfer to PCI capable hospital as soon as possible (especially if high risk)
Convalescent (including pre-discharge)	• Post-infarction angina pectoris. • Provocable myocardial ischemia—exercise or pharmacologic (dipyridamole, adenosine, dobutamine) stress testing (radionuclide wall motion or perfusion scans/2-dimensional echocardiography). • Non-ST segment elevation MI (conservative noninvasive strategy of risk stratification vs. aggressive invasive approach remains unsettled). • Persistent LV dysfunction (ejection fraction <40%). • Recurrent ventricular tachycardia or ventricular fibrillation despite antiarrhythmic therapy. • Young patients, especially those with physically demanding jobs and active life styles. • Non-infarct artery PCI may be considered at time of primary PCI, or as a staged procedure prior to discharge, in select patients with ST elevation MI and multivessel CAD. Late PCI of occluded infarct related artery, however, has not been shown to be of benefit.

FIGURE 11-24

**Comparison of Thrombolysis and Direct Percutaneous Coronary Intervention
for ST Segment Elevation Myocardial Infarction**

Thrombolysis	Percutaneous Coronary Intervention
Universally available	Available only in specialized centers with 24 hr cath lab capability and skilled interventional personnel
Easy, rapid administration	Technologically demanding, time delay to perform. Single-stage procedure. Clot and plaque addressed at same time.
Higher bleeding and stroke risk	Lower bleeding and stroke risk
Higher rates of reocclusion and recurrent ischemia	Lower rates of early reocclusion and ischemia
Many contraindications	Few contraindications. Allows reperfusion when thrombolytics are contraindicated
Lower vessel patency rates (TIMI-3 flow rates 55%–60%)*	Higher vessel patency rates (TIMI-3 flow rates >90%)*
Longer length of hospital stay	Shorter length of hospital stay. Improved survival in high risk patients. Greater efficacy for cardiogenic shock.
	Provides additional information regarding coronary artery anatomy and left ventricular function. Allows risk stratification.**

*Note: Angiographic assessment of coronary blood flow can be semiquantitated using the grading method of the Thrombolysis in Acute MI (TIMI) investigators. TIMI-0 = no flow past obstruction, TIMI-1 = incomplete filling of vessel, TIMI-2 = slow but complete filling of vessel, TIMI-3 = brisk filling of vessel.

**After administration of thrombolytic therapy, all patients, especially those at high risk (extensive ST segment elevation, previous MI, new onset LBBB, tachycardia, or hypotension), should be transferred to a PCI-capable hospital as soon as possible so that PCI can be performed as needed.

---

beneficial in the early treatment or secondary prevention of acute MI. These agents may promote reflex tachycardia and hypotension and thereby exacerbate ischemia, and are not considered part of the routine management of MI patients. (Exception: The rate-slowing non-dihydropyridine calcium channel blocker diltiazem has been shown to reduce recurrent MI in patients with a first non-ST elevation (non-Q wave) MI who have intact LV function). Nifedipine and other short-acting formulations may increase morbidity and mortality. Diltiazem and verapamil should be used with caution, if at all, in patients with LV dysfunction, because they reduce ventricular contractility.

The role of routine magnesium sulfate in patients with acute MI is uncertain. It should be given to the patient with hypomagnesemia, especially if polymorphic VT associated with QT prolongation ("torsades de pointes") is present (since hypomagnesemia prolongs the QT interval and predisposes to torsade de pointes).

Complications of acute MI should be managed appropriately and expeditiously. For example:

- Patients with *CHF* should be treated with ACE inhibitors/ARBs, beta blockers (as tolerated), diuretics, and aldosterone antagonists.

- Symptomatic *ventricular arrhythmias* should be treated with beta blockers (lidocaine is no longer recommended prophylactically due to potentially detrimental effects). If refractory, they should be treated with the antiarrhythmic agent amiodarone, procainamide, or lidocaine, and/or ICD implantation (in patients at high risk of sudden cardiac death).

- *Supraventricular arrhythmias* should be treated with beta blockers (e.g., IV esmolol), diltiazem, verapamil, digoxin.

- *Cardiogenic shock* is the most common cause of death in hospitalized patients with acute MI. Prompt restoration of coronary blood flow (preferably by PCI) can increase survival. IABP can be used in the interim for hemodynamic stabilization.

- *Surgery* or *percutaneous* intervention may be indicated, particularly for acute MR and VSD.

- Nitroglycerin should be used cautiously, if at all, in patients with *inferior MI* who have concomitant *RV infarction,* since profound hypotension may result. Furthermore, nitroglycerin (or nitrates) should not be administered to patients with chest pain who have taken drugs for erectile dysfunction, e.g., *sildenafil* (Viagra), *vardenafil* (Levitra), or *tadalafil* (Cialis) within the previous 24-48 hours. A marked drop in BP and even death may occur. Viagra is also potentially hazardous in patients with CHF and borderline low BP, including patients on multiple antihypertensive drug therapy.

Note: Consider the use of cocaine in a young person who presents with chest pain, particularly following a party. Cocaine may induce coronary spasm, leading to acute MI. The management of *cocaine-induced* MI differs from that of classic MI. Beta blockers, e.g., metoprolol, should be avoided acutely, as these agents may lead to unopposed α-mediated vasoconstriction and worsen myocardial ischemia. Labetalol and carvedilol, however, have combined (alpha)-and (beta)-blocking properties, and can be considered. Benzodiazepines can be used as an anxiolytic to reduce tachycardia and hypertension, along with antiplatelet and antithrombotic therapy, nitrates, calcium channel blockers, and phentolamine (an α-blocker) to relieve coronary spasm. Immediate angiography with PCI (if appropri-ate) should be considered if chest pain and ST segment elevation persists. PCI is the preferred reperfusion strategy in these patients, as there are usually comorbid features (e.g., seizures, dissection, severe hypertension) that preclude the use of thrombolytic therapy.

Complications of Acute MI

During the hours following initiation of therapies for acute ST segment elevation MI, the patient should be observed closely for the development of acute complications. A variety of electrical and/or mechanical complications can occur, even when treatment is initiated promptly. The nature, diagnosis and treatment strategies for these complications are presented in the following section.

Electrical Complications of Acute MI

Cardiac arrhythmias and conduction disturbances are the most common complications of acute MI (**Figure 11-25**).

FIGURE 11-25

Management of Electrical Complications of Acute Myocardial Infarction

I. VENTRICULAR TACHYCARDIA/FIBRILLATION

  A. Acute Phase (First 48 Hours)
- If hemodynamically unstable - electrical cardioversion/defibrillation/cardiopulmonary resuscitation.
- If hemodynamically stable – IV amiodarone (preferred), procainamide, or lidocaine may be used. Lidocaine reduces primary ventricular fibrillation; however routine prophylaxis no longer recommended for all patients since toxicities (increased fatal asystolic events) tend to offset antifibrillatory benefit.
- Beta blockers—reduce incidence of ventricular tachycardia and fibrillation.
- Correct electrolyte imbalance ($\downarrow$ K$^+$, $\downarrow$ Mg^{++}), acid-base disturbances, hypoxemia, adverse drug effects.

  B. Convalescent Phase (After 48 Hours)
- Beta blockers and amiodarone
- Consider non-drug methods (e.g., wearable defibrillator or ICD, ventricular aneurysm resection, ablation of arrhythmogenic foci, antitachycardia pacemakers, with or without CABG).

II. SUPRAVENTRICULAR TACHYARRHYTHMIAS
- Beta blockers (esmolol), adenosine, verapamil, diltiazem, digoxin—slows ventricular rate.
- Class IA antiarrhythmics (e.g., procainamide) or class III (e.g., sotalol, amiodarone) or
- Synchronized DC electrical cardioversion, if clinically or hemodynamically unstable—restores sinus rhythm.

III. BRADYARRHYTHMIAS AND CONDUCTION DISTURBANCES
- Atropine
  - If symptomatic or hemodynamically unstable (excessive increase in heart rate may worsen ischemia, extend infarction, or promote ventricular tachycardia/ventricular fibrillation).
- Temporary external transcutaneous or transvenous pacemaker.
  - Mobitz Type II 2nd degree AV block
  - Complete heart block
  - New bifascicular block including alternating right and left bundle branch block (LBBB), new RBBB with left anterior or posterior hemiblock, new LBBB with first degree AV block in anterior MI.

With initiation of early reperfusion therapy, both brady- and tachyarrhythmias will often develop after restored patency of the infarct-related coronary artery (so-called "reperfusion arrhythmias"). The most common rhythm disorder seen after reperfusion with thrombolytic therapy or PCI is an accelerated idioventricular rhythm (AIVR—**Figure 3-34**), so-called "slow VT", occurring at a rate of 60–100 beats/min, which is well tolerated hemodynamically in most patients. It is transient, and usually does not require specific treatment.

Ventricular Arrhythmias

Ventricular arrhythmias (i.e., PVCs, VT or VF) are the most frequently observed rhythm disturbances in acute MI. They reflect the electrical instability of the damaged ischemic myocardium and occur in >90% of patients during the first 72 hours. Electrolyte imbalance (e.g., hypokalemia, hypomagnesemia), hypoxemia, adverse drug effects, and increased sympathoadrenal discharge may also play a role.

PVCs and nonsustained (<30 seconds) VT not associated with hemodynamic compromise, are not indicative of increased risk of sudden cardiac death and do not require specific therapy in the acute phase of MI.

Early-onset or "primary" sustained VT is common in the first hours and days after MI, and does not appear to be associated with an increased risk for subsequent mortality if the arrhythmia is rapidly terminated. Late-onset or "secondary" sustained VT occurring after 24–48 hours, however, is associated with a marked increase in mortality. These late-onset ventricular arrhythmias reflect a transmural infarct of substantial size with advanced LV dysfunction and portend a far more ominous prognosis.

Patients with VF (which may occur without any warning arrhythmias) or sustained VT associated with symptoms or hemodynamic compromise should undergo defibrillation or electrical cardioversion immediately. Underlying ischemia and electrolyte abnormalities ($\downarrow$ K$^+$, $\downarrow$ Mg^{++}) should be addressed and corrected. IV amiodarone remains an effective agent for the treatment of symptomatic VT or VF. *Although it reduces primary VF, lidocaine is no longer used as a prophylactic measure,* since the overall incidence of primary VF (in this era of reperfusion therapy and beta blockade) appears to be decreasing, and recent studies have demonstrated a disturbing trend toward an increased number of fatal bradycardic and asystolic cardiac arrests in lidocaine-treated patients. Persistent ventricular arrhythmias (despite the use of IV amiodarone therapy), however, may necessitate the administration of another antiarrhythmic agent, e.g., IV procainamide or lidocaine and/or a more aggressive invasive (i.e., cardiac catheterization, EPS) management strategy (for those who may benefit from revascularization and/or implantation of an ICD).

Supraventricular Arrhythmias

Supraventricular arrhythmias (i.e., PACs, paroxysmal SVT, atrial fibrillation and/or flutter) may be manifestations of the left atrial distension and pressure rise resulting from LV failure, and as such are associated with an increased infarct size and mortality. These arrhythmias may also occur with pericarditis, excessive sympathetic stimulation, electrolyte disturbances, hypoxia, or atrial infarction. Sinus tachycardia is the most common supraventricular arrhythmia. If it occurs secondary to another cause (e.g., anemia, fever, CHF), the primary problem should be treated first. However, if it appears to be due to sympathetic overstimulation (e.g., fever, pain, anxiety), then treatment with a beta blocker is indicated. PACs occur in 15–30% of patients and usually do not require specific therapy. They are often harbingers of more severe grades of atrial tachyarrhythmias. Atrial fibrillation occurs in up to 15% of patients early after MI, with atrial flutter and paroxysmal SVT occurring much less frequently.

Management of supraventricular arrhythmias in the setting of acute MI is similar to the management in other settings; however the threshold for cardioversion should be lower and the urgency with which the rapid ventricular response is controlled should be greater. When the ventricular response is rapid, an increase in myocardial oxygen demand and decrease in diastolic filling time may produce hemodynamic instability and exacerbate ischemia. Atrial fibrillation or flutter associated with a rapid ventricular response, therefore, should be treated promptly with electrical cardioversion. Pharmacologic agents, e.g., beta blockers, calcium channel blockers, and digoxin, increase the AV block and slow the ventricular rate. Beta blockers are generally the first line agents in acute MI, to control the rapid ventricular response. Diltiazem and verapamil are appropriate alternatives in patients without CHF or significant LV systolic dysfunction, and digoxin for patients with concomitant LV dysfunction. If spontaneous conversion to normal sinus rhythm does not occur, IV unfractionated or SQ low molecular weight heparin therapy (in patients not already receiving it) along with Class IA antiarrhythmic agents (e.g., procainamide) or Class III agents (e.g., amiodarone) (**Figure 7-5**) should be considered. Of the antiarrhythmic agents available, amiodarone is probably the safest in the peri-infarct setting.

Bradyarrhythmias and Conduction Disturbances

Bradyarrhythmias and conduction disturbances are common during the course of acute MI. They are encountered 2–3 times more frequently in inferior than in anterior MIs, and may be due to increased vagal tone or ischemia and/or infarction of conduction tissue. Prognosis and treatment vary greatly, depending on the size and location of infarct, the ventricular response, the degree of AV block, and the patient's clinical status (**Figure 11-26**). The most common brad-

---

FIGURE 11-26

AV Conduction Disturbances in Acute Myocardial Infarction

	INFERIOR	ANTEROSEPTAL
QRS width	Narrow	Wide
Site of block	Proximal to His (AV junction)	Distal to His
Compromised arterial supply	Right Coronary Artery (80%)	Left Anterior Descending Coronary Artery
	Left Circumflex Coronary Artery (20%)	
Extent underlying MI	Mild to moderate	Usually severe
Development of complete heart block	Stepwise (Wenckebach-Mobitz I)	Often abrupt (Mobitz II)
Escape rhythm	Satisfactory	Often none or very unstable
Reversibility	Almost always	May be permanent
Response to atropine	Frequent	Rare
Indication for permanent pacemaker	Almost never (usually transient)	Usually

---

yarrhythmia associated with acute MI is sinus bradycardia which is seen in 20–25% of patients. It is particularly common early in the course of acute inferior MI, or after reperfusion of the right coronary artery. In most patients with acute MI, sinus bradycardia is asymptomatic and requires no treatment. If the heart rate is extremely low (<40 beats/min) or if systemic hypotension is present, IV atropine should be considered. Atropine should be used sparingly and appropriately, however, because of the protective effect of vagal stimulation against VF in the setting of acute MI.

AV block of some degree occurs in 15–25% of patients with acute MI. Heart block in inferior infarction often progresses in a step-wise gradual fashion, from first degree AV block to Mobitz Type I second degree (Wenckebach) AV block to complete heart block (**Figure 3-51**) and is usually transient. The AV block in acute MI is due to ischemia of the AV node and is accompanied by a QRS complex of normal duration and an adequate rate of junctional escape rhythm. Most of these patients are asymptomatic and are hemodynamically and electrically stable. Since return to normal AV conduction is the rule, cardiac pacing is rarely required.

Mobitz Type II second degree AV block is much less common than Mobitz Type I block. In contrast to Mobitz Type I block, Mobitz Type II block is more frequently associated with anterior MI and is due to a defect below the His bundle. Complete heart block may develop suddenly, with an unstable, wide complex, slow ventricular escape rhythm and a high incidence of asystole. Cardiac pacing, therefore, is indicated. Although complete heart block may occur with either inferior or anterior MI, the implications differ considerably depending on the location of the infarct. Complete heart block in the presence of an *inferior MI* is usually transient and well tolerated. The escape rate is often stable and requires only that the patient be connected to a standby transcutaneous pacemaker. A permanent pacemaker is rarely required. In the setting of an *anterior MI,* however, complete heart block is usually a result of extensive myocardial necrosis that involves the bundle branches. The escape rhythm is usually unstable and the AV block permanent. Mortality is extremely high and permanent pacing should be performed unless there are contraindications. Because of the overwhelming effect of the extent of myocardial damage on prognosis, pacing in this setting has not been shown to lessen mortality. It is likely however, that pacing will benefit those patients with severe slowing of the heart rate but without extensive myocardial necrosis.

Bundle branch block, right more often than left, occurs in 10–15% of patients with acute MI. These patients tend to be older, have larger infarcts, more extensive LV dysfunction and higher morbidity and mortality rates. Patients with anteroseptal MI and new bifascicular blocks, including alternating right and left bundle branch block, new RBBB with left anterior or posterior hemiblock, and new LBBB, particularly with first degree AV block or Mobitz Type II (distal) second degree AV block, are at increased risk for progression to complete heart block. Prophylactic temporary transcutaneous and/or transvenous pacing should be considered. If Mobitz Type II second degree AV block or complete heart block, transient or permanent, develops during the course of an anterior MI with bundle branch block, a permanent pacemaker is indicated.

Mechanical Complications of Acute MI

Prompt recognition and attention to serious life-threatening arrhythmias and conduction disturbances that complicate acute MI by modern cardiac care units, along with early restoration of coronary artery patency by aggressive reperfusion strategies, have significantly reduced the in-hospital mortality to 5–10%. The current mortality is almost entirely due to LV systolic dysfunction ("pump failure") and the mechanical complications resulting from the infarction (**Figure 11-27**).

Left Ventricular (LV) Systolic Dysfunction

Patients with an acute MI may come to medical attention with worsening heart failure, proportionate to the extent of myocardial necrosis, but exacerbated by preexisting dysfunction and ongoing ischemia. In general, damage to ≥25% of the myocardium results in LV systolic dysfunction. In patients with massive LV systolic dysfunction (i.e., damage to ≥40% of the myocardium), shock may occur. Four subgroups of patients with acute MI have been classified from low (*Class I*) to high (*Class IV*) mortality risk on the degree of LV systolic dysfunction by clinical examina-

---

FIGURE 11-27

Management of Mechanical Complications of Acute Myocardial Infarction

I. HYPOTENSION

- Right Ventricular Infarction
  - Administer IV fluids to augment RV filling pressure.
  - Avoid diuretics and nitrates.
  - Add positive inotropic agents (e.g., dobutamine or dopamine) if low cardiac output persists.
  - Institute temporary pacing, if high grade AV block and hemodynamic compromise is present (AV sequential pacing may be required to restore atrial transport).

II. HYPERTENSION

- Adequate analgesics and sedation to relieve pain and anxiety.
- Nitroglycerin, especially if ongoing ischemic chest pain, LV failure; Nitroprusside–potential "coronary steal" effect.
- Beta blockers, particularly useful if hyperadrenergic state.
- Diuretics, if volume depletion not present.
- ACE inhibitors/ARBs, particularly if high-risk groups (e.g., anterior MI, CHF, ejection fraction < 40%).
- Calcium channel blockers (after the acute phase), if LV failure (ejection fraction < 40%) not present.

III. PUMP FAILURE AND CARDIOGENIC SHOCK

- Initiate invasive hemodynamic monitoring (to keep MAP > 60 mmHg, CI (CO/BSA) > 2.2 L/min/m², and PCWP ~ 14-18 mmHg)*.
- Administer pharmacologic support–optimize LV filling pressure and cardiac output.
  - Diuretics (e.g., furosemide, bumetanide, torsemide) to reduce pulmonary capillary wedge pressure.
  - Inotropic drugs (e.g., dopamine, dobutamine, or milrinone) to improve contractility.
  - Vasodilators (IV nitroglycerin, nitroprusside, and ACE inhibitors/ARBs (if ACE inhibitor intolerant [e.g., cough]), or ARNI [if not hypotensive]) to reduce preload and afterload.
- Assure adequate ventilation and oxygenation.
- Correct metabolic abnormalities.
- Control tachy- and brady-arrhythmias.
- Initiate mechanical circulatory assistance.
  - Intra-aortic balloon pump (IABP), percutaneous left ventricular assist device (LVAD), or extracorporeal membrane oxygenation (ECMO)-bridge to surgery.
- Identify surgically correctable mechanical complications (ventricular septal rupture, acute mitral regurgitation, LV aneurysm).
- Primary ("direct") PTCA/stenting within initial hours of acute MI.

---

*Note: There is little evidence that the routine use of PA catheters in CHF patients improves clinical outcomes. Invasive hemodynamic monitoring, however, can be useful in acutely ill patients with decompensated CHF who have persistent symptoms despite standard therapies, whose fluid status or perfusion is uncertain, and in whom the measurements obtained are expected to guide therapy or influence management decisions.

FIGURE 11-28

Killip Classification of Acute Myocardial Infarction

Class	Clinical Evidence of LV Dysfunction	Mortality
I	No heart failure (uncomplicated)	3–5%
	Absence of S3 gallop and pulmonary rales.	
II	Mild to moderate heart failure.	6–10%
	Mild to moderate orthopnea.	
	S3 gallop	
	Bibasilar rales confined to ≤50% of both lung fields.	
	Radiographic evidence of pulmonary venous congestion.	
III	Pulmonary edema.	20–30%
	Severe respiratory distress.	
	Rales heard over >50% of both lung fields.	
	Radiographic evidence of interstitial and alveolar pulmonary edema	
IV	Cardiogenic shock	> 80%
	Hypotension (systolic BP <90 mmHg)	
	Tachycardia	
	Signs of diminished peripheral perfusion:	
	• Skin—cold, clammy, cyanotic.	
	• CNS—mental confusion, agitation, obtundation.	
	• Kidney—oliguria	

---

tion (so-called *Killip classification*) (**Figure 11-28**). The therapy of the patient with an acute MI and resultant LV systolic dysfunction depends on the extent of such dysfunction. In most patients with symptoms and signs of Class II LV systolic dysfunction, CHF is transient, and usually responds to bed rest, salt restriction, and medical therapy, i.e., IV nitroglycerin, diuretics, ACE inhibitors, or angiotensin receptor blockers, and beta blockers.

In patients with more severe CHF unresponsive to medical therapy, as well as in those with pulmonary edema, hypotension, or evidence of systemic hypoperfusion, invasive hemodynamic monitoring may be necessary. Such measures include the Swan-Ganz catheter, along with vasopressors, inotropes, insertion of an IABP or percutaneous LVAD, transthoracic or transesophageal echo and/or cardiac catheterization (with emergency PCI or even CABG) looking for a potentially correctable cause (e.g., acute MR, VSD). The therapeutic interventions used in the different hemodynamic subsets are listed in **Figure 11-29.**

Note: An increasingly recognized condition mimicking acute MI that causes acute reversible balloon-like LV systolic dysfunction, typically in the absence of obstructive CAD, is *stress cardiomyopathy*, also called *tako-tsubo car-*

diomyopathy, transient LV apical ballooning, and *broken heart syndrome*. This disorder is often precipitated by sudden emotional or physical stress and occurs primarily in postmenopausal women. Despite the frequent occurrence of CHF or even cardiogenic shock, most patients recover completely within 1–4 weeks, and recurrence is rare.

Acute Ventricular Septal Defect and Papillary Muscle Rupture

Several complications of MI may interfere with the mechanical function of the heart, including perforation of the ventricular septum (resulting in an acute VSD), and rupture of the papillary muscle (causing acute MR). During the hours, or more commonly days, after the onset of an acute MI, the patient should be observed closely for the development of these complications.

If a patient with an acute MI develops sudden onset of pulmonary edema, respiratory distress and/or shock, together with a new systolic murmur heard best long the left sternal border, and also at the apex, consider the diagnosis of an acute VSD vs. papillary muscle rupture. Keep in mind that these conditions are life-threatening. **Figure 11-30** summarizes clues that may help distinguish acute VSD from

---

FIGURE 11-29

Therapeutic Intervention in Acute Myocardial Infarction

Hemodynamic Subset	Intervention
Normal	Aspirin and/or clopidogrel (if aspirin contraindicated), ticagrelor, or prasugrel (if PCI planned); heparin or enoxaparin; nitrates (except in patients with suspected RV infarction and hypotension); beta blockers (if not contraindicated)*; thrombolytic therapy or percutaneous coronary intervention (PCI) if within 6–12 hrs of symptoms and onset of ST segment elevation MI; GP IIb/IIIa platelet receptor antagonists are given to high risk patients with unstable angina or non ST elevation MI, and patients undergoing PCI. Bivalirudin (if PCI planned) and fondaparinux (if no PCI planned) may be acceptable alternatives to heparin or enoxaparin.
Hyperdynamic state	Beta-blockers, then normal subset protocol.
Hypoperfusion (due to hypovolemia)	Fluid challenge, then normal subset protocol.
Congestive heart failure	Diuretic + ACE inhibitor/ARB + beta-blocker* + aldosterone blocker (eplerenone).
Cardiogenic shock	IV nitroglycerin, nitroprusside, dopamine, dobutamine, diuretic, circulatory assistance (IABP, LVAD), angioplasty/stenting or surgical revascularization and/or correction of mechanical complication (e.g., acute VSD, papillary muscle rupture).

IABP = intraaortic balloon pump, LVAD = left ventricular assist device (e.g., TandemHeart, Impella).

***Note:** Early (<24 hr) use of IV beta blockers may increase risk of cardiogenic shock and should be avoided in patients with signs of CHF, evidence of low output state, or other risk factors, e.g., age > 70 yrs, systolic BP < 120 mmHg, sinus tachycardia > 110/min., heart rate < 60/min. or delayed presentation after symptom onset. In the absence of contraindications, oral beta blockers should be continued for up to 3 years after uncomplicated MI, and indefinitely in patients with LV systolic dysfunction.

---

acute MR. Prompt diagnosis along with hemodynamic stabilization by means of IABP counterpulsation (**Figure 11-10**) and early surgical (or percutaneous) intervention can be life-saving. Acute MR more often causes severe dyspnea and pulmonary edema. The JVP is usually elevated with acute VSD, but may not be elevated with MR. Inferior MI favors MR (because of papillary muscle dysfunction), whereas anterior MI favors acute VSD (because anterior MI commonly involves a large portion of the septum).

Right Ventricular Infarction

The right coronary artery supplies blood to both the inferior wall of the LV and the RV wall. When a patient with prolonged retrosternal chest discomfort accompanied by nausea and vomiting exhibits hypotension, bradycardia, distended neck veins increasing during inspiration (Kussmaul's sign), and clear lung fields, strongly consider the possibility of an inferior wall MI with concomitant RV infarction. Don't forget that "heartburn" may be one of the most common symptoms of an inferior wall MI!

Although evidence of RV infarction can be detected in up to 30–50% of patients with an inferior MI, hemodynamically significant RV dysfunction is present in less than 10% of patients with this complication. **Figure 11-18** summarizes the clinical features of right ventricular infarction.

Treatment should be directed at rapidly reperfusing the occluded coronary artery (via thrombolytic therapy, or direct PCI, particularly in high-risk patients with severe RV infarction). Patients should also receive volume expansion (i.e., saline infusions) directed toward increasing left heart filling so that cardiac output and arterial BP are restored to levels that sustain systemic perfusion. Inotropic therapy (e.g., dobutamine or dopamine) may also be required when hypoperfusion persists, to stimulate RV contractility.

It is important to keep in mind that nitrates, morphine, and/or diuretics can aggravate the condition by causing preload reduction and hypotension. In fact, if a patient with inferior MI develops profound hypotension upon initiation of these agents (especially nitroglycerin), the practitioner should strongly consider the diagnosis of right ventricular infarction. Patients with RV infarction have a stiff, noncompliant ventricle that depends on high filling pressures; thus, these patients may not tolerate the reduction in preload or venodilation induced by nitrates, morphine, and/or diuretics. Since a high venous filling pressure is required, if the elevated JVP is misconstrued to represent CHF (and diuretics and/or nitrates administered), there may be further compromise in the patient's clinical condition.

FIGURE 11-30

Ventricular Septal Defect vs Papillary Muscle Rupture in Acute Myocardial Infarction

	VENTRICULAR SEPTAL DEFECT	PAPILLARY MUSCLE RUPTURE
Location	Anterior MI (apical portion of septum) or inferior MI (basal portion of septum)	Inferior-posterior MI (posteromedial papillary muscle)
Clinical Presentation	Left and right heart failure–cardiogenic shock	Left heart failure– *Pulmonary edema– Cardiogenic shock–
Murmur		
• Type	Harsh, holosystolic (crescendo-decrescendo)	Early to holosystolic (decrescendo) or absent
• Palpable thrill	Common (>50%)	Rare
• Location	Left sternal border (90%)	Apex (50%)
• Intensity	Loud, does not get louder with respiration	May be faint or silent
2-D Echocardiogram and Color Doppler	Visualize VSD and L→R Shunt	Visualize flail mitral apparatus and systolic regurgitant jet into left atrium
Cardiac catheterization and LV angiography	Oxygen step-up from RA to RV (or pulmonary artery) Visualize septal defect and concomitant coronary artery disease	Large regurgitant "V" waves on PCW tracing Visualize and quantitate severity of mitral regurgitation and concomitant coronary artery disease
Management	Vasodilator Rx, inotropic support, IABP Early ventricular septal defect repair (+/− CABG) for acute VSD	Vasodilator Rx, inotropic support, IABP Early mitral valve repair/replacement (+/− CABG) for severe MR

*Note: A new systolic murmur with the patient lying flat suggests acute VSD, whereas a new systolic murmur with the patient sitting bolt upright and short of breath suggests acute MR due to papillary muscle rupture.

Figure 3-33. ECG tracing showing acute inferior MI with RV infarction in a patient with severe "indigestion", hypotension and elevated neck veins. Note the ST segment elevation in leads II, III, aVF with reciprocal ST segment depression in leads I and aVL. ST segment elevation is present in the right sided chest leads (V4R-V6R) indicative of coexisting RV involvement.

Left Ventricular Aneurysm

Ventricular aneurysms are a common mechanical complication of acute MI, occurring in ~10–15% of patients. Typically, patients have sustained a large anterior wall MI resulting from persistent total occlusion of the proximal portion of a poorly collateralized left anterior descending coronary artery.

Many strokes are caused by cerebral emboli. Clots that form in the heart can break off and travel through the bloodstream, blocking blood supply to the brain. Whenever a patient with a recent anterior MI develops a stroke several days later, always consider the possibility of a cerebral embolus from a mural thrombus located within a ventricular aneurysm. *A ventricular aneurysm may be suspected if a systolic impulse ("bulge") is palpated above and medial to the cardiac apex (the "ectopic" area) and persistent ST segment elevation on the ECG,* (**Figure 3-44**), *along with distortion of the left heart border on the CXR* (**Figure 4-5**), *is present.* An echo can confirm the diagnosis, as can radionuclide imaging and cardiac catheterization with left ventriculography. Keep in mind that ventricular aneurysms rarely rupture, but that intractable CHF and ventricular arrhythmias may also occur. Surgical resection may be indicated, perhaps with CABG and/or electrophysiologic mapping, in patients with refractory CHF, life-threatening ventricular arrhythmias, or recurrent systemic embolization despite adequate anticoagulation therapy.

A neurologic deficit occurring at the time of onset of chest pain is a clue to aortic dissection until proven otherwise. To confirm your clinical suspicion, search for other clues to dissection, e.g., unequal blood pressure and/or pulses in the extremities, a new diastolic murmur of aortic regurgitation (louder along the right sternal border than the left), dilated aortic root on chest x-ray.

LV Free Wall Rupture and Pseudoaneurysm

Rupture of the LV free wall is a life-threatening complication of acute MI, accounting for ~15% of deaths and occurring about 10 times more often than septal or papillary muscle rupture. This dread complication is most likely to occur in older female patients days after a first anterior Q-wave MI. The incidence of rupture appears to be increased in patients with pre-existing or persistent hypertension, and in those receiving antiinflammatory drugs, e.g., steroids, NSAIDs (which may impair infarct healing) or in those who receive thrombolytic therapy many hours after the onset of chest pain. In the majority, acute rupture is catastrophic, leading to the sudden loss of BP despite continued electrical activity on the ECG (so-called pulseless electrical activity or EM dissociation). Although death usually ensues rapidly within minutes, salvage is possible with prompt resuscitation, immediate pericardiocentesis for cardiac tamponade, and surgical repair of the defect.

Clinical clues to subacute rupture include persistent or recurrent chest pain, repetitive nausea and vomiting, restlessness and agitation followed by abrupt dyspnea, hypotension, neck vein distension and pericardial tamponade. A rare patient may develop a slow leak of blood into the pericardial space, producing a chamber or a false sac referred to as a *pseudoaneurysm*. The resulting hematoma is contained within fibrous pericardial adhesions or organized fibrotic clot and is connected to the LV through a narrow neck. Clinical examination may reveal a low pitched rumbling systolic and diastolic, to and fro type murmur in and out of the narrow neck. Two-dimensional Doppler-echo and TEE may help confirm the diagnosis. Unlike true LV aneurysms, thin-walled pseudoaneurysms are devoid of myocardial tissue and have a high risk of rupture and should be repaired surgically.

Pericarditis

Pericarditis is a common complication of acute ST segment elevation MI. The patient may present with sharp chest pain, aggravated by deep inspiration and lying supine, relieved when sitting upright and leaning forward. The pain typically radiates to the left shoulder and trapezius ridge. *The appearance of concave ST segment elevation (particularly in leads expected to reveal "reciprocal" ST segment depression) along with PR segment depression in a patient with acute MI are clues to superimposed pericarditis.* The correct identification of pericarditis as the cause of recurrent chest pain is important, since treatment with aspirin is indicated. Failure to recognize pericarditis may lead to the erroneous diagnosis of recurrent ischemic chest pain with resultant inappropriate use of anticoagulants, nitrates, beta blockers or coronary angiography. Anticoagulation therapy potentially could cause tamponade in the presence of pericarditis and therefore should not be used unless there is a compelling indication. Often, no treatment is required, but aspirin will usually relieve the pain. Nonsteroidal antiinflammatory agents and steroids are generally avoided since they may inhibit healing of the infarct.

Dressler's (post-MI) syndrome is an immunologic phenomenon characterized by pericardial pain, generalized malaise, fever, elevated white blood cell count and erythrocyte sedimentation rate, and pericardial effusion. It occurs several weeks to months after MI. As in acute pericarditis, aspirin should be given as primary therapy, while steroids and nonsteroidal antiinflammatory agents should be avoided if possible until at least one month has elapsed since MI.

Secondary Prevention: Pharmacologic Therapy, Risk Factor Modification, and Cardiac Rehabilitation

The goals of therapy for patients with acute MI are to limit infarct size, increase myocardial oxygen supply, decrease myocardial oxygen demand, promote electrical stability, and prevent or manage mechanical complications. Early recognition and appropriate treatment of these electrical and mechanical complications are essential to reduce morbidity and mortality.

In general, the foundation of care in acute coronary syndromes has undergone remarkable evolution over the past several years. Recent data from numerous well-designed clinical trials have shed considerable light on the optimal therapeutic approach (**Figure 11-31**). An overall summary of beneficial and non-beneficial measures in the acute and long-term treatment of MI is presented in **Figure 11-32**. In addition to aggressive reperfusion strategies (e.g., thrombolytic agents, "direct" PCI), aimed at rapid and complete restoration of coronary blood flow through the infarct-related artery, adjunctive pharmacologic therapies have been shown to improve survival and reduce the incidence of re-infarction. These adjunctive therapies include beta blockers, aspirin, P2Y12 inhibitors, statins, heparin, warfarin, ACE inhibitors/ARBs, and aldosterone blockers, particularly in patients with diminished LV function (ejection fraction <40%).

The ischemic and thrombotic benefit but increased bleeding risk of ticagrelor and prasugrel over clopidogrel (particularly the latter in patients who have a prior stroke or TIA, are >75 years of age, or weigh <60 kg), the potentially harmful effects of the short-acting dihydropyridine calcium channel blockers (e.g., nifedipine), the limited role of the rate-slowing non-dihydropyridine calcium channel blockers (e.g., diltiazem, verapamil) in the setting of non ST elevation MI and intact LV function, the lack of mortality benefit of routine magnesium in a large clinical "megatrial", the lack of benefit of routine late PCI of an occluded infarct-related artery in stable patients days to weeks after MI and the trend

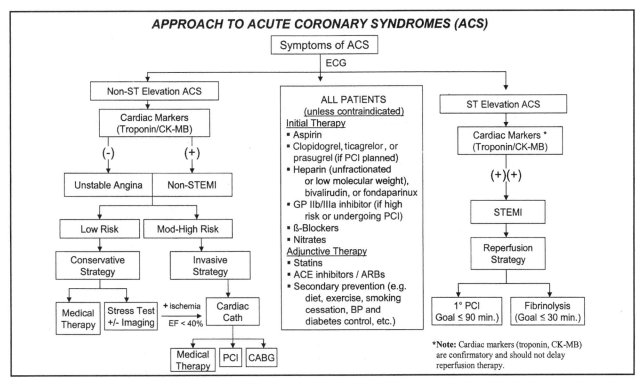

APPROACH TO ACUTE CORONARY SYNDROMES (ACS)

Symptoms of ACS
ECG

Non-ST Elevation ACS
Cardiac Markers (Troponin/CK-MB)
(−) (+)
Unstable Angina | Non-STEMI
Low Risk | Mod-High Risk
Conservative Strategy | Invasive Strategy
Medical Therapy | Stress Test +/− Imaging | + ischemia / EF < 40% | Cardiac Cath
Medical Therapy | PCI | CABG

ALL PATIENTS (unless contraindicated)
Initial Therapy
- Aspirin
- Clopidogrel, ticagrelor, or prasugrel (if PCI planned)
- Heparin (unfractionated or low molecular weight), bivalirudin, or fondaparinux
- GP IIb/IIIa inhibitor (if high risk or undergoing PCI)
- ß-Blockers
- Nitrates
Adjunctive Therapy
- Statins
- ACE inhibitors / ARBs
- Secondary prevention (e.g. diet, exercise, smoking cessation, BP and diabetes control, etc.)

ST Elevation ACS
Cardiac Markers * (Troponin/CK-MB)
(+)(+)
STEMI
Reperfusion Strategy
1° PCI (Goal ≤ 90 min.) | Fibrinolysis (Goal ≤ 30 min.)

*Note: Cardiac markers (troponin, CK-MB) are confirmatory and should not delay reperfusion therapy.

Note: In non-ST elevation ACS (unstable angina, non- STEMI) an early invasive strategy (cath and possible revascularization) is advised in high risk patients. Primary PCI is preferred over fibrinolysis is STEMI patients if it is available within 90 minutes (120 minutes if transferring to a PCI-capable hospital) Unless contraindicated, the more potent P2Y12 inhibitors ticagrelor and prasugrel (at the time of PCI) are preferred over clopidogrel in ACS, except in STEMI patients undergoing fibrinolysis, or in those at high risk of bleeding.

Figure 11-31

toward a higher incidence of cardiovascular events within the first year of initiation of hormone (estrogen/progesterone) replacement therapy in older postmenopausal women, the potentially detrimental effects of routine prophylactic lidocaine, the "proarrhythmic" effects of empiric class I antiarrhythmic agents, and the survival advantage of ICD therapy in patients 40 days or more post-MI who have an LV ejection fraction of 30% or less, have also been noted.

In more recent times, a new wave of clot-specific thrombolytics (e.g., alteplase [t-PA], reteplase [r-PA], tenecteplase [TNK-tPA]), antithrombotics (e.g., UFH, enoxaparin, fondaparinux, bivalirudin), and antiplatelet agents (e.g., GP IIb/IIIa blockers, clopidogrel, prasugrel, ticagrelor, vorapaxar) have come into the limelight. The appropriate choices of treatment is dictated the type, location and severity of MI, the extent of accompanying ischemia, the degree of LV dysfunction, and the presence of supraventricular and ventricular arrhythmias and conduction disturbances, mural thrombus formation, and other associated complications.

In this era of fascination with new technologies and innovative treatment strategies, the practitioner must not neglect the importance of secondary prevention measures including risk factor modification. These risk factor modifications include smoking cessation, proper diet, lipid-lowering therapy, hypertension and diabetes control, weight reduction (if appro-

priate), stress management techniques, supervised exercise, and cardiac rehabilitation. These measures aim to halt the progression or enhance the regression of atherosclerotic cardiovascular disease, as part of the contemporary management scheme. In terms of cholesterol lowering, patients should be treated with high dose statins as tolerated. In addition to lowering LDL-cholesterol, early administration of high dose HMG CoA reductase inhibitors ("statins") have been shown to be beneficial in reducing vascular inflammation, improving endothelial function, stabilizing impending plaque rupture, and reducing CAD events and mortality (so-called "pleiotropic effects"). Serum markers of inflammation e.g., high sensitivity C-reactive protein (CRP) levels may help to identify those patients at risk who will benefit most from statin therapy (<1 mg/L = low risk, 1–3 mg/L = intermediate risk, >3 mg/L = high risk). Although recent studies suggest an association between improved clinical outcomes and lower CRP levels after statin treatment, there is no definitive evidence that lower CRP levels *per se* prevent vascular events. While optimal risk reduction strategies are of paramount importance, it must be realized that an optimistic attitude on the part of the practitioner and the entire health-care team from the outset, along with continued reassurance as to the patient's ultimate recovery and return to normal activities, are essential requisites to an improved quality of life and overall clinical outcome.

FIGURE 11-32

Modern Treatment of Acute Myocardial Infarction

	ACUTE	LONG-TERM
Significant benefit	• Reperfusion therapy (if ST elevation MI) —Thrombolytic agents (e.g., TPA, rPA, TNK-TPA, SK) —Primary PCI, "rescue" PCI (if thrombolysis fails), or routine early PCI (after successful fibrinolysis) in PCI-capable centers • Aspirin (chewed, oral) and/or clopidogrel, ticagrelor, or prasugrel (with PCI). • GP IIb/IIIa antagonists-if non STEMI or in high risk patients (e.g., large thrombus burden) undergoing PCI • Heparin —IV unfractionated with PCI or fibrin selective thrombolytic agents (e.g., TPA, rPA, TNK-TPA) to maintain coronary patency • IV unfractionated or Sub Q low molecular weight heparin (e.g., enoxaparin [Lovenox], dalteparin [Fragmin]), in anterior MI to reduce risk of mural thrombus and systemic embolization. Recent trials support use of enoxaparin or fondaparinux in the setting of thrombolysis. —Low dose Sub Q to prevent deep venous thrombosis and pulmonary embolism (especially if elderly, obesity, congestive heart failure or prolonged immobilization) • Beta blockers (IV, oral), if no contraindication —with or without thrombolysis • ACE inhibitors (oral) —especially large anterior MI without hypotension • Acute nitrates —If ischemic chest pain, LV dysfunction, or hypertension is present • IABP —To enhance thrombolytic efficacy, reduce reocclusion after PCI, or as "bridge" to surgery • Emergency CABG —If failed reperfusion (PCI), left main or severe 3 vessel CAD.	• Aspirin and/or clopidogrel, prasugrel, or ticagrelor, if aspirin intolerant. Both for non STEMI/STEMI and PCI. • Beta blockers —especially high-risk patient with large or anterior MI and recurrent ischemia, LV dysfunction or complex ventricular ectopy • ACE inhibitors (or ARBs or ARNI) —if asymptomatic patient with LV ejection fraction $< 40\%$ or symptomatic heart failure • Risk factor modification —Smoking cessation; BP, lipid, and glucose control; treatment of obesity; and moderate physical activity —HMG CoA reductase inhibitors ("statins") to reduce LDL cholesterol $> 50\%$, if tolerated • Warfarin —Following IV heparin if large anterior MI, apical dyskinesis, LV thrombus or systemic embolization • Rate-limiting calcium channel blockers (diltiazem, verapamil) —Following non STEMI with preserved LV function • Aldosterone blocker (eplerenone) —in patients with LV systolic dysfunction and CHF receiving standard therapy (e.g., beta blockers and ACE inhibitors/ARBs) • Implantable cardioverter-defibrillator in patients with VT/VF or EF $\leq 30\%$ at least 40 days post-MI
Doubtful efficacy or Potentially harmful	• Calcium channel blockers —Especially immediate-release dihydropyridines • Routine prophylactic lidocaine (decreases risk of primary VF but also increases risk of fatal asystolic events) is no longer recommended —Reserved for sustained/ symptomatic ventricular tachycardia, ventricular fibrillation, or "complex" (frequent, multifocal) PVCs • Nitrates for RV MI (preload dependent) • Magnesium sulfate —Not recommended routinely, however, may be beneficial for post-infarction ventricular arrhythmias and torsades de pointes, especially if hypomagnesemia is present. • Beta blockers in cocaine-induced MI (may potentiate coronary spasm) • Fibrinolytics in unstable angina/non STEMI	• Class I antiarrhythmic agents (proarrhythmic effect-torsades de pointes) • Calcium channel blockers —If severe LV dysfunction or heart failure is present • Hormone therapy during first year in older postmenopausal women • Nitrates within 24–48 hours of sildenafil (Viagra), vardenafil (Levitra), or tadalafil (Cialis). • Late PCI of an occluded infarct-related artery in stable patients days to weeks after MI • NSAIDs, nonselective or COX-2 selective

CHAPTER 12.   APPROACH TO THE PATIENT WITH HEART FAILURE

Heart failure is a complex clinical syndrome resulting from a structural or functional abnormality that impairs the ability of the ventricles to eject or fill with blood. It is commonly termed "congestive" heart failure (CHF), since signs and symptoms of increased pulmonary and/or systemic venous pressure are often prominent. Although CHF is common, it is not a specific diagnosis in and of itself, but rather is the result of some underlying cardiac or occasionally noncardiac disorder. This chapter will review the practical clinical approach to the evelation and treatment of the patient who presents with *chronic* or *acute* heart failure with LV *systolic* (reduced EF) or *diastolic* (preserved EF) *dysfunction*.

ETIOLOGY AND PATHOPHYSIOLOGY

Heart failure is a clinical condition (not a disease) in which the output of blood from the heart is insufficient to meet the metabolic needs of the body. Patients with this clinical syndrome may be asymptomatic or present with dyspnea (with exertion and at rest), fatigue, and fluid retention, with pulmonary and systemic venous congestion.

In general, CHF can be divided into two main categories: *systolic dysfunction* (due to reduced LV contractility), which is most common, and *diastolic dysfunction* (due to impaired LV relaxation and filling).

Systolic dysfunction is characterized by:

- LV dilatation
- Reduced LV contractility (either generalized or localized depending on the etiology)
- Diminished *ejection fraction* (<40%) (i.e., that fraction of end-diastolic blood volume ejected from the ventricle during each systolic contraction). In failing hearts, the LV end-diastolic volume (or pressure) may increase as the stroke volume (or cardiac output) decreases.

On the other hand, in *diastolic dysfunction:*

- The cavity size is normal or small
- Contractility is normal or hyperdynamic
- Ejection fraction is normal (≥50%) or near normal
- The LV is usually hypertrophied; however, there is impaired LV relaxation and filling to such an extent that left atrial pressure rises and CHF develops.

Both forms of heart failure can lead to identical degrees of elevation of left atrial pressure, severe pulmonary congestion and even pulmonary edema. In some patients there may be a combination of both systolic and diastolic dysfunction (e.g., CAD, hypertension, aortic valve disease).

Figure 12-1. Ventricular function (Frank-Starling) curves in a normal person and a patient with CHF relating cardiac output (a measure of LV performance) to left ventricular end-diastolic pressure (LVEDP) or volume (preload). In heart failure, the curve is displaced downward, so that at a given LVEDP, the cardiac output is lower than in a normal individual. Diuretics and venodilators (e.g., nitrates) reduce LVEDP (preload), but do not change the position of the curve; the output is still low. Pulmonary congestion improves, but cardiac output may fall. Inotropic therapy and afterload reduction (e.g., vasodilator therapy) displaces the curve upward toward normal so that at any LVEDP, the cardiac output is higher. Radiographically evident pulmonary redistribution and edema correlate with elevated LVEDP as noted.

Figure 12-2. Schematic diagram comparing the echocardiographic features of systolic and diastolic heart failure. In *systolic dysfunction,* LV dimension is increased; LV wall thickness is decreased, normal, or increased; and LV ejection fraction is decreased. Mitral valve regurgitation is common, and pulmonary artery systolic pressure is moderately elevated. In *diastolic dysfunction,* LV dimension is normal or decreased, LV wall thickness is increased, and LV ejection fraction is preserved. Mitral regurgitation is uncommon, and pulmonary artery systolic pressure is mildly elevated.

LEFT VENTRICULAR SYSTOLIC DYSFUNCTION

It is estimated that more than 5 million Americans have CHF, and approximately 500,000 new cases are diagnosed each year. CHF due to LV systolic dysfunction is a common complication of many types of heart disease, e.g.:

- CAD with ischemic LV damage (i.e., acute MI, acute MR/VSD, LV aneurysm, "ischemic cardiomyopathy")
- Chronic systemic arterial hypertension
- Dilated cardiomyopathy
- Valvular heart disease with its pressure (e.g., AS) and/or volume (e.g., MR, AR) overloading of the heart.

In fact, CHF is the most frequently used (and most expensive) cardiovascular hospital diagnosis-related group (DRG) discharge diagnosis in the United States today. CAD is the underlying cause of CHF in ~2/3 of patients with LV systolic dysfunction. The remainder have nonischemic causes e.g., hypertension, valvular heart disease, myocar-

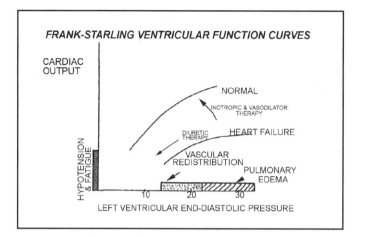

Figure 12-1

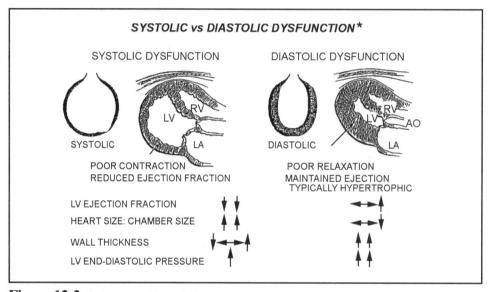

Figure 12-2 (* also termed heart failure with *reduced* EF **[HFrEF]** vs *preserved* EF [HFpEF]).
Note: A new term, **HFmrEF**, has recently been introduced for heart failure with *mid-range* EF (40-49%).

dial toxins (i.e., alcohol or doxorubicin), myocarditis, or no identifiable cause, e.g., idiopathic dilated cardiomyopathy.

The clinical history, physical examination, ECG, CXR, and selected laboratory tests (e.g., two-dimensional Doppler-echo) are essential components of the initial evaluation of the heart failure patient. The "five finger" approach to the clinical evaluation of the patient with heart failure is summarized in **Figures 12-3 and 12-4.** In general, left heart failure can be diagnosed with a high degree of certainty when a patient presents with progressive symptoms of dyspnea, orthopnea, paroxysmal nocturnal dyspnea, dry, non-productive cough (due to pulmonary vascular congestion) along with weakness, fatigue and a decrease in exercise tolerance (due to a low cardiac output). Typically, dyspnea occurs with progressively lesser amounts of exercise and finally develops at rest as CHF

worsens. Patients often unconsciously restrict their activity to avoid this unpleasant sensation, and should, therefore, be questioned closely concerning effort intolerance. While the presence and severity of symptoms can be graded according to NYHA functional class as asymptomatic (**class I**), symptomatic with moderate activity (**class II**), symptomatic with mild activity (**class III**), or symptomatic at rest (**class IV**), patients can also be classified according to the American Heart Association by their stage in the course of their illness, beginning with patients at high risk for CHF (**stage A**), and progressing to those who have asymptomatic LV dysfunction (**stage B**), symptomatic CHF (**stage C**), or advanced, refractory CHF (**stage D**). In severe CHF, patients may spend the entire night sleeping in a chair to breathe more comfortably. Other respiratory symptoms that can accompany CHF include

History	Dyspnea on exertion (or at rest), orthopnea, paroxysmal nocturnal dyspnea, fatigue, cough, weight gain.
Physical examination	Sinus tachycardia, pulsus alternans, elevated JVP, pulmonary rales, wheezes, decreased breath sounds (pleural effusion), cardiomegaly, S4 and S3 gallops, murmurs consistent with regurgitation due to papillary muscle dysfunction and/or other valvular heart disease, hepatomegaly, ascites, peripheral edema.
Electrocardiogram	LA enlargement, LV hypertrophy, LBBB, ST-T changes and/or Q waves (myocardial ischemia/infarction pattern), arrhythmias (e.g., atrial fibrillation, VT), low voltage (infiltrative cardiomyopathy e.g., amyloid, pericardial effusion, hypothyroidism).
Chest X-Ray	Cardiomegaly (in systolic dysfunction, not in diastolic), increased pulmonary vascularity, interstitial edema, alveolar pulmonary edema, pleural effusion
Diagnostic Laboratory Blood tests	Elevated BNP or NT-pro BNP (B-type or brain natriuretic peptide)*; elevated BUN/creatinine (due to renalhypoperfusion); elevated cardiac enzymes e.g., CK-MB, troponin (markers of myocardial necrosis); complete blood count (anemia may aggravate CHF); abnormal thyroid function (thyroid disease may worsen CHF); fasting blood glucose (diabetes mellitus); lipid profile (hyperlipidemia); electrolyte abnormalities (hypokalemia may result from diuretic therapy, hyponatremia is a poor prognostic finding); abnormal liver function tests (due to congestive hepatopathy in patients with right sided CHF).
Echocardiogram, including 2D Doppler and tissue Doppler imaging	Systolic dysfunction: dilated LV, global or regional wall motion abnormalities, reduced EF Diastolic dysfunction: normal LV, LV hypertrophy, dilated LA, normal or near normal EF, abnormal LV filling pattern – transmitral Doppler inflow E/A ratio < 1 (impaired relaxation), 1-2 (pseudonormal), > 2 (restrictive), and transmitral E to mitral annular tissue Doppler é (E/é) ratio > 15 (indicates elevated LA/LV filling pressures).** Signs of mitral and tricuspid regurgitation (due to papillary muscle dysfunction) or other valvular heart disease (e.g., aortic stenosis, aortic regurgitation).
Cardiac Catheterization	Hemodynamic abnormalities, confirm status of LV function, presence and severity of valvular heart disease and/or CAD.

Note: A history of MI, an S3 gallop, Q waves on the ECG and cardiomegaly on the CXR favor systolic dysfunction. Hypertension, an S4 gallop, LV hypertrophy on the ECG and a normal heart size on the CXR favor diastolic dysfunction.

*BNP may be helpful in confirming or excluding the diagnosis of CHF (i.e., BNP <100 pg/ml = CHF unlikely, BNP 100–500 pg/ml = indeterminate ["grey zone"], BNP >500 pg/ml = CHF likely). Similarly, for NT-pro BNP, age-specific cut-offs for the diagnosis of CHF are NT-pro BNP <300 pg/ml = CHF unlikely, and NT-pro BNP >450 pg/ml (age <50 years), NT-pro BNP >900 pg/ml (age 50–75 years), and NT-pro BNP >1800 pg/ml (age >75 years) = CHF likely. However, BNP and NT-pro BNP can be elevated in acute coronary syndromes, pulmonary embolism, renal failure, sepsis, older age, and in women, and can be decreased in obesity and during the first 1–2 hours of flash pulmonary edema (since it takes time for BNP to rise). Of note, BNP and NT-proBNP cannot be used to differentiate between HFrEF and HFpEF. BNP and NT-pro BNP, therefore, are not stand-alone tests and should be used as an adjunct to, and not a substitute for, a careful clinical evaluation.

**The transmitral Doppler E wave reflects the rate of blood flow from the LA into the LV. The mitral annular tissue Doppler é wave reflects how rapid the LV relaxes. The E/é ratio increases if the LA pressure "pushing" blood into the LV is relatively greater than the rate of relaxation.

wheezing ("*cardiac asthma*") and Cheyne-Stokes respiration (periods of hyperpnea alternating with apnea), especially in patients with cerebral atherosclerosis and low cardiac output. On physical examination, the patient with CHF may have an increased respiratory rate and tachycardia. The practitioner should gently palpate the radial artery and feel for alternating strong and weak arterial pulse pressures (so-called pulsus alternans), an immediate and often subtle clue to the presence of LV systolic dysfunction. Alternation of heart sounds (particu-

larly S2) and heart murmurs, along with a ventricular (S3) diastolic gallop at the cardiac apex, will also be detected if specifically searched for (**Figures 12-4 and 12-5**).

Figure 12-5. Left. A patient with dilated cardiomyopathy and congestive heart failure. Note patient is short of breath, sitting upright with 2–3 pillow orthopnea and has distended neck veins, a protuberant abdomen (ascites), and pitting peripheral edema. The clinical appearance may resemble that of a patient with constrictive pericarditis. **Right. (*Insert*)**

FIGURE 12-4

Clinical Signs of Left vs. Right Heart Failure

Clue	Clinical Significance
Symptoms	
Dyspnea on exertion or at rest, orthopnea	
Paroxysmal nocturnal dyspnea, dry cough	
Physical Findings	
Tachypnea, tachycardia, diaphoresis	
Pulmonary rales (crackles), wheezes, decreased breath sounds, dullness to percussion (pulmonary venous congestion and pleural effusion)	Left Heart Failure and Pulmonary Venous Hypertension
Pulsus alternans, heart sound and murmur alternans ⎫	
Left-sided S3 gallop ⎬ LV systolic	
Paradoxical splitting of S2 ⎬ dysfunction	
Displaced LV apical impulse ⎬	
MR murmur ⎭	
Loud P2 (due to pulmonary hypertension)	
S4 gallop ⎫ LV diastolic	
Sustained LV apical impulse ⎬ dysfunction	
Symptoms	
Ankle swelling, weight gain	
Abdominal distention, pain and nausea (due to hepatic enlargement).	
Physical Findings	
Elevated JVP with prominent V-waves	Right Heart Failure and Systemic Venous Congestion
Positive hepatojugular reflux	
Right-sided S3 gallop	
Palpable RV heave, TR murmur	
Peripheral (ankle/sacral) edema	
Ascites	
Congestive hepatomegaly	
Symptoms	
Fatigue	
Decreased exercise tolerance	
Altered mental status	
Physical Findings	Low Cardiac Output
Hypotension	
Tachycardia (due to decreased stroke volume)	
Decreased pulse pressure	
Cold blue extremities	
Muscle wasting, cachexia	

Note pulsus alternans (alternating strong and weak arterial pulse) which can often be detected by gentle palpation of the radial arterial pulse. It represents an important sign of LV systolic dysfunction. Alternation in intensity of heart sounds and murmurs, along with an S3 gallop, is frequently present.

Moist crackles (rales), a classic auscultatory sign of left heart failure (resulting from elevated pulmonary ve-nous and capillary pressure along with transudation of fluid into the alveolar spaces) generally begins at the lung bases and progresses up both lung fields in proportion to the severity of pulmonary congestion. In patients with chronic CHF, rales may be absent, even when pulmonary capillary wedge pressure is markedly elevated (due to increased lymphatic drainage with chronic CHF).

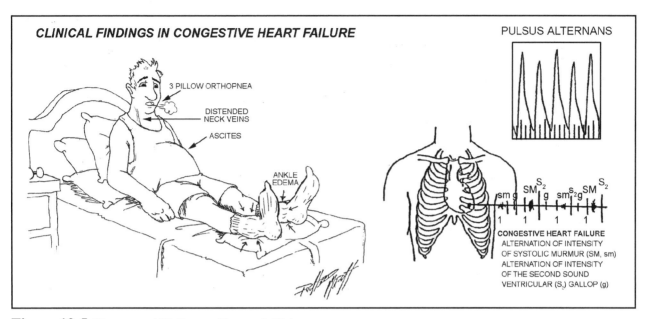

Figure 12-5 (Courtesy of W. Proctor Harvey, M.D.)

DILATED CARDIOMYOPATHY (A FORM OF SYSTOLIC DYSFUNCTION)

Cardiomyopathies are defined as diseases of the myocardium associated with mechanical and/or electrical dysfunction. Cardiomyopathies either are confined to the heart (primary) or are part of generalized systemic disorders (secondary). The traditional classification of cardiomyopathies divides them into three main groups:

1. *Dilated cardiomyopathy* (systolic dysfunction*)*
2. *Hypertrophic cardiomyopathy* (diastolic dysfunction)
3. *Restrictive (or obliterative) cardiomyopathy* (diastolic dysfunction) (e.g., amyloidosis, sarcoidosis, hemochromatosis, scleroderma)

Each cardiomyopathy can be further classified using a 5 letter code: M (morphofunctional phenotype), O (organ involvement), G (genetic inheritance pattern), E (etiology), and S (stage of CHF) — so-called *MOGES classification*.

Figure 12-6. The morphologic types of cardiomyopathy. In the normal heart, the LV chamber is cone shaped, tapering at the apex. In dilated cardiomyopathy, the LV chamber becomes dilated with only mild hypertrophy, and nearly spherical in diastole. In hypertrophic cardiomyopathy, the LV cavity is small in diastole, demonstrates significant LV hypertrophy, often asymmetrically involving the septum, and becomes slit shaped and partly obliterated in systole. In restrictive cardiomyopathy, due to infiltration or fibrosis of the myocardium, the LV cavity is smaller than normal.

Dilated cardiomyopathy, the most common form of cardiomyopathy, is characterized by LV or biventricular dilatation, impaired contractility, and systolic dysfunction. Symptoms and signs of CHF are common in patients with dilated cardiomyopathy. (**Figure 12-7**) While some cases have specific known causes, many are idiopathic (of unknown cause). Specific secondary causes should be strongly entertained: in the clinical setting of a previous "flu-like" illness or other viral infection (e.g., parvo B19, human herpes 6, coxsackie, echo, human immunodeficiency virus [HIV]), CAD, heavy alcohol consumption, illicit drug use (e.g., cocaine), chemotherapy (e.g., doxorubicin [Adriamycin]), connective tissue diseases (e.g., periarteritis, systemic lupus erythematosus), the pregnant or postpartum state, thyroid disease (either hypo- or hyperthyroidism), sleep apnea, emotional or physical stress, or chronic persistent tachycardia (usually supraventricular). At present, most cases of cardiomyopathy are considered idiopathic, and presumed to be either familial (genetic) or an autoimmune response to a previous insult to the myocardium, most commonly (but not necessarily) viral. A relatively uncommon, but frequently overlooked cause of "idiopathic" dilated cardiomyopathy is LV hypertrabeculation/noncompaction (also called "spongy myocardium"), thought to be either a genetic (embryologic defect) or an acquired morphologic trait. It is important to exclude secondary causes, however, since certain conditions (e.g., CAD, alcohol, sleep apnea, thyroid disease, tachycardia or stress) may be "curable" or at least partially reversible.

Keep in mind that excessive alcohol consumption may exacerbate cardiomyopathy, and that alcoholic cardiomyopathy can result from what would be considered

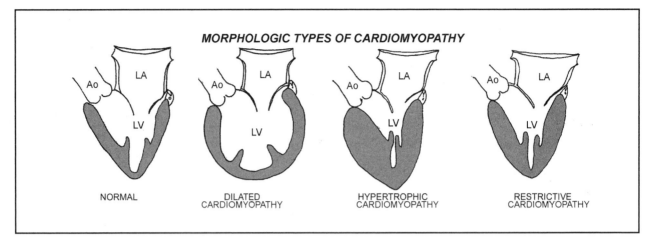

MORPHOLOGIC TYPES OF CARDIOMYOPATHY

NORMAL | DILATED CARDIOMYOPATHY | HYPERTROPHIC CARDIOMYOPATHY | RESTRICTIVE CARDIOMYOPATHY

Figure 12-6

in some circles to be "socially acceptable" chronic levels of drinking. There is ~35% chance that a cardiomyopathy due to heavy alcohol intake will resolve if the patient can abstain from drinking. The prognosis of peripartum cardiomyopathy is better than in other idiopathic dilated cardiomyopathies. Patients who show a significant reduction in heart size after 6 months of treatment (50%) have a good chance of total recovery. Women who do not recover completely should be advised against additional pregnancies, since post-partum cardiomyopathy may recur with subsequent pregnancies. The prognosis of stress-induced (tako-tsubo) cardiomyopathy, a reversible cardiomyopathy that mimics acute MI in the absence of CAD, seen primarily in postmenopausal women, is generally favorable. Complete resolution of the balloon-like LV apical wall motion abnormalities typically occurs within 1–4 weeks. In patients with LV systolic dysfunction due to severe CAD (so-called "ischemic cardiomyopathy"), CABG surgery may improve LV function if hypokinesis is due to substantial hibernating myocardium (where damage is potentially reversible). If a patient is receiving chemotherapy, e.g., doxorubicin (Adriamycin), look for signs of systolic LV dysfunction (e.g., pulsus alternans, heart sound and/or murmur alternans, S3 gallop) due to a dilated cardiomyopathy as a result of the

---

FIGURE 12-7

Clinical Approach to Dilated Cardiomyopathy

Pathophysiology	Dilated LV with systolic dysfunction
History	Fatigue, weakness, dyspnea, orthopnea, paroxysmal nocturnal dyspnea, chest pain on exertion (~10% of cases, even without CAD), palpitations, embolic episodes
Physical Examination	Pulmonary rales, S3 and S4 gallops, pulsus alternans, functional MR and TR murmurs, diffuse laterally displaced LV impulse. If RV failure present, elevated JVP, hepatomegaly, peripheral edema.
Electrocardiogram	Non specific ST-T abnormalities, sinus tachycardia, Q waves, LBBB, low voltage, atrial fibrillation, ventricular arrhythmias.
Chest X-Ray	Cardiomegaly, pulmonary vascular congestion.
Laboratory	
Echocardiogram	Dilated, poorly contractile LV (↓ ejection fraction) +/− mural thrombus.
Cardiac Catheterization	Diffusely dilated hypokinetic LV, low ejection fraction, +/− mitral regurgitation, low cardiac output
Treatment	Standard therapy for CHF (ACE inhibitor/ARB [or ARNI], β-blocker [if not in decompensated CHF], diuretic, digoxin, aldosterone antagonist), +/- ivabradine (if sinus rhythm ≥ 70 beats / min), +/− anticoagulation (if atrial fibrillation, LV thrombus, low EF), +/- vasopressin antagonist (if severe refractory hyponatremia), +/− amiodarone/ICD (for symptomatic/recurrent VT/VF and/or if poor LV function). If necessary, tailored hemodynamic therapy (+/− implantable PA pressure monitoring device); cardiac resynchronization therapy (biventricular pacing), if refractory symptoms, LBBB and a widened QRS complex (≥ 150 msec); left ventricular assist device (LVAD); cardiac transplantation.

drug. Standard medical therapy for dilated cardiomyopathy includes removal of any potential myocardial toxin, along with treatment of systolic LV dysfunction, e.g., ACE inhibitor or ARB, beta blocker, diuretic (including aldosterone antagonist), digoxin, other vasodilators, e.g., nitrates, hydralazine, and anticoagulants as indicated.

The clinical course of dilated cardiomyopathy is often insidious, without any history of a precipitating factor (**Figure 12-8**). Unrecognized mild myocardial disease may exist for years and produce no noticeable symptoms. Sudden onset of palpitations and syncope (due to ventricular arrhythmias or heart block), embolic phenomenon, e.g., stroke (from a left atrial or ventricular thrombus), and even sudden death may be the first clue. An alternate presentation is the patient who denies symptoms but has been identified on CXR (or echo) to have an unexplained enlarged (or poorly functioning, i.e. low ejection fraction) heart. Sometimes an abnormal ECG, e.g., LV hypertrophy, LBBB, pseudo-infarction Q waves due to extensive fibrosis, ST-T abnormalities, PACs, PVCs, and VT, are the first evidence of the disease in an asymptomatic patient. In Chagas disease, caused by the protozoan Trypanosoma cruzi, RBBB may be a helpful clue.

However, the diagnosis of dilated cardiomyopathy usually is made when patients seek medical attention when progression of the disease finally produces symptoms due to CHF, namely, fatigue (caused by a low cardiac output), dyspnea and weight gain (often with venous and hepatic congestion). At this stage, the physical examination may reveal pulsus alternans and an S_3 gallop reflective of significant LV systolic dysfunction. Palpitations due to sinus tachycardia and arrhythmias (particularly PVCs, VT, and atrial fibrillation) are common, and the apical impulse is diffuse, displaced and may also alternate in intensity (*precordial alternans*). The chest x-ray may demonstrate cardiomegaly along with pulmonary congestion, pulmonary venous hypertension, and pleural effusion (right > left). (**Figures 4-6B and 4-10**). However, these findings are present in only 50% of patients with increased pulmonary capillary wedge pressure (PCWP). Thus, the absence of radiographic findings does not exclude pulmonary venous hypertension.

Certain blood chemistries may be altered in the patient with dilated cardiomyopathy and left heart failure. A complete blood count may indicate that anemia is an aggravating factor. The serum sodium concentration may be low (due to increased water retention), the BUN may be disproportionately increased relative to the serum creatinine (due to reduced renal perfusion), and liver enzyme levels may be elevated (due to hepatic congestion). An elevated BNP (B-type or brain natriuretic peptide) level has recently been shown to be helpful in identifying CHF as the cause of acute dyspnea. BNP levels track closely with pulmonary capillary wedge pressure, rising and falling quickly as the severity of CHF changes. Other biomarkers, e.g., cardiac troponin, may be elevated in CHF, even in the absence of ACS, and is associated with a higher risk of adverse outcomes.

Because both the CXR and 12 lead ECG are insensitive and nonspecific, neither should be used alone to determine the basis for the specific cardiac abnormality responsible for the development of CHF. Furthermore, although the history and physical examination may provide important clues, identification of the structural abnormality leading to CHF generally requires noninvasive or invasive imaging of the cardiac structures. *Echo-Doppler is the single most useful diagnostic test in the evaluation of patients with dilated cardiomyopathy and CHF.* (**Figure 5-4D**). It not only allows the clinician to estimate the LV ejection fraction, but also helps identify dilated LV dimensions, along with global hypokinesis and, at times, LV thrombi. However, an echo study does not make the diagnosis of CHF, despite the fact that LV dysfunction is

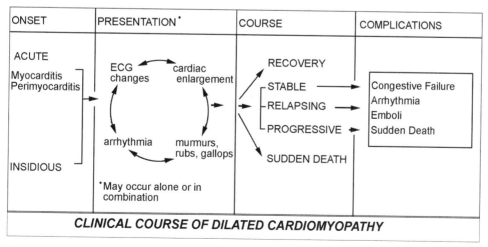

CLINICAL COURSE OF DILATED CARDIOMYOPATHY

Figure 12-8

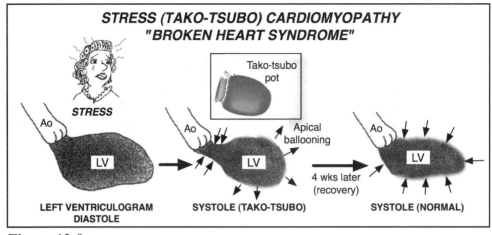

**STRESS (TAKO-TSUBO) CARDIOMYOPATHY
"BROKEN HEART SYNDROME"**

Figure 12-9

observed. Clinical signs and symptoms must be present to make the clinical diagnosis of CHF.

Although segmental wall motion abnormalities usually suggest underlying CAD, they may be present in patients with dilated cardiomyopathy and do not necessarily imply the presence of coronary atherosclerosis. Transient wall motion abnormalities, in the absence of CAD, also occur in stress (tako-tsubo) cardiomyopathy and generally involve the apical and/or mid ventricular segments **(Figure 12-9)**.

Figure 12-9. Postmenopausal woman under extreme emotional stress with stress (tako-tsubo) cardiomyopathy or "broken heart syndrome". Note left ventriculogram showing LV apical ballooning during systole that resembles the shape of the Japanese fisherman's octopus pot—the "tako-tsubo" (insert) which resolves within 4 weeks. Coronary angiography typically shows no obstructive CAD.

Doppler-echo may be used to estimate the severity of associated functional MR and TR (commonly present in severe biventricular failure) and to estimate pulmonary artery systolic pressure. Radionuclide ventriculography (MUGA scan), and cardiac MRI can also provide reproducible assessment of ejection fraction, end-systolic and end-diastolic volume. Biventricular dilatation with a global decrease in contractility is typical in dilated cardiomyopathy. Exercise or pharmacologic stress myocardial perfusion imaging may suggest the possibility of underlying CAD. Cardiac catheterization helps to confirm the diagnosis (i.e., elevated filling pressures, decreased cardiac output and ejection fraction) and identifies the presence or absence of coexistent CAD, especially in patients with chest pain, CAD risk factors, and/or segmental wall motion abnormalities on noninvasive imaging.

The clinical course of the patient with CHF usually is characterized by periods of relatively stable symptoms interrupted by exacerbations that require changes in medication and/or hospitalization. In some of these patients, the clinical features of right heart failure and systemic venous congestion may predominate. These clinical features include neck vein distention, right-sided gallop sounds, systolic murmur and jugular venous V waves ("no-no" sign) of TR, hepatomegaly, increased abdominal girth (ascites), weight gain and dependent edema. (**Figure 12-6**). Tender hepatomegaly (due to increased venous pressure transmitted via the hepatic veins) and a pulsatile liver (due to TR) is a quite specific and useful sign. A small, weak arterial pulse, peripheral cyanosis and cool extremities are findings that suggest a low cardiac output and peripheral vasoconstriction. Patients with chronic severe heart failure sometimes develop anorexia and marked muscle wasting ("*cardiac cachexia*").

It is a mistake to consider pulmonary rales (or peripheral edema, for that matter) the hallmark of congestive heart failure. There is truth to the saying that "most patients with rales don't have heart failure, and most of those with heart failure don't have rales". Never assume that the lack of rales (or radiographic evidence of edema) means that left-sided CHF is not present. In order for heart failure to produce pulmonary rales, it is usually very severe and there must be a markedly elevated pulmonary venous pressure to cause intra-alveolar edema. It is far more common for rales to be due to chronic lung disease or atelectasis, whereby pulmonary secretions partially obstruct the airways. This makes rales a rather nonspecific and insensitive sign of CHF. Likewise, peripheral edema is commonly caused by local venous, hepatic, or renal disease, or the side effect of medication (e.g., calcium channel blockers).

In assessing a patient with the above clinical findings, the astute practitioner must be certain that the patient is not presenting with a dilated cardiomyopathy "look-alike". A number of other cardiac diseases may present with signs and symptoms that can mimic the disease. Those look-alike diseases include severe end-stage valvular heart disease, where the typical findings are masked (i.e., the respective murmurs are faint or even absent due to very low cardiac output and blood flow through the affected valves), or constrictive pericarditis.. The diagnosis of dilated cardiomyopathy can be confirmed by echo (or radionuclide ventriculography), which may reveal cardiomegaly and decreased LV function (low EF). It should be noted that approximately 10% of patients with dilated cardiomyopathy may have chest pain.

Patients with newly diagnosed CHF with LV systolic dysfunction should undergo an ischemic workup. When it is not possible to distinguish between CAD (ischemic cardiomyopathy) and idiopathic dilated cardiomyopathy on clinical grounds, coronary angiography should be performed to confirm the presence or absence of severe CAD, especially in patients who are candidates for intervention. Although cardiac catheterization remains the "gold standard" for the diagnosis for CAD, myocardial perfusion imaging (or coronary CT angiography) may be considered initially in patients with a low-to-intermediate pretest probability of ischemia. Endomyocardial biopsy may be useful to "rule-out" giant cell myocarditis, especially in patients with acute, rapidly progressive CHF, in whom the diagnosis is suspected. It is often essential that the diagnosis be established early, so that immunosuppressant therapy can begin as soon as possible, since the more severe the involvement the less the chance of survival. Spontaneous improvement with a resolution of symptoms and recovery of cardiac function may occur in up to 25% of patients with recent onset dilated cardiomyopathy. Approximately 50% of patients with acute (viral) myocarditis recover cardiac function within 6-12 months. Peripartum cardiomyopathies show significant improvement within 6 months in ~50% of cases, alcoholic cardiomyopathy is largely reversible with complete abstinence from drinking, and stress-induced cardiomyopathy usually resolves within 1–4 weeks.

Treatment of dilated cardiomyopathy consists of the standard approach to LV systolic dysfunction and includes *ACE inhibitors/ARBs or ARNI (see below), beta blockers, diuretics, digoxin,* and *aldosterone antagonists. Long term anticoagulation* with warfarin is advisable (if no contraindications exists) for patients with severe LV dysfunction, established or paroxysmal atrial fibrillation, a history of previous thromboembolism, or echo evidence of intracardiac thrombi, because of the high incidence of systemic and pulmonary embolization. Implantation of a cardioverter defibrillator has been shown to be more efficacious than antiarrhythmic drug therapy in patients with mild to moderate (NYHA class II-III) CHF and poor LV function (EF ≤35%), and those with sustained VT or sudden cardiac death (due to the proarrhythmic drug effects of antiarrhythmic drug therapy, i.e., potential to aggravate arrhythmias). Some patients with severe underlying CAD may have a significant amount of viable (stunned or hibernating) myocardium and may benefit from coronary artery bypass graft (CABG) surgery. Certain patients with advanced cardiomyopathy, particularily those with LBBB and a wide QRS complex ≥ 150 msec (which reflects LV dyssynchrony) may benefit from cardiac resynchronization therapy with biventricular pacing, which uses 3 leads: one lead in the right atrium, one in the right ventricle, and a third through the coronary sinus into a cardiac vein on the lateral wall of the left ventricle. Beneficial effects include reverse remodeling (decreased heart size and ventricular volumes, improved ejection fraction, and decreased mitral regurgitation). Other patients with end-stage disease and symptoms refractory to medical therapy may require cardiac transplantation. Implantable LV assist devices appear to have a role as a bridge to transplantation.

Dietary restriction of sodium is one of the most important aspects of treatment of a patient with congestive heart failure. It is also one of the most neglected. Many patients are told to "cut down" on salt, but no specific dietary education and counseling is provided. In fact, many patients say they're on a sodium-restricted diet but upon further questioning about where and what they ate, quickly identify no significant restriction at all. Beware of hidden sodium (e.g., in packaged, convenience, "fast", and canned foods). Advise your patients to be "heart-smart" and avoid eating such foods as pickles, chips and processed meats (e.g., ham, lunch meats). A "trick of the trade": You can tell that the patient is not adhering to a low-sodium diet if he or she states "The food 'tastes good' (i.e., contains too much salt) when I eat out (e.g., fast-food, delicatessen, Chinese or Italian restaurant)".

Mechanical heart support therapies, e.g., implantable LV assist devices, may also have a role as permanent or "destination" therapy. The prognosis for patients with dilated cardiomyopathy and advanced CHF is poor, with an average 5 year survival rate of <50%. The current 5 and 10 year survival rates after transplantation are ~75% and 55%, respectively. Because of the scarcity of donor hearts, however, fewer than 2500 transplants (out of the 20,000 patients who could potentially benefit) are performed in the United States each year.

LEFT VENTRICULAR DIASTOLIC DYSFUNCTION

LV diastolic dysfunction is usually associated with *LV hypertrophy* (due to hypertension, valvular AS or HOCM), CAD (ischemia, acute MI), small vessel disease (e.g., diabetes mellitus), *restrictive cardiomyopathy* (e.g., amyloidosis, sarcoidosis, hemochromatosis, scleroderma), or the aging process. Although LV contractility is normal, there is impaired LV relaxation and filling to such an extent that heart failure and even acute ("flash") pulmonary edema may result (e.g., with the onset of rapid atrial fibrillation). Diastolic dysfunction is responsible for approximately 50% of all heart failure episodes, particularly in patients with associated CAD and/or hypertension. Its incidence increases with age and is higher in women than in men. An atrial (S4) gallop is the major auscultatory finding in these patients. *Unlike the S3 gallop, the S4 gallop does not by itself denote ventricular decompensation. Instead, it is a clinically useful sign of LV diastolic dysfunction ("stiff LV").* It can be detected, if carefully searched for, over the cardiac apex using light pressure on the bell of the stethoscope with the patient in the left lateral position. The resting ECG is often quite helpful in the assessment of these patients:

- Evidence of LV hypertrophy with repolarization abnormalities (e.g., ST segment abnormalities) (in the absence of pathologic Q waves), and a normal heart size on CXR, are clues to *diastolic dysfunction* as the underlying cause of CHF.
- Conversely, diffuse low voltage (in the absence of COPD, pericardial effusion), and poor R wave progression or Q waves on the ECG along with cardiomegaly on the CXR, suggests the *systolic dysfunction* as the dominant mechanism.

Two-dimensional echo reveals the presence of preserved systolic function without LV dilatation. Many patients with diastolic dysfunction exhibit abnormal LV filling dynamics, such that small changes in volume result in large increments in filling pressure. This mechanism is the cause of "flash" pulmonary edema when such patients are administered excess volume too rapidly (e.g., post-operative fluid overload) or develop myocardial ischemia secondary to CAD superimposed on baseline abnormal LV compliance.

The goals in treating diastolic dysfunction include controlling hypertension and/or ischemia, maintaining normal sinus rhythm, avoiding tachycardia (with beta blockers, rate-slowing calcium channel blockers), and managing the congestive state (with diuretics, salt and fluid restriction, ACE inhibitors, or ARBs).

* * *

Summary:

Congestive heart failure can result from two major underlying pathophysiologic mechanisms:

1. *Systolic dysfunction* (low ejection fraction, usually <40%) caused by *CAD with LV damage, dilated cardiomyopathy, "burned out" hypertension,* and *valvular heart disease.*
2. *Diastolic dysfunction* (normal or near normal ejection fraction with impaired relaxation, which results in a stiff, noncompliant LV) caused by *CAD with ischemia, hypertension with LV hypertrophy, valvular AS, HOCM, small vessel disease* (e.g., diabetes mellitus), and *restrictive cardiomyopathy* (e.g., amyloidosis, sarcoidosis, hemochromatosis, scleroderma). Although up to 50% of patients may have isolated diastolic dysfunction, evidence of both is common.

Clinical clues to *systolic dysfunction* include:

- A history of MI
- Cardiomegaly on physical examination and CXR
- Poor R wave progression or Q waves on the ECG
- Pulsus alternans
- A murmur of MR

- S3 gallop: signifies elevated LA and LV filling pressures

Clinical clues to *diastolic dysfunction* include:

- The presence of hypertension
- LV hypertrophy on ECG (exception is amyloid, where the ECG shows low voltage [due to infiltrative process] despite LV hypertrophy on echo)
- A normal cardiac size on chest x-ray
- S4 gallop: reflects impaired LV relaxation and compliance

Acute myocardial ischemia and/or infarction should be considered as a precipitating cause in all patients with new onset of CHF or acute pulmonary edema (especially in the absence of cardiomegaly). The sudden onset of acute pulmonary edema with a normal (or nearly normal) sized heart, should also suggest other possible acute events. These may include acute AR or MR, or the abrupt onset of rapid atrial fibrillation in a patient with LV outflow tract obstruction (e.g., valvular AS, HOCM) or mitral stenosis. Rupture of the chordae tendineae of the mitral valve may be caused by endocarditis, trauma, or occur spontaneously, as a result of myxomatous degeneration (MVP). Acute AR may also be caused by endocarditis, trauma, as well as aortic dissection, annuloaortic ectasia, or aortic root dilatation, associated with Marfan's syndrome. Diastolic dysfunction should also be suspected in a patient with heart failure who has a normal-sized heart.

The CXR in acute ischemic LV dysfunction can lag behind the clinical picture by up to several hours, therefore, early in the case it may be normal. Although an S4 gallop, along with ECG evidence of LV hypertrophy, are useful clinical clues to diastolic dysfunction, echo findings, e.g., a normal ejection fraction and an abnormal LV filling (mitral Doppler inflow) pattern, may be helpful in confirming the diagnosis (**Figure 5-6A**). The goals of therapy are to maintain normal sinus rhythm, lower filling pressure (e.g., with diuretics and nitrates), reduce heart rate (e.g., with beta-blockers, verapamil, diltiazem) and treat hypertension and/or myocardial ischemia.

* * *

TREATMENT OF CHRONIC HEART FAILURE

Effective management of CHF focuses on searching for and correcting the predisposing risk factors and underlying cause, if possible. These include identifying and treating CAD, hypertension, diabetes mellitus, dyslipidemia, anemia, or thyroid disease; repairing or replacing a significantly regurgitant or stenotic heart valve; restoring blood flow to an obstructed coronary artery (by PCI or CABG); correcting a persistently fast heart rate or restoring sinus rhythm (as in atrial fibrillation, SVT); eliminating alcohol intake (alcohol may cause a cardiomyopathy); and avoiding drugs (if possible) that may aggravate the condition. Such drugs include NSAIDs, steroids, and thiazolidinediones (which cause fluid retention), and the anticancer drug doxorubicin, which causes cardiomyopathy. Many types of medications exist to help reduce the symptoms of systolic CHF and potentially prolong life. In contrast to systolic dysfunction, no medications are approved yet to reduce mortality in patients with diastolic dysfunction.

The "ABCs" of the pharmacologic treatment of systolic LV dysfunction include:

A: ACE inhibitors e.g., captopril (Capoten), enalapril (Vasotec), lisinopril (Zestril, Prinivil), ramipril (Altace), fosinopril (Monopril), quinapril (Accupril) benazepril (Lotensin), trandolapril (Mavik). These drugs help reduce symptoms and increase survival, in all patients with LV EF < 40% and/or

Angiotensin II receptor-blockers (ARBs), e.g., losartan (Cozaar), irbesartan (Avapro), candesartan (Atacand), valsartan (Diovan), olmesartan (Benicar), telmisartan (Micardis), eprosartan (Teveten) especially if intolerant to side effects of ACE inhibitors (e.g., cough, angioneurotic edema)

Angiotensin receptor neprilysin inhibitor (ARNI), e.g., valsartan/sacubitril (Entresto), in place of ACE inhibitor or ARB, to reduce mortality and hospitalization.

Aldosterone antagonists, e.g., spironolactone (Aldactone), in patients with advanced CHF, and eplerenone (Inspra), in post-MI patients with CHF. These drugs reduce mortality, but may cause hyperkalemia (especially if combined with ACE inhibitors/ARBs).

B: Beta blockers, e.g., carvedilol (Coreg, Coreg-CR), long-acting metroprolol succinate (Toprol-XL), bisoprolol (Zebeta), as tolerated. These drugs help reduce symptoms and increase survival (starting with a low dose and building up gradually over a period of weeks).

B-type or Brain Natriuretic Peptide i.e., IV nesiritide (Natrecor), for acutely decompensated CHF

C: Combination therapy e.g., hydralazine (Apresoline), a pure arterial vasodilator, and nitrates, a venodilating agent, should also be considered if intolerant to ACE inhibitors or ARBs (particularly if renal insufficiency or hyperkalemia are limiting factors), or in African-Americans.

Coumadin (warfarin), especially if severe dilated cardiomyopathy, atrial fibrillation, mechanical heart valves, or previous history of systemic or pulmonary embolism are present.

Cardiac Inotropes i.e., IV sympathomimetic amines e.g., dopamine (Intropin), dobutamine (Dobutrex), and phosphodiesterase inhibitors e.g., milrinone (Primacor), for severe and/or end-stage CHF

D: Diuretics, help reduce symptoms and decrease hospitalization rates. The goal is to achieve a "dry weight" as determined by reducing the elevated JVP and the abnormal abdominojugular reflux, along with other signs of fluid retention (e.g., rales, peripheral edema). A simple bedside scale with routine recording of weight is a helpful tool to determine diuretic response. *Avoid overly vigorous diuresis*. An excessive reduction of blood volume may actually reduce cardiac output, interfere with renal function, and produce profound weakness and lethargy. Exercise caution when using diuretics in patients with "restrictive filling" hemodynamics (e.g., HOCM, constrictive pericarditis). Remember to avoid diuretics (and nitrates) in patients with RV infarction (since they decrease preload, while the stiff RV needs higher intraventricular pressure to function).

Digoxin (Lanoxin), improves symptoms and decreases hospitalization rates (but has no survival benefit). It may be beneficial when rapid atrial fibrillation is present. (**Note:** It is important to avoid a low potassium level. Hypokalemia can precipitate potentially dangerous ventricular arrhythmias, particularly in patients who are receiving digoxin. You should lower digoxin dose when taking verapamil, quinidine, amiodarone and dronedarone. These drugs raise digoxin levels.)

Diet (restrict sodium and limit fluid intake)—to reduce fluid accumulation (edema) in the lungs, liver, abdomen and legs. Abstain from alcohol (because of its myocardial depressant effects).

Diuretics may be more effective, however, on the days when there is less physical activity. Many patients have little or no diuretic response during busy weekdays, but on a quiet, more restful weekend have a prompt and/or significant response (due to increased preload to the heart when the patient is at rest that improves cardiac output and renal perfusion). Thiazides, e.g., hydrochlorothiazide (HydroDIURIL), chlorothiazide (Diuril), chlorthalidone (Hygroton), and indapamide (Lozol), are standard therapy for chronic CHF (without renal insufficiency) when edema is mild to modest. Effectiveness is limited by intense proximal tubular reabsorption of sodium in more advanced stages of CHF (thiazides work in the distal tubule). With more advanced degrees of CHF (or when renal insufficiency is present, i.e., creatinine >2 mg/dL) the stronger loop diuretics and/or combinations of diuretics may be needed. Such drugs may include thiazide or thiazide-like agent metolazone (Zaroxolyn) and an intravenous loop diuretic e.g., furosemide (Lasix), bumetanide (Bumex), torsemide (Demadex). Torsemide and bumetanide have greater bioavailability and may be considered in patients with significant right-sided CHF, where absorption of furosemide is frequently unpredictable. A short course of IV diuretics may improve absorption and effectiveness of oral agents by helping to reduce gut edema. Spironolactone (Aldactone), a potassium-sparing diuretic (when added to an ACE inhibitor and a loop diuretic, with or without digoxin) has been shown to improve CHF symptoms and reduce mortality rates (spironolactone is an aldosterone antagonist that counteracts the adverse effects of excess aldosterone on ventricular remodeling). A newer aldosterone antagonist, eplerenone (Inspra), also appears effective in preventing LV remodeling and has been shown to improve survival in post-MI patients with CHF.

Even if the patient has responded favorably to a diuretic, treatment with an ACE inhibitor (and/or ARB) and a beta blocker should be initiated and maintained unless these drugs are not tolerated or their use is contraindicated. Vasodilators are important treatment in patients with CHF. *ACE inhibitors are clearly the vasodilator of choice. ACE inhibitors, along with beta blockers and aldosterone antagonists, prolong life, whereas loop and thiazide diuretics as well as digoxin just relieve symptoms.*

The combination of a pure *arterial vasodilator* (e.g., *hydralazine* [Apresoline]) and a strong *venodilating agent* (e.g., *nitrates*) can reduce afterload, improve forward flow (cardiac output), decrease filling pressure (preload), improve congestive symptoms, and has been shown to reduce mortality. This combination was used for many years in patients with CHF before the advent of ACE inhibitors. Although this potent vasodilator pair improves survival, studies have shown that ACE inhibitors do so to an even greater extent. In patients who cannot tolerate ACE inhibitors (or ARBs), however, or when symptoms persist despite aggressive therapy with ACE inhibitors and diuretics, the combination of hydralazine and nitrates remains a viable option. Of note, the combination of isosorbide dinitrate (a nitric oxide donor) and hydralazine (an antioxidant that inhibits destruction of nitric oxide) (BiDil) has been shown to be particularly beneficial in African-Americans with CHF (who may have a less active renin-angiotension system and a lower bioavailability of nitric oxide).

Therapy with digoxin may be initiated at any time to reduce symptoms or to slow the ventricular response in patients with rapid atrial fibrillation. It may seem paradoxical that beta blockers can exacerbate or worsen CHF (negative inotropic effect) and are now considered first-line treatment for CHF, but both are true. There is mounting clinical evidence that if stable patients are initiated on low doses of a beta blocker e.g., carvedilol, long-acting metoprolol succinate (not short-acting tartrate), or bisoprolol (added to standard CHF therapy) with gradual upward titration, they may derive significant benefit. The mechanism of this benefit may relate to blunting of the cardiotoxic effects of excess circulating catecholamines and improvement in LV size and shape (so-called reverse-remodeling). Following several weeks of therapy, beta blockers have been consistently shown to increase ejection fraction by 5 to 10 points (e.g., from an ejection fraction of 20% to 25–30%). Furthermore, data suggest that beta blockers slow the progression of CHF, reduce hospitalization and the need for adjustments of other CHF medications and heart transplantation, and they reduce mortality.

Of note, a novel heart rate lowering agent, ivabradine (Corlanor), that acts by selectively inhibiting the I_f ("funny") current in the sinoatrial node, has recently been approved as add-on therapy to reduce the risk of hospitalization (but not mortality) for worsening heart failure in patients with chronic stable, symptomatic CHF with reduced ejection fraction

$\leq$35%, who are in sinus rhythm with a resting heart rate $\geq$ 70 beats per minute, and who are on maximum tolerated doses of beta blockers or have a contraindication to their use. Unlike beta blockers, ivabradine has no effect on myocardial contractility (i.e., no negative inotropic effect).

Worthy of mention, a new class of drug called angiotensin receptor neprilysin inhibitor (ARNI), combines an ARB (valsartan) with a neprilysin inhibitor (sacubitril) and blocks both the angiotensin (ATI) receptor and the enzymatic breakdown of endogenous natriuretic and vasodilatory peptides. This novel combination drug (Entresto) has been shown to be more effective than an ACE inhibitor (enalapril) in reducing cardiovascular mortality and hospitalization and holds promise as a first line treatment of CHF.

Selected patients with severe CHF also may benefit symptomatically from ultrafiltration (which reduces fluid overload) and the periodic IV infusion of inotropic agents, such as:

- the sympathomimetic amines including dopamine (Intropin) (which at low dosages stimulates dopaminergic receptors in the renal vascular bed causing increased renal blood flow which facilitates diuresis, and at moderate doses increases inotropy by stimulating cardiac β -1 receptors
- dobutamine (Dobutrex), a synthetic analog of dopamine that preferentially stimulates β-1 receptors in addition to β -2 and α receptors
- milrinone (Primacor), a phosphodiesterase -3 inhibitor, which increases calcium uptake, myocardial contractility, stroke volume, ejection fraction and sinus rate, while decreasing peripheral resistance (and thus act as an "inotropic dilator")

Dobutamine must be used with caution in patients with systolic blood pressure less than 100 mmHg because it can worsen hypotension. Since dobutamine and milrinone may adversely affect survival (due to increased incidence of ventricular tachyarrhythmias), these agents should be reserved for short-term administration in patients with end-stage CHF refractory to conventional therapy.

Nitroprusside (Nipride) remains the primary intravenous vasodilator for the hospitalized CHF patient (especially in the setting of hypertension). This balanced venous and arterial dilator reduces pulmonary and systemic vascular resistance with improved hemodynamics and enhanced diuresis. Side effects include excess hypotension, paradoxical oxygen desaturation due to AV shunting, coronary steal, and cyanide toxicity. IV *nesiritide* (Natrecor), a genetically engineered recombinant form of human BNP approved for the treatment of acute decompensated CHF, acts as a potent vasodilator and natriuretic factor that reduces ventricular filling pressure, enhances diuresis, and improves cardiac output. Nesiritide has not been shown to provide a clear clinical benefit over standard therapy, however, and its use is not routinely recommended.

In some situations, however, the heart becomes so weak that conventional medical treatment has little impact. In selected patients with a widened QRS complex, resynchronization therapy with *biventricular pacing* appears to induce an improvement in symptoms and survival. *Left ventricular assist devices* and *heart transplantation* may need to be considered for those patients with end-stage CHF refractory to all other therapeutic measures. Contraindications to heart transplantation include old age, pulmonary hypertension, infection (including HIV), co-morbid conditions that significantly limit life expectancy, unresolved alcohol and/or drug abuse, and a noncompliant patient.

When using potent diuretics, normal serum potassium (and magnesium) levels need to be carefully maintained. Taking potassium-sparing diuretics (e.g., spironolactone), potassium supplements, eating potassium-rich foods, and/or monitoring serum potassium levels are precautionary measures. Keep in mind that hyperkalemia may result when potassium-sparing diuretics and/or supplements are administered to patients taking ACE inhibitors (which can cause hyperkalemia) and in patients with renal insufficiency, particularly if diabetic.

It is important to emphasize that patients who are symptomatic with dyspnea at rest or who are hemodynamically unstable should not be started on beta blocker therapy. Patients receiving beta blocker therapy may need a dose reduction or discontinuance if clinically significant cardiac decompensation develops. Decompensation may, however, respond to an increase in diuretic dose without requiring beta blocker withdrawal. The clinician should always try to ascertain if there is a history of high sodium and fluid intake or medication noncompliance when decompensation occurs. One of the most common causes of an acute exacerbation of CHF is inadvertent or inappropriate reduction in therapy. This may occur through noncompliance on the part of the patient with compensated CHF and mild symptoms or through changes in medications made by other practitioners.

In the "real world", patients often discontinue medication or fail to renew their prescriptions ("I ran out of my pills") because they are taking too many drugs, too many each day, are spending too much money, and have too many side effects. Whenever possible, therefore, try to keep it simple. Prescribe long-acting and/or combination preparations (if possible). Keep in mind that the cost of multiple drug therapy is an extremely important concern to patients, particularly those who are retired, or on disability programs with fixed incomes and limited insurance coverage (**Figure 12-10**).

Ambulatory patients with CHF should adhere to a restricted sodium diet. Limiting total fluid intake to 1500–2000 ml/day (or less if hyponatremia is present) is a reasonable guideline for most patients with CHF. Some patients may need to be overdiuresed in order to prevent congestive symptoms.

The "ABCs" of treating diastolic dysfunction:

A: Avoid digoxin (Lanoxin), unless systolic LV dysfunction and/or rapid atrial fibrillation is also present (digoxin acts by increasing systolic contractility, which is not needed in diastolic dysfunction). Especially avoid digoxin in HOCM, where an increased LV contractility can worsen the outflow tract gradient.

ACE inhibitors (effect on ventricular remodeling), e.g., captopril (Capoten), enalapril (Vasotec), lisinopril (Zestril, Prinivil), ramipril (Altace), fosinopril (Monopril), quinapril (Accupril). **Note: ARBs** may be used if ACE intolerant.

Aldosterone antagonists, e.g., spironolactone (Aldactone), may reduce hospitalization for CHF and cardiovascular mortality (controversial)

B: Beta blockers, e.g., propranolol (Inderal), metoprolol (Lopressor, Toprol-XL), atenolol (Tenormin), nadolol (Corgard), acebutolol (Sectral). Beta blockers and calcium channel blockers (particularly verapamil and diltiazem) enhance diastolic relaxation (in addition to decreasing systolic contractility) (especially in hypertrophic cardiomyopathy) and decrease heart rate, which in turn increases diastolic filling time (a key goal in patients with CHF and LV hypertrophy).

C: Calcium channel blockers, e.g., dihydropyridines (nifedipine [Procardia, Adalat], amlodipine [Norvasc], felodipine [Plendil], isradipine [DynaCirc], nisoldipine [Sular]), and nondihydropyridines (verapamil [Isoptin, Calan, Verelan], and diltiazem [Cardizem, Tiazac, Dilacor]).

D: Diuretics, e.g., furosemide (Lasix), bumetanide (Bumex), torsemide (Demadex) for symptoms of fluid overload, to reduce the congestive state. (**Note:** Monitor diuretic effects carefully since excessive administration may result in a drop in cardiac output, hypotension and prerenal azotemia.)

Diet (low sodium)

When treating patients with diastolic dysfunction, it is important to keep in mind the importance of correcting the underlying remediable causes and exacerbating factors, e.g., by:

- Valve replacement in aortic stenosis
- Preventing tachycardia (with beta blockers, calcium channel blockers, catheter ablation and pacing) and maintaining atrial contraction (by electrical or pharmacologic cardioversion)
- Controlling hypertension (with antihypertensive agents)
- Treating myocardial ischemia (with nitrates, beta blockers, calcium channel blockers, PCI, or CABG) that may impair LV relaxation.

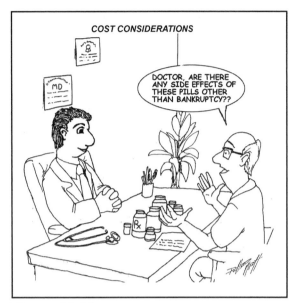

Figure 12-10

TREATMENT OF ACUTE HEART FAILURE AND PULMONARY EDEMA

Acute heart failure may develop suddenly in a previously asymptomatic patient (e.g., with an ACS, a hypertensive crisis, or acute AR/MR), or it may complicate chronic compensated CHF following a precipitating event (e.g., dietary indiscretion, medication noncompliance, intercurrent illness or infection, arrhythmias, e.g., rapid atrial fibrillation or VT, anemia, thyroid disease, alcohol, or drugs, e.g., NSAIDs, steroids, thiazolidinediones) and toxins (e.g., cocaine, anthracyclines). The patient's volume status (wet vs. dry) and adequacy of tissue perfusion (cold vs. warm) should be assessed.

Patients presenting with acute pulmonary edema require immediate stabilization. The goal of therapy is to improve oxygenation and reduce elevated left heart filling pressure. The patient should be placed in a sitting position with legs dangling over the side of the bed to reduce venous return and ease breathing. Supplemental oxygen should be delivered by face mask (to maintain O_2 sat > 90 %), and morphine sulfate given intravenously to reduce preload as well as patient anxiety (through its action on opiate receptors in the brain). Watch for respiratory depression. Loop diuretics (e.g., furosemide, bumetanide, torsemide) are administered intravenously (either as a bolus or continuous infusion), without delay, and in addition to their diuretic properties, also produce venodilation, thereby reducing LV preload. Vasodilators, e.g., nitroglycerin (sublingual and/or intravenous), or nesiritide, titrated by clinical and blood pressure response, reduce both preload and afterload and are especially useful in the presence of hypertension and myocardial ischemia. Intravenous nitroprusside (with careful

monitoring) in patients with severe MR or AR, and inotropic drugs (e.g., dopamine, dobutamine, milrinone) may be considered for hemodynamic support. For patients with symptomatic hypotension and end-organ dysfunction (cardiogenic shock) despite IV vasoactive therapy, mechanical support (e.g., IABP, LVAD, ECMO) should be considered. The patient should be monitored by continuous pulse oximetry and if respiratory failure ensues, intubated and mechanical ventilation begun.

During resolution of the acute event, attention should be directed at identifying and treating the underlying cause.

* * *

Pearls:

- In patients with symptomatic CHF or asymptomatic LV dysfunction, the presence of an elevated JVP or S_3 gallop predicts mortality and hospitalization for CHF.
- Unless contraindicated, patients with CHF with reduced ejection fraction should take an ACE inhibitor (or ARB) and a beta blocker to reduce mortality, and if volume overloaded, a diuretic to decrease symptoms.
- Addition of an aldosterone antagonist can reduce mortality and hospitalization for CHF.
- The combination of hydralazine and isosorbide dinitrate has been shown to reduce mortality and symptoms of CHF in African Americans.
- Digoxin can decrease symptoms and lower the rate of hospitalization for CHF, but does not reduce mortality.
- A new class of drug, ARNI, which combines an ARB with a neprilysin inhibitor, has been shown to be superior to an ACE inhibitor in reducing mortality and hospitalization for CHF.
- In patients with advanced CHF with reduced ejection fraction ≤ 35%, LBBB and a wide QRS complex ≥ 150 msec, device therapy with ICD and CRT (biventricular pacing) can improve symptoms and reduce hospitalization and mortality for CHF.
- There is little evidence that drug treatment improves clinical outcomes in patients with HFpEF (with the exception of an aldosterone antagonist [controversial]).
- Keep in mind the *mnemonic* "**LMNOP**" in the management of acute pulmonary edema.
  - **L**oop diuretics
  - **M**orphine
  - **N**itroglycerin
  - **O**xygen
  - Upright **P**osition

* * *

248

CHAPTER 13. APPROACH TO THE PATIENT WITH SYSTEMIC ARTERIAL HYPERTENSION

PRIMARY AND SECONDARY FORMS OF HYPERTENSION

Hypertension is a powerful risk factor for acute MI, CHF, stroke, renal failure, aortic aneurysm and/or dissection. It is the most common disease-specific reason for practitioner visits in the United States today. According to updated guidelines issued by the American Heart Association, nearly half of the adults in the United States (~100 million) are now considered to have hypertension, redefined as a BP ≥ 130/80 mmHg (down from the previous standard of 140/90 mmHg), and up to three times as many African-Americans have an elevated BP than does the general population. It has also been reported that of the 70% of adults who are aware of their diagnosis, only one third to one half are being adequately treated.

The great majority (95%) of patients have no identifiable cause and are said to have essential or primary hypertension. Although the specific cause is unknown, familial patterns of primary hypertension are common. In addition, environmental factors e.g., obesity, alcohol consumption, sedentary lifestyle, salt intake, and psychogenic stress may play a role. If hypertension is unresponsive to medical therapy or hypertension is in an accelerated phase, you should evaluate the patient for the possibility of an underlying curable secondary cause.

This chapter will review the practical clinical approach to the patient with systemic arterial hypertension.

CLINICAL MANIFESTATIONS OF HYPERTENSION

Most patients with systemic hypertension have no specific complaints or clinical manifestations other than an elevated systolic and/or diastolic blood pressure (i.e., "silent killer"). Some, however, complain of morning occipital headache (which is less frequent than commonly assumed), epistaxis, or blurred vision if hypertension is severe. Systolic hypertension, without diastolic hypertension, accounts for as many as one half of the cases of hypertension in the elderly, and also leads to an increased incidence of MI, CHF and stroke. In fact, more recent data suggest that the level of systolic BP in persons older than 50 years may be a more important cardiovascular disease risk factor (and the more difficult component to control) than that of the diastolic BP.

The clinical history should include a review of the family history for hypertension and heart disease, previous measurements of the BP, symptoms suggestive of secondary hypertension (**Figure 13-1**) and other cardiovascular risk factors (e.g., cigarette smoking, hyperlipidemia, obesity, diabetes mellitus). Hypertensive patients should be carefully questioned about symptoms that suggest the presence of CAD, cerebrovascular disease, CHF, peripheral vascular disease, diabetes mellitus, and chronic renal disease. In women, obtain any history of previous hypertension associated with pregnancies or the use of oral contraceptives. Also inquire about the use of alcohol or certain medications, e.g., steroids, NSAIDs (volume expanders), monoamine oxidase inhibitors, and cyclosporine (vasoconstrictors).

Instead of the gradual onset of elevated BP as seen in patients with essential hypertension, patients with secondary hypertension usually have a relatively abrupt onset of hypertension. The new onset of elevated BP in an individual < age 30 years or > age 50 years should alert you to the possibility of renovascular hypertension.

When an elevated BP reading is detected, it should be measured at least twice during two separate examinations after the initial screening. Transient elevation of BP caused by excitement or apprehension does not constitute hypertensive disease but may indicate a propensity toward its evolution. A progressive and linear relationship exists between increasing BP and cardiovascular risk, beginning at a BP of 115/75 mmHg and doubling with each increment of 20/10 mmHg. Defining a precise cutoff point at which BP is considered "high", therefore, is somewhat arbitrary. Although hypertension in adults has been traditionally defined as a BP ≥ 140/90 mmHg, recent clinical trial data have identified groups of patients at increased cardiovascular risk in whom BPs below this value may be associated with improve outcomes. Accordingly, recently revised quidelines now define a "normal BP" as a BP < 120/80 mmHg; an "elevated BP" (previously termed "prehypertension") as a BP 120-129/< 80 mmHg; "stage 1 hypertension" as a BP 130-139/80-89 mmHg; and "stage 2 hypertension" as a BP ≥ 140/90 mmHg. A "hypertensive crisis" is defined as a severe elevation in BP (BP > 180/120 mmHg) with (hypertensive emergency) or without (hypertensive urgency) evidence of new or worsening target organ damage or dysfunction. (**Figure 13-2**).

Figure 13-2. Updated classification of BP for adults aged ≥ 18 years.

Most patients with mild or moderate hypertension have no physical findings referable to their disease early in the course of the illness. Abnormalities generally involve the target organs (i.e., heart, brain, kidneys, eyes, and peripheral arteries) and develop over time. A careful physical examination focuses on the presence or absence of such target organ damage and should include an evaluation of the

---

FIGURE 13-1

Clinical Clues to Hypertension

Clue	Clinical significance
Family history of hypertension	Essential hypertension (~95%)
Hypokalemia (in the absence of diuretics), muscle weakness and cramps	Primary aldosteronism
Truncal obesity, moon face, buffalo hump, acne, purple striae, hirsutism, easy bruising	Cushing's disease/syndrome
Morbid obesity, male gender (90%), nocturnal snoring, daytime hypersomnolence	Sleep apnea
Resistant, accelerated, or malignant hypertension; early onset (< age 30) or late onset (> age 50); abdominal or flank bruit; atherosclerosis at other sites; "flash" pulmonary edema; worsening of renal function with the use of ACE inhibitor or ARBs	Renovascular hypertension
The 5 P's: palpitations, pallor, head pain, perspiration, paroxysmal hypertension and postural hypotension	Pheochromocytoma
Bilateral (abdominal or flank) palpable masses	Polycystic kidneys
Delayed or decreased femoral pulses (radial-femoral delay); blood pressure higher in arms than legs; rib notching on chest x-ray	Coarctation of the aorta
Flank pain, frequency, dysuria, hematuria, history of renal disease, volume overload, anemia	Renal parenchymal disease
Non-steroidal antiinflammatory drugs, steroids, alcohol or cocaine abuse, oral contraceptives, nasal decongestants, cyclosporine	Drug-induced
Symptoms of excess thyroid hormone, tachycardia, goiter, exophthalmos, lid lag, stare	Thyrotoxicosis

---

optic fundi for hypertensive changes, e.g., arteriolar narrowing with focal constrictions, hemorrhage and exudates, and papilledema (acute changes) , that may occur immediately if the BP is very high, as well as the more chronic changes of arteriovenous nicking, copper and silver wiring, that may take years to develop if the BP is poorly controlled.

Figure 13-3. Retinal changes in acute and chronic hypertension (A, artery; V, vein) (From Goldberg S: Ophthalmology Made Ridiculously Simple, MedMaster, Inc. 2001).

Examination of the neck may reveal carotid bruits and thyromegaly, and the cardiac examination may demonstrate signs of LV hypertrophy and diastolic dysfunction (sustained PMI, palpable and audible S4 gallop) and/or LV systolic dysfunction (inferolaterally displaced PMI, S3 gallop). The abdominal examination may uncover expansile (aneurysm) or palpable (kidney) masses (**Figure 13-4**).

The ECG may show LV hypertrophy (a poor prognostic sign, particularly if ST-T wave changes are also present).

(**Figure 3-38**). An apical S4 gallop (due to decreased LV compliance), is frequently heard in the presence of a loud "tambour" A2 (over the aortic area). There may also be an aortic systolic murmur and on occasion a "functional" diastolic murmur of AR caused by dilatation of the aortic ring (which may lessen in intensity or even disappear coincident with reduction in BP from antihypertensive drug therapy). These auscultatory sounds and murmurs can be the earliest clinical findings detected in patients with hypertensive heart disease and often precede ECG and other signs of LV hypertrophy. As LV hypertrophy becomes more evident, a palpable sustained LV lift may be evident. When the LV can adapt no further to an increase in afterload, an S3 gallop (along with pulsus alternans) appears on clinical examination, denoting the presence of LV systolic dysfunction.

The chest x-ray may help detect LV enlargement and pulmonary vascular congestion, as well as involvement of other thoracic structures (e.g., aortic dilatation and rib notching with aortic coarctation). Echocardiogra-

FIGURE 13-2

Classification of Blood Pressure for Adults Aged ≥ 18 Years*

BP Category	Systolic BP, mmHg	Diastolic BP, mmHG
Normal BP	< 120	< 80
Elevated BP	120-129	< 80
Stage 1 hypertension	130-139	80-89
Stage 2 hypertension	≥ 140	≥ 90
Hypertensive crisis** (emergency/urgency)	≥ 180	>120

***Note:** Blood pressure (BP) is categorized as normal, elevated, and stage 1 or 2 hypertension, based on an average of ≥ 2 careful readings obtained on ≥ 2 occasions. Individuals with systolic BP and diastolic BP in 2 categories should be designated to the higher BP category.
****Hypertensive crises are divided into 2 types, emergencies or urgencies, based on the presence or absence of new or worsening target organ damage or dysfunction, respectively.

Adapted from Whelton PK, Carey RM, Aronow WS, et. al., ACC/AHA Guideline for the Prevention, Detection, Evaluation, and Management of High Blood Pressure in Adults; A Report of the American College of Cardiology/American Heart Association Task Force on Clinical Practice Guidelines. Hypertension, 2017.

phy is more sensitive then either the physical examination, ECG or CXR in identifying whether LV hypertrophy is present, and in determining the functional status of the myocardium, but it is expensive. It is of particular value, however, when one is concerned about the progression of cardiac involvement in a patient with hypertensive heart disease, and when there is a question as to the structural or functional effect of antihypertensive drug therapy on LV mass, wall thickening and function. Although Doppler-echo may detect hemodynamically insignificant AR in 10–20% of patients, its primary role is in the evaluation of patients with clinical symptoms and/or signs of heart disease.

Some baseline laboratory tests may also be helpful for the initial evaluation of a patient with hypertension, e.g., urinalysis (to search for hematuria, proteinuria, and casts), BUN and creatinine (to assess renal function), serum potassium levels (to screen for mineralocorticoid excess, or as a baseline for diuretic therapy), fasting blood sugar levels (to detect diabetes mellitus), and plasma lipid panel (an indicator of atherosclerotic risk and an additional target for therapy). It is neither cost-effective nor rewarding to perform a thorough work-up on every patient with hypertension to search for a secondary cause. Since most hypertension is primary, few

studies are necessary beyond those mentioned above. If conventional therapy is unsuccessful or if symptoms and/or signs suggest a secondary, potentially curable cause (**Figure 13-1**), further studies (e.g., renal ultrasound, CT scan, MRI, or angiography) may be indicated.

TREATMENT OF HYPERTENSION

Currently, up to 30% of those with hypertension remain undiagnosed and only one third to one half of those known to have high blood pressure are adequately controlled. Institution of early antihypertensive therapy will not only prevent the development of hypertensive heart disease but will also reduce the morbidity and mortality from CAD, CHF, kidney disease and stroke.

Hypertension control begins with proper detection and diagnosis. There is both overdiagnosis e.g., *"white coat"* (office) *hypertension,* whereby the stress of visiting the practitioner may sometimes lead to falsely elevated BP readings, as well as underdiagnosis (due to lack of taking BP or poor BP technique). Proper diagnosis requires correct BP measurement techniques (automated vs manual [auscultatory]) and confirmation of high blood pressure with repeat measurements on at least two separate occasions before establishing a diagnosis and the need for treatment. Be aware of circumstances that temporarily raise blood pressure in the absence of disease (e.g., anxiety, rushing to make the appointment on time, bladder distention, recent cigarette smoking, alcohol or caffeine intake, improper technique, such as wrong cuff size).

In deciding if and when to treat your patient with hypertension, have him or her keep a log of their blood pressure readings at home. Although it remains controversial, hypertension may be defined by repeated home BP readings that average ≥ 130/80 mmHg. Ambulatory 24-hour BP monitoring may be a useful adjunct to home or office BP measurements in evaluating patients with marked discrepancies in BP readings, e.g., *"white coat"* (isolated office) hypertension, or *"masked"* (isolated home) hypertension, and in identifying individuals at increased cardiovascular risk, e.g., those without a normal "dip" in BP at night (nocturnal hypertension), or who have a steep surge in BP in the morning or during stress (intermittent hypertension). A diary should be kept as to whether or not stress or problems had occurred on a particular day. It is important to recognize that *BP decreases postprandially* and that this can affect interpretation of the BP reading. Review of the log at the end of several weeks usually identifies the individual who needs treatment, and may help eliminate those who may not require treatment. After starting treatment, the patient should continue to keep a log for you to review. Necessary adjustments in therapy may become evident.

The most important early treatment recommendations should include lifestyle modifications, e.g., weight loss (if overweight), moderation of alcohol consumption, regular physical activity, reduction in sodium intake, and smoking cessation (to reduce cardiovascular risk, not necessarily BP), along with a diet rich in fruits and vegetables (high potassium), and low-fat dairy products (high calcium), with a reduced content of saturated and total fats (DASH diet). (**Figure 13-5**)

Practitioners may differ as to when to start antihypertensive therapy in a patient having milder degrees of blood pressure elevation. Previous practice guidelines set the threshold for beginning pharmacologic treatment at a BP ≥ 140/90 mmHg in most patients with hypertension, and a BP ≥ 150/90 mmHg in older hypertensive adults. However, based on recent clinical trial data, updated guidelines now recommend initiation of antihypertensive therapy at a BP ≥ 140/90 mmHg in all hypertensive patients, and a BP ≥ 130/80 mmHg in individuals at higher risk, i.e., those with known cardiovascular disease, diabetes, chronic kidney disease, or a 10 year ASCVD risk of ≥ 10% (see below). The magnitude of BP elevation should be used to guide the number of antihypertensive agents to start with when implementing drug therapy. For patients

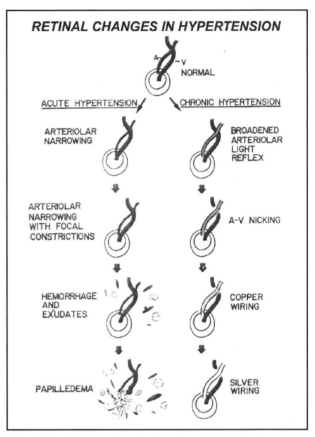

Note: Moderate to severe hypertensive retinopathy is defined as severe hypertension with retinal hemorrhages, exudates, or papilledema, with or without hypertensive encephalopathy.

Figure 13-3

with moderate to severe hypertension, more intensive pharmacologic therapy may be warranted, especially if target organ damage is present. The presence of an S4 can be one of the earliest signs of target organ damage, and is a "clue" that the heart has already been affected. In addition to an S4 gallop, if a tambour S2 (particularly with higher levels of BP) and an aortic systolic murmur are also present, they may provide further justification for treatment. Keep in mind that lifestyle modification may be all that is necessary in patients with milder degrees of elevated BP. For example, what is often not recognized is that obese patients may have a return to a normal blood pressure reading once the excess weight is lost. Remember that spurious high blood pressure readings can be recorded in obese individuals if the wrong cuff-size is used. If a larger (more appropriate) size cuff is used, it may reveal a normal blood pressure. Several blood pressure recordings should be recorded on each patient in a given visit. It is not unusual for a drop of 10 to 15 mm Hg in systolic pressure and 5 to 10 mm Hg in diastolic pressure to occur over a period of 5 to 10 minutes. Take the blood pressure in both arms. If a

---

FIGURE 13-4

Clues to Target Organ Damage in Hypertension*

Clues	Target Organ
Clinical, ECG, CXR, or echo evidence of:	
LV hypertrophy	Heart
LV systolic and diastolic dysfunction or heart failure	
Myocardial ischemia and/or infarction	
Transient ischemic attack or stroke	Brain
Aortic aneurysm and/or dissection	Aorta and peripheral vasculature
Peripheral arterial disease—absence of one or more pulses in the extremities, intermittent claudication	
Carotid bruits	
Nephrosclerosis	Kidney
Renal failure—elevated serum creatinine, proteinuria, microalbuminuria	
Retinopathy—arterial narrowing, hemorrhages, exudates, papilledema, AV nicking, copper and silver wiring	Eye

***Note:** The evaluation of the patient with hypertension should include a careful search for clinical and laboratory clues that suggest the presence of target organ damage. The major target organs affected by the destructive effect of chronic hypertension are the heart, brain, aorta, peripheral vasculature, kidneys, and eyes.

---

discrepancy exists on the second arm examined, go back to recheck the first arm.

The challenge in the evaluation and treatment of hypertension is identifying the minority (5%) of patients who have potentially curable forms of secondary hypertension and establishing the best BP control regimen for the vast majority of patients with primary hypertension. The extent to which cardiac output, peripheral vascular resistance, intravascular volume, sympathetic nervous system stimulation, and the renin-angiotensin-aldosterone system influence BP differs from patient to patient. Therapy should be individualized as much as possible for each patient. Although essential hypertension has no cure, dietary restriction of sodium and alcohol intake along with lifestyle modifications (including exercise, weight reduction, and stress management) can often control it, especially in early, mild cases. If the BP remains elevated, especially if target organ damage or cardiovascular risk factors are present, the use of one or more of the various antihypertensive drugs currently available may be helpful (**Figure 13-5**).

Ideally, treatment should begin before damage to a vital organ takes place. The vital organs affected by hypertension are the heart, brain, aorta, peripheral vasculature,

kidneys, and eyes. Left untreated, ~ 50% of hypertensive patients die from CAD or CHF, ~ 33% from stroke, and ~ 10–15% from complications of renal failure. There are several major categories of drugs available to control hypertension. Keep in mind that the blood pressure (BP) is the product of the cardiac output (CO) and the peripheral vascular resistance (PVR) (BP = CO × PVR). Since the key factors that regulate BP are cardiac output (stroke volume × heart rate) and the peripheral vascular resistance (particularly as mediated through blood vessel constriction), all anti-hypertensive drugs act by reducing either the CO and/or the PVR.

BP can be reduced by:

1. *Diuretics,* which decrease volume overload, particularly thiazide diuretics, e.g., hydrochlorothiazide (HydroDIURIL) and potassium-sparing agents (plus thiazide), e.g., spironolactone (Aldactazide), Dyrenium (Dyazide, Maxzide), amiloride (Moduretic). Loop diuretics, e.g., furosemide (Lasix), bumetanide (Bumex), torsemide (Demadex) are effective in patients with renal insufficiency (serum creatinine >2 mg/dL) and in those with CHF.

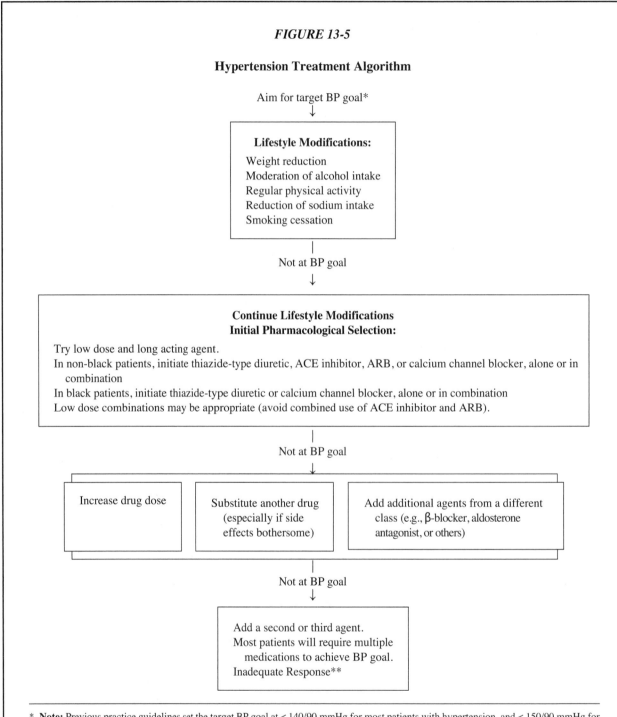

FIGURE 13-5

Hypertension Treatment Algorithm

Aim for target BP goal*
↓

Lifestyle Modifications:

Weight reduction
Moderation of alcohol intake
Regular physical activity
Reduction of sodium intake
Smoking cessation

Not at BP goal
↓

Continue Lifestyle Modifications
Initial Pharmacological Selection:

Try low dose and long acting agent.
In non-black patients, initiate thiazide-type diuretic, ACE inhibitor, ARB, or calcium channel blocker, alone or in combination
In black patients, initiate thiazide-type diuretic or calcium channel blocker, alone or in combination
Low dose combinations may be appropriate (avoid combined use of ACE inhibitor and ARB).

Not at BP goal
↓

| Increase drug dose | Substitute another drug (especially if side effects bothersome) | Add additional agents from a different class (e.g., β-blocker, aldosterone antagonist, or others) |

Not at BP goal
↓

Add a second or third agent.
Most patients will require multiple medications to achieve BP goal.
Inadequate Response**

* **Note:** Previous practice guidelines set the target BP goal at < 140/90 mmHg for most patients with hypertension, and < 150/90 mmHg for older hypertensive adults. However, based on recent clinical trial data, updated guidelines now recommend pharmacologic treatment at a target BP goal of < 140/90 mmHg for all hypertensive patients, and a lower BP goal of < 130/80 mmHg for individuals at higher risk, i.e., those with known cardiovascular disease, diabetes, chronic kidney disease, or a 10 year ASCVD risk of ≥ 10%.
**If not at goal BP, consider referral to a hypertension specialist.

2. *Beta blockers,* which block adrenergic receptors in the heart (reduces heart rate and work load), e.g., propranolol (Inderal), metoprolol (Lopressor, Toprol-XL), atenolol (Tenormin), nadolol (Corgard), acebutolol (Sectral), esmolol (Brevibloc).

3. *Centrally acting anti-adrenergic agents,* which reduce sympathetic (adrenergic) outflow from the brain (activates inhibitory α-2 receptors), e.g., clonidine (Catapres), methyldopa (Aldomet). Side effects include drowsiness, dry mouth, fatigue, and orthostatic hypotension. Clonidine is available as a transdermal patch that makes once-a-week dosing possible.

Dilating blood vessels with:

4. α-blockers (blocks α$_1$ mediated vasoconstrictors), e.g., terazosin (Hytrin), prazosin (Minipress), doxazosin (Cardura)—not a first choice agent (may induce significant postural hypotension; therefore, first dose should be taken at bedtime).

5. *Alpha-beta-blockers,* e.g., labetalol (Normodyne), (Trandate), carvedilol (Coreg).

6. *ACE inhibitors* (suppresses the synthesis of angiotensin II, a potent vasoconstrictor), e.g., captopril (Capoten), enalapril (Vasotec), lisinopril (Zestril, Prinivil), ramipril (Altace), fosinopril (Monopril), quinapril (Accupril).

7. *ARBs* (antagonizes the angiotensin II receptor of vascular muscle), e.g., losartan (Cozaar), irbesartan (Avapro), candesartan (Atacand), valsartan (Diovan), telmisartan (Micardis), eprosartan (Teveten), especially if intolerant to side-effects of ACE inhibitors (e.g., cough, angioneurotic edema).

8. *Calcium channel blockers* (blocks calcium entry into smooth muscle cells of arterial walls, thereby preventing contraction). These include the dihydropyridines, e.g., nifedipine (Procardia, Adalat), amlodipine (Norvasc), felodipine (Plendil), isradipine (DynaCirc), nisoldipine (Sular), nicardipine (Cardene), clevidipine (Cleviprex), and the non-dihydropyridines, e.g., verapamil (Isoptin, Calan, Verelan), and diltiazem (Cardizem, Tiazac, Dilacor).

9. *Direct renin inhibitors* (blocks the action of renin which decreases the production of angiotensin and promotes vasodilation), e.g., aliskiren (Tekturna).

10. *Direct vasodilators* (relaxes smooth muscle cells which surround blood vessels), e.g., hydralazine (Apresoline), minoxidil (Loniten). Hydralazine may cause a lupus-like syndrome; minoxidil may cause unwanted hair growth. Reflex tachycardia (palpitations) and fluid retention (edema) are also common. These agents can worsen angina in patients with CAD.

In the uncomplicated patient, thiazide-type diuretics, ACE inhibitors, ARBs, or calcium channel blockers, alone or in combination, should be considered as initial therapy for most. Additional drug choices (e.g., β-blockers, aldosterone antagonists, or others) may be used based on the response to the initial therapy and/or as dictated by concomitant medical conditions and the drug's safety, tolerability, cost, and other lifestyle issues (**Figure 13-5** and **13-6**). In certain clinical conditions, there may be compelling indications for specific agents as the initial treatment. For example:

- ACE inhibitors and ARBs in patients with Type I and Type II diabetes with proteinuria (these agents slow the progression of nephropathy in patients with diabetes mellitus)
- Hypertension in African-Americans tends to respond better to diuretics or calcium channel blockers than to beta blockers or ACE inhibitors.
- CHF due to systolic LV dysfunction (ACE inhibitors, diuretics [including spironolactone], beta blockers, e.g., carvedilol [Coreg] as tolerated, and ARBs)
- CHF due to diastolic dysfunction (beta blockers, diuretics, and calcium channel blockers)
- CAD (beta blockers and long-acting calcium channel blockers)
- Isolated systolic hypertension in the elderly (diuretics and long-acting dihydropyridine calcium channel blockers)
- Benign prostatic hypertrophy (alpha blockers, e.g., doxazosin [Cardura], terazosin [Hytrin])
- Aortic regurgitation (ACE inhibitors and nifedipine)
- Migraine headaches (beta blockers and calcium channel blockers [especially verapamil])

While younger patients and those with specific comorbidities (e.g., CAD, CHF, tachyarrhythmias) may exhibit net benefit from using beta blockers as antihypertensive agents, older patients with primary hypertension appear to accrue less benefit and can potentially have an increased risk for stroke.

It is important to consider the patient's lifestyle when prescribing antihypertensive therapy. The adverse physical, mental and metabolic side effects of hypertensive therapy (e.g., fatigue, depression, and erectile dysfunction from beta blockers) may result in nonadherence to prescribed regimens.

FIGURE 13-6

Tailored Pharmacologic Therapy for Hypertension

Indication	Drug Therapy
Types I and II diabetes mellitus with proteinuria	ACE inhibitor Angiotensin II receptor blocker (ARB)
Heart failure	ACE inhibitor Diuretic Beta blocker Angiotensin II receptor blocker (ARB) Aldosterone antagonist
Isolated systolic hypertension (older patient)	Diuretic (preferred) Long-acting dihydropyridine calcium channel blocker
Myocardial infarction	Beta blocker ACE inhibitor or ARB (with systolic dysfunction)
Angina pectoris	Beta blocker Calcium channel blocker (long-acting)
Atrial tachycardia and fibrillation	Beta blocker Non-dihydropyridine calcium channel blocker
Benign prostatic hyperplasia	α -blocker
Essential tremor	Beta blocker (noncardioselective)
Hyperthyroidism	Beta blocker
Migraine	Beta blocker (noncardioselective)
Renal insufficiency	ACE inhibitor Diuretic Calcium channel blocker (non-dihydropyridine)

The majority of patients with primary hypertension will require 2 or more medications to achieve target BP goal. Most of these regimens include a thiazide-type diuretic (unless absolutely contraindicated). A minority of patients require 3 or more medications in combination. Patients who are compliant with their regimen and who do not respond should be evaluated for secondary causes.

HYPERTENSIVE CRISES: EMERGENCIES/URGENCIES AND OTHER CONSIDERATIONS

An occasional patient with primary or secondary hypertension may enter an accelerated phase characterized by severe arterial hypertension and papilledema, a condition known as *malignant hypertension*. Many of these patients also have headache, vomiting, visual disturbances, paralyses, seizures, stupor, or even coma (*hypertensive encephalopathy*). These conditions are termed *hypertensive emergencies*. The patient with a hypertensive emergency may also present with severe hypertension complicated by evidence of acute target organ dysfunction, e.g., unstable angina, acute MI, pulmonary edema, aortic dissection, preeclampsia-eclampsia, or rapidly deteriorating renal function. Although the actual BP level may not be as important as the rate of BP rise, most end-organ damage is noted with systolic BP > 180 mmHg and/or diastolic BP > 120 mmHg. Management of hypertensive emergencies is often performed in the hospital and by means of intravenous drugs, to reduce the BP as rapidly and safely as possible. The mean arterial BP should be reduced by no more than 25% initially, and then, if the patient is stable, to a BP goal of 160/100-110 mmHg over the next several hours. Larger reductions in BP may worsen target organ dysfunction, particularly in the brain. An exception to this rule is aortic dissection which demands that the BP be reduced quickly to a lower target goal (systolic BP <100-120 mmHg) if tolerated. A growing number of agents are available for management of acute hypertensive syndromes. The appropriate therapeutic approach varies according to the clinical presentation (**Figure 13-7**):

- Drugs available for treatment of hypertensive emergencies include parenteral antihypertensives e.g., nitroprusside (Nipride); nitroglycerin; labetalol (Normodyne, Trandate)—combination beta and alpha blocking effects; esmolol (Brevibloc); enalaprilat (Vasotec); fenoldopam (Corlopam); nicardipine (Cardene); clevidipine (Cleviprex); and phentolamine (Regitine).
- Nitroprusside in combination with a beta blocker is especially useful in patients with aortic dissection. Thiocyanate levels should be monitored when using nitroprusside, since cyanide toxicity may occur with high doses, prolonged infusion, or when hepatic or renal impairment is present.
- With myocardial ischemia, IV nitroglycerin or an intravenous beta blocker, e.g., labetalol or esmolol, is preferable.
- ACE inhibitors (and ARBs) slow the progression of nephropathy in patients with diabetes mellitus, and are first line agents in this setting. The practitioner should keep in mind that the dosage of ACE inhibitors needs to be reduced in the presence of renal failure and that these agents (along with ARBs) are contraindicated in pregnancy because they may cause adverse effects on the fetus.
- Methyldopa is the drug of choice in pregnancy because of its proven safety. Hydralazine, labetalol, and calcium channel blockers are also safe and can be used as alternative agents.

Patients with less severe hypertensive syndromes, i.e., *hypertensive urgencies,* have no evidence of acute target organ dysfunction and can often be treated with oral therapy. When the BP has been brought under control, combinations of oral antihypertensive agents can be substituted as parenteral drugs are tapered off.

Antihypertensive medication must be used with caution in certain settings. For example:

- Beta blockers may induce bronchospasm in patients with lung disease.
- ACE inhibitors may worsen renal function, especially with renal artery stenosis (In renal artery stenosis, the kidney needs a high efferent glomerular arteriolar resistance for successful filtration; ACE inhibitors reduce the arteriolar resistance and may result in renal failure).
- Thiazide diuretics are ineffective when the serum creatinine is >2.5 mg/dL.
- Spironolactone may induce hyperkalemia when combined with ACE inhibitors/ARBs or if marked renal insufficiency is present.
- Alpha blockers may induce postural hypotension and should be used with caution in the elderly.
- ACE inhibitors, ARBs, and direct renin inhibitors should be avoided in pregnancy.
- Abruptly stopping clonidine may lead to rebound hypertension.
- Beta blockers may precipitate a hypertensive crisis in patients with pheochromocytoma if given alone or before alpha blockers by leaving α-adrenergic stimulation unopposed.
- The combination of obesity, hypertension, hyperglycemia (adult onset [type II] diabetes mellitus), elevated triglycerides and low HDL cholesterol levels are clues to the *metabolic or insulin resistance syndrome.* Thiazide diuretics should be used with caution since they may exacerbate insulin resistance, and as a result, raise serum glucose levels. Keep in mind that beta blockers may raise triglyceride levels, lower HDL cholesterol levels, promote weight gain, and increase the incidence of new onset diabetes (compared with other antihypertensive drugs).

FIGURE 13-7

Treatment of Hypertensive Emergencies

- **Myocardial ischemia**
  —Nitroglycerin, and beta-blockers
- **Pulmonary edema**
  —Loop diuretic, nitroprusside, nitroglycerin
- **Aortic dissection**
  —Type A–surgery
  —Type B–labetalol, or nitroprusside with a beta-blocker (Avoid medications that predispose to reflex tachycardia)
- **Hypertensive encephalopathy**
  —Sodium nitroprusside, or labetalol
- **Pheochromocytoma** (a catecholamine-secreting tumor)
  —Phentolamine (an alpha blocker)

Hypertension therapy should start with a low dose of a long-acting once-daily drug (preferably a thiazide-type diuretic) and titrate the dose to manage side effects and maximize compliance. If no response, or bothersome side effects occur, another drug from another class should be substituted. If the response is inadequate, but the drug is well tolerated, a second agent from a different class should be added. Although updated BP goals for older hypertensive patients are the same as for younger patients, it is advisable to "start low and go slow".

- Drugs that may exaggerate postural hypotension or cause cognitive dysfunction should be used with caution.
- The peripheral vasodilator SL nifedipine (Procardia) should be avoided due to its unpredictable, and often dramatic and precipitous decrease in BP, along with the reflex increase in heart rate and its attendant threat of damage to the brain or myocardium from hypoperfusion. Elderly patients and those with volume depletion are at particular risk of hypotension during treatment.

BLOOD PRESSURE GOAL AND CHOICE OF DRUG THERAPY

Considerable controversy surrounds the optimal BP goal for the treatment of hypertension. Previous practice guidelines set the BP goal for most adults with hypertension at <140/90 mmHg, irrespective of age, and <130/80 mmHg (based largely on expert opinion) for those with diabetes or chronic kidney disease. Observational studies demonstrated that lower BP is better than higher, and many trials have confirmed that treatment of hypertension is beneficial. Over the years, however, clinical trial data called into question the concept of "lower is better", and failed to show evidence of significant clinical benefit of "intensive" over "standard" BP control in reducing cardiovascular event rates (with the exception of a small reduction in the risk of stroke), and suggested the potential for harm with overly aggressive therapy (so-called "J curve" phenomenon). Accordingly, an expert panel of the eighth Joint National Committee (JNC 8) on the management of hypertension in adults issued updated "evidence – based" guidelines that recommended a less stringent BP goal of <140/90 mmHg for patients with diabetes or chronic kidney disease, the same as for the general population of adults under the age of 60. A slightly more relaxed (and controversial) BP goal of < 150/90 mmHg was recommended for patients age 60 or older, based on prior evidence showing little additional benefit

from achieving a lower BP target. However, not all experts agreed with the revised BP goal for patients over the age of 60, arguing that the evidence does not support the change, and that a less aggressive BP goal may lead to harmful consequences. Other U.S. and international practice guidelines set similar, less intensive BP goals of <140/90 mmHg for "high risk" patients (i.e., those with diabetes, chronic kidney disease or ASCVD) and < 150/90 mmHg for older hypertensive adults, however, the age cutoff (80 years as opposed to 60 years) is higher in some than in the JNC 8 guidelines, and according to many experts, better reflects when treatment-related adverse events, e.g., dizziness and falls, are more likely to occur. Caution is advised against lowering diastolic BP to below 60 mmHg, particularly in CAD patients over the age of 60, since it may reduce coronary perfusion and worsen myocardial ischemia.

Adding more fuel to the debate are the results of a recent "landmark" clinical trial that has shown a beneficial effect of an aggressive systolic BP goal of < 120 mmHg as compared to <140 mmHg in reducing cardiovascular event rates (CHF, but not MI or stroke) and mortality, albeit at a cost of additional medication side effects, e.g., hypotension, syncope, and acute kidney injury, in "high risk" non-diabetic hypertensive adults age 50 years and older. Of note, BP measurements in this trial were taken unattended (to minimize "white-coat" effect) using an automated device, which tend to be 5-10 mmHg lower than if taken manually (auscultatory method). As a result, updated guidelines now recommend a more intensive manual (auscultatory) BP target of <130/80 mmHg in patients with, or at high risk for, cardiovascular disease, if it can be achieved without producing significant medication side effects. Regardless of the BP goal, BP reduction should be gradual and treatment individualized ("one size does not fit all"), and should be accompanied by appropriate lifestyle modifications and management of other cardiovascular risk factors.

As primary preventive therapy, β-blockers are less effective than other antihypertensive agents at reducing the risk of stroke, lack cardiovascular morbidity and mortality benefit, and have adverse metabolic effects. Therefore, for non-black patients with uncomplicated hypertension without known CAD, preference should be given to ACE inhibitors, ARBs, calcium channel blockers, and thiazide-type diuretics. For black patients, initial therapy should include a thiazide-type diuretic or calcium channel blocker. For patients with chronic kidney disease, initial (or add-on) therapy should include an ACE inhibitor or ARB (not both combined), to preserve renal function, with close monitoring of potassium and serum creatinine levels. The combination of an ACE inhibitor plus a calcium channel blocker has recently been shown to be effective initial therapy, possibly superior to the combination of an ACE inhibitor (or a β-blocker) and a thiazide diuretic. However, chlorthalidone is longer acting than hydrochlorothiazide, provides greater 24 hour BP reduction, and may be associated with better clinical outcomes. For the management of hypertension in patients with established CAD (stable or unstable angina, non ST or ST elevation MI), β-blockers along with ACE inhibitors or ARBs are the treatment of choice. If further BP lowering is needed, a thiazide diuretic and/or a dihydropyridine calcium channel blocker, e.g., amlodipine, can be added. If a β-blocker is contraindicated or not tolerated, a non-dihydropyridine calcium channel blocker, e.g., diltiazem or verapamil, can be substituted. If there is LV systolic dysfunction, recommended therapy consists of an ACE inhibitor or ARB, a β-blocker, and either a thiazide or loop diuretic. In patients with more severe heart failure, an aldosterone antagonist and direct-acting vasodilators, e.g., hydralazine/isosorbide dinitrate (in African American patients) should be considered.

RESISTANT HYPERTENSION

Resistant hypertension is defined as a BP that remains elevated despite the use of 3 or more antihypertensive medications (including a diuretic) at optimal dosages. Successful treatment of patients with resistant hypertension requires consideration of lifestyle factors that contribute to treatment resistance, e.g., obesity, dietary salt intake, and alcohol consumption; diagnosing and treating secondary causes of hypertension, e.g., drug-related causes (NSAIDs, steroids, oral contraceptives, decongestants, diet pills, cocaine, licorice, amphetamine-like stimulants, ephedra, cyclosporine, and erythropoietin), obstructive sleep apnea, chronic kidney disease, primary aldosteronism, and renal artery stenosis; and using multiple drug treatments with different mechanisms of action effectively. In this regard, a generally useful strategy for most patients with resistant hypertension is to combine an ACE inhibitor or ARB, together with a long acting calcium channel blocker (e.g., amlodipine), and a thiazide-like diuretic (preferably chlorthalidone). If the BP remains uncontrolled despite an optimized 3-drug regimen, other antihypertensive medications e.g., an aldosterone antagonist (spironolactone, eplerenone), vasodilating β-blocker (combined α-/β-blocker [e.g., carvedilol, labetalol] or nebivolol), pure α-blocker (e.g., terazosin, doxazosin), central acting antiadrenergic agent (e.g., clonidine), and direct vasodilator (e.g., hydralazine, minoxidil) can be added as needed. Among specific classes of antihypertensive medications, diuretics are the most useful (and most underused) agents in the man-

agement of resistant hypertension. Medications that antagonize mineralocorticoid receptor actions i.e., aldosterone antagonists, e.g., spironolactone, can further reduce BP among patients receiving multiple antihypertensive medications, particularly those with primary aldosteronism (which is found in ~20% of patients with resistant hypertension). Loop diuretics should be considered in patients with chronic kidney disease and/or those receiving potent vasodilators (e.g., minoxidil).

Evaluation of patients with resistant hypertension should be directed at confirming true treatment resistance. Excluding "pseudo-resistance" due to poor patient adherence to therapy (one of the leading causes of uncontrolled hypertension) or a "white-coat" effect may require more frequent office visits and home, work, or 24 hour ambulatory BP monitoring. The central acting alpha 2 agonist clonidine is a poor choice in intermittently compliant patients due to sudden rebound hypertension that may result if the drug is abruptly stopped. Since complex dosing regimens are associated with poor patient compliance, prescribed regimens should be simplified as much as possible. Dosing some antihypertensive medications at night may reduce BP to a greater degree than dosing during the day. If the BP remains uncontrolled after 6 months of treatment or a specific secondary cause of hypertension is suspected, referral to an appropriate specialist is recommended.

It should be noted, however, that despite focused efforts on lifestyle modification and aggressive pharmacological treatment strategies, a significant number of patients with resistant hypertension fail to achieve adequate BP control, even under expert-guided care, and remain at high risk for a major cardiovascular event. (**Note:** Cardiovascular risk doubles with each increment of 20/10 mmHg in BP). Evidence suggests that treatment failure in these patients may be due, at least in part, to over-activation of the sympathetic nervous system. Recently developed interventional therapies targeting excess sympathetic neural activity, either directly by radiofrequency catheter ablation of the renal artery sympathetic nerves (*renal sympathetic denervation*), or indirectly by electrical activation of the carotid baroreflex via a surgically implantable pacemaker-like baroreceptor stimulation device (*carotid baroreflex activation*), are currently undergoing active investigation. Although results from preliminary clinical trials have been promising, more recent clinical trial data has failed to show a significant benefit of renal sympathetic denervation in lowering BP when compared to a placebo. As a result, the future role of these novel device-based therapies in the management of treatment-resistant hypertension is uncertain.

CHAPTER 14.   APPROACH TO THE PATIENT WITH DYSLIPIDEMIA

Atherosclerotic cardiovascular disease (ASCVD) is the leading cause of morbidity and mortality in the United States. Dyslipidemia, i.e., elevated serum levels of total and LDL cholesterol, low HDL cholesterol, and/or high triglycerides, is a powerful risk factor for atherosclerosis, and its proper identification and treatment, particularly LDL cholesterol reduction with a statin, the cornerstone in the primary and secondary prevention of CAD. This chapter will provide an overview of plasma lipids, their role in the pathogenesis of atherosclerosis, and the practical approach to the patient who presents with dyslipidemia.

LIPIDS AND ATHEROSCLEROSIS

Lipids, e.g., cholesterol and triglycerides, are transported around the body by particles called lipoproteins. These lipoproteins contain surface proteins, known as apoproteins (apo), that help guide lipid transport and metabolism. Lipoproteins can be classified as high density lipoprotein (HDL), intermediate density lipoprotein (IDL), low density lipoprotein (LDL), very low density lipoprotein (VLDL), and chylomicrons. All lipoprotein fractions play a role in atherogenesis. Two major apo B containing lipoproteins, cholesterol-rich LDL (especially small, dense LDL) and its genetic variant, lipoprotein (a), and triglyceride-rich VLDL, promote atherosclerosis, whereas apo A-1 containing HDL cholesterol inhibits the process due to HDL's ability to transport lipids away from the vessel walls back to the liver for disposal (so-called "reverse cholesterol transport"). The development of atherosclerosis is a complex interaction between genetic predisposition, CAD risk factors, endothelial dysfunction, lipid accumulation (mainly oxidized LDL), vascular inflammation, and arterial thrombosis. Dyslipidemia has emerged as a major modifiable risk factor and clinical trials have clearly demonstrated the benefits of pharmacologic lipid reduction, especially LDL cholesterol lowering with a statin, in patients with or at risk for CAD. The lipid "hypothesis", therefore, is no longer a theory, it is a fact! Numerous primary and secondary prevention studies have demonstrated a nearly 30% reduction rate in CAD death or non-fatal MI with statin therapy.

The most important prognostic feature of CAD is the stability or instability of the coronary atherosclerotic plaque. A previously unstable (but nonobstructive and noncalcified) lipid-rich and inflammatory plaque can rupture with sudden partial or total occlusion from coronary thrombosis, resulting in an acute coronary syndrome (unstable angina, acute MI) or sudden cardiac death. These unstable plaques that are vulnerable to rupture are usually not large and appear on coronary angiography to obstruct <70% of the arterial lumen. This explains why a patient may have no symptoms, a normal resting ECG, exercise stress test, and cardiovascular examination, and even a negative EBCT scan, and have a heart attack soon thereafter! The stability or instability of a coronary plaque is not discernible by EBCT or routine coronary angiography. Elevated serum LDL-cholesterol levels, however, are a major contributor to the development of the unstable coronary plaque. HMG-coenzyme A reductase inhibitors ("statins"), for example, can lower LDL cholesterol, decrease lipid deposition in the arterial wall, reduce inflammation (as measured by reduction in C-reactive protein), improve endothelial dysfunction, stabilize the plaque and make it less likely to rupture. (**Note:** A 1% reduction in LDL cholesterol level correlates with ~1% reduction in CAD rates.) Aggressive lipid-lowering therapy with a statin should be strongly encouraged in both the primary (patients without evident CAD) and secondary (patients with known vascular disease) prevention of CAD. Beta blockers and ACE inhibitors can also stabilize plaques. A ruptured plaque may heal or result in clot formation, often with more severe stenosis. Keep in mind that aspirin helps to prevent clot formation and is effective in reducing primary and secondary coronary events.

THERAPEUTIC CONSIDERATIONS

Dyslipidemia is usually asymptomatic, but may on rare occasion be discovered when physical signs of hyperlipidemia (e.g., xanthelasmas, corneal arcus, xanthomas) or more commonly when abnormal lipid levels are detected during routine examination or evaluation of a patient. Therapeutic lifestyle changes, e.g., diet and exercise, are mainstays of lipid management. Lifestyle changes alone, however, rarely reduce LDL cholesterol more than 10–20%. As an adjunct to lifestyle interventions, there are seven major classes of drugs that are used to treat lipid disorders (**Figure 14-1**). Before starting lipid therapy, however, a potentially reversible secondary cause of dyslipidemia, e.g., hypothyroidism, poorly controlled diabetes, obesity, excess alcohol use, or drugs (e.g., thiazide diuretics, β-Blockers, estrogens, steroids, protease inhibitors) should be searched for and corrected if possible. In general, the higher the overall CAD risk, the lower should be the LDL-cholesterol.

According to previous practice guidelines, risk factors that modify treatment goals for LDL cholesterol include:

- Cigarette smoking
- Hypertension

FIGURE 14-1

Treatment of Dyslipidemia

Drug	LDL	HDL	TG	Side Effects
HMG-CoA reductase inhibitors (Statins) **Lovastatin (Mevacor)** **Pravastatin (Pravachol)** **Simvastatin (Zocor)** **Atorvastatin (Lipitor)** **Fluvastatin (Lescol)** **Rosuvastatin (Crestor)** **Pitavastatin (Livalo)**	↓ 18–55%	↑ 5–15%	↓ 7–30%	Hepatotoxicity ⎫ dose-dependent (especially Myopathy ⎭ high dose simvastatin)* Small ↑ risk of new onset diabetes and cognitive dysfunction (outweighed by ↓ CAD events and ↓ mortality) Potential drug interactions
Bile acid sequestrants (Resins) **Cholestyramine (Questran)** **Colestipol (Colestid)** **Colesevelam (Welchol)**	↓ 15–30%	↑ 3–5%	may ↑	GI distress, constipation, bloating
Fibrates **Gemfibrozil (Lopid)** **Fenofibrate (Tricor)** **Fenofibric acid (Trilipix)**	↓ 5–20%	↑ 10–35%	↓ 20–50%	GI distress, nausea, gallstones Myopathy (when with statin)— especially gemfibrozil
Nicotinic acid (Niacin)	↓ 5–25%	↑ 15–35%	↓ 20–50%	Flushing (may be relieved by aspirin), pruritus, GI distress, exacerbates peptic ulcer disease, hyperglycemia, hyperuricemia (or gout), hepatotoxicity
Cholesterol absorption inhibitors **Ezetimibe (Zetia)**	↓ 18–20%	↑ 1–5%	↓ 5–11%	Generally well tolerated. Slightly more fatigue, GI distress, muscle and back pain compared to placebo Hepatotoxicity (when with statin)
Omega-3 fatty acids **Fish oil (Lovaza)**	may ↑	↑ 5–10%	↓ 20–50%	GI distress, nausea, fishy after taste, may increase bleeding when used with antiplatelet or anticoagulant agents.
PCSK9 inhibitors **Alirocumab (Praluent)** **Evolocumab (Repatha)**	↓ 40-65%	↑ 5–10%	↓ 15–25%	Myalgias, rash, urticaria, cognitive effects, mild injection-site reactions

*****Note:** Risk of myopathy increases significantly with 80 mg dose of simvastatin (avoid unless dose already tolerated > 12 months).

- Low HDL (<40 mg/dL); High HDL (≥60mg/dL) is a "negative" risk (subtract 1 risk factor)
- Positive family history of coronary artery disease (Men, first degree relative <55 years) (Women, first degree relative < 65 years)
- Age (Men ≥45 years)(Women ≥55 years)

The cholesterol-lowering agents have long been used to achieve a primary goal target LDL cholesterol level of:

- <160 mg/dL if no CAD and 0–1 risk factors
- <130 mg/dL if no CAD and ≥ 2 risk factors
- <100 mg/dL if CAD, PAD, AAA, carotid artery disease, and/or diabetes mellitus is present. Those with ACS, CAD and multiple risk factors or diabetes are at very high risk and a target LDL cholesterol level of <70 mg/dL has been the goal.

For individuals who have a low HDL cholesterol and a high triglyceride level, secondary goals have included a target HDL cholesterol of >40 mg/dL, a triglyceride level of < 150 mg/dL, a "non-HDL" cholesterol (total cholesterol − HDL cholesterol) level 30 mg/dL higher than the target LDL cholesterol goals, and an apo B level (a measure of the total number of atherogenic lipoprotein particles) of <90 mg/dL (or <80 mg/dL if at very high risk).

CAD is preventable. In concert with reduction of other CAD risk factors (e.g., cigarette smoking, hypertension, diabetes mellitus), all patients over age 20 should be screened for elevated total and LDL-cholesterol, reduced HDL-cholesterol, and elevated triglycerides at least once every 5 years. Keep in mind that when you order a lipid profile, the usual lipids measured directly are total cholesterol, HDL cholesterol and triglycerides. In general, the higher the HDL (so-called "good") cholesterol (which protects the arteries against the build-up of fatty deposits) and the lower the triglycerides, the better. The level of LDL cholesterol (referred to as "bad" cholesterol since it causes fatty deposits to build up in the arteries) is a valuable clue to determining the risk for ASCVD. Another lipoprotein, Lp(a), is associated with increased risk for CAD, but treatment with statins does not lower Lp(a) levels or risk. Small LDL particles and HDL subfractions are related to CAD, but are not superior to LDL or HDL in predicting risk. Measurement of these other lipoproteins is not routinely indicated.

Although LDL cholesterol can be measured directly, it is more commonly calculated indirectly by clinical laboratories using the following formula: *LDL cholesterol =* total cholesterol − HDL cholesterol − *(triglyceride/5).* (**Note:** If the triglyceride level is >400 mg/dL, this formula will not be accurate.) Total cholesterol and HDL cholesterol levels can be measured at any time of the day in the non-fasting state, but triglyceride levels should be measured only from fasting patients (at least 12–14 hours after eating) because triglycerides increase after a fatty meal. It is important to keep this in mind since *the higher the triglycerides, the lower the calculated LDL cholesterol.* Thus, LDL cholesterol may be falsely low in the non-fasting state, rather than elevated (as is sometimes assumed). Cholesterol levels measured within the first 24 hours post-MI reflect pre-event lipid values. Cholesterol values fall markedly (and triglyceride levels rise), however, in the week post-MI and remain low for up to 1 month. Patients who recently had a MI, therefore, should be tested at a later time. Lipid determinations are best carried out in stable ambulatory patients.

For the past decade, practice guidelines have focused primarily on reducing LDL cholesterol by at least 30–40%, particularly with a statin. The exception is the case of very high triglycerides (>500–1000 mg/dL) which requires urgent correction to prevent acute pancreatitis. If adequate LDL cholesterol lowering can not be achieved with statin therapy alone, either ezetimibe, a bile acid sequestrant, or niacin may be added; however, proof of clinical benefit for the latter two is lacking. In patients with triglyceride levels >200 mg/dL, non-HDL cholesterol (a surrogate marker of apo B) has been the next target, and the clinician may consider adding a fibrate or niacin to statin therapy. Although high triglycerides and low HDL cholesterol are associated with an increased risk for CAD, there is no clearcut evidence of cardiovascular benefit from treating these disorders. Since elevated triglycerides are often associated with

other lipid abnormalities, e.g., low HDL cholesterol levels and small dense LDL particles (atherogenic dyslipidemia), along with a cluster of other risk factors (e.g., abdominal obesity, hypertension, and fasting hyperglycemia) as part of the *metabolic syndrome*, treatment of high risk patients with niacin, a fibrate, or fish oil in addition to statin therapy seems reasonable. **(Figure 14-2)** Both fibrates and niacin lower triglycerides, raise HDL cholesterol, and can shift small, dense ("pattern B") LDL particles that are highly atherogenic to larger, more buoyant and fluffy ("pattern A") LDL particles which are less atherogenic. Refractory cases of hypertriglyceridemia may benefit from omega-3 fatty acids (fish oil supplements) which, by reducing VLDL production, can lower the triglyceride level by 20–50%. If multiple drug therapy is being considered, lipid levels, along with liver enzymes, e.g., transaminases and creatinine kinase (clues to hepatotoxicity and myopathy, respectively) should be monitored as needed.

It should be realized, however, that the target lipid levels that have long been recommended by practice guidelines have not been based on solid clinical trial evidence. Furthermore, despite improvements in the lipid profile, no currently available lipid controlling drugs with the exception of ezetimibe, have been shown to offer significant cardiovascular benefit over statin therapy alone. Accordingly, the American Heart Association has issued updated "evidence-based"

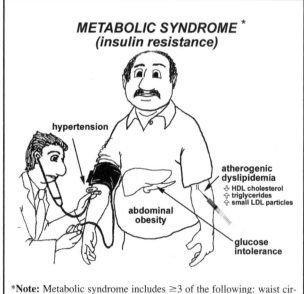

METABOLIC SYNDROME *
(insulin resistance)

hypertension

atherogenic dyslipidemia
⇩ HDL cholesterol
⇧ triglycerides
⇧ small LDL particles

abdominal obesity

glucose intolerance

*Note: Metabolic syndrome includes ≥3 of the following: waist circumference >40 in. (men) or >35 in. (women); triglycerides >150 mg/dL; HDL cholesterol <40 mg/dL (men) or <50 mg/dL (women); BP >130/85 mmHg; fasting glucose >100 mg/dL.

Figure 14-2

FIGURE 14-3

Treatment of Blood Cholesterol to Reduce Atherosclerotic Cardiovascular Risk in Adults

Patient Groups		Treatment
With atherosclerotic cardiovascular disease and ≥ 21 years of age	≤ 75 years of age	High intensity statin
	> 75 years of age	Moderate intensity statin
With an LDL cholesterol level of ≥ 190 mg/dL	— — — — — —	High intensity statin
With a 10 year ASCVD risk of ≥ 7.5%	— — — — — —	High intensity statin
With type 1 or 2 diabetes and ages 40-75 years	— — — — — —	Moderate intensity statin
With a 10 year ASCVD risk of ≥ 7.5% and ages 40–75 years	— — — — — —	Moderate to high intensity statin

Note: High intensity statin lowers LDL cholesterol by ≥50%; moderate intensity statin lowers LDL cholesterol by 30-50%.

Adapted from Stone, NJ, Robinson J, Lichtenstein AH, et al. AHA/ACC guidelines on the treatment of blood cholesterol to reduce atherosclerotic cardiovascular risk in adults J Am Coll Cardiol, 2013.

guidelines on cholesterol management that has shifted the focus away from treatment to specific LDL (and non-HDL) cholesterol targets to reduction in overall cardiovascular risk with therapeutic lifestyle changes, along with the use of moderate to high intensity statin therapy which, by virtue of its LDL-cholesterol lowering (by at least 30-50%) and pleiotropic (e.g., antiinflammatory, antithrombotic) effects, has been shown to be beneficial in the primary and secondary prevention of atherosclerotic cardiovascular disease (ASCVD). Four groups of patients who derive the most benefit from statin therapy, regardless of the baseline lipid levels, have been identified. These include patients who already have ASCVD (CAD, stroke/TIA, PAD); those with an LDL-cholesterol of ≥ 190 mg/dL (i.e., familial hypercholesterolemia); individuals aged 40 to 75 years with diabetes; and those who have an estimated 10 year risk of ASCVD of at least 7.5%, based on a new risk calculator (which some experts claim may overestimate risk) that factors in age, gender, race, cholesterol levels, BP, diabetes and smoking status. If risk remains unclear, other factors, e.g., family history of premature ASCVD, high sensi-

tivity C-reactive protein (a marker of inflammation), coronary calcium score, and ankle brachial index may be considered (**Figure 14-3**). Due to the lack of clinical trial evidence, non-statin therapies, alone or in combination with a statin, are not recommended as first line treatment to reduce ASCVD risk. However, non-statin lipid controlling agents e.g., ezetimibe, may be considered in patients who have an inadequate response to statin therapy or are statin-intolerant since recent clinical trial data has shown that the addition of ezetimibe to a statin in high risk ACS patients provides incremental cardiovascular benefit over statin therapy alone. Novel cholesterol lowering therapies, e.g., injectable (subcutaneous) monoclonal antibodies (alirocumab [Praluent], evolocumab [Repatha]) that inhibit the function of proprotein convertase subtilisin-kexin type 9, so-called *PCSK9 inhibitors*, lower LDL cholesterol substantially more than ezetimibe (by 40–70%). These agents have recently been approved as an adjunct to statin therapy for high risk patients with heterozygous familial hypercholesterolemia or known ASCVD, and hold promise as alternative therapy for patients who are statin-intolerant. Results from preliminary clinical trials have been encouraging. Long term cardiovascular outcome data will help establish the role of these powerful (and more costly) new cholesterol lowering agents in ASCVD risk management.

* * *

Pearls:

- In addition to therapeutic lifestyle changes, statins (by virtue of their LDL cholesterol lowering and pleiotropic effects) are the drugs of choice for primary and secondary prevention of ASCVD.

- Four groups of patients who derive the most benefit from statin therapy include those with ASCVD, an LDL cholesterol ≥190 mg/dL, diabetes mellitus (ages 40–75 years), and an estimated 10 year ASCVD risk ≥7.5%.

- When considering the "cluster" of risk factors in the patient with metabolic syndrome, keep in mind the mnemonic **"HOLD"** (**H**ypertension, **O**besity, **L**ipid disorders, **D**iabetes).

- Although low HDL cholesterol and high triglycerides (atherogenic dyslipidemia) are linked to increased ASCVD risk, no lipid controlling therapy, with the exception of ezetimibe, has been shown to offer significant cardiovascular benefit over a statin alone.

- In patients intolerant to high dose statins, lower doses or a different statin may be tried on alternate days (or with coenzyme Q10), before switching to other cholesterol lowering drugs.

* * *

CHAPTER 15.   APPROACH TO THE PATIENT WITH VALVULAR HEART DISEASE

Valvular heart disease (VHD) is one of the major types of cardiac disease encountered in clinical practice. With the declining incidence of acute rheumatic fever, mitral valve prolapse and congenital bicuspid aortic valve are now the most common valvular lesions. Updated guidelines classify VHD into four stages: at risk **(stage A)**, progressive (mild to moderate) and asymptomatic **(stage B)**, asymptomatic severe **(stage C)**, with normal (C1) or abnormal (C2) LV or RV function, and symptomatic severe **(stage D)**. In its earliest stages, valvular dysfunction may be detected by a specific heart murmur (produced by stenosis or regurgitation) and later by the symptoms and/or signs that are characteristic of the natural history of the disease. There are five steps the practitioner should take in the clinical evaluation of the patient with VHD.

- Correctly diagnosing the affected valve(s)
- Estimating the severity of the lesion
- Judging its effect on the myocardium
- Deciding on the need (or lack thereof) for infective endocarditis (or antistreptococcal) prophylaxis*
- Deciding on the advisability and/or timing of surgical (or catheter-based) intervention

*Note: Antibiotic prophylaxis is no longer recommended for patients with VHD unless the patient has a history of previous endocarditis, or has undergone a valve replacement or repair using prosthetic material.

AORTIC STENOSIS (AS)

Aortic stenosis (AS) is the most common fatal valvular heart lesion in adults. In the older population (i.e., those over 65 years of age), "degenerative" calcification of a normal trileaflet aortic valve (aortic sclerosis), now considered to be an inflammatory process related to atherosclerosis, has emerged as the most common cause. Younger adults (particularly males) with isolated aortic stenosis most often have a congenitally bicuspid valve traumatized by abnormal turbulent flow patterns, which over years to decades produced fibrosis and calcification by a process of "wear and tear". Rheumatic heart disease may also cause AS but is infrequent without associated mitral valve involvement.

Figure 15-1 summarizes the clinical approach to severe valvular aortic stenosis.

Clinical Recognition of AS

AS may be recognized in a variety of ways. The disease is often discovered during a routine clinical examination when a heart murmur is heard or an abnormal ECG is noted for the first time. In other instances, the patient may present with angina pectoris, exertional dyspnea, episodes of effort-related lightheadedness, or a true syncopal spell. Initial clinical evaluation of all patients, therefore, must include a careful detailed history with particular focus on these cardinal symptoms. It should be noted, however, that the disease is marked initially by a long, latent asymptomatic period which precedes the onset of these classic symptoms. Most patients with mild to moderate valvular AS are asymptomatic and develop symptoms only when the valve obstruction becomes severe.

The cardiac physical examination will generally reveal the severity of the underlying valvular lesion. The hallmark of valvular AS is a harsh, grunting (similar to the sound of clearing one's throat), crescendo-decrescendo systolic ejection murmur best heard over the aortic area, radiating into the neck (carotids), over the clavicles (bone conduction) and down to the apex, where it may have a high frequency musical quality (so-called "*Gallavardin phenomenon*"), especially in the elderly, or in barrel-chested individuals with COPD. (**Figures 15-2 and 15-3**).

Figure 15-2. Left. Schematic diagram showing the morphologic features of a degenerative trileaflet aortic valve. Note focal cuspal fibrous thickening and calcific deposits. **Right.** Clinical findings in severe valvular aortic stenosis. Note the loud late peaking crescendo-decrescendo aortic systolic ejection murmur accompanied by an S4 gallop. The carotid pulse tracing demonstrates a slow rate of rise along with palpable coarse systolic vibrations ("shudder") on the upstroke.

Figure 15-3. Schematic diagram illustrating the clinical findings in a middle-aged male with valvular AS who is experiencing symptoms of chest pain, shortness of breath and near-syncopal episodes on exertion. Note the loud late peaking aortic systolic ejection murmur associated with a palpable systolic thrill, radiating toward the right shoulder and neck regions. The murmur is well heard across the precordium to the apex, where it has a musical quality. LV hypertrophy with "strain" pattern is noted on the ECG (**Figure 3-38**) along with aortic valve calcification and post stenotic dilatation of the ascending aorta on the chest x-ray. (**Figure 4-7B**). A systolic gradient of 100 mmHg is present on Doppler echo. Cardiac catheterization confirms the presence of severe AS with no associated coronary artery disease.

The length of the murmur is key. The murmur of aortic sclerosis and/or mild stenosis is not very long and does not peak late. As the severity of the stenosis increases with time, the murmur becomes loud and prolonged, peaking later in systole; it is then accompanied by an S4 gallop (due to enhanced atrial contraction against a stiff, noncompliant hypertrophied LV); a single (absent A2) or paradoxically

FIGURE 15-1

Clinical Approach to Severe Valvular Aortic Stenosis

Etiology	History	Physical Exam	ECG	Chest X-Ray	Lab Tests	Timing of Surgical Intervention
(Congenital, degenerative, rheumatic) If isolated lesion (e.g., congenital bicuspid valve, calcified trileaflet valve) most commonly seen in older males.	Angina, CHF, syncope (prone to sudden death).	Harsh late-peaking systolic ejection murmur radiating to neck (murmur may ↓ as cardiac output ↓), palpable systolic thrill, weak and slow rising carotid pulse, sustained LV impulse, S2 single (absent A2) or paradoxical split, S4 gallop.	LV hypertrophy, LBBB also common. Heart block (rare) from calcific involvement of conduction system.	Aortic valve calcification, Post-stenotic dilatation of aorta, LV prominence without dilation.	Echo: calcified aortic valve, mean Doppler gradient ≥ 40 mmHg, LV hypertrophy, aortic valve area ≤ 1.0 cm² Cath: confirms LV-aortic gradient >50 mmHg (lower if LV dysfunction due to decreased flow) and aortic valve area ≤ 1.0 cm², and documents concomitant CAD (present in 50%).	Aortic valve replacement as soon as possible in symptomatic patients (Percutaneous balloon valvuloplasty for temporary [6 months] relief of symptoms or TAVR in those at intermediate to high surgical risk). Asymptomatic patients with LV dysfunction (EF <50%) may also be candidates for surgery.

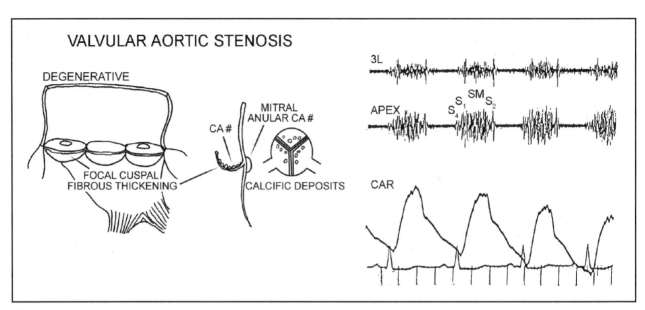

Figure 15-2

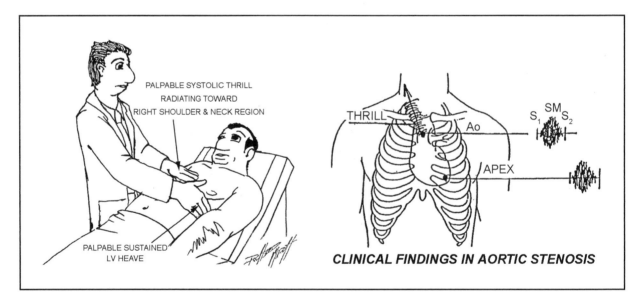

Figure 15-3 (Courtesy of W. Proctor Harvey, M.D.)

split S2 (secondary to prolongation of LV ejection due to severe outflow obstruction); a palpable systolic thrill directed towards the right clavicle; and a small, weak, slow-rising, late-peaking (*pulsus parvus et tardus*) arterial pulse, often with a palpable carotid shudder, a forceful, slow and sustained LV apical heave, and an apical-carotid or brachioradial delay.

The duration of the murmur is more important than intensity as an indicator of the severity of the obstruction. If advanced LV failure is present, however, the systolic murmur may become short or even absent, consequent to the marked decrease in cardiac output and reduced forward flow across the aortic valve. Furthermore, the signs of severity of valvular AS are less reliable in the elderly. Older patients often have stiff, less compliant carotid vessels, resulting in a more rapid pulse transit time to the neck (pseudonormalization of the upstroke), thereby masking the arterial pulse findings of hemodynamically significant valvular AS. The arterial pulse may then feel normal or show a normal or slightly increased pressure.

Laboratory studies can be quite helpful in assessing the severity of AS. The ECG may show evidence of LV hypertrophy with strain when the LV is significantly pressure loaded, and LBBB (due to calcific invasion of the conduction system) is not uncommon as AS progresses. Valve calcification (best seen on the lateral view) along with post-stenotic dilatation of the aorta may be noted on the CXR. In general, the absence of calcium in the aortic valve in patients over 35 indicates the absence of severe AS. Echo is most helpful in confirming the diagnosis, documenting valve calcification, and estimating the aortic valve area and gradient. Invasive testing should be reserved for those patients being considered for surgery in whom conflicting clinical and echocardiographic findings exist and to rule-out coexisting CAD. Cardiac catheterization delineates the severity (measures the systolic pressure gradient between the LV and aorta, along with aortic valve area) and documents the presence of concomitant CAD (~50% of cases), which may require a combination of aortic valve replacement and coronary bypass at the time of surgery (if severe AS, i.e., aortic valve area ≤ 1.0 cm² is found) (**Figures 15-1, 15-4, and 15-5**).

Figure 15-4. Left. M-mode echocardiogram in a patient with severe calcific valvular aortic stenosis. Note aortic valve opening is markedly reduced with multiple dense echoes (arrow) consistent with sclerotic and heavily calcified aortic valve. **Right.** Continuous wave Doppler flow recording across aortic valve in a patient with severe valvular AS. Peak aortic flow velocity is 5 meters per second. Applying the modified Bernoulli equation (peak transaortic gradient $[P] = 4 \times V^2$), the estimated peak pressure gradient would be 100 mmHg.

Figure 15-5. Left. Left ventricular (LV) and aortic (Ao) pressure tracings in severe aortic stenosis. **Right.** Note the large systolic pressure gradient (~100 mmHg) across the aortic valve with delayed upstroke of the arterial pulse.

Isolated valvular AS in young and middle-aged adult males is most often due to a congenital bicuspid aortic valve. Consequently, the disease may be manifested as an aortic ejection sound heard best at the aortic area and cardiac apex, not varying with respiration, along with a systolic murmur and in some cases, an early high-pitched blowing diastolic murmur of AR (**Figure 15-6**). An S4 gallop in these young individuals (without other reasons for LV hypertrophy) usually indicates a hemodynamically significant degree of stenosis. The patient may remain completely asymptomatic for several decades during which time stenosis progresses in severity. Later in the course of the disease, often by age 40–50, the cardinal symptoms of angina (related to the imbalance between myocardial oxygen supply and demand), syncope (due to decreased cerebral perfusion in the setting of a fixed cardiac output), and CHF (due to elevated filling pressures in the stiff hypertrophied LV [diastolic dysfunction]) emerge, heralding a rapidly progressive

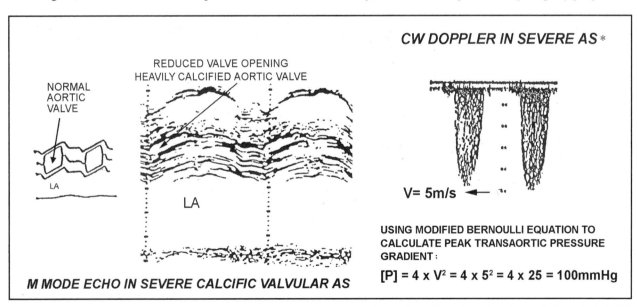

CW DOPPLER IN SEVERE AS *

NORMAL AORTIC VALVE

LA

REDUCED VALVE OPENING
HEAVILY CALCIFIED AORTIC VALVE

LA

V= 5m/s ◄

USING MODIFIED BERNOULLI EQUATION TO CALCULATE PEAK TRANSAORTIC PRESSURE GRADIENT:

$[P] = 4 \times V^2 = 4 \times 5^2 = 4 \times 25 = 100mmHg$

M MODE ECHO IN SEVERE CALCIFIC VALVULAR AS

*Note: Severe AS is defined as a valve area ≤ 1.0 cm² (normal 3 to 4 cm²), a mean gradient ≥ 40 mmHg, and a peak aortic jet velocity ≥ 4 m/s (which corresponds to a peak gradient ≥ 64 mmHg). Patients with LV systolic dysfunction and reduced cardiac output may have lower pressure gradients, but severe AS by calculated valve area. If AS is truly severe, increasing the cardiac output during dobutamine stress echo will increase the gradient but the valve area will remain ≤ 1.0 cm². If dobutamine increases the valve area to >1 cm² but the gradient does not change, "pseudo-severe AS" is said to be present. The absence of any change in valve area or gradient indicates that contractile reserve is poor and benefit from surgery is unlikely.

Figure 15-4

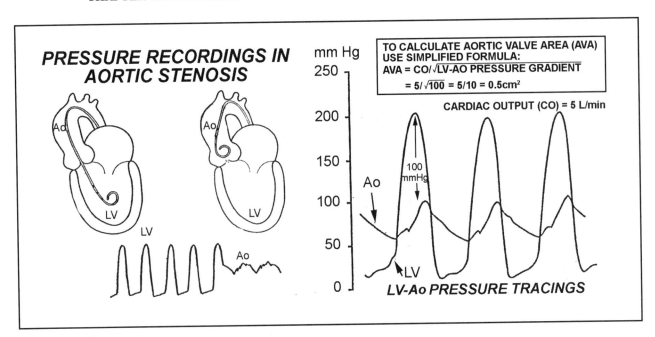

Figure 15-5

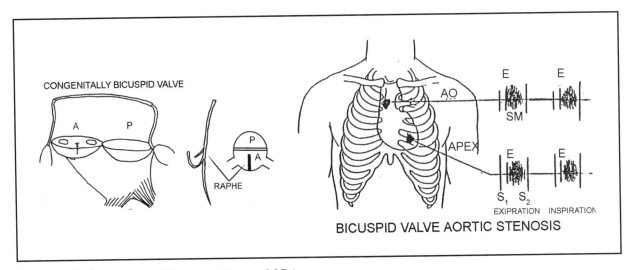

Figure 15-6 (Courtesy of W. Proctor Harvey, M.D.)

downhill course along with a substantial risk of sudden death that is unresponsive to medical management alone. Surgery is clearly indicated in these patients.

Figure 15-6. Left. Morphologic features of a congenitally bicuspid aortic valve. **Right.** A patient with congenital bicuspid aortic valve stenosis. The ejection sound (E) is unchanged by respiration and is well heard over the aortic area and apex. The ejection sound is not eliminated with firm pressure of the stethoscope, as would be the case with an S4 gallop. (Courtesy of Dr. W. Proctor Harvey).

Figure 15-7. Left. Schematic illustration of a congenital bicuspid aortic valve. **Right.** Two-dimensional echo, parasternal short axis view, demonstrating bicuspid aortic valve.

Figure 15-8. Left. Schematic diagram of calcific bicuspid and tricuspid aortic valve stenosis. **Right.** The natural history of valvular aortic stenosis. There is a long, latent asymptomatic period during which stenosis progresses in severity and survival is nearly normal. When symptoms of angina, syncope, or heart failure occur, there is a dramatic increase in mortality along with a substantial increased risk

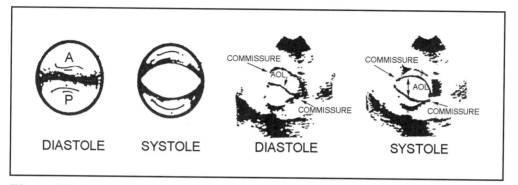

Figure 15-7

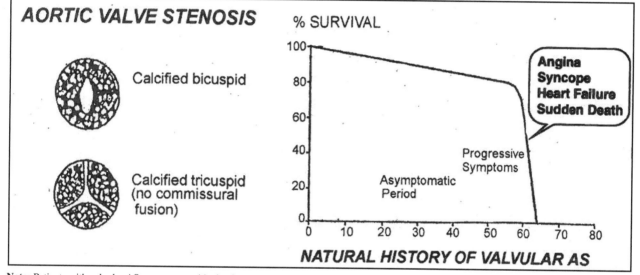

Note: Patients with valvular AS can present with classic symptoms, which can be remembered by the mnemonic **"SAD"**: **S**yncope **A**ngina, and **D**yspnea (i.e., heart failure). AVR is indicated once symptoms occur since survival is limited and there is an increased risk of sudden death.

Figure 15-8

of sudden death unless aortic valve replacement is performed.

Management of AS

The question of surgical intervention in asymptomatic patients with significant AS remains controversial. The asymptomatic patient with valvular AS may generally be treated medically until symptoms develop. The risk of sudden death in asymptomatic patients is extremely low (<1%). Patients should be advised to report the onset of symptoms as soon as they occur. Once symptoms of angina, syncope, or CHF develop, survival is likely limited to 5 years, 3 years, or 2 years, respectively, unless surgery is performed. Aortic valve replacement in the symptomatic patient with significant valvular AS, therefore, should be strongly recommended without delay.

While "watchful waiting" is generally considered safe in asymptomatic patients with valvular AS, some experts suggest that asymptomatic patients with critical AS (aortic valve area < 0.6 cm², mean gradient > 60 mmHg) and an expected low operative risk (<1%), and those who have LV dysfunction (EF <50%), develop symptoms or hypotension during closely supervised exercise testing, or have a high likelihood of rapid progression (e.g., age, severe calcification, CAD) may benefit from surgery.

Although vasodilator therapy has become the mainstay of treatment for patients with CHF, these agents can produce hypotension, syncope, and even death in a patient with severe aortic stenosis in the setting of a fixed cardiac output and, thus, are best avoided. The possibility of halting the progression of aortic valve sclerosis (along with CAD) with lipid-lowering therapy ("statins") is an intriguing but as yet unproven prospect for the management of this disease.

Operative mortality rate in elective surgery is ~3–5% and increases with age and with worsening hemodynamic status. The overall response to aortic valve replacement is excellent. If LV function is depressed, an improvement can be anticipated after surgery once the obstruction is relieved.

Once symptoms of chest pain, dyspnea, dizziness, or syncope occur, aortic valve replacement (AVR) should be strongly considered. There is an ~75%, 3-year mortality for symptomatic patients who do not undergo surgery, but a nearly normal post-operative survival rate. This makes the decision to perform aortic valve replacement in symptomatic patients with severe valvular AS an obvious choice in the absence of surgical contraindications. A patient having symptoms related to severe aortic stenosis, therefore, should be promptly referred for surgical intervention. The next episode of syncope could be the last!

In general, a mechanical prosthesis is recommended if the patient is young or middle-aged, and if there is no reason to withhold anticoagulation. A bioprosthetic tissue valve from a human (homograft) or animal (heterograft, e.g., porcine, bovine pericardial) is recommended for older patients (>75 years of age) with limited life expectancy, bleeding tendency, or anticipated difficulty with anticoagulation (i.e., warfarin). Lifelong anticoagulation with warfarin is required for mechanical prostheses but is not essential with bioprosthesis after the first 3 months (unless additional risk factors for emboli, e.g., atrial fibrillation, LV dysfunction, previous thromboembolism, are present). Approximately 30–50% of heterograft valves need replacing within 10 years after implantation. Some centers have begun performing the *Ross procedure,* which entails switching the patient's pulmonary valve to the aortic position and placing a bioprosthesis in the pulmonary position, since they do not deteriorate as fast on the right side of the heart. Percutaneous balloon valvotomy for AS is not the preferred approach because improvement in aortic valve area is limited (frequently <1 year) due to a high incidence of restenosis. (**Figure 8-5**). It may be useful, however, as a temporary measure, in patients with serious severe comorbidity, patients requiring urgent noncardiac surgery, and as a bridge to AVR in hemodynamically unstable patients with cardiogenic shock or severe CHF. Although patients with valvular AS are at increased risk for developing infective endocarditis, recent guidelines no longer recommend prophylactic antibiotics before dental and other invasive procedures unless there is a past history of endocarditis or prior prosthetic valve replacement. Patients with degenerative calcific AS have an increased incidence of lower GI bleeding, often related to right-sided colonic angiodysplasia (Heyde's syndrome). AVR in these patients often prevents recurrent bleeding.

Presently, the risks of surgery and prosthetic valve complications in the asymptomatic patient with normal LV function outweigh the benefits of preventing sudden cardiac death and prolonging survival. Asymptomatic patients with severe valvular AS and declining LV function (EF < 50%), or those with moderate-severe AS undergoing CABG or surgery on the aorta or another heart valve, should be considered for aortic valve replacement. The surgical mortality is acceptable (~10%) among elderly patients and those with concurrent LV systolic dysfunction. Transcatheter aortic valve replacement (TAVR) is a viable alternative to surgery for intermediate to high risk or inoperable patients with severe symptomatic AS. Keep in mind that as surgical and percutaneous techniques continue to improve, patients with significant AS may become candidates for valve replacement earlier in the course of the disease.

AORTIC REGURGITATION

Chronic AR

There are multiple etiologies for chronic aortic regurgitation (AR). In an age of declining incidence of rheumatic fever and syphilis, degenerative disorders of the aortic root and cusps are the most common causes. AR frequently results from dilatation of the ascending aorta (ascending aortic aneurysm, cystic medial necrosis of the aorta, aortic dissection) and/or severe long-standing hypertension. Pure AR may be due to primary valve disease (bicuspid aortic valve, calcific degeneration, endocarditis, rheumatic). It can also be caused by rheumatoid arthritis, ankylosing spondylitis, and systemic lupus erythematosus. Recent studies have shown an association between the use of weight reduction drugs (*Phen-Fen*) and an increased prevalence of AR.

Clinical Recognition of Chronic AR

Early in the course of the disease, the patient may have symptoms attributable to an augmented stroke volume, i.e., a forceful heartbeat and prominent arterial pulsations in the neck. When clinical deterioration occurs, patients may present with symptoms of left heart failure (fatigue, weakness, exertional dyspnea, orthopnea, PND), night sweats, or angina (due to decreased coronary artery flow secondary to the low diastolic pressure in the aorta).

Figure 15-9. The natural history of chronic aortic regurgitation. Patients with chronic aortic regurgitation usually remain asymptomatic for decades, often until the fourth or fifth decade of life, before signs and symptoms of heart failure occur. (Courtesy of Dr. Gordon A. Ewy)

The physical examination reveals a high-frequency blowing decrescendo diastolic murmur best heard with the diaphragm applied firmly along the left sternal border with the patient in the sitting position leaning forward with breath held in deep expiration. A wide arterial pulse pres-

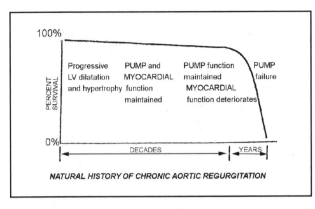

Figure 15-9

sure, i.e., high systolic and very low diastolic BP (<40 mmHg and which can sometimes be heard down to 0 mmHg), may be present when AR is severe. Other characteristic physical findings relate to the wide pulse pressure, e.g., head bobbing (so-called *deMusset's* or *"yes-yes" sign*), visible (bounding) neck pulsations, quick rising ("flip") or collapsing arterial pulses (so-called *water-hammer* or *Corrigan pulse*) often with a double (*bisferiens*) contour, subungual capillary pulsations (so-called *Quincke's pulses*), and *Duroziez's sign* (a diastolic murmur heard over a partially compressed peripheral artery, commonly the femoral). A diffuse, inferolaterally displaced LV apical impulse and a low frequency apical diastolic rumble (*Austin-Flint murmur*) may also be noted when the degree of AR is severe. The Austin-Flint murmur is caused by turbulent flow across the mitral valve, which is partially closed by the regurgitant jet from the incompetent aortic valve. A systolic ejection murmur along the left sternal border (due to increased forward flow across the aortic valve) often is present and does not necessarily imply concomitant aortic stenosis.

Figure 15-10 summarizes the clinical approach to severe aortic regurgitation.

In a patient with chronic AR, an aortic *systolic* murmur (due to the large LV stroke volume) followed by the typical early blowing aortic diastolic murmur can also be heard (the characteristic "to and fro" murmurs of AR). The systolic murmur in some patients can be loud (≥ grade 4) and accompanied by a palpable systolic thrill and resemble valvular AS. It is important to realize that, in such a patient, if peripheral signs of AR exist, e.g., a wide pulse pressure on the BP readings (160–170/40–30 down to 0), no matter how loud the systolic murmur or how faint the diastolic murmur, there is no AS present, only significant regurgitation. The severity of AR correlates better with the duration of the diastolic murmur rather than with its intensity.

In patients with severe chronic AR, marked LV dilatation ("boot-shaped" heart) may be seen on CXR (**Figure 4-6A**) along with LV hypertrophy on the ECG. Dilation of the ascending aorta points to patients with aortic dissection, Marfan's syndrome, or cystic medial necrosis. Doppler-echo and cardiac catheterization with left ventriculography and supravalvular aortography, can confirm the diagnosis, estimate the severity of the leak, and assess LV size and function, a critical determinant for the timing of aortic valve replacement. (**Figures 5-4E, 5-6, and 5-23**).

Acute AR

Clinical Recognition of Acute AR
Acute AR can result from aortic dissection, infective endocarditis or trauma. The patient with acute AR usually has marked symptoms of left heart failure, which often begins abruptly and progresses rapidly to full-blown pulmonary edema (since the sudden severe leak of the aortic valve does not allow time for the LV to adapt). On physical examination, many of the peripheral signs of chronic AR may be absent, since they have had insufficient time to develop (see **Figure 15-10**).

In contrast with chronic AR, in acute AR the pulse pressure may not be widened, the diastolic blood pressure may be low normal, and the "to and fro" systolic (due to increased forward flow and not necessarily associated stenosis) and diastolic murmurs, usually heard along the left sternal border, are shorter in duration; S1 is faint or absent (an important clue to premature mitral valve closure), and there is marked sinus tachycardia, often in the setting of acute pulmonary edema (with a normal sized heart on chest x-ray). As S1 intensity diminishes or disappears, S2 may be mistaken for the absent S1, the aortic diastolic murmur misinterpreted as a systolic murmur, and AR missed completely. Chest or back discomfort (especially in a patient with a Marfanoid appearance) and unequal pulses are clues to aortic dissection. With infective endocarditis, fever, petechiae, purpura, and arterial embolic events, may be seen. Echo can document the severity of AR, confirm mitral valve preclosure, and may reveal the underlying cause of the regurgitant flow (e.g., vegetation on the aortic valve in infective endocarditis or an intimal tear in aortic dissection).

Figure 15-11. Morphologic features of infective endocarditis on a trileaflet aortic valve. Note presence of vegetation and perforation of valve leaflet, causing aortic regurgitation. Auscultatory findings in an acutely ill patient who presents with pulmonary edema due to infective endocarditis of the aortic valve include a short diastolic murmur (DM) in addition to systolic murmur (SM).

FIGURE 15-10

Clinical Approach to Severe Aortic Regurgitation

Etiology	History	Physical Exam	ECG	Chest X-Ray	Lab Tests	Timing of Surgical Intervention
Chronic Aortic root dilatation (e.g., hypertension, cystic medial necrosis, aortic ectasia), rheumatic, congenital bicuspid aortic valve	Late and insidious onset of dyspnea, angina, fatigue	Wide pulse pressure, low diastolic pressure, bounding (quick rise) arterial pulses, inferolaterally displaced LV impulse; long decrescendo diastolic murmur along LSB (valvular) or RSB (aortic root); systolic ejection murmur, Austin-Flint rumble at apex, S3 gallop	LV hypertrophy If isolated lesion, NSR common.	Cardiomegaly, LV enlargement ("boot-shaped" heart), dilatation of the ascending aorta	Echo: dilated LV and aorta, Doppler shows large color flow regurgitant jet Cath: confirms diagnosis, shows severe aortic → LV reflux, LV function	Aortic valve replacement when symptoms develop, ejection fraction <50% or LV end-systolic dimension >50 mm or LV end-diastolic dimension >65 mm on echo (if surgical risk is low)
Acute (Endocarditis, Aortic dissection, ruptured sinus of Valsalva, prosthetic valve)	Sudden onset of pulmonary edema	Short diastolic murmur, faint S1	Not helpful	Normal heart size, pulmonary congestion	Echo: Prolapsing aortic leaflets, vegetation, aortic dissection (TEE) Cath: confirms diagnosis	AVR, often urgent when acute AR caused by aortic dissection or infective endocarditis

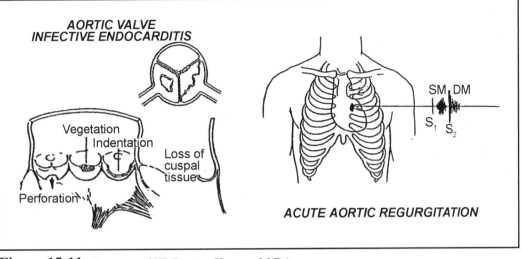

Figure 15-11 (Courtesy of W. Proctor Harvey, M.D.)

Surgical intervention is indicated. (Courtesy of Dr. W. Proctor Harvey).

Management of Chronic and Acute AR

AR can be treated either medically or surgically, depending on the acuteness of presentation, symptoms, and LV size and function.

If hypertension is present in patients with chronic AR, treatment with afterload reducing agents (e.g., dihydropyridine calcium channel blockers, ACE inhibitors/ARBs, hydralazine) should be initiated. Theoretically, beta-blockers should be avoided, because they slow the heart rate, prolong diastole, and thus may worsen AR. Vasodilator therapy (ACE inhibitors/ARBs) along with the cautious use of beta-blockers (which may exert beneficial effects on LV dilatation and remodeling) may be considered, however, in symptomatic patients with severe AR, those with LV systolic dysfunction (to improve hemodynamics before proceeding with AVR), and those who are not surgical candidates (because of comorbidities).

Data on the benefits of medical treatment in asymptomatic severe AR are controversial. There are no recommendations for vasodilator therapy in patients with severe, chronic AR who are asymptomatic with normal LV systolic function and have no hypertension.

Beta-blockers (by reducing aortic wall stress) and vasodilating agents, e.g., ARBs (by blocking TGF-beta) may slow the rate of aortic dilatation in patients with Marfan's syndrome.

Although at increased risk for acquiring infective endocarditis, antibiotic prophylaxis is no longer recommended in patients with AR unless there is a previous history of endocarditis. Asymptomatic patients with normal LV function may participate in all kinds of activities. However, strenuous isometric exercise should be avoided.

Aortic valve replacement is advised in patients with chronic AR when symptoms appear, the ejection fraction is <50%, or the end-systolic dimension is >50 mm or the end-diastolic dimension is >65 mm on echo (if surgical risk is low). Early LV dysfunction will probably reverse with aortic valve replacement. AR due to aortic root disease requires repair or replacement of the root as well as the aortic valve (Bentall procedure), which is a more difficult operation.

At present, TAVR is not approved for use in the U.S. in patients with native AR (due to concerns over the lack of valvular calcification that may prevent secure anchoring). Transcatheter "valve-in-valve" replacement, or insertion of a vascular plug (occluder device), however, may be an option in anatomically suitable patients with bioprosthetic paravalvular AR.

Because of the embolic and anticoagulation risks of prosthetic aortic valves, the goal is to delay surgery without subjecting the patient to an irreversible loss of LV function. At the present time, it seems prudent to intervene surgically as soon as asymptomatic patients demonstrate a clear, persistent deterioration in LV function (even if mild). Following surgery, LV size usually decreases and LV function improves, except when dysfunction has been present chronically.

Acute AR can be catastrophic. In patients with acute AR, prompt recognition, appropriate antibiotic therapy (if infective endocarditis is the cause), and emergent surgical intervention (in patients with acute AR due to dissection or trauma and/or who are hemodynamically unstable) can be lifesaving.

MITRAL REGURGITATION (MR)

With the decline of rheumatic fever, MVP has become the most common cause of valvular mitral regurgitation (MR) (~65% of cases). Myxomatous degeneration of the mitral valve is a very common cause of mild MR in adults (especially in women) and the severity may increase with age (particularly in men) so that significant MR may supervene. The reasons for this gender/age distribution are not known. MVP may be associated with ASD (secundum type),

HOCM, and Marfan's syndrome. Anorectic drugs (*Phen-Fen*) also have been reported to cause MR. The clinical approach to severe mitral regurgitation is summarized in **Figure 15-12.** See the CD on Heart Sounds for further description of mitral regurgitation and the special case in which MR is due to MVP.

Chronic MR
Clinical Recognition of Chronic MR
Figure 15-13. Natural history of chronic mitral regurgitation. (Courtesy of Dr. Gordon A. Ewy)

Patients with mild to moderate chronic MR are relatively symptom-free for decades or life. LV systolic performance is satisfactory until late in the course, at which time LV function begins to deteriorate. The patient with chronic MR may then present with a slow, insidious onset of CHF (exertional dyspnea, orthopnea, PND, cough, weakness and fatigue [due to a low cardiac output state]) as the valvular leak becomes progressively more severe ("MR begets MR"). Ankle swelling (edema) is a late finding.

Enlargement of the LA can lead to irregular heart rhythms (e.g., atrial fibrillation) and may cause palpitations. The murmur of chronic MR is typically high frequency and blowing in quality, heard best at the apex, radiating laterally and posteriorly in a "band-like" fashion into the axilla, left infrascapular area and back, and at times, up the spine to the top of the head (when the anterior leaflet is involved). In general, the severity of MR is not reflected in the intensity of the systolic murmur, but rather by the accompanying diastolic events. A late systolic murmur or holosystolic murmur with a late systolic accentuation usually is a clue to mild MR, especially when an S3 gallop is absent. When hemodynamically significant, the holosystolic murmur is accompanied by an S3 gallop and a short diastolic "flow rumble" at the cardiac apex (**Figure 2-63**). It should be noted, however, that in patients with significant MR due to acute MI with severe LV systolic dysfunction, hypotension and a low cardiac output, or a prosthetic perivalvular leak, or in those who have

marked emphysema, obesity or thick chest walls, the systolic murmur may be barely audible or even absent ("silent MR").

In chronic MR, the ECG may show evidence of LA enlargement, LV and RV hypertrophy, and atrial fibrillation. The CXR may reveal evidence of marked LA and LV enlargement. The lung fields may be clear if pulmonary vascular pressures are not sufficiently high to produce clinically overt pulmonary edema. The so-called giant LA is seen in chronic severe MR (usually when combined with mitral stenosis.) Doppler-echo confirms the diagnosis and estimates the severity of the regurgitant jet. (**Figure 5-6**). Serial echos help in the decision-making process regarding timing of surgery. TEE may reveal the cause of MR and identify candidates for valvular repair. A small degree of clinically insignificant (so-called "physiologic") MR can be detected on Doppler-echo in as many as 80% of normal healthy individuals. Care should be taken not to over-interpret this finding as clinically significant. Cardiac catheterization is performed to confirm the diagnosis and to assess LV function and pulmonary artery pressure. (**Figure 15-12**). The rate and intensity of opacification of the left atrium provide an assessment of the severity of regurgitation (graded 1+ to 4+). (**Figure 5-23**). Coronary angiography is often indicated to determine the presence of CAD prior to valve surgery.

Management of Chronic MR
Mild-to-moderate MR usually causes no symptoms and has an excellent prognosis unless infective endocarditis or spontaneous chordal rupture occurs. Although patients with MR are at increased risk for acquiring infective endocarditis, recent guidelines no longer recommend routine antibiotic prophylaxis, unless there is a history of previous endocarditis or prior prosthetic valve replacement/repair. Congestive symptoms are improved with dietary restriction of sodium, along with diuretics and vasodilator therapy (e.g., ACE inhibitors/ARBs). There are no long-term studies to indicate that vasodilators are beneficial in asymptomatic patients with normal LV function. Atrial fibrillation is a late occurrence (usually denotes marked LA enlargement) and requires rate control (with beta blockers, calcium channel blockers, digitalis) and anticoagulation therapy with warfarin (to achieve a target INR of 2-3). Electrical cardioversion is rarely successful on a long-term basis.

Because progressive and irreversible deterioration of LV function may occur prior to the onset of symptoms, early operation is indicated even in asymptomatic patients with chronic MR when the ejection fraction is declining (≤60%) or LV dilation (end systolic dimension ≥40 mm on echo) is present. Surgical intervention should be considered when symptoms develop as long as the ejection fraction is >30% and/or the LV end systolic dimension is <55mm. **Note:** An ejection fraction of <30% indicates severely reduced LV function. The ejection fraction

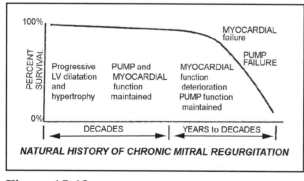

Figure 15-13

FIGURE 15-12

Clinical Approach to Severe Mitral Regurgitation

Etiology	History	Physical Exam	ECG	Chest X-Ray	Lab Tests	Timing of Surgical Intervention
Chronic MVP, CAD, LV dilatation of any cause, rheumatic.	Late onset of left heart failure (dyspnea, fatigue), later right heart failure. Middle aged with equal sex incidence.	Quick rise arterial pulse, dilated LV, late parasternal lift (LA "rock"), apical holosystolic murmur radiating to axilla, with S3 gallop and diastolic flow rumble, and wide-split S2	Left atrial enlargement, LV hypertrophy, atrial fibrillation common.	Cardiomegaly, LV and LA enlargement	Echo: LV and LA dilatation, marked mitral leaflet prolapse, Doppler shows large color flow regurgitant jet Cath: shows severe LV → LA mitral regurgitation and LV function (EF supranormal in compensated states. EF <60% with severe MR and LV impairment).	Mitral valve repair preferred, mitral valve replacement if necessary. As soon as possible when more than mild symptoms develop on diuretics, and afterload reduction (e.g., ACE inhibitors) or when LV dysfunction develops (ejection fraction ≤60% or LV end-systolic dimension ≥40 mm).
Acute Endocarditis, (ruptured chordae, perforation of leaflet, prosthetic valve), papillary muscle rupture.	Acute pulmonary edema Usually older males.	Quick rise arterial pulse, decrescendo systolic murmur radiates to neck (posterior leaflet) or back (anterior leaflet), S4 gallop, loud P2, widely split S2.	NSR. (Acute MI, if present)	Pulmonary edema, normal heart size	Echo: flail mitral leaflet or vegetation hyperdynamic LV, normal size LV and LA Cath: large V waves in PCWP tracing, shows MR on LV angiogram.	Acute MR due to infective endocarditis or torn chordae tendineae may require urgent surgical repair.

should normally be ≥65% in MR.) The onset of atrial fibrillation or pulmonary hypertension (PA pressure >50mmHg) is also an indication for surgery. With improved surgical techniques, mitral valve repair (valvuloplasty) now is being performed earlier (and in preference to valve replacement) than in the past, as the operative risk is lower and LV function better preserved when the subvalvular structures can be maintained intact after surgery. Advances in mitral valve surgery (including minimally invasive and robotically assisted valve repair and valve replacement with chordal preservation) have improved perioperative and long-term outcomes in patients with MR. Percutaneous approaches to valve repair, e.g., the edge-to-edge mitral clip, can be considered when the LV ejection fraction is <30% and the operative risk is high. However, due to the high incidence of residual MR, surgical repair (if feasible) remains the intervention of choice in patients who are acceptable candidates for operation.

Acute MR

Clinical Recognition and Management of Acute MR
Acute MR (caused by spontaneous chordae tendineae rupture, infective endocarditis, or papillary muscle rupture in the setting of acute MI) is a potentially lethal condition characterized by the abrupt onset of pulmonary edema and severe perfusion failure. Hemodynamic disturbances are profound because the regurgitant flow is suddenly imposed on a normal LA. The inability of the LA to acutely dilate and increase compliance results in marked increases in LA pressure, leading to the pulmonary edema.

Figure 15-12 summarizes the key features of acute mitral regurgitation. See CD on Heart Sounds for further details on the murmur of MR.

On physical examination, the patient is tachypneic and dyspneic and often prefers the upright to the supine position. In contrast to chronic MR, the murmur of acute MR is louder in early to mid systole, tapers off well before S2 (as left atrial pressure rises rapidly and decreases regurgitant flow), tends to radiate anteriorly and upward to the base and, at times, even into the neck (when the posterior leaflet is involved) where it can be mistaken for the murmur of valvular aortic stenosis. In the acute form (predominantly in middle-aged or older males), normal sinus rhythm (rather than atrial fibrillation) and a prominent S4 gallop (normal-sized, vigorously contracting left atrium) are the rule. The ECG is usually normal and the CXR typically reveals a normal size heart with evidence of pulmonary edema. Echo studies may reveal the cause of acute valve dysfunction e.g., ruptured chordae tendineae, vegetation, flail leaflet, etc. At the time of cardiac catheterization, MR is visualized on left ventriculography. If the regurgitation is severe, pulmonary capillary wedge pressure is elevated with especially prominent regurgitant V waves. (**Figure 5-27**).

Because the patient with acute severe MR tolerates the lesion poorly, immediate surgical repair may be required following stabilization with inotropic agents, vasodilators (if tolerated), and IABP counterpulsation.

MITRAL VALVE PROLAPSE (MVP) (FIGURE 15-16)

Clinical Recognition of MVP

The most common mitral valve abnormality is mitral valve prolapse (MVP), affecting up to 2 to 3% of the population. There are two distinct clinical subsets of patients with this disorder. The first group is characterized by mitral leaflet abnormalities with little MR on echo and a mid systolic click with or without a late systolic murmur on physical examination. Young women (20 to 50 years of age), especially those with a thin, lean body habitus, constitute the majority of individuals affected. Most of these patients are asymptomatic. Patients with MVP in the first group generally have a good prognosis. Sudden death is an extremely rare occurrence.

The second group of patients with MVP is characterized by considerable leaflet thickening and MR on echo. Most of these patients are men (40 to 70 years of age) and have a high likelihood of having progressive MR that necessitates mitral valve surgery. Another problem is that chordal rupture can cause a sudden increase in the severity of MR and an abrupt onset of severe symptoms. Patients with severe MR are at increased risk of sudden death (most often caused by ventricular arrhythmias).

Figure 2-48 illustrates the squatting maneuver in a young female with mitral valve prolapse who presented with atypical chest pain and palpitations. Maneuvers that reduce ventricular volume (e.g., standing) make the click and murmur earlier, whereas those that increase ventricular volume (e.g., squatting) delay the click and murmur. Note the systolic click (C) and murmur move closer to the first heart sound (S1) on standing and closer to the second heart sound (S2) with squatting.

In the hands of an experienced clinician, the stethoscope is the best instrument to diagnose MVP. Although echo is very useful in identifying MVP, it is not needed in the great majority of patients to make the diagnosis. (**Figure 5-4A**). In fact, the systolic click may be heard even when MVP can not be demonstrated on echo. Echo may be helpful, however, in the patient suspected of having MVP with normal or classic auscultatory findings to determine the thickness of the mitral valve, its movement characteristics, degree of regurgitation, and annulus size. Such information can be of help to determine the likelihood of complications of MVP. Improper use and/or inaccurate interpretation of echo may lead to the diagnosis of MVP in patients who do not have the syndrome, or the failure to document MVP when it is unequivocally present (i.e., the echo may be normal in patients with clinical evidence of a mid-systolic click and/or a late systolic murmur). The ECG may demonstrate ST segment depression and/or T wave abnormalities in the inferior or lateral leads (and lead to an erroneous diagnosis of CAD), QT prolongation, and premature atrial and ventricular contractions. Although the great majority of patients with MVP remain asymptomatic and have no serious complications (normal life expectancy), significant MR can occur from rupture of a chordae tendineae, either spontaneously or as a result of infective endocarditis.

Figure 15-14. Morphologic features of ruptured chordae in mitral valve prolapse causing acute mitral regurgitation. Rupture of the chordae tendineae can result in a dramatic change in the auscultatory findings of mitral valve prolapse from multiple mid systolic clicks and/or late apical systolic murmur (sm) to the sudden onset of a loud holosystolic murmur (SM) that decreases in the latter part of systole, typical of acute severe mitral regurgitation. Surgery may be necessary for correction of the leak.

Figure 15-15. Spectrum of auscultatory findings in mitral valve prolapse. Note the wide variety of clicks (C), systolic murmurs (SM), and click-murmur complexes that may be found in patients with mitral valve prolapse. Auscultatory findings may even vary from time to time in the same patient. The second and third sketches on the bottom line represent decrescendo tapering of a holosystolic murmur, typical of a ruptured chordae tendineae. (Courtesy of Dr. W. Proctor Harvey)

Management of MVP

Severe MVP (with valve leakage) is the most common heart condition associated with infective endocarditis. Endocarditis may also occur in the milder forms of MVP. Although MVP is the most common underlying condition that predisposes to the acquisition of infective endocarditis, the absolute incidence of endocarditis for the entire population with MVP is extremely low. Furthermore, MVP is not usually associated with the highest risk of an adverse outcome from infective endocarditis as are other higher risk cardiac conditions. Thus routine antibiotic prophylaxis is no longer recommended in these patients when undergoing dental, GI, or GU tract procedures (see chapter 17).

Beta blockers may be tried in symptomatic patients (e.g., palpitations, chest pain, and anxiety or panic attacks). Sudden death (most often caused by ventricular arrhythmias) is a rare occurrence. Most patients with MVP (~90%) have neither symptoms nor a high-risk profile. Patients with MVP should be reassured that their prognosis is generally excellent. The incidence of complications is very low and is usually associated with an increase in mitral valve leaflet thickness or hemodynamically significant MR. In general, complications increase with age and are more common in males than in

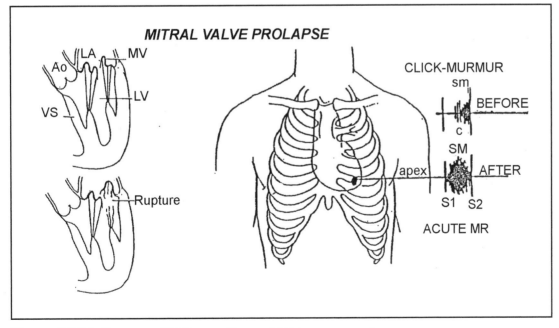

Figure 15-14 (Courtesy of W. Proctor Harvey, M.D.)

females. Often, quiet reassurance of the benign prognosis and explanation of the disease entity is all that is required.

Patients with severe MR unresponsive to drug therapy, e.g., afterload reduction (ACE inhibitors, hydralazine and nitrates), may require valve repair and/or replacement. Restriction from competitive sports may be required for patients with MVP who have significant MR with LV enlargement and/or dysfunction, uncontrolled tachyarrhythmias, prolonged QT intervals, a history of unexplained syncope, aortic root enlargement, and a family history of sudden cardiac death (**Figure 15-16**).

RHEUMATIC MITRAL STENOSIS (MS) (FIGURE 15-17)

Clinical Recognition of Rheumatic MS

Rheumatic fever is the major cause of mitral stenosis. Although we witnessed a dramatic decline in acute rheumatic fever in the United States (due to control of group A streptococcal infection), strep infections and acute rheumatic fever have recently re-emerged as clinical problems. Rheumatic

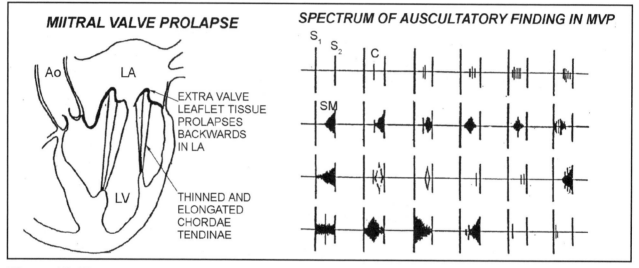

Figure 15-15 (Courtesy of W. Proctor Harvey, M.D.)

FIGURE 15-16

Clinical Approach to Mitral Valve Prolapse

History	Asymptomatic, or "atypical" chest pain, palpitations, autonomic dysfunction, shortness of breath, fatigue, anxiety and/or panic attacks, transient ischemic attacks.
Physical Examination	Mid to late systolic click (or clicks) and/or apical late systolic or holosystolic murmur or "whoop" of MR.
Electrocardiogram	Non diagnostic ST-T abnormalities in the inferolateral leads, premature atrial and/or ventricular contractions.
Chest X-Ray	Normal heart size, chest wall deformity (straight back, pectus excavatum, pectus carinatum, kyphoscoliosis).
Laboratory Echocardiogram	Thickened, redundant mitral valve leaflets with superior systolic displacement (in the parasternal long axis view) +/− chordal rupture, Doppler MR. (MVP can be overdiagnosed in the apical 4 chamber view).
Cardiac Catheterization	Visualize mitral valve prolapse and document severity of MR.
Treatment	Infective endocarditis prophylaxis (even with MR and/or thickened leaflets) is no longer recommended. Beta blockers for symptomatic patients (e.g., palpitations, chest pain). Aspirin to prevent emboli. Mitral valve replacement or repair for severe MR.

FIGURE 15-17

Clinical Approach to Severe Mitral Stenosis

Etiology	History	Physical Exam	ECG	Chest X-Ray	Lab Tests	Timing of Surgical Intervention
Rheumatic heart disease (but ~50% of patients give no history of having had rheumatic fever).	Symptoms of left heart failure (dyspnea, fatigue), palpitations, and later right heart failure.	Long diastolic rumble at apex, short S2-OS interval, signs of pulmonary hypertension (loud P2, palpable RV heave)	LA enlargement, RV hypertrophy, atrial fibrillation frequent	Kerley lines, pulmonary venous congestion, LA enlargement, mitral valve calcification, RV enlargement	Echo: reduced valve area ≤ 1.5 cm^2 and high velocity inflow by Doppler, high PA systolic pressure, large left atrium Cath: confirms diagnosis, quantifies transmitral gradient (severe stenosis = mean gradient of > 5 mmHg).	Usually when more than mild symptoms develop or evidence of pulmonary hypertension, right heart failure, mitral valve area ≤ 1.5 cm^2. Consider percutaneous mitral balloon valvuloplasty when mitral valve area ≤ 1.5 cm^2 (in pliable, non-calcified valve if left atrial thrombus, and/or significant MR is not present).

valvular disease affects the mitral valve most frequently, followed next by the aortic valve and, least frequently, the tricuspid valve. MS may be present for a lifetime with few or no symptoms. In most cases, there is a long asymptomatic phase, followed by subtle limitation of activity. Pregnancy (and its associated increase in blood volume) and the onset of rapid atrial fibrillation often precipitate symptoms.

Figure 15-18. Natural history of rheumatic mitral valve disease. Significant mitral stenosis typically develops years to decades after the initial attack of acute rheumatic fever (that may have been unrecognized up to 50% of the time, or forgotten).

Clinical features of MS include chronic fatigue, decreasing exercise tolerance, and dyspnea with progressively less provocation. The astute clinician should conduct a careful search for clinical signs of MS when a patient with a previous history of acute rheumatic fever in childhood (especially a middle-aged female with a prior history of dyspnea during the third trimester of her pregnancy) develops progressive symptoms of dyspnea on exertion, orthopnea, PND with cough (as the mitral valve area diminishes from the normal 4–6 cm^2 to ≤ 1.5 cm^2), abrupt onset of palpitations (from atrial fibrillation), acute pulmonary edema, a systemic embolism (e.g., stroke), hemoptysis (rarely, due to rupture of a bronchial vein or pulmonary emboli), or hoarseness (compression of the left recurrent laryngeal nerve by an enlarged pulmonary artery).

Figure 2-79 shows the clinical findings in a patient with rheumatic mitral stenosis. Note the loud first heart sound (S1), opening snap (OS), and diastolic murmur (DM). To best detect a diastolic rumble (DM) turn the patient to the left lateral position. Palpate to feel the point of maximal impulse of the left ventricle and place the bell of the stethoscope lightly over this area. If a diastolic rumble of mitral stenosis is present, it is almost always heard over this localized spot. In general, the closer the opening snap is to S2 (the higher the LA pressure), and the longer the diastolic rumble, the greater the severity of the stenosis.

As the disease progresses, pulmonary hypertension develops (which worsens the prognosis and increases the operative mortality), along with symptoms of fatigue (due to a low cardiac output), nausea, anorexia, and right upper quadrant pain and signs of RV failure, including ascites and peripheral edema. Findings on ECG (LA enlargement or atrial fibrillation, RV hypertrophy and right axis deviation if pulmonary hypertension is present), CXR (LA and RV enlargement, mitral valve calcification, pulmonary vascular congestion), and lab tests (specifically Doppler-echo, which shows mitral calcification, and allows estimation of transvalvular diastolic gradient and mitral valve area) **(Figures 15-17 and 5-24)** may also point to mitral stenosis. Most patients are asymptomatic. When symptoms develop, they are most often the

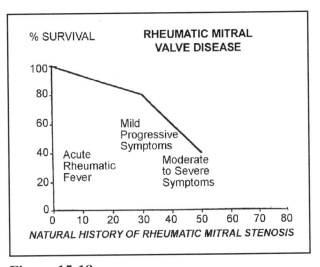

Figure 15-18

result of mitral valve dysfunction, atrial arrhythmias, heart block, calcific thromboembolism and infective endocarditis.

Specifically ask patients about a history of *rheumatic fever* (RF). Many patients with rheumatic heart disease have no history of acute rheumatic fever, whereas other patients give histories of clear-cut, well-documented episodes of *carditis, arthritis, rash, subcutaneous nodules,* and *chorea,* the major manifestations of RF (*Jones criteria*). Inquiry about various *RF "equivalents"*, e.g., "growing pains" (arthritis), St. Vitus' dance (chorea), frequent sore throats (streptococcal infections), nosebleeds, or prolonged febrile illness as a child may provide clues if the patient denies a history of RF. A patient who was put to bed for a long period of time as a child may well have had RF. Conversely, questions regarding features of the illness are important even when a patient states he or she has had RF, since many patients have been told that they "had rheumatic fever" based on the presence of a heart murmur heard many years later, when in fact there never was a clinically apparent episode. Remember, RF is unusual before the age of 4 years. Fortunately, in most sections of the United States today, the incidence of RF has declined greatly. Note the *"50% rule"*: If there is a history of rheumatic fever, there is a 50% chance of having rheumatic valvular heart disease. Conversely, only 50% of patients with rheumatic MS have a history of rheumatic fever. Keep in mind the following *rheumatic "triad": rheumatic fever, MS, atrial fibrillation.* When the first two are present, the third will also be evident or probably forthcoming.

Patients with rheumatic mitral valve disease comprise a spectrum of abnormalities ranging from pure mitral stenosis to pure MR.

Figure 15-19. Auscultatory findings in mitral stenosis and combined mitral stenosis and mitral regurgitation. In the patient with mitral stenosis, the first heart sound (1) is loud and

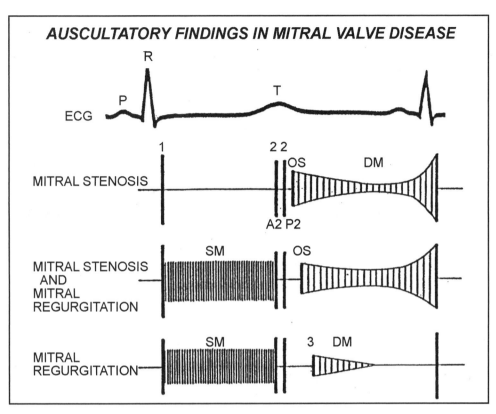

Figure 15-19

sharp, the second heart sound is split into aortic (A2) and pulmonic (P2) components, and an early opening snap (OS) introduces a mid-diastolic and late-diastolic murmur (BM) with presystolic accentuation. Combined mitral stenosis and regurgitation is suggested by a holosystolic murmur (SM) and a late opening snap. The patient with mild mitral stenosis and severe regurgitation has the findings of a holosystolic (SM), wide splitting of the second heart sound, a third heart sound (3), and a short mid-diastolic murmur (DM) of increased left ventricular filling. (Courtesy of Dr. Bernard L. Segal)

Management of Rheumatic MS

- Preventive measures against rheumatic fever, including administration of either penicillin (or sulfadiazine or erythromycin, if allergic), are suggested in all patients for at least 10 years after the last RF episode, or until age 40 in those patients with frequent exposure to streptococcal infection, e.g., teachers and day-care workers. Recent guidelines, however, no longer recommended prophylactic antibiotics against infective endocarditis. Patients with MS should be managed medically unless symptoms persist despite such therapy.
- Systemic thromboembolism is a serious complication of MS, and anticoagulation should be strongly

considered in these patients (especially those with atrial fibrillation).
- Rate control (e.g., beta blockers, calcium channel blockers, digoxin) is indicated for atrial fibrillation. Electrical cardioversion should be attempted.
- Correction usually requires surgical intervention (valve replacement), but percutaneous balloon valvuloplasty may be considered a treatment option in symptomatic patients with MS and an orifice area of ≤ 1.5 cm^2 if they have suitable mitral valve morphology on echo, i.e., thin, mobile, noncalcified leaflets, with little subvalvular involvement (favorable "Wilkins score"), and minimal or no MR and no LA clot. Problems associated with prosthetic valves include thrombosis, perivalvular leak, endocarditis, and degenerative changes in tissue valves.

* * *

Tips regarding indications for valve surgery:

When considering the optimal timing of surgery in valvular heart disease, clues derived from the cardiac clinical examination, along with an objective and quantitative measure of LV contractile function (e.g., by echo) can be most helpful. Keep in mind the following:

- In hemodynamically significant *valvular AS* (valve area ≤1.0 cm²), it's time to operate once symptoms of CHF, syncope or angina develop. Surgery may be considered in asymptomatic patients when LV dysfunction (LV ejection fraction <50%) or an adverse response to exercise is present.
- In patients with *chronic AR,* consider surgery when symptoms (dyspnea, angina) develop or when objective signs of LV dilatation and/or dysfunction (LV ejection fraction <50% or LV end-systolic dimension >50 mm or LV end-diastolic dimension >65 mm) are present.
- In patients with *chronic MR* consider valve repair or replacement for symptoms or decline of LV function into the low-normal range (LV end systolic dimension ≥40 mm or ejection fraction 30-60%), or if new onset atrial fibrillation or pulmonary hypertension (PA pressure > 50mmHg) is present.
- In patients with severe *rheumatic MS* (valve area ≤ 1.5 cm²), consider mitral balloon valvuloplasty (if pliable, noncalcified valve) or valve replacement if symptoms or pulmonary hypertension is present.

Keep in mind that any patient with significant valvular regurgitation (e.g., MR, AR) should be followed carefully with attention to the possibility of insidious myocardial dysfunction. As mentioned earlier, normalization of the ejection fraction from a previously "supranormal" level means that significant myocardial functional loss has occurred and that the time for surgical intervention has probably arrived. Because the patient with acute severe MR and AR generally tolerates the lesion poorly, urgent surgical intervention may be required.

* * *

TRICUSPID REGURGITATION (TR)

Clinical Recognition of TR

Organic tricuspid valve disease may result from various etiologies including rheumatic heart disease, infectious endocarditis, myxomatous degeneration, metastatic carcinoid, tumor, RV infarction (papillary muscle rupture), severe blunt trauma, and right atrial myxoma. Significant "functional" tricuspid regurgitation (TR) may also result from pulmonary hypertension of any cause or RV failure. TR can be recognized by:

- A holosystolic murmur best heard at the left lower sternal border, becoming louder during inspiration (Carvallo's sign), accompanied by a right-sided S3 gallop and "flow rumble", prominent "V" waves in the neck veins, with a rapid "Y" descent, and systolic pulsations of the liver.
- Signs and symptoms of systemic venous hypertension in all patients with moderate to severe TR.
- Right-sided heart failure, which may result in anorexia, nausea, vomiting, abdominal distension (ascites) and edema.
- Doppler-echo shows retrograde flow from the RV into the RA as well as systolic flow reversal in the hepatic veins and can estimate the severity of TR. (**Figure 5-6**).

Most normal individuals have very mild ("physiologic") TR on Doppler-echo, which is not significant and goes undetected by auscultation. High pulmonary artery pressures are generally associated with secondary TR.

TR may also result from infective endocarditis due to IV injections of contaminated narcotics. In a febrile IV drug abuser with tricuspid valve endocarditis and septic pulmonary emboli, the systolic murmur may be unimpressive, or heard only on inspiration, not on expiration. Prolapse of the tricuspid valve can occur just as it does with the mitral valve.

One very rare but important cause of tricuspid (and pulmonic) valve regurgitation (and/or stenosis) is carcinoid. Acute coronary syndromes may lead to TR. Mechanisms include ischemic papillary muscle dysfunction and papillary muscle infarction with rupture.

Management of TR

Although patients with TR caused by an abnormal tricuspid valve are at increased risk for infective endocarditis, as with other forms of valvular heart disease, recent guidelines no longer recommend prophylactic antibiotics based solely on lifetime risk (see chapter 17). The basic principle of management of TR is to treat the underlying condition (e.g., infective endocarditis, cardiomyopathy, pulmonary hypertension). TR may decrease in severity if appropriate medical therapy improves global or right heart function, or results in a decrease in pulmonary artery pressure or resistance. Surgical intervention is usually unnecessary for primary organic TR without pulmonary hypertension. If TR is severe and refractory, valve repair or annuloplasty may be indicated and is often preferable to valve replacement. In the patient with mitral and/or aortic valve disease requiring valve surgery, decisions regarding the state of tricuspid valve function and the need for tricuspid annuloplasty or valve repair may require intraoperative TEE.

CHAPTER 16. APPROACH TO THE PATIENT WITH HYPERTROPHIC CARDIOMYOPATHY

Hypertrophic cardiomyopathy is a primary disorder of the heart muscle characterized by marked LV hypertrophy, with or without outflow tract obstruction, in the absence of an identifiable cause (e.g., hypertension, valvular AS). This chapter will review the clinical approach to the patient with hypertrophic obstructive cardiomyopathy along with the risk factors for sudden cardiac death.

CLINICAL RECOGNITION OF HYPERTROPHIC OBSTRUCTIVE CARDIOMYOPATHY (HOCM)

Hypertrophic obstructive cardiomyopathy (HOCM—previously called idiopathic hypertrophic subaortic stenosis [IHSS]) is a genetic heart muscle disease that occurs in about 1 out of 500 births. It is a common cause of sudden death in young athletes who die in the course of heavy exercise. There is a thickening of the ventricular walls, particularly the ventricular septum; the myocardial fibers are in histological disarray. Although there is good ventricular systolic contraction, the ventricular wall is stiff and noncompliant, resulting in poor diastolic ventricular filling and high ventricular diastolic pressure that is not due to systemic hypertension or aortic stenosis. The thickened septum along with anterior displacement of the mitral valve can cause LV outflow tract obstruction and mitral regurgitation.

A patient with HOCM may be asymptomatic or present with shortness of breath and chest discomfort, as well as palpitations, lightheadedness or syncope with exertion (due to dynamic LV outflow tract obstruction). Symptoms may begin at any age and often do not appear until mid-life (30s or 40s). Symptoms can develop at different rates, with long periods of stability, and often vary from day to day. Unfortunately, HOCM may cause no symptoms until the tragic episode of sudden cardiac death occurs (due to VT and VF that most likely originate from the disorganized heart muscle or small scars, or result from a sudden increase in LV outflow obstruction).

Figure 16-1. Hypertrophic obstructive cardiomyopathy. Asymmetric septal hypertrophy along with systolic anterior motion of the anterior mitral valve leaflet may cause dynamic LV outflow tract obstruction with MR. Note "quick rise" carotid arterial pulse with "spike and dome" configuration, and murmur, peaking in mid systole, along left sternal border, becoming louder on standing (or Valsalva maneuver, e.g. blowing on finger in mouth) and fainter on squatting. Also note the LV apical impulse which often demonstrates prominent presystolic and double systolic movement ("triple ripple"). Additional auscultatory findings not shown include paradoxical splitting of S2 and a systolic murmur of MR at the cardiac apex. The murmur can be faint and unimpressive, mimicking an "innocent" systolic murmur or systolic ejection murmur across a sclerotic aortic valve, or loud and long, and be mistaken for the murmur of MR or VSD. If performing the Valsalva maneuver, keep in mind that the maneuver should not be held for more than 10 seconds. The decreased cardiac output and drop in BP may result in syncope (**Figure 16.2**).

Figure 16-3 summarizes the clinical approach to hypertrophic cardiomyopathy.

Family members of an affected person should always be screened for this condition (since ~50% of the time it is transmitted genetically as an autosomal dominant trait). A mutation in one of the genes that encode cardiac muscle sarcomere proteins (i.e., β-myosin heavy chain, myosin-binding protein C, and cardiac troponins) is responsible for this disorder. In sporadic cases, especially in middle-aged and older persons, however, the condition is often benign and rarely causes syncope, or, even less likely, sudden cardiac death.

Figure 16-4. Harvey's "1, 2, 3, 4" diagnosis of hypertrophic obstructive cardiomyopathy:

1. A quick rise in the arterial pulse (radial or carotid most frequently used) is noted.
2. Aortic regurgitation is suspected as a possibility; however, no aortic diastolic murmur (DM) is present.
3. Instead, a systolic murmur is heard.
4. On squatting, the systolic murmur (SM) becomes fainter or disappears. On standing, the systolic murmur becomes significantly louder. This maneuver should be repeated several times because the characteristic change in the murmur might not occur until the third or fourth time. (**Figure 2-49**).

Following these clues, the diagnosis of hypertrophic obstructive cardiomyopathy can be made or strongly suspected.

Although the vast majority of patients with symptoms of exertional-related chest pain have underlying CAD, keep in mind that those with "muscle-bound" hearts (e.g., valvular AS and HOCM) can also have myocardial ischemia despite the presence of normal coronaries. Also note that patients with angina pectoris due to CAD alone rarely have ECG signs of LV hypertrophy. When LV hypertrophy is noted on the ECG, search for a cause other than (or in addition to) CAD. HOCM is frequently misdiagnosed as CAD (i.e., angina and/or MI) or as valvular AS.

The diagnosis of HOCM can be readily confirmed with Doppler-echo (demonstrating small hypercontractile LV with

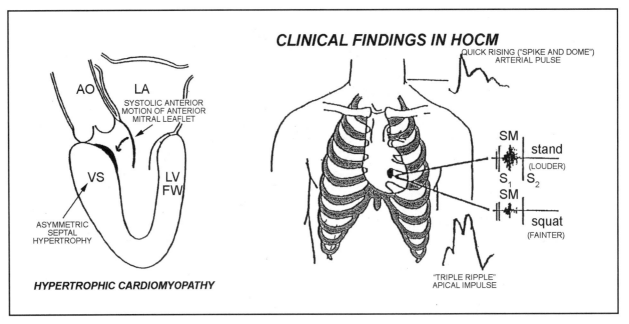

Figure 16-1 (Courtesy of W. Proctor Harvey, M.D.)

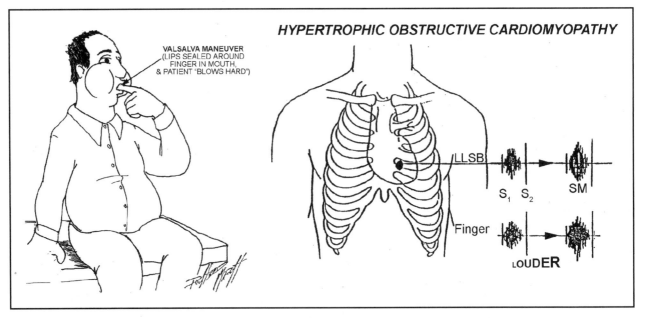

Note: Keep in mind the diagnosis of hypertrophic obstructive cardiomyopathy in a young athlete who presents with substernal chest pain, shortness of breath, and dizziness, along with a harsh systolic murmur that increases with Valsalva maneuver or from squatting to standing.

Figure 16-2 (Courtesy of W. Proctor Harvey, M.D.)

asymmetric septal hypertrophy [ASH], systolic anterior motion [SAM] of mitral valve, dynamic LV outflow tract gradient, and MR). Doppler echo is also a useful diagnostic tool to screen relatives of patients with known disease. (**Figure 5-4C**). Cardiac catheterization demonstrates the outflow tract gradient, hypertrophic LV with vigorous systolic function and cavity obliteration, and the presence of associated MR. The outflow tract obstruction in HOCM is "dynamic", i.e., its magnitude may vary between examinations and even from beat to beat and can be provoked by pharmacologic interventions that reduce LV volume or chamber size (e.g., nitrates, diuretics) or enhance LV contractility (e.g., digitalis, other inotropic agents). Therefore, a history of worsening chest pain in a patient receiving these medications should alert the astute

---

FIGURE 16-3

Clinical Approach to Hypertrophic Cardiomyopathy

Pathophysiology	Genetic disease characterized by marked LV hypertrophy (often asymmetric) with diastolic dysfunction +/− dynamic LV outflow tract obstruction.
History	Dyspnea on exertion, chest pain (angina-like), syncope, palpitations, sudden death (particularly young adult males with a history of previous syncope and/or family history of sudden death).
Physical Examination	S4 gallop, systolic ejection murmur, loudest along left sternal border (↑ with Valsalva and standing, ↓ with squatting) if dynamic LV outflow obstruction present, accompanied by MR, paradoxical splitting of S2, "quick-rise" arterial pulse.
Electrocardiogram	LV hypertrophy, deep septal Q waves, anterolateral and inferior "pseudo" infarction pattern, +/− apical giant T wave inversions (apical variant).
Chest X-Ray	Normal heart size or cardiomegaly
Laboratory	
Echocardiogram	LV hypertrophy (≥15 mm), often more pronounced in septum (asymmetric septal hypertrophy), systolic anterior motion of mitral valve, with LV outflow tract gradient +/− MR.
Cardiac Catheterization	Supranormal ejection fraction, +/− LV outflow tract obstruction +/− MR
Treatment	Beta-blockers, calcium channel blockers (verapamil), disopyramide, DDD pacemaker, ICD, amiodarone (in patients at high risk for sudden cardiac death), alcohol septal ablation, surgery (myo-myectomy for refractory obstructive symptoms, mitral valve replacement/repair for MR). Avoid strenuous activity, dehydration, digoxin, diuretics (may be used with caution for CHF), and vasodilator therapy. Infective endocarditis prophylaxis is no longer recommended. Rate control and anticoagulant therapy for atrial fibrillation.

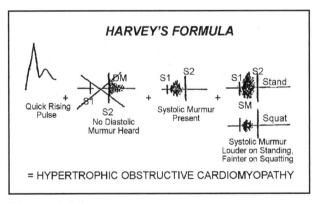

Figure 16-4 (Courtesy of W. Proctor Harvey, M.D.)

Right. Simultaneous aortic and LV pressure recordings demonstrating the dynamic LV outflow tract obstruction in a patient with HOCM. Note the increase in the LV-aortic pressure gradient, along with the characteristic decrease in aortic pulse pressure (*Brockenbrough sign*) and "spike and dome" configuration (due to the rapid upstroke of the arterial pulse in early systole with a second peak in late systole due to dynamic LV outflow tract obstruction) of the aortic pressure recording, after a premature ventricular contraction (PVC).

TREATMENT OPTIONS FOR HOCM

Medical treatment attempts to reduce the outflow tract obstruction, relax the ventricle, and avoid rhythm disturbances that may be associated with this condition:

- Beta blockers are the initial treatment of choice in symptomatic patients. Calcium channel blockers (e.g., verapamil) may also be useful in relieving symptoms (to allow more time for diastolic filling).
- If atrial fibrillation supervenes, every effort should be made to restore normal sinus rhythm (and preserve

clinician to the diagnosis. (**Figure 16-5**). In general, these drugs should be avoided.

Figure 16-5. Pressure recordings in hypertrophic obstructive cardiomyopathy. **Left.** Schematic diagram illustrating the subaortic systolic pressure gradient between the LV cavity and the LV outflow tract during a catheter "pullback" from deep in the LV chamber to the ascending aorta. No gradient between the LV outflow tract and aorta is present.

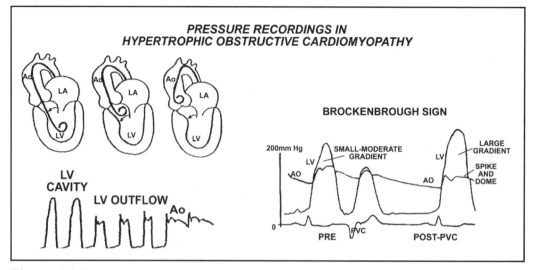

Figure 16-5

"atrial kick"). Frequent paroxysms or established atrial fibrillation indicate the need for long-term anticoagulation.
- Although at increased risk for infective endocarditis, recent guidelines no longer recommend antibiotic prophylaxis based solely on lifetime risk (see chapter 17).
- Certain anti-arrhythmic agents, e.g., disopyramide (due to its negative inotropic effects) and amiodarone, may be effective forms of therapy.

Surgical relief of the outflow tract gradient by myotomy and myectomy of the hypertrophied septum (when symptoms persist despite intensive pharmacologic treatment), or mitral valve replacement (reserved for the few in whom severe MR develops) provide mechanical solutions to the problem of dynamic LV outflow tract obstruction. In experienced hands, myectomy has a low operative mortality (~1–2%) and most patients have long-lasting improvement in their clinical outcome. Percutaneous transcoronary septal reduction with alcohol, along with dual chamber pacing (to reduce outflow tract gradient), and implantable cardioverter defibrillators (ICDs) may also be considered in the treatment strategy, and now provide additional forms of therapy for those patients who are refractory to medical therapy. The ICD is the most reliable and effective treatment for patients at high risk, particularly those who survive a cardiac arrest. Long-term results of these newer procedures, however, are under investigation. Recent studies have cast doubt on the value of dual chamber pacing and suggest that improvement is often largely due to a placebo effect. Furthermore, follow-up of patients after septal ablation is relatively brief and there is some concern that the permanent scar produced within the septum may eventually generate serious rhythm disturbances and actually increase risk for sudden death.

RISK OF SUDDEN DEATH

The most alarming aspect of this disease is the risk of sudden death. Unlike with valvular AS, reduction or abolition of the systolic pressure gradient across the obstruction (by surgical or other treatments) does not abolish this risk. Analyses suggest that the risk of sudden death is not as high as previously believed, only ~ 1% per year. The risk of sudden cardiac death increases in patients with malignant ventricular arrhythmias, syncope, a family history of sudden death, severe LV hypertrophy (≥30 mm), high risk mutations, a blunted or hypotensive blood pressure response to exercise, and is more common in children and young adults (particularly athletes). The presence of a resting LV outflow tract gradient of ≥ 30 mmHg in patients with HOCM is a strong independent predictor of progression to severe symptoms of CHF and/or death. Although symptoms due to outflow obstruction may be relieved by drugs with negative inotropic properties (e.g., beta blockers, verapamil, disopyramide), these agents do not prevent sudden arrhythmic death. Patients with malignant ventricular arrhythmias and unexplained syncope in the presence of a positive family history for sudden death are probably best managed with an ICD. Since sudden cardiac death (due to ventricular tachyarrhythmias) usually occurs during heavy exertion, patients with HOCM should not participate in any strenuous exercise or high-intensity competitive sports. First-degree relatives of an affected individual should undergo periodic clinical screening with ECG and echo (since the timing of onset of HOCM is variable), along with genetic testing, if a definite pathogenic mutation has been identified.

CHAPTER 17. APPROACH TO THE PATIENT WITH INFECTIVE ENDOCARDITIS

Infective endocarditis occurs when infective organisms invade the endothelial (particularly the valvular) surfaces of the heart, causing tissue destruction and vegetations. Despite medical and surgical advances, the mortality rates remain high. This may be due to the fact that infective endocarditis is now occurring in older individuals, in patients unaware of having heart valve disease, in those with prosthetic valves or other intracardiac devices, and is being caused by aggressive organisms, e.g., staphylocci. This chapter will review the diagnosis, treatment, and prevention of this complex, commonly missed, and potentially lethal disease.

ETIOLOGY AND RISK FACTORS

Although bacteria remain the most common cause, virtually all organisms (including viruses, fungi, and rickettsia) can cause endocarditis. The species of infecting organisms relates to whether intravenous drug abuse is involved and whether infection affects a native or a prosthetic valve. The portal of entry may also give the clue to the type of organism. Infections with *viridans streptococci* (normal inhabitants of the oropharynx) are the most common causative organisms (from dental procedures) and usually attack prosthetic or previously damaged valves. Strains of *enterococci,* the next most frequent cause, particularly occur in older men after GU infection. *Streptococcus bovis,* another common pathogen, is particularly prevalent in elderly patients with colonic polyps or GI malignancy. *Staphylococcus aureus,* which is particularly virulent and can attack previously normal valves, is the most common organism in IV drug use and prosthetic valve infection. *Staphylococcus epidermidis* is a common cause of "early" prosthetic valve endocarditis (occurring <60 days following implantation).

CLINICAL PRESENTATION OF INFECTIVE ENDOCARDITIS

The clinical syndrome may be acute or subacute, depending on the causative organisms. *Subacute* disease (as commonly occurs with *Strep viridans* infection) denotes a form, often of insidious onset, with slow development of the characteristic lesions and absence of marked toxicity for a long period of time. The patient may complain of fever, but its magnitude and pattern may vary considerably. In contrast, *acute* infective endocarditis (e.g. from *Staph aureus*) may present as a fulminant infection, with abrupt onset, high fever, and a rapid downhill course with respect to both valve destruction and systemic toxicity. CHF (due to valvular regurgitation) and arterial emboli (from the infective valvular vegetations) are the most common complications and result in significant morbidity and mortality.

The classic triad of *fever, heart murmur,* particularly regurgitant (e.g., MR, AR, TR), and *positive blood cultures* (present in >95% of cases) should alert the clinician to the possibility of infective endocarditis. *Regurgitant lesions are more prone to infections than stenotic lesions.* **Figure 17-1** summarizes the clinical criteria for diagnosis of infective endocarditis, while **Figure 17-2** summarizes how the manifestations of the condition have changed over the past few decades.

Risk factors include a history of valvular heart disease, the presence of a prosthetic heart valve, and IV drug use. Degenerative aortic and mitral valve disease and MVP are the most common substrates for endocarditis. MVP is associated with more than one third of cases of endocarditis of the mitral valve. Endocarditis most frequently occurs in mild lesions (e.g., mild MR, AR), rather than a severely damaged valve. Infection of a bicuspid aortic valve accounts for 20% of cases in persons >60 years of age, whereas a secundum ASD rarely becomes infected (because it is a low pressure system). Additional risk factors are HOCM and Marfan's syndrome associated with AR and MVP. IV drug users have a unique propensity to develop infective endocarditis of the tricuspid valve and often present with septic pulmonary emboli.

A patient with unexplained fever and a heart murmur should be viewed as having infective endocarditis until proven otherwise. Approximately 15% of patients with infective endocarditis, however, do not have a heart murmur. In a patient with a "fever of unknown origin", infective endocarditis should be considered even with no murmur. A symptom pattern that may provide a useful clue is that of a vague illness over several weeks or months that responds transiently to courses of outpatient antibiotics, but recurs shortly after they are discontinued. Fever may be absent, however, in the elderly, and in those who are severely debilitated or with renal failure. Other symptoms, e.g., anorexia, weight loss, myalgias, and arthralgias are also frequent.

Over 50% of patients will have some form of peripheral vasculitic lesion, including *petechiae* (conjunctiva, mucosa, skin), *splinter hemorrhages* (beneath the nail beds), *Osler's nodes* (painful, tender erythematous nodules on the

---

FIGURE 17-1

Clinical Criteria for Diagnosis of Infective Endocarditis

Definite	Possible	Reject

• 2 major criteria
  —1 major and 3 minor criteria, or
  —5 minor criteria
	• 1 major and 1 minor criteria, or
	• 3 minor criteria
		• Firm alternative diagnosis

MAJOR	MINOR

• Positive blood cultures (either)
  —typical organisms*
  —persistently positive (at least 12 hrs apart)
• Echocardiographic (either)
  —oscillating mass (vegetation)
  —abscess
  —dehiscence of prosthetic valve
• New valvular regurgitation (increase or change in preexisting murmur not sufficient)
	• Predisposing clinical conditions e.g., prosthetic heart valve, IV drug use, previous endocarditis
	• Fever greater than 38°C
	• Vascular phenomena, e.g., septic embolus, Osler's nodes, Janeway lesions, conjunctival petechiae
	• Immunologic phenomena, e.g., glomerulonephritis, positive rheumatoid factor, and C-reactive protein
	• Microbiologic evidence (one positive culture with a typical organism)

*Note: Typical organisms include streptococcus viridans, streptococcus bovis, enterococcus, staphylococcus or the "HACEK" group (Haemophilus, Actinobacillus, Cardiobacterium, Eikenella, and Kingella species). Positive Q fever (Coxiella burnetti) serology is now considered major criterion.

Adapted from Duke criteria. Source: AHA/ACC Guidelines. Diagnosis and management of infective endocarditis and its complications. Circulation 1998, 99: 2936–2948.

---

fingers and toes), *Janeway lesions* (non-tender, hemorrhagic macular lesions on the palms and soles), and *Roth spots* (retinal hemorrhages with white centers), which are caused by large or small emboli that tear loose from the vegetations of endocarditis. Other clinical findings, e.g., wasting, clubbing, splenomegaly, pallor (secondary to anemia), are related in part to the duration of infection. Cerebral emboli may lead to hemiplegia, ataxia, aphasia, or change in mental status. A young person with an acute stroke, therefore, should be evaluated for possible infective endocarditis.

Figure 17-3. Morphologic features of infective endocarditis on the tricuspid valve. Note the vegetation and ruptured chordae resulting in acute tricuspid regurgitation. Auscultatory findings in a young IV drug abuser with tricuspid valve endocarditis reveal the systolic murmur (SM) of acute tricuspid regurgitation, which, although not holosystolic, is best heard over the left lower sternal border (llsb) and gets louder with inspiration (insp). (Courtesy of Dr. W. Proctor Harvey).

The most important laboratory test for endocarditis is the blood culture (taken three times for assurance), since it confirms the diagnosis and guides appropriate therapy. A small number of patients with infective endocarditis have negative blood cultures, though, as a result of prior treatment of the infection with antibiotics or the presence of certain types of infections that do not culture well. These infections include fastidious gram negative bacilli such as the HACEK group (Haemophilus, Actinobacillus, Cardiobacterium, Eikenella, and Kingella) or fungi, such as Candida or Aspergillus from an indwelling IV catheter, which tend to produce larger vegetations than bacteria, and often embolize. Histologic study of these septic emboli may be the first clue to the presence of fungal endocarditis.

The ECG may demonstrate progressive heart block, which is an ominous sign indicating that an abscess has formed in the myocardium (particularly the interventricular septum) and that the conduction system is involved.

Examine the CXR for signs of heart failure. Patients with right-sided endocarditis may demonstrate multiple pulmonary infiltrates secondary to septic embolism to the lungs.

Echo, especially TEE, is an essential noninvasive imaging study for diagnosing vegetations (the classic lesion of endocarditis) and revealing the presence and severity of valvular regurgitation. Transthoracic echo reveals vegetations in about 50–60% of patients. TEE is a very sensitive (>95%) technique for identifying valvular vegetations (particularly in those with prosthetic valves). Vegetations

FIGURE 17-2

Changing Characteristics of Infective Endocarditis

CHARACTERISTICS	OLD TYPE	NEW TYPE
Fever	Weeks	Days
Murmur	Obvious	Subtle
Splenomegaly	Common	Rare
Peripheral Manifestations:		
Osler's Nodes	Common	Rare
Janeway Lesions	Common	Rare
Arthritis	Common	Rare
Arterial Emboli	Common	Not infrequent
Roth Spots	Common	Rare
Culture Negative	Rare	5% to 10%
Abnormal Urinalysis	Common	Infrequent
Organism	Streptococci	Strep/Staph
Valve	Native	Native/Prosthetic
IV Drug Abuse	Rare	Not Infrequent
Prognosis	Very Poor	Fair-to-Good

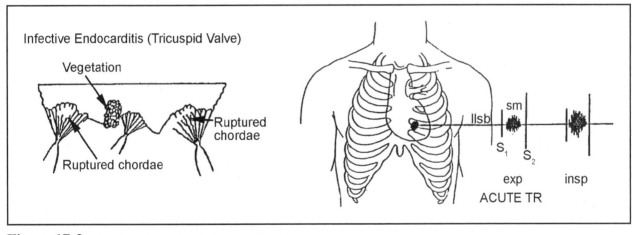

Figure 17-3 (Courtesy of W. Proctor Harvey, M.D.)

may first appear two weeks after the diagnosis and persist for months after clinical cure. Unfortunately, a negative echo does not exclude the diagnosis.

Invasive diagnostic procedures should be undertaken with great care because of the fear of dislodging material from a vegetation with resultant embolism.

Figure 17-4 summarizes the clinical approach to infective endocarditis.

Some of the more classic manifestations of endocarditis (e.g., petechiae, splinter hemorrhages, Osler's nodes, Janeway's lesions) represent late signs of untreated disease.

Clues to the diagnosis of infective endocarditis in the elderly include fever with unexplained heart failure, stroke, progressive renal failure, low back pain, weight loss, anemia, and systemic embolism. Elderly patients and patients taking steroids or NSAIDs may be afebrile.

THERAPY AND PREVENTION OF INFECTIVE ENDOCARDITIS

Antibiotic therapy in patients with suspected infective endocarditis should begin after at least 3 sets of blood cultures are

---

FIGURE 17-4

Clinical Approach to Infective Endocarditis

History	Fever (80–90%), chills, sweats, anorexia, weight loss, fatigue, malaise. History predisposing condition, e.g., prosthetic heart valve, acquired or congenital valvular heart disease. History previous dental work (including teeth cleaning), indwelling intravascular catheter, IV drug abuse.
Physical Examination	New valvular regurgitation murmurs (due to fenestrated valve or ruptured chordae), muffled prosthetic valve sounds, pericardial friction rub, pallor (anemia), Janeway lesions (non-tender hemorrhagic macules on palms or soles), Osler's nodes (tender nodules on pads of fingers and toes), petechiae (conjunctiva, palate), Roth spots (retinal hemorrhage with pale center), tender splenomegaly, splinter hemorrhages on nail beds, neurologic signs of stroke (secondary to emboli), hemiplegia, seizures, coma.
Electrocardiogram	May be normal, or show findings of preexisting cardiac disease, e.g., LA/LV or RA/RV hypertrophy or enlargement, new conduction abnormalities (secondary to septal abscess), acute MI (due to coronary artery embolus).
Chest X-Ray	May be normal, or show signs of increasing CHF (especially if native valve or prosthetic valve involved), multiple pulmonary infiltrates secondary to tricuspid valve involvement with septic embolism to lungs.
Laboratory	
Blood cultures	Positive blood cultures (before initiation of antibiotics), at least 3 sets (aerobic and anaerobic bottles). May be negative (often as a result of prior treatment of infection with antibiotics).
Blood tests	Anemia, elevated sedimentation rate, positive Rheumatoid factor, white blood cell count may be elevated, normal, or low.
Echocardiogram	Transthoracic echo (or TEE if non-diagnostic or negative but endocarditis strongly suspected or prosthetic valve). Detects vegetations and/or location and severity of valvular regurgitation (TEE more sensitive than transthoracic echo).
Treatment	Antibiotic therapy for 4–6 weeks. Empiric therapy (before culture results available) in acutely ill patients: Native valve bacterial endocarditis (Vancomycin + Ceftriaxone or Vancomycin + Gentamycin). Prosthetic valve endocarditis (Vancomycin + Gentamycin + Rifampin). Surgery for refractory CHF, persistent or refractory infection, worsening conduction defect, prosthetic valve malfunction or dehiscence, or staph aureus infection, recurrent emboli, fungal infection.

---

obtained. Empiric therapy should cover the most likely pathogens, including streptococci, staphylococci, enterococci and HACEK group. Pathogen directed therapy should be initiated once the causative organism has been identified. Prolonged intravenous antimicrobial therapy (for 4 to 6 weeks or longer) may be needed to eradicate the infection, sterilize the vegetation, and prevent recurrence. Valve replacement is often indicated when a staph aureus or fungal infection is present, a prosthetic valve is infected, complications (e.g., myocardial abscess or acute valvular dysfunction associated with CHF) has developed, medical therapy has failed, or a large vegetation or more than one embolic event has occurred (**Figure 17-5**). Device-related (pacemaker/ICD) endocarditis generally requires removal of the entire system, including the leads, with reimplantation, if needed, on the contralateral side.

For decades, it has been a commonly held belief that antimicrobial prophylaxis before procedures that may cause transient bacteremia can prevent infective endocarditis in patients at increased risk for this disorder. The effectiveness of this common practice, however, has never been established by controlled trials in humans. Experts now believe that infective endocarditis is much more likely to develop secondary to random bacteremias associated with daily activities, e.g., chewing food, brushing teeth, and flossing, than from transient bacteremia caused by a dental, gastrointestinal (GI) or genitourinary (GU) tract procedure. Furthermore, even if antimicrobial prophylaxis were 100% effective, it would only prevent an exceedingly small number of cases of infective endocarditis. In addition, the risk of antibiotic-associated adverse events would exceed the benefit, if any, from the use of antibiotics.

Accordingly, the American Heart Association has issued updated guidelines on the prevention of infective endocarditis. Whereas previous guidelines recommended

---

FIGURE 17-5

Clinical Indications for Surgery in Infective Endocarditis

- Acute aortic or mitral regurgitation associated with CHF
- Continuing ("refractory") CHF (despite maximal medical therapy)
- Persistent or refractory infection (e.g., positive blood culture after one week of appropriate IV antibiotic therapy)
- Invasive infection (e.g., ring abscess, new heart block or conduction defects)
- Prosthetic valve, especially with valve malfunction or dehiscence, or staph aureus or gram negative infection not responding to antibiotic therapy.
- Recurrent systemic emboli.
- Fungal infection
- "Very large" mobile vegetations

FIGURE 17-6

Endocarditis Prophylaxis Is Recommended For:

Cardiac Conditions*

- Prosthetic cardiac valves (including transcatheter valves) or prosthetic material used for valve repair
- Previous endocarditis
- Unrepaired, recently repaired (within 6 months), or partially repaired cyanotic congenital heart disease
- Cardiac valvulopathy following heart transplantation

Procedures

- Dental procedures that involve manipulation of gingival tissue or the periapical region of teeth or perforation of the oral mucosa (e.g., teeth extractions and cleanings)
- Invasive respiratory tract procedures involving incision or biopsy of the respiratory mucosa (e.g., tonsillectomy and adenoidectomy)
- Surgical procedures that involve infected skin or musculoskeletal structures

---

Adapted from Wilson W, Taubert, KA, Gewitz, M, et al. Prevention of Infective Endocarditis. Guidelines from the American Heart Association. A Guideline from the American Heart Association Rheumatic Fever, Endocarditis, and Kawasaki Disease Committee, Council on Cardiovascular Disease in the Young, and the Council on Clinical Cardiology, Council on Cardiovascular Surgery and Anesthesia, and the quality of Care and Outcomes Research Interdisciplinary Working Group. Circulation 115: 2007.

*Note: Antimicrobial prophylaxis is recommended only in patients with cardiac conditions associated with the highest risk of adverse outcome from endocarditis, not in patients solely at increased risk of acquiring infective endocarditis.

---

prophylaxis for individuals at increased lifetime risk for acquiring infective endocarditis, the revised guidelines emphasize prophylaxis only for patients with cardiac conditions associated with the highest risk for adverse outcome from infective endocarditis. "High risk" patients include those with prosthetic heart valves (including transcatheter valves) or prosthetic material used for valve repair; previous infective endocarditis; unrepaired, recently repaired (within 6 months), or partially repaired cyanotic congenital heart disease; and cardiac valvulopathy following heart transplantation.

Even for these "high risk" patients, prophylaxis is recommended only before dental procedures that involve manipulation of gingival tissue, or the periapical region of teeth, or perforation of the oral mucosa; invasive respiratory tract procedures involving incision or biopsy of the respiratory mucosa; or surgical procedures that involve infected skin or musculoskeletal structures. Infective endocarditis prophylaxis is no longer recommended for GU or GI tract procedures, even in these high risk patients. Antibiotic prophylaxis is also not recommended for other common procedures including ear and body piercing, tattooing, vaginal delivery, and hysterectomy.

Since the revised guidelines no longer recommend antimicrobial prophylaxis solely to prevent infective endocarditis, patients with MVP and mitral regurgitation or thickened valve leaflets, a congenital bicuspid aortic valve, calcific AS, rheumatic heart disease, or structural disorders, e.g., VSD and HOCM, are no longer considered candidates for prophylaxis. Routine prophylaxis is also not recommended prior to cardiac catheterization, or in patients with cardiac pacemakers, implanted defibrillators, coronary stents, or in those who have had CABG surgery. Although dental disease may increase the risk of infective endocarditis, the revised guidelines shift emphasis away from antimicrobial prophylaxis for dental procedures to meticulous oral health and hygiene and improved dental care in patients with conditions that carry an increased risk for the infection.

The revised (and somewhat controversial) prophylaxis recommendations are given in **Figures 17-6 to 17-8**.

FIGURE 17-7

Infective Endocarditis Prophylaxis Is Not Recommended For:

Cardiac Conditions

- Mitral valve prolapse with mitral regurgitation or leaflet thickening
- Bicuspid aortic valve
- Rheumatic or acquired valvular heart disease
- Hypertrophic obstructive cardiomyopathy
- ASD, VSD, and PDA
- Cardiac catheterization, including PCI
- Coronary stents, cardiac pacemakers, implanted defibrillators
- Coronary artery disease or previous coronary bypass surgery

Procedures*

- Dental procedures that involve routine anesthetic injections through noninfected tissue, taking dental radiographs, placement of removable prosthodontic or orthodontic appliances, adjustment of orthodontic appliances, placement of orthodontic brackets, shedding of deciduous teeth, and bleeding from trauma to the lips or oral mucosa
- Bronchoscopy (without incision or biopsy of respiratory tract mucosa)
- GU (e.g., cystoscopy, urethral dilatation) or GI tract procedures, including endoscopy or colonoscopy
- Ear and body piercing, and tattooing
- Vaginal delivery and hysterectomy

Adapted from Wilson W, Taubert, KA, Gewitz, M, et al. Prevention of Infective Endocarditis. Guidelines from the American Heart Association. A Guideline from the American Heart Association Rheumatic Fever, Endocarditis, and Kawasaki Disease Committee, Council on Cardiovascular Disease in the Young, and the Council on Clinical Cardiology, Council on Cardiovascular Surgery and Anesthesia, and the quality of Care and Outcomes Research Interdisciplinary Working Group. Circulation 115: 2007.

*Note: In the case of a procedure that involves infected tissues, it may be necessary to provide appropriate doses of antibiotics for treatment of the established infection.

FIGURE 17-8

Endocarditis Prophylaxis Regimens

Situation	Agent
	(single dose 30-60 min before procedure)
Oral prophylaxis	Amoxicillin*
Parenteral prophylaxis	Ampicillin
	or
	Cefazolin or Ceftriaxone
	or
	Clindamycin

---

*Note: For penicillin-allergic individuals, cephalexin, cefadroxil, clindamycin, or azithromycin-clarithromycin may be used. Cephalosporins should not be used, however, in those with immediate-type hypersensitivity reaction (e.g., urticaria, angioedema, or anaphylaxis) to penicillin.

Adapted from Wilson W, Taubert, KA, Gewitz, M, et al. Prevention of Infective Endocarditis. Guidelines from the American Heart Association. A Guideline from the American Heart Association Rheumatic Fever, Endocarditis, and Kawasaki Disease Committee, Council on Cardiovascular Disease in the Young, and the Council on Clinical Cardiology, Council on Cardiovascular Surgery and Anesthesia, and the quality of Care and Outcomes Research Interdisciplinary Working Group. Circulation 115: 2007.

CHAPTER 18.   APPROACH TO THE PATIENT WITH AORTIC AND PERIPHERAL ARTERIAL DISEASE

Diseases of the aorta and its branches may present as one of three clinical conditions: *aortic dissection, aortic aneurysm, and peripheral arterial disease*. This chapter will discuss the diagnosis and management of these common vascular diseases.

AORTIC DISSECTION

Acute *aortic dissection* and its variants, *intramural hematoma* and *penetrating atherosclerotic ulcer*, are part of a spectrum of acute, life-threatening aortic events termed *"acute aortic syndromes"*. Classic aortic dissection results when blood gains entry into the media of the vessel wall from a primary tear in the intima, producing a so-called false lumen that propagates distally (or sometimes antegrade) for some distance. An aortic intramural hematoma results when bleeding occurs within the media (from rupture of vasa vasorum) without evidence of an intimal tear. A penetrating aortic ulcer is an erosion of an atherosclerotic plaque into the media, which results in a localized hematoma.

- *Type A* dissections originate in the ascending aorta, usually within a few centimeters of the aortic valve, and either extend around the aortic arch into the descending aorta (type 1) or are limited to the ascending aorta (type 2).
- *Type B* (or type 3) dissections (which are less common than Type A) involve only the descending aorta and originate just distal to the origin of the left subclavian artery. Type B dissections have the best prognosis. (**Figure 18-1**).

Proximal dissections may involve the aortic valve, resulting in acute AR. The aorta may rupture into the pericardium and cause cardiac tamponade (*hemopericardium*) or into the left pleural cavity with exsanguination (*hemothorax*). The hematoma may compress the aortic branches, causing acute myocardial ischemia or infarction due to occlusion of the coronary ostium (right coronary artery most commonly involved), stroke, paraplegia (spinal cord ischemia), abdominal pain (mesenteric ischemia), or limb pain (ischemia of the extremities), depending on the vessels occluded. Some patients with cystic medial necrosis have progressive dilatation of the ascending aorta and AR without dissection (so-called *annuloaortic ectasia*). *Aortic dissection is most common in middle-aged to older males with a history of hypertension*. Patients with a history of cocaine use, connective tissue disorders, e.g., *Marfan's, Loeys-Dietz, and Ehlers-Danlos syndromes*, and women in their last trimester of *pregnancy* are also at increased risk.

Coarctation of the aorta and a *bicuspid aortic valve* are less common predisposing risk factors. *Iatrogenic trauma* from cardiac catheterization procedures or cardiac surgery (particularly aortic valve replacement) may also cause aortic dissection.

The abrupt onset of severe chest pain, "ripping" or "tearing" in quality, radiating to the back (interscapular area), should lead the astute practitioner to consider aortic dissection. In contradistinction to the discomfort of MI, which begins as a mild sensation and gradually builds in intensity, the pain of aortic dissection is maximal in intensity at its onset. Patients may present with complaints secondary to obstruction of an artery to the heart, brain, or extremities. Dyspnea secondary to the development of acute AR may be prominent.

The following are all clues to an acute (type I) aortic dissection:

- A new high frequency diastolic blowing murmur of AR, heard best along the right sternal border (third and fourth intercostal spaces) as compared to the left (which is usually the case for murmurs of valvular AR)
- Unequal or absent pulses
- A neurological deficit (e.g., stroke) from cut-off of blood supply to the brain, spinal cord or limb
- A syncopal episode

Such patients often appear pale and sweaty (shock-like) but generally have moderate to severe hypertension. A pericardial friction rub that develops under these circumstances

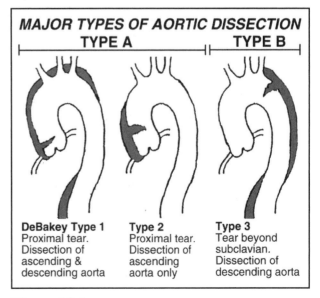

Figure 18-1

signifies bleeding into the pericardial sac and is, therefore, an ominous finding. Patients may present with acute pericardial tamponade (manifest by hypotension, pulsus paradoxus, jugular venous distention, and muffled heart sounds).

Keep in mind the following formula: *Chest pain (radiating through to the interscapular region)* + hypertension + right-sided aortic regurgitation murmur = dissection of the first portion of ascending aorta (Harvey's sign). This can provide a valuable clue to the diagnosis and thus enable prompt life-saving surgical intervention (**Figure 2-77**).

The chest x-ray finding of a widened mediastinum, especially if it is new, along with increased distance (greater than 1 cm) from aortic intimal calcification to the outer edge of the aortic shadow, is highly suggestive of aortic dissection. (**Figure 4-7A**). The ECG findings are usually nonspecific (e.g., sinus tachycardia, ST-T changes) but may reveal LV hypertrophy from long-standing hypertension. A rare patient may develop obstruction of a coronary artery (particularly the right) with resultant ECG findings of acute (usually inferior) MI. The extent of dissection usually can be visualized with TEE, CT scan with contrast, MRI, and aortography. The preference of the cardiothoracic surgeon may influence the study chosen. In the hemodynamically unstable patient with suspected aortic dissection, TEE is generally the study of choice because of its high sensitivity and specificity and because it can be performed rapidly and at the bedside.

Surgical consultation should be obtained as soon as aortic dissection is suspected.

- For patients with proximal dissection, the immediate goal of treatment is to lower BP, first with IV beta blocker therapy, e.g., esmolol, labetalol (which also reduces shear stress by lowering the BP) and then with IV nitroprusside, while awaiting emergent surgical repair. *Misdiagnosis of aortic dissection as acute MI can have disastrous consequences should the patient receive anticoagulants or thrombolytic therapy.* Thrombolytic therapy can lead to exsanguination in this setting, and is therefore contraindicated. Pericardial tamponade may result and is generally a terminal event.
- For type A dissection, the ascending aorta and, if necessary, the aortic valve and arch are replaced with reimplantation of the coronary and brachiocephalic vessels. Aspirin, heparin, and thrombolytics are contraindicated. Following successful surgery, chronic beta blocker therapy and annual imaging (CT scan or MRI) are indicated to evaluate for the development of progressive aortic dilatation or recurrent dissection.
- For type B (distal) dissection, long term pharmacologic therapy with beta blockers (or, if contraindicated, verapamil or diltiazem) is recommended as

long as the patient remains stable. Surgical treatment, after several weeks of pharmacologic therapy, is advised by some authorities who believe that the majority of type B dissections will ultimately develop an indication for surgical intervention, e.g., increasing aortic size, an enlarging saccular aneurysm, compromise of major branches of the aorta, or symptoms related to their chronic dissection. Catheter-based repair with endovascular stent-grafts is currently being employed as an alternative to surgery.

AORTIC ANEURYSM

An *aortic aneurysm* is a localized ≥50% dilatation ("bulge") of the aorta involving all three layers of the vessel wall (intima, media, adventitia). The most common location for aneurysm formation is the infrarenal abdominal aorta, followed by the ascending thoracic aorta. Ascending thoracic aortic aneurysms (TAAs) are generally caused by cystic medial necrosis (as may be seen in Marfan's, Loeys-Dietz, and Ehlers-Danlos syndromes, bicuspid aortic valve, aortitis, and hypertension), whereas abdominal aortic aneurysms (AAAs) are primarily associated with atherosclerosis and its risk factors, i.e., advanced age, hypertension, smoking, dyslipidemia, male gender, and family history. The pathogenesis of AAA involves a combination of inflammation, a proteolytic breakdown in the structural proteins elastin and collagen, and biochemical stresses which lead to weakening of the vessel wall.

Most aortic aneurysms are asymptomatic. Chest, abdominal, or back pain may be produced by expanding aneurysms, which is often a harbinger of impending rupture. Acute rupture, however, may occur without warning, and is always life-threatening. The triad of hypotension, abdominal or back pain, and a pulsatile abdominal mass is diagnostic of a ruptured AAA. Pressure on adjacent structures from a TAA may produce hoarseness (laryngeal nerve), respiratory symptoms (trachea), dysphagia (esophagus), and facial edema (superior vena cava). Extremity pain may result from embolization of mural thrombi. Ascending TAAs may present with CHF due to AR. Chest and abdominal X-rays may reveal an enlarged aorta outlined by calcification. Ultrasonography (abdominal or TEE), CT, MRI, and aortography, can localize and assess the size of the aneurysm.

Unstable patients with a ruptured aneurysm require immediate operation. Elective surgical or endovascular aortic repair (EVAR) is advisable for aneurysms that are large, i.e., > 5.5 cm (AAA or ascending TAA), or > 6 cm (descending TAA), symptomatic, or are growing rapidly. Patients with smaller aneurysms can be managed conservatively (risk factor modification, BP control, beta blockade) and followed by abdominal ultrasound (US) or CT scan every 6 to 12 months. Ultrasound screening for AAA is recommended for men age 65 to 75 who have smoked, and for those > 60 years with a family history of AAA.

Figure 18-2 summarizes the clinical approach to aortic dissection and aortic aneurysm.

PERIPHERAL ARTERIAL DISEASE

Peripheral arterial disease (PAD) generally refers to atherosclerotic occlusive disease in the arteries of the lower extremities. Mild PAD may be asymptomatic or cause intermittent claudication, a cramping pain in the legs induced by exercise and relieved by rest. Pain in the buttocks and thighs (+/- erectile dysfunction) suggests aortoiliac disease (Leriche syndrome), whereas calf muscle pain implies femoropopliteal

disease. Severe PAD may cause rest pain with skin atrophy, hair loss, cyanosis, ischemic ulcers, and gangrene. Diminished or absent pulses, along with arterial bruits may be present. The diagnosis may be confirmed by the ankle-brachial index (ABI), i.e., the ratio of the ankle to the brachial systolic BP (ABI < 0.9 = mild PAD; < 0.4 = severe PAD). Doppler ultrasound can detect abnormal blood flow caused by arterial stenoses.

Treatment of PAD includes risk factor modification, exercise, and antiplatelet therapy (aspirin, clopidogrel, vorapaxar). Cilostazol (Pletal), a phosphodiesterase inhibitor-vasodilator with platelet inhibiting properties, has been shown to relieve symptoms and improve walking distance, and is recommended (if no CHF) in patients with intermittent claudication. Severe PAD usually requires percutaneous or surgical intervention, and as a last resort, amputation if critical limb ischemia is present. The prognosis for lower extremity PAD itself is generally good, although the mortality rate remains high because CAD and cerebrovascular disease often coexist.

FIGURE 18-2

Clinical Approach to Aortic Dissection and Aortic Aneurysm

History	Sudden onset severe "ripping" or "tearing" anterior chest pain, maximal at onset, radiating to the back in aortic dissection.
	Most aortic aneurysms are asymptomatic. Chest, abdominal, or back pain occurs when aneurysm enlarging. Pressure on surrounding structures may cause hoarseness, respiratory symptoms, dysphagia, and facial edema (TAA). Extremity pain may result from embolization of mural thrombus.
Physical Examination	In aortic dissection, a new diastolic murmur of AR (with proximal dissection involving aortic root), pericardial friction rub (due to rupture into pericardial sac), unequal BP or pulses, neurologic deficits, shock-like state with moderate or severe hypertension may be present.
	Pulsation in sternal notch and right-sided diastolic murmur of AR (ascending TAA). Pulsatile, expansile, abdominal mass (AAA). Triad of hypotension, abdominal/back pain, and pulsatile mass = ruptured AAA.
Electrocardiogram	May be normal. If dissection involves coronary ostia, MI (particularly inferior) may occur.
Chest X-Ray	Mediastinal widening or increase in aortic diameter. Aortic calcification may be visualized.
Laboratory TEE and US CT Scan MRI Aortography	Reveals false lumen (intimal tear) in aortic dissection. Detects and assesses size of aortic aneurysm.
Treatment	Short term in aortic dissection: IV nitroprusside and beta-blocker to ↓ BP and shear stress. Immediate surgery for proximal (Type A) dissection. Long term medical therapy: Beta-blockers after surgery or for distal (Type B) dissection. Endovascular stent-grafts are currently being employed as an alternative to surgery in Type B dissection.
	Elective open or endovascular aortic repair (EVAR) for aneurysms that are large (> 5.5 cm AAA or ascending TAA, > 6 cm descending TAA), symptomatic, or growing rapidly. Risk factor modification, BP control with beta-blockers, and surveillance imaging (US, CT) for small asymptomatic aneurysms.

CHAPTER 19. APPROACH TO THE PATIENT WITH PERICARDIAL DISEASE

Diseases of the pericardium can produce a variety of clinical findings that may mimic many other organ system diseases e.g., pulmonary or liver disease, and be mistaken for other cardiac diagnoses, e.g., acute myocardial ischemia or infarction and chronic CHF. In this modern era of reperfusion therapy and aggressive intervention for acute coronary syndromes, investigation into such conditions as pericardial disease that are at especially high risk for developing hemorrhagic complications if inadvertently treated with thrombolytic agents and/or anticoagulant drugs is of the utmost importance. The clinical diagnosis of pericardial disease can usually be made using the "five-finger" approach. Knowledge of the multiple etiologies of pericarditis and their clinical presentations, along with an understanding of the physiology of pericardial tamponade and constriction enables the astute clinician to determine the cause, evaluate the severity of these complications, and direct appropriate therapy. This chapter will highlight the clinical presentation and evaluation of these common manifestations of pericardial heart disease.

ACUTE PERICARDITIS

Pericarditis is an inflammation of the visceral and/or parietal pericardium. It has numerous etiologies and the natural history depends to a great extent on the specific cause. The 5-finger description of acute pericarditis is presented in **Figure 19-1.**

The most common cause is idiopathic, although the majority of these cases are likely due to viruses (e.g., Coxsackie A or B virus, influenza, HIV). Pericarditis may also result from an underlying malignancy (especially lung, breast, lymphoma), non-penetrating (e.g., steering wheel) chest injury, connective tissue disease (e.g., systemic lupus erythematosus, rheumatoid arthritis), certain medications (e.g., hydralazine, procainamide), and end-stage renal disease (uremic pericarditis). Pericarditis may also arise after an acute MI (early-contiguous, or late [10–14 days, *Dressler's syndrome*]), or cardiac injury (*post-pericardiotomy syndrome*).

Pericardial friction rubs may occur when a transmural (Q wave) infarction has extended to the pericardium and as such, denotes an infarct that is larger in size. The friction rub and fever usually occur a day or more after the onset of pain.

The development of chest pain after cardiac surgery (particularly after CABG) can present a challenge to the clinician. The return of typical angina raises the possibility of graft occlusion, but pleuritic-type chest pain suggests post-pericardiotomy syndrome. Cardiac isoenzymes (e.g., CK-MB, cardiac troponins) may be increased if pericarditis is accompanied by myocarditis. Therefore, cardiac enzymes cannot be used to definitively distinguish myopericarditis from an acute MI.

The pericardial friction rub, although pathognomonic of pericarditis, may be missed on auscultation since it can

---

FIGURE 19-1

Clinical Approach to Acute Pericarditis

History	Sharp chest pain, typically retrosternal, radiating to left trapezius ridge, aggravated by deep breathing and lying supine, relieved by sitting up and leaning forward.
Physical Examination	Two or three component pericardial friction rub (variable and evanescent), fever.
Electrocardiogram	Diffuse concave ST segment elevation (without reciprocal depression), PR segment depression.
Chest X-Ray	May be normal. Enlarged cardiac silhouette (if pericardial effusion is present).
Laboratory	
Echocardiogram	+/− pericardial effusion.
Blood studies	Elevated erythrocyte sedimentation rate, leukocytosis, +/− CK-MB or troponin (if myopericarditis is present).
Treatment*	Aspirin (preferred after acute MI) or nonsteroidal antiinflammatory agents. Colchicine for acute and/or recurrent cases, or steroids (only as last resort) for refractory cases.

*Note: Most patients with acute pericarditis can be managed on an outpatient basis. Hospitalization is indicated for high risk patients with fever > 38° C, subacute onset, immunodepression, trauma, oral anticoagulant therapy, myopericarditis, large pericardial effusion, cardiac tamponade, or medical failure.

be remarkably evanescent. Its absence, therefore, does not exclude the diagnosis. When a rub is not heard initially in a suspected case of pericarditis, frequent, repeated auscultation using the diaphragm of the stethoscope applied firmly along the lower left sternal border with the patient sitting upright and leaning forward can be rewarding in its detection. As a rule, it is wise never to diagnose a "one-component pericardial friction rub". Unless 2 or 3 components, corresponding to atrial systole, ventricular systole (most common), and early diastolic filling of the ventricle (least common) are heard, the diagnosis of a pericardial friction rub should be withheld since most one-component sounds are usually scratchy systolic murmurs. A pericardial effusion does not always cause the heart sounds to be reduced in intensity and may not eliminate the presence of a pericardial friction rub. Rubs can be heard even in the presence of large pericardial effusions. It should be noted, however, that the diagnosis of acute pericarditis is made by documenting the clinical syndrome of chest pain, a pericardial friction rub and characteristic ECG abnormalities, rather than by the presence of a pericardial effusion. In fact, acute pericarditis may be present without significant (or any) pericardial effusion on echo, and conversely, pericardial effusion may occur in conditions other than acute pericarditis (e.g., myxedema, CHF, or volume overload states). Echo, therefore, is useful for confirming the diagnosis when it shows even a small pericardial effusion, but the absence of effusion does not exclude the diagnosis. (**Figure 5-4F**).

Figure 19-2. Chest pain in a patient with acute pericarditis is worse lying down, relieved when sitting up. Typically, there is a three component pericardial friction rub (as, vs, vd), which generally gets louder with inspiration. To detect a pericardial friction rub, listen along the left sternal border, exerting firm pressure on the diaphragm of the stethoscope with the patient sitting upright, breath held in deep expiration. The ventricular systolic component (vs) in this patient is loud and has a musical quality.

Figure 19-3. Typical 12 lead ECG tracing in a patient with acute pericarditis. Note the concave upward ST segment elevation with PR segment depression.

The vast majority of cases of pericarditis are self-limited and uncomplicated. About 15–30% experience recurrences. The pain and inflammation is usually relieved by anti-inflammatory agents, e.g., aspirin or NSAIDs (e.g., ibuprofen, indomethacin), with or without colchicine (to reduce recurrence). Steroids are not used routinely (because of their significant side effects) but may be reserved for uncontrolled pericarditis. Although they provide rapid and effective relief, steroids must be used cautiously, since an increased risk of recurrent pericarditis may develop when drug therapy is discontinued. Anticoagulation is not recommended due to the increased risk of pericardial hemorrhage and tamponade.

CARDIAC TAMPONADE

In pericardial tamponade, fluid accumulates in the pericardial space, compresses the heart, and impairs diastolic filling and cardiac function. In "*slow tamponade*", the patient may not appear acutely ill. Typically, the major complaint is dyspnea. Other symptoms include dizziness and a feeling of fullness in the head. Conversely, in sudden massive tamponade, patients having rapid deterioration may not be able to complain of symptoms, and precipitous hypotension and death may occur. Cardiac tamponade is often rapid in onset and is frequently related to chest trauma (blunt or penetrating),

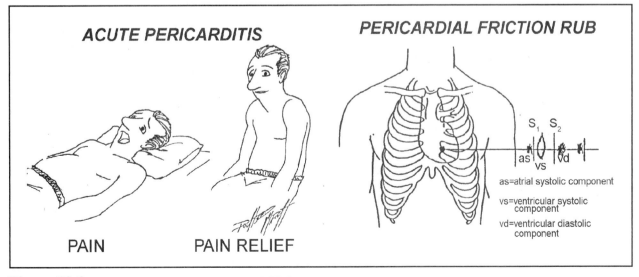

Figure 19-2 (Courtesy of W. Proctor Harvey, M.D.)

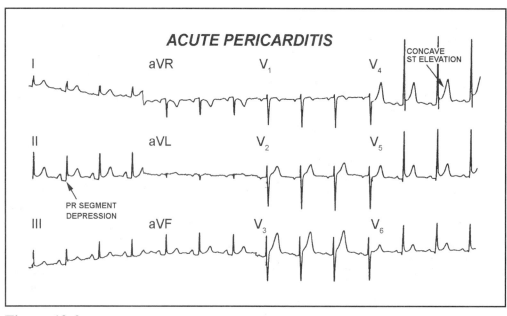

Figure 19-3

infectious, uremic, or neoplastic disease. It may also occur during the first few days following cardiac surgery (intrapericardial bleeding). The degree of tamponade and hemodynamic embarrassment is related to the rapidity of fluid accumulation, not the quantity of fluid. Acute tamponade may occur with small pericardial effusions (even small amounts of fluid may cause significant elevation of pressure if the pericardium is noncompliant and stiff).

Figure 19-4 summarizes the 5-finger approach to cardiac tamponade. Pericardial tamponade should always be suspected in a patient who presents in shock with hypotension, distended neck veins (with blunted "Y" descent), and distant heart sounds (Beck's triad) and a paradoxical (an inspiratory decrease of >10 mmHg) arterial BP and pulse. The ECG often shows low QRS voltage and, rarely, total electrical alternans of the P, QRS and T waves (virtually pathognomonic of cardiac tamponade, often due to metastatic cancer). This ECG phenomenon represents the swinging movement of the heart within the effusion and results in beat-to-beat changes in the electrical axis. The clinician should note whether the Korotkoff sounds disappear during inspiration as the BP cuff pressure is reduced a few millimeters at a time from the top systolic level (**Figure 2-23**). A palpable paradoxus is a clinically significant paradoxus. The presence of pulsus paradoxus indicates impending hemodynamic compromise and should be considered a cardiac emergency. Significant pulsus paradoxus is usually detectable, but may be masked when severe hypotension is present, or if there is elevation of the diastolic pressure of either ventricle.

The chest x-ray shows an enlarged cardiac silhouette with a "*water-bottle*" configuration if a large (250 cc) pericardial effusion is present (which need not be the case if the effusion develops rapidly). (**Figure 4-8**). Echo delineates the effusion and its hemodynamic significance, e.g., right atrial and RV diastolic collapse (a sign of right-sided chamber compression from elevated intrapericardial pressure).

Figure 19-5. Electrical alternans in precordial ECG leads. This finding is highly specific for a large pericardial effusion with cardiac tamponade. When the cardiac wall swings anteriorly, the QRS voltage is high; when it swings posteriorly, it is low ("*swinging heart*" pattern). Remember, however, that rapid accumulation of 100 cc of fluid (e.g., post-cardiac surgery and/or trauma with hemopericardium) can produce tamponade, yet a slow accumulation of a large quantity of fluid (e.g., hypothyroidism) may not interfere with cardiac function.

Urgent treatment by draining the pericardial fluid by needle (pericardiocentesis), or surgery (creating a pericardial window) is required to relieve cardiac compression. Removal of a small amount of fluid can be lifesaving.

Figure 19-6. Needle ECG-guided pericardiocentesis in a patient with cardiac tamponade. Note a current of injury pattern ("contact" current) with an elevated ST segment on the ECG when the needle tip touches the epicardium. The needle should be withdrawn slightly. Removal of only a small amount of fluid can result in dramatic clinical improvement. Following removal of fluid, there

---

FIGURE 19-4

Clinical Approach to Cardiac Tamponade

History	Dyspnea, cough, chest pain, weakness, fatigue. History of connective tissue disease, uremia, malignancy, post-MI (especially if thrombolytic agent or anticoagulant therapy administered), post-cardiac surgery, trauma, proximal aortic dissection with rupture.
Physical Examination	Elevated neck veins with blunted "Y" descent, hypotension, tachycardia, pulsus paradoxus, distant heart sounds.
Electrocardiogram	Electrical alternans, low voltage (due to large pericardial effusion).
Chest X-Ray	Large cardiac silhouette (due to pericardial effusion). May be normal (if effusion develops rapidly)
Laboratory	
Echocardiogram	Pericardial effusion with diastolic collapse of RA or RV.
Cardiac catheterization	Equalization of diastolic pressures in all four cardiac chambers.
Treatment	Volume resuscitation, emergency pericardiocentesis (with echo-directed guidance), surgical pericardiectomy.

---

may be a prompt rise to normal of arterial pressure with disappearance of pulsus paradoxus.

CONSTRICTIVE PERICARDITIS

Constrictive pericarditis is characterized by a thick, rigid, scarred, pericardium that restricts filling of all four chambers of the heart. It is usually a chronic consequence of acute or viral pericarditis, but may occur with carcinoma (especially breast and bronchogenic), prior radiation therapy to the chest for malignancy, and particularly following previous cardiac surgery. The clinical features include signs and symptoms of circulatory failure and systemic and pulmonary venous congestion. **Figure 19-7** summarizes the clinical features. Important clues to distinguishing CHF from constrictive pericarditis center on the common finding of normal LV function in constrictive pericarditis, and include the absence of pulmonary edema, normal heart size on chest x-ray, no significant heart murmurs, normal LV function on echo, the absence of BBB or LV hypertrophy on ECG, and a normal or nearly normal BNP level.

Always consider the possibility of constrictive pericarditis whenever there are:

- Ascites (developing earlier or disproportionate to peripheral edema)
- Distended neck veins with prominent "X" and "Y" descents (When the neck veins are overlooked, these patients are often mistakenly diagnosed as having cirrhosis of the liver.) (**Figure 2-16**).

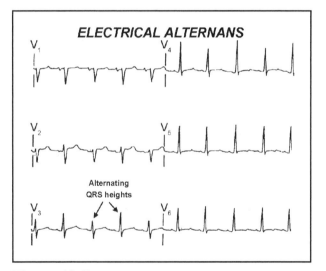

Figure 19-5

- Kussmaul's sign (an inspiratory rise in mean JVP) (**Figure 2-14**) and the absence of pulsus paradoxus, which help distinguish constrictive pericarditis (has Kussmaul's sign) from pericardial tamponade (has pulsus paradoxus). (**Figure 2-23**).
- Pericardial knock. The knock occurs early in diastole and is usually heard best along the left sternal border with the diaphragm of the stethoscope.

Figure 19-8. Constrictive pericarditis. Distended neck veins and a high-pitched early diastolic pericardial

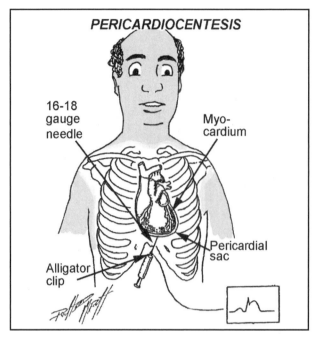

PERICARDIOCENTESIS

16-18 gauge needle

Myo-cardium

Alligator clip

Pericardial sac

Note: Pericardial effusions can range from asymptomatic to life-threatening (tamponade). Moderate to large effusions in which the cause is critical to diagnosis (e.g., infection, malignancy), or in which hemodynamic compromise is present, should be "tapped" immediately. If no cause can be found in an otherwise healthy patient with an effusion that persists >3 months, diagnostic pericardiocentesis can be considered on an elective basis. Post-pericardiocentesis, pericardial fluid should be sent for cell count, glucose, protein, culture, and cytology.

Figure 19-6

knock (K) sound along with pericardial calcification (upper right) on the lateral CXR (as may occur in ~50% of cases) are clues to the diagnosis of constrictive pericarditis.

Calcification may not be seen if enough time has not elapsed since prior cardiac surgery. Echo can demonstrate a thickened or calcified pericardium and exclude significant LV or RV systolic dysfunction as the cause of the heart failure. MRI or CT scan (both of which can image the pericardium and measure its thickness) may be more helpful in confirming the diagnosis. Cardiac catheterization is the definitive technique for documenting the elevation and equalization of right and left ventricular diastolic pressures along with the characteristic "*dip and plateau*" or "*square root sign*" (due to the rigid constricting pericardium limiting both left and right ventricular filling) (**Figure 19-9**).

Figure 19-9. Simultaneous right ventricular (RV) and left ventricular (LV) pressure waveforms in a patient with constrictive pericarditis. The characteristic "dip and plateau" (or "square root sign") contour in both ventricles along with equalization and elevation of diastolic pressures throughout most of diastole results from the rigid and non-distensable pericardium abruptly limiting both left and right ventricular filling.

Acute treatment usually includes gentle diuresis, whereas definitive therapy is surgical stripping of the pericardium.

FIGURE 19-7

Clinical Approach to Constrictive Pericarditis

History	Fatigue, dyspnea, weight gain, abdominal discomfort and distention, edema. History of tuberculosis, cardiac surgery, radiation therapy, infection, uremia, malignancy.
Physical Examination	Distended neck veins with prominent "X" and "Y" descents increasing with inspiration (Kussmaul's sign), early diastolic sound (pericardial knock), edema, ascites (often disproportionate to pedal edema).
Electrocardiogram	+/− low voltage, non specific ST-T changes, atrial fibrillation.
Chest X-Ray	Normal sized heart, pericardial calcification in 25–30% (best seen in the lateral view).
Laboratory	
Echocardiogram	Thickened pericardium with normal LV function, septal bounce during early diastole.
CT Scan, MRI	More sensitive in revealing thickened pericardium
Cardiac Catheterization	Early diastolic dip followed by diastolic plateau in ventricular pressures ("square root sign"), equalization of diastolic pressures in all cardiac chambers.
Treatment	Acute therapy: gentle diuresis
	Definitive therapy: surgical stripping of the pericardium

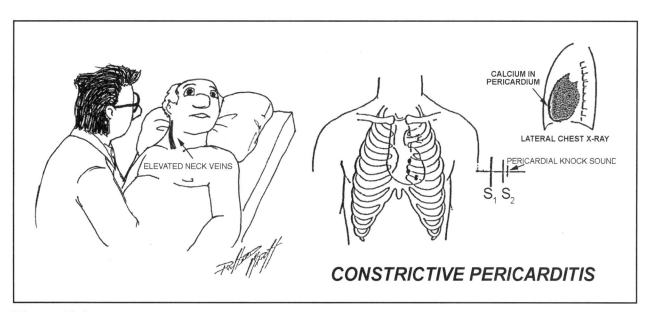

Figure 19-8 (Courtesy of W. Proctor Harvey, M.D.)

Of note, constrictive pericarditis may be difficult to distinguish from restrictive cardiomyopathy (e.g., due to amyloid). This distinction is important because surgical pericardiectomy may be "curable" for constrictive pericarditis, whereas treatment for restrictive cardiomyopathy is palliative and rarely, if ever, effective. The findings of restrictive cardiomyopathy may mimic constrictive pericarditis, but with subtle differences. Both conditions present with predominantly right sided CHF and an elevation in LV and RV diastolic pressures, along with the characteristic dip and plateau ("square root sign"). The hemodynamic differences relate to the fact that in restrictive cardiomyopathy, the left ventricle is usually more involved than the right, whereas in constrictive pericarditis there is equal involvement of both ventricles. As a result, in constrictive pericarditis, there is nearly identical elevation in LV and RV diastolic pressures (within 5 mmHg), pulmonary arterial pressures are normal or only modestly elevated (<55 mmHg), and there is discordant change in RV and LV systolic pressures with inspiration (RV rises, LV falls)—so-called *"ventricular interdependence"*. In restrictive cardiomyopathy, the LV diastolic pressure is usually higher than the RV diastolic pressure (by more than 5 mmHg), pulmonary arterial pressures are significantly elevated (>55 mmHg), and there is a concordant change in LV and RV systolic pressures with respiration.

Before a thoracotomy is undertaken in the face of uncertainty about the diagnosis, it may be useful to perform an endomyocardial biopsy, particularly to rule out cardiac amyloidosis, the condition most likely to simulate constrictive pericarditis.

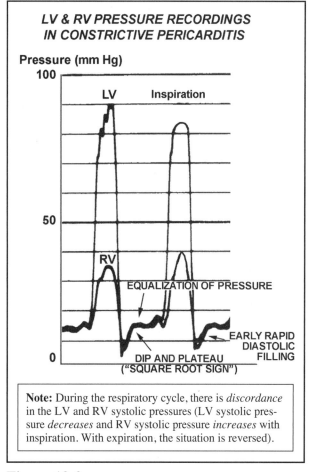

Figure 19-9

CHAPTER 20.   APPROACH TO THE PATIENT
WITH PULMONARY HYPERTENSION

GENERAL CONSIDERATIONS

Pulmonary hypertension is defined as a hemodynamic state in which there is an elevation in mean pulmonary artery pressure of ≥ 25 mmHg at rest. Pulmonary artery pressure may increase secondary to:

- Progressive obliteration of small pulmonary arteries and arterioles (i.e., idiopathic or primary)
- An increase in pulmonary venous (left atrial) pressure caused by mitral valve disease or left heart failure (most common)
- Pulmonary parenchymal disease (hypoxemia)
- A reduction in the cross-sectional area of the pulmonary vascular bed (e.g., multiple pulmonary emboli)
- Miscellaneous disorders (multifactorial mechanisms)

Pulmonary hypertension can be classified into one of five types: *arterial, venous, hypoxic, thromboembolic*, or *miscellaneous*. This chapter will focus on the clinical approach to the diagnosis and management of the patient who presents with idiopathic or primary pulmonary arterial hypertension.

CLINICAL RECOGNITION OF IDIOPATHIC (PRIMARY) PULMONARY HYPERTENSION

Idiopathic (primary) pulmonary hypertension is an intrinsic, obstructive disease of the small pulmonary arteries and arterioles. It most commonly affects young and middle-aged (otherwise healthy appearing) women during the third or fourth decade of life. Progressive exertional dyspnea, angina-like chest pain (presumably due to RV ischemia), fatigue, weakness, dizziness and syncope are the most typical presentations. Hoarseness may occur as a result of compression of the left recurrent laryngeal nerve between the aorta and the enlarged left pulmonary artery (*Ortner's syndrome*). **Figure 20-1** summarizes the 5-finger approach and treatment.

Although idiopathic (primary) pulmonary hypertension occurs in the absence of identifiable cause (e.g., pulmonary emboli, lung disease, CHF, or congenital heart disease), genetic (e.g., mutations in the bone morphogenic protein receptor-2 [*BMPR2*] gene) and environmental factors (e.g., HIV infection, cocaine, and anorexigen use) may play a role. An association with the appetite-suppressant drug *Phen-fen* has been demonstrated. If a young woman (in her 20's to 30's) with Raynaud's phenomenon develops shortness of breath, fatigue, chest pain, or syncope with exertion, always consider the possibility of idiopathic (primary) pulmonary hypertension. Diagnosis is confirmed by:

- A large A wave in the jugular venous pulse (poor RV compliance)
- Palpable systolic pulsation in the second left intercostal space (dilated pulmonary artery)
- Sustained impulse along the left parasternal area (RV hypertrophy)
- An abnormally loud, closely split P2 (easily heard at the apex)
- Systolic (and/or diastolic) murmur due to pulmonic flow (and/or regurgitation), and pulmonic ejection sound (decreasing with inspiration)
- Elevated JVP, hepatomegaly, ascites, and peripheral edema are noted once RV failure ensues.
- RV hypertrophy and RA enlargement on the ECG (**Figure 3-39**)
- A large pulmonary artery on chest x-ray (**Figure 4-11**)

Transthoracic echocardiography with Doppler and agitated saline injection is the preferred test for the initial evaluation of suspected pulmonary hypertension. Pulmonary artery systolic pressure (PASP) can be estimated by measuring the velocity (V) of the TR jet (PASP = $4 \times V^2$ + RA pressure). Signs of RV pressure overload include RA and RV enlargement, abnormal septal flattening, and TR.

Additional studies may be useful in excluding secondary causes of pulmonary hypertension. These include pulmonary function tests (obstructive or restrictive lung disease), ventilation-perfusion lung scanning and CT pulmonary angiography (chronic thromboembolic disease), overnight oximetry or polysomnography (obstructive sleep apnea), and laboratory testing, e.g., antinuclear antibody and other connective tissue serologies, HIV antibodies, and liver function tests. Of note, there is no specific test to diagnose idiopathic (primary) pulmonary hypertension. The diagnosis is one of exclusion.

The definitive diagnosis of pulmonary hypertension is made during right heart catheterization with direct measurement of pulmonary arterial pressures. Right heart catheterization can also be used to determine the severity of the hemodynamic impairment, test pulmonary vasoreactivity, and guide therapy.

Figure 20-2. Auscultatory findings in a young female with idiopathic (primary) pulmonary hypertension who experienced a syncopal episode. Note the closely split second heart sound (S2) with a loud pulmonic closure (P). The pulmonic ejection sound (E) becomes fainter with inspiration (Insp). There is also a palpable RV impulse and a palpable P2.

Figure 20-3. Schematic representation of flow-directed, balloon tipped (Swan Ganz) catheter being floated

FIGURE 20-1

Clinical Approach to Idiopathic (Primary) Pulmonary Hypertension

Pathobiology

Pulmonary vascular remodeling resulting from an imbalance in vasoactive mediators ($\uparrow$ vasoconstrictors: endothelin-1, thromboxane A_2; $\downarrow$ vasodilators: nitric oxide, prostacyclin) which leads to vasoconstriction, smooth muscle and endothelial cell proliferation, and thrombosis in situ. May be familial (mutation in the *BMPR2* gene) or sporadic (HIV infection, cocaine, anorexigen use).

History

Dyspnea, exertional syncope (hypoxia, $\downarrow$ cardiac output), chest pain (RV ischemia), fatigue, palpitations, sudden death. Rule out secondary causes, e.g., congenital heart disease, connective tissue disease, chronic pulmonary thromboemboli, COPD and hypoxemia, left sided heart failure, mitral valve disease, anorexic agents.

Physical Examination

Young and healthy appearing (women more often than men), loud P2, right sided S4 and S3, RV heave, pulmonic flow murmur, TR and PR murmurs, +/− RV failure: $\uparrow$ JVP with large A and/or V waves, + HJR, ascites, peripheral edema.

Electrocardiogram

Right axis deviation, RBBB, RA enlargement ("P pulmonale"), RV hypertrophy.

Chest X-Ray

Dilatation and "pruning" of pulmonary arteries, RA and RV enlargement.

Laboratory
Echocardiogram
Cardiac Catheterization

Doppler estimation of elevated pulmonary pressures, abnormal septal motion, TR, PR. $\uparrow$ PA pressures (mean PA pressure $\geq$ 25 mmHg at rest), $\uparrow$ pulmonary vascular resistance ($\geq$ 3 Woods units), normal pulmonary capillary wedge pressure ($\leq$15 mmHg). Assesses acute response to pulmonary vasodilator (e.g., IV adenosine, inhaled nitric oxide, IV epoprostenol)*.

Treatment

Oxygen (maintain O_2 sat > 90–92%), diuretics (cautious diuresis since RV is preload dependent), digoxin (empirical, but may counteract potential negative inotropic effects of calcium channel blockers), vasodilators (e.g., oral calcium channel blockers, IV prostacyclin therapy, prostacyclin analogs, endothelin receptor antagonists, phosphodiesterase inhibitors, soluble guanylate cyclase stimulators, prostacyclin receptor agonists), anticoagulation (oral warfarin may improve survival), atrial septostomy, lung transplantation.

*Note: A $\downarrow$ of $\geq$10 mmHg in mean PA pressure to a value of < 40 mmHg without a $\downarrow$ in cardiac output predicts a response to long-term calcium channel blockers.

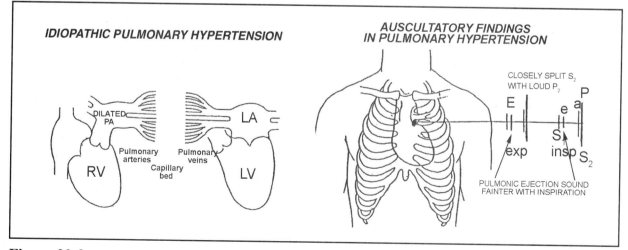

Figure 20-2 (Courtesy of W. Proctor Harvey, M.D.)

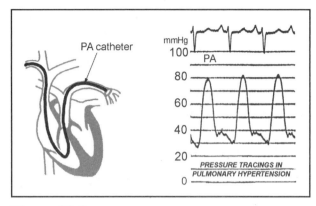

Figure 20-3

into the pulmonary artery. Note elevated pulmonary arterial pressure in a patient with pulmonary hypertension. The peak systolic pressure measures 80 mmHg.

MANAGEMENT OF PULMONARY ARTERIAL HYPERTENSION

Treatment is rapidly evolving. Therapy may include:

- Cautious use of *vasodilators* (oral calcium channel blockers [in pulmonary vasodilator responders]) or continuous IV infusion of the vasodilator prostacyclin may relieve the pressure in the pulmonary circulation and benefit some patients. Prostacyclin analogs or other vasodilators, e.g., endothelin antagonists, or phosphodiesterase 5 inhibitors may be considered (in non-responders).
- Chronic *anticoagulation* therapy with warfarin (for in situ pulmonary thrombi) may also increase life expectancy.
- Portable *oxygen* (for marked hypoxemia at rest or during exercise testing) to maintain O_2 saturation at >90–92% (reduces hypoxic vasoconstriction).
- *Diuretics* for those with clinical signs of right-sided venous hypertension (elevated JVP, ascites, edema). Cautious diuresis since RV is preload dependent.
- *Digoxin,* often administered empirically, may counteract the potential negative inotropic effects of calcium channel blockers. Dobutamine can be used short term for decompensated pulmonary hypertension.
- *Balloon atrial septostomy* (R → L shunt causes ↑ cardiac output, ↓ arterial oxygen saturation, net ↑ tissue oxygen delivery).
- *Lung transplant* if the disease progresses despite maximal therapy. Heart-lung transplant needed if Eisenmenger physiology.

Vasodilator therapy particularly applies to those who respond favorably to a vasodilator challenge (e.g., IV prostacyclin, IV adenosine, inhaled nitric oxide) during right heart catheterization. Complications of pulmonary vasodilator therapy include systemic hypotension, hypoxemia, and even death. The most effective vasodilator is IV prostacyclin (epoprostenol [Flolan]), which is also the most complicated to administer (requires continuous infusion via a permanent venous catheter using a portable IV pump). This agent has been shown to decrease symptoms, increase exercise capacity, and decrease mortality in patients with idiopathic (primary) pulmonary hypertension. Current therapies for pulmonary arterial hypertension include vasoactive agents e.g., prostacyclin analogues (e.g., SQ, inhaled treprostinil [Remodulin, Tyvaso], inhaled iloprost [Ventavis]), endothelin-receptor antagonists (e.g., oral bosentan [Tracleer], oral ambrisentan [Letairis] oral macitentan [Opsumit]), phosphodiesterase 5 inhibitors (e.g., oral sildenafil [Revatio], oral tadalafil [Adcirca]), soluble guanylate cyclase stimulators (e.g., oral riociguat [Adempas]), and prostacyclin receptor agonists (e.g., oral selexipag [Uptravi]) which decreases pulmonary vascular resistance.

Overall, the outlook for patients with untreated idiopathic (primary) pulmonary hypertension remains poor (median survival 2.8 years). The prognosis is markedly improved if the patient responds to vasodilator therapy (up to 95% survival at 5 years). The outlook for patients with secondary pulmonary hypertension depends on the course of the underlying disease. The prognosis is generally favorable when pulmonary hypertension is detected early and the underlying cardiac and/or pulmonary diseases leading to it are treated appropriately. Patients with chronic thromboembolic disease may be considered for pulmonary thromboendarterectomy. Predictors of a poor prognosis include advanced functional class, poor exercise capacity (as measured by a 6-minute walk test), high RA and PA pressure, low cardiac output, significant RV dysfunction, and an elevated BNP or NT-pro BNP level. Death in pulmonary arterial hypertension is most commonly due to right heart failure. In advanced stages, pulmonary artery pressures decline as the RV fails to generate enough blood flow to maintain high pressure. In select patients with advanced, refractory pulmonary hypertension, percutaneous balloon atrial septostomy may be considered as a bridge to lung transplantation or as a palliative treatment option. Creation of an intraatrial right-to-left shunt decompresses the failing right ventricle, increases LV filling, and improves cardiac output. Despite the decrease in arterial oxygen saturation that results, there is a net increase in tissue oxygen delivery. Improvement in survival and quality of life have been reported, but the procedure-related mortality remains high. Lung transplantation should be considered if recurrent syncope and/or severe RV failure, refractory to medical therapy, are present. The 5 year survival rate following lung transplantation is ~45–55%.

CHAPTER 21. APPROACH TO THE PATIENT WITH A HEART MURMUR

Careful and accurate clinical evaluation of the patient with a heart murmur is one of the most common and important tasks that a clinician is called on to perform in the daily practice of medicine. Proper interpretation will enable the experienced examiner to make appropriate and cost-effective management decisions regarding the need for further diagnostic laboratory studies, medical and/or surgical intervention, antibiotic prophylaxis for endocarditis, risk of non-cardiac surgery, pregnancy, competitive and/or recreational sports, job-related activities, and eligibility for military service or life insurance. This chapter will provide a practical approach to the patient with a heart murmur, with an emphasis on clinical examination skills, especially cardiac auscultation, and the appropriate, cost-effective use of Doppler echocardiography.

EVALUATION OF A HEART MURMUR: AN INTEGRATED APPROACH

The evaluation of the patient with a heart murmur may vary greatly, depending on its timing in the cardiac cycle (systolic, diastolic, or continuous), intensity, location, radiation, and response to dynamic maneuvers. Also of importance is the presence or absence of symptoms and signs that provide clues as to whether the murmur may be "significant" (pathologic), and requires additional testing, or "innocent" (benign), and needs no further work-up **(Figure 21-1)**.

Although the increasing availability and use of Doppler-echo studies threatens to deemphasize the importance of cardiac auscultatory skills, it remains true that the simple stethoscope, when used properly, is an inexpensive and expedient diagnostic tool that often enables the well-trained clinician to correctly identify the cause and significance of many heart murmurs with fewer, if any, additional laboratory tests.

Nevertheless, there is an unfortunate (and expensive) trend today to obtain an echo study on an indiscriminate basis, simply because a heart murmur is heard, or worse, to "rule-out" a heart murmur, suggesting that the practitioner did not even take the time to listen. All too commonly, the notation "no murmurs, rubs, or gallops" appears on the medical record which, in many cases, means that virtually no cardiac auscultatory exam took place. The practitioner can be trapped into this approach when inadequate time is allotted for a careful clinical evaluation. The responsible clinician, however, should employ Doppler-echo studies (as well as other laboratory tests) to confirm the clinical diagnosis of heart disease and quantitate its severity, not in the

---

FIGURE 21-1

Clinical Clues to Significant Systolic Murmurs

- **Presence of clinical symptoms**
  - Ischemic-type chest pain, congestive heart failure, syncope
- **Associated auscultatory findings**
  - Loud in intensity (grade 3 or greater)
  - Long in duration (mid or late-peaking or holosystolic)
  - Prominent radiation to axilla or neck (carotids)
  - Changes in intensity during physiologic maneuvers (e.g., Valsalva, squatting)
  - Associated diastolic murmur
  - Abnormal heart sounds
    - Loud S1; wide, "fixed" or paradoxical split S2; loud A2 or P2, S4 or S3 gallops; mid-systolic click; aortic or pulmonic ejection sounds; opening snap; pericardial knock
- **Other physical examination findings:**
  - *Abnormal jugular venous pulse*
    - Elevated mean venous pressure
    - Large A or V waves
  - *Abnormal arterial pulse/blood pressure*
    - Wide pulse pressure
    - Pulsus alternans
    - Pulsus paradoxus
    - Brisk, rapid-rising pulse
    - Small, weak or slow-rising pulse
    - Cardiac arrhythmia (atrial fibrillation)
  - *Abnormal precordial movements*
    - Sustained LV apical or RV parasternal lift or heave (hypertrophy)
    - Diffuse, inferolaterally displaced impulse (LV enlargement)
    - Bifid LV apical impulse
    - "Ectopic" bulge (LV aneurysm)
- **ECG Findings**
  - Left or right ventricular hypertrophy
  - Pathologic Q-waves or ST-T-wave changes
  - Arrhythmias and/or conduction abnormalities
- **Chest X-ray Findings**
  - Cardiomegaly
  - Valve calcification
  - Abnormal pulmonary vasculature
  - Pulmonary venous congestion or edema

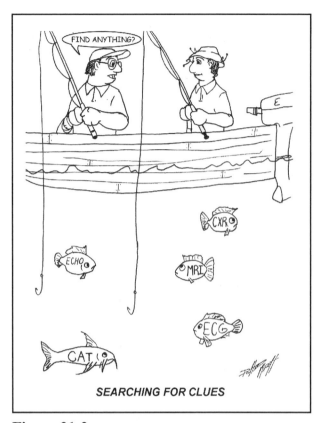

Figure 21-2

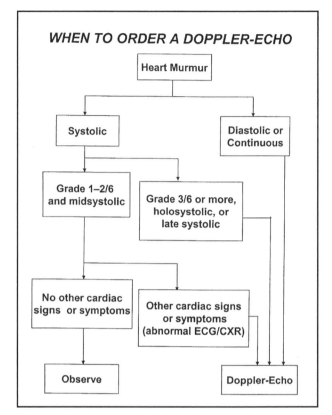

Figure 21-3

manner of a "fishing expedition" simply to establish its presence (**Figure 21-2**).

Over-utilization of echo imaging techniques wastes time and financial resources. The use of Doppler-echo as a screening tool is not cost-effective and may lead to mistakes by an inexperienced observer unaware of the normal variants of heart structure and function. The echo transducer is no substitute for the stethoscope and often renders a false diagnosis of heart disease in a patient who has no murmur and only trivial to mild ("physiologic") valvular regurgitation (so-called "echocardiographic heart disease"). Furthermore, grading of the severity of valvular regurgitation by color flow Doppler imaging remains qualitative and subjective. The echo can overdiagnose severe MR when, in fact, the degree of leak is mild to moderate (i.e., the patient has no symptoms, LA and LV dimensions and function are normal, and only a faint, grade 1-2/6 apical mid-to-late or holosystolic murmur with no S3 or diastolic flow rumble is heard). Misleading echo data can be worse than no information at all.

Color-Doppler echo is a highly operator dependent imaging modality that should aid and not replace the cardiac clinical examination. A thorough cardiac examination

should be the rate-limiting step in the decision-making process as to whether or not one should obtain an echo study. Echo is best applied and interpreted in the context of a given clinical presentation, i.e. when specific questions raised are addressed and when the information discovered is likely to impact on further patient management decisions, alter the therapeutic strategy, and improve clinical outcome.

Indications for Doppler-Echo

Although Doppler-Echo can provide important information about patients with heart murmurs, it is not a necessary test for all patients, and often adds little but cost to the evaluation of asymptomatic patients with short, grade 1-2/6 mid-systolic ("innocent") murmurs and no other signs of cardiac disease. According to current guidelines, Doppler-echo is indicated in the assessment of patients with diastolic, continuous, holosystolic, late or loud systolic murmurs, or in patients with murmurs and signs or symptoms of CHF, ischemia, syncope, infective endocarditis, or thromboembolism. If an ECG or CXR is obtained and is abnormal, echo is also indicated (**Figure 21-3**).

Figure 21-3. Strategy for evaluating heart murmurs based on whether the murmur is likely "innocent" and needs only observation, or "significant" (pathologic) and requires further investigation, e.g., Doppler-echo.

Echo is most cost-effective when it is clinically goal-directed and when the findings are concordant with the clinical assessment. To some extent, a decision whether or not to order an echo depends on the practitioner's comfort with characterizing murmurs and categorizing them as "innocent". It is estimated that ~20–25% of echos ordered by primary care practitioners today could be avoided if a skilled clinical evaluation had been performed first.

Clues from the Cardiac Clinical Exam

The cardiac clinical examination, in addition to demonstrating a heart murmur, provides useful clues to the etiology and severity of underlying heart disease. For the experienced examiner, the findings on the basic clinical evaluation often predict what will be noted on the echo study. The following examples serve to illustrate:

- If one hears a short, grade 1-2/6, early to mid-systolic murmur (and a normal S1 and S2, no extra systolic sounds or diastolic murmur) in a healthy-appearing young person with an otherwise normal cardiac examination, and whose clinical history, ECG, and CXR is otherwise unremarkable, the clinician can make the diagnosis of an "innocent" or functional systolic murmur with confidence. An echo is unlikely to yield any additional clinically useful information, and it is not necessary to order one to "prove" the clinician correct. In older adults, differentiating a benign from a pathologic murmur may be more difficult, since some of these patients often have some degree of aortic valve thickening (sclerosis). While progression of aortic sclerosis to significant AS may occur in elderly patients with an asymptomatic systolic murmur, clinical outcome remains excellent until symptom onset.
- When conducted properly, the cardiac clinical examination is the optimal method for diagnosing MVP, and the stethoscope, the best instrument in its detection. The young female patient with a high-frequency mid or late systolic click (or clicks) followed by a faint, grade 1-2/6, late apical systolic murmur (which becomes longer and often louder on standing from squatting) with no S3 gallop or di-

astolic flow rumble, a normal arterial pulse, and a normal apical impulse (along with a normal ECG and CXR), has MVP with trivial to mild MR. An echo will likely reveal nothing further.
- An athletic individual with a family history of sudden cardiac death, exertional chest pain, increasing effort-related dyspnea, a quick rising arterial pulse, a palpable presystolic and double systolic apical impulse ("triple ripple"), a paradoxically split S2, and a harsh systolic murmur loudest at the left sternal border, that decreases with a prompt squat and increases on standing and during the Valsalva maneuver (along with LV hypertrophy and pseudo infarction Q waves in the inferolateral ECG leads), has hypertrophic obstructive cardiomyopathy (the most common cause of sudden death in young athletes below the age of 30) until proven otherwise.
- A patient with a sharp, high-frequency (ejection) sound immediately following S1, heard best at the cardiac apex and base (not varying with respiration), along with a harsh aortic systolic murmur radiating to the neck and apex, a preserved aortic

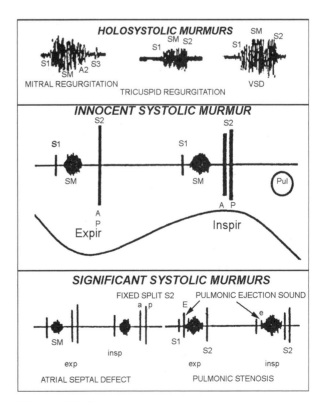

Figure 21-4 (Courtesy of W. Proctor Harvey, M.D.)

second sound, and a faint aortic diastolic murmur, likely has congenital bicuspid aortic valve disease.

- In a patient with chest pain, dyspnea on exertion and dizziness, the presence of a palpable small volume, slow-rising arterial pulse, a pre-systolic and sustained, forceful LV apical impulse with an apical-carotid delay, a loud, late-peaking systolic ejection murmur radiating to the carotids, an S4 gallop, and a paradoxically split S2 (along with LV hypertrophy and strain on the ECG, and a prominent ascending aorta with calcification of the aortic valve on CXR), strongly supports the diagnosis of severe valvular AS.

- In an active patient with quick-rising and collapsing (bounding) peripheral arterial pulses, a wide pulse pressure, a diffuse, forceful LV apical impulse displaced inferolaterally, a medium-frequency to harsh but brief systolic ejection murmur and a loud high-pitch blowing diastolic murmur (heard best during full expiration with a patient sitting up and leaning forward), a faint S_1 and a prominent diastolic (*Austin-Flint*) rumble (along with LV enlargement on the ECG and CXR), severe AR can be diagnosed with a high degree of certainty.

- In a young patient with a grade 2/6 early to midsystolic murmur heard at the pulmonic area and left sternal border, the presence of wide "fixed" splitting of S2 during inspiration and expiration, prominent jugular venous A and V waves, a palpable pulmonary artery impulse, and an RV lift (along with an RSR[1] in lead V1 in the ECG and prominent pulmonary "shunt" vascularity on the CXR) provide clues to the diagnosis of an atrial septal defect

Figure 21-4. Innocent vs. significant murmurs. **Top.** Three causes of holosystolic murmurs—mitral insufficiency, tricuspid insufficiency, ventricular septal defect (VSD). **Middle.** Innocent systolic murmur in early to mid systole. Note normal splitting of second heart sound (S2), single with expiration (Expir) and split (A-P) with inspiration (Insp). **Bottom Left.** Atrial septal defect. Note the second sound remains widely split with both expiration (exp) and inspiration (insp). **Bottom Right.** Pulmonic stenosis. Note the ejection sound (e) on expiration becomes fainter with inspiration. (Courtesy of Dr. W. Proctor Harvey).

Figure 21-5. Auscultatory findings in various cardiac conditions. **A)** Innocent systolic murmur with normal splitting of the second heart sound; **B)** Bicuspid valve aortic stenosis with long late-peaking crescendo-decrescendo systolic murmur and ejection sound well heard at the aortic area and apex that does not vary with respiration; **C)** Mitral valve prolapse

with mid systolic clicks and late apical systolic murmur; **D)** Severe aortic regurgitation with "to and fro" systolic and diastolic murmurs along left sternal border and Austin Flint rumble at apex; **E)** Systolic murmur of hypertrophic obstructive cardiomyopathy, increasing in intensity on standing, decreasing in intensity on squatting; **F)** Systolic murmur of atrial septal defect with wide "fixed" splitting of the second heart sound with respiration. (Courtesy of Dr. W. Proctor Harvey).

These examples represent but a few of the many practical applications of the cardiac clinical examination in the evaluation of patients with heart disease. Although heart disease may not always be detectable or accurately quantifiable on clinical examination, much of the information which is now being obtained by sophisticated echo imaging techniques can also be obtained safely, more conveniently and less expensively by a careful clinical cardiovascular evaluation. Furthermore, when making serial observations, the practitioner cannot routinely order an echo each and every time he or she sees a patient. The astute clinician should look for changes in the patient's condition (e.g., signs of stability, improvement or deterioration) on the basis of a careful clinical evaluation.

Many management decisions can evolve from a properly performed clinical examination. For example, if a patient with a recent MI develops shortness of breath, along with pulsus alternans, an S3 gallop, and pulmonary rales, he or she is in CHF. Treatment need not be delayed awaiting confirmation by an echo. Moreover, what is often lost sight of is that considerable variation in technical and interpretative skills exists among various echo laboratories providing the service. An unwary practitioner might at times be misled by errors in the reported findings. Even in the best of hands, the echo may over-diagnose (i.e., false-positive) or under-diagnose (i.e., false-negative) certain conditions. The inability to demonstrate MVP by echo in some patients with typical systolic clicks, for example, should not cast doubt on the diagnostic reliability of the click, but rather highlight the shortcomings of the technique (which may fail to adequately visualize such a complex structure as the mitral valve). Doppler-echo is an excellent diagnostic test. The inexperienced practitioner, however, often equates the Doppler color flow signals (which are based on velocity) to what is seen on angiography (which is based on volume). In many patients, high velocity small volume valvular regurgitant jets may look significant on color flow Doppler, but are not clinically significant at all. Conversely, in some patients with clinically significant AS, a falsely low gradient may be detected on the echo when the Doppler beam is not well aligned with the velocity jet. As valuable as echo may be, a high-quality cardiac clinical examination provides a much

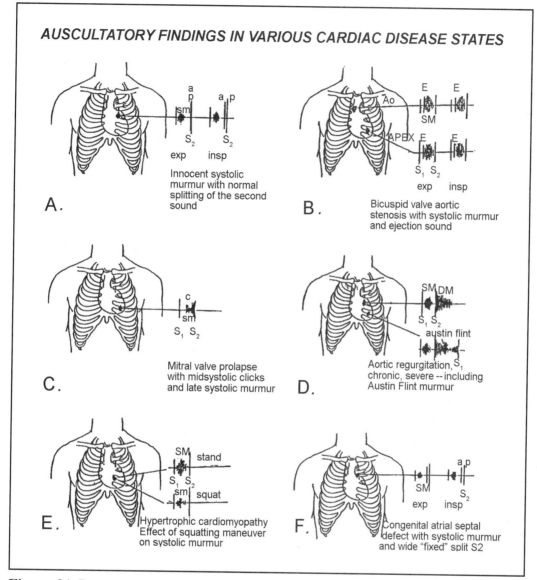

Figure 21-5 (Courtesy of W. Proctor Harvey, M.D.)

needed safeguard against a poor quality echo study. The ability of the basic clinical evaluation to provide an added level of quality control, may be even more important than the potential cost-savings that result. As handheld echo becomes more ubiquitous, there is a risk that cardiac auscultation will become further marginalized. Despite its imperiled status, cardiac auscultation still remains the most appropriate clinical method of screening for heart disease. When used properly, the time-honored stethoscope remains a powerful, reliable and cost-effective tool in the clinical evaluation of the cardiac patient, often allowing the seasoned clinician, skilled in the art of auscultation, to arrive at a definitive and accurate physiologic and anatomic diagnosis in the office or at the bedside.

CHAPTER 22.   APPROACH TO THE PATIENT WITH CARDIAC ARRHYTHMIAS AND CONDUCTION DISTURBANCES

Electrical disturbances of the heart result from abnormal impulse formation and/or conduction, and may range from a benign, incidental finding, to a potentially life-threatening condition. This chapter will present a practical clinical approach to the diagnosis and management of the patient who presents with a cardiac arrhythmia or conduction abnormality, with an emphasis on the most common rate and rhythm disorders encountered in daily practice.

GENERAL CONSIDERATIONS

A patient's awareness of palpitations (and of regular or irregular cardiac rhythm) varies significantly. Some patients perceive slight variations in their heart rhythm with great accuracy, whereas others are oblivious even to sustained episodes of VT. Still others complain of palpitations when they actually are in normal sinus rhythm. What is palpitation to one patient, therefore, may not be to another. Some patients may be able to use their hand to "tap out" what they feel (or recognize the beat "tapped out" by the clinician's hand) and thus identify their arrhythmia.

Figure 22-1. Using your hand to tap out the heart beat is a useful technique to help simulate and diagnose various arrhythmias. Note the clinician's hand is moving up and down rapidly to indicate a tachycardia. **A)** Premature ventricular contraction (3rd beat); **B)** Supraventricular tachycardia; **C)** Atrial flutter; **D)** Atrial fibrillation; **E)** Ventricular tachycardia.

- A quick beat, followed by a pause, can simulate a premature beat (e.g., PAC, PVC); more than one quick motion can simulate two or three or more premature beats in a row. Bigeminal or trigeminal rhythm (regular alternation of a PVC with one or two normal cardiac cycles, respectively) can also be easily reproduced.
- A rapid and irregularly irregular rhythm may be a clue to *atrial fibrillation*. Atrial fibrillation has an atrial rate of 350–600/min, but the rate of QRS generation and ventricular contraction is much less due to variable transmission of atrial depolarization to the ventricles.

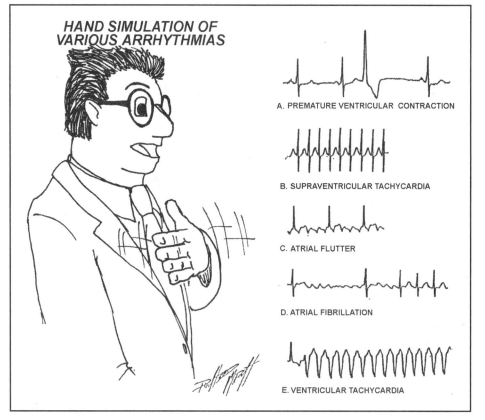

HAND SIMULATION OF VARIOUS ARRHYTHMIAS

A. PREMATURE VENTRICULAR CONTRACTION

B. SUPRAVENTRICULAR TACHYCARDIA

C. ATRIAL FLUTTER

D. ATRIAL FIBRILLATION

E. VENTRICULAR TACHYCARDIA

Figure 22-1

- A rapid and regular rhythm at a rate of 150 beats per minute may indicate atrial flutter with 2:1 conduction. (Atrial flutter typically has 250–350 atrial waves/min., but not all atrial waves get through to the ventricles.) Sinus tachycardia, which originates from rapid firing of the SA node, is any sinus-originating rhythm >100 min.
- A rapid and regular rhythm at a rate greater than 150 beats per minute suggests *paroxysmal supraventricular tachycardia* (most commonly *AV nodal reentrant tachycardia,* which originates in dual pathways in the AV junction) or VT. In a young, otherwise healthy individual, it suggests paroxysmal SVT. In an older patient with underlying heart disease and near-syncope or syncope, it suggests VT. As a general rule, SVTs are less likely to cause pre-syncopal or syncopal events than is VT.
- A regular and slow rhythm suggests sinus bradycardia in a young person (particularly in a trained athlete due to increased vagal tone), or heart block in an older person with underlying heart disease.

Although the ECG may provide more extensive and specific information, the patient may be seen initially in a setting where the recording of an ECG is not possible, and clinical clues to the diagnosis can be very helpful. For example, absent A (fibrillatory) waves in the neck veins, along with a variable intensity of S1 suggests atrial fibrillation. A variable intensity of S1 with intermittent cannon A waves in the neck veins is a clue to VT (fast heart rate) or complete heart block (slow heart rate). A paradoxically split S2 suggests LBBB, and a widely physiologically split S2 provides a clue to RBBB.

Carotid sinus massage is a simple and useful vagotonic maneuver to diagnose and/or treat various tachyarrhythmias. Before commencing with this maneuver, however palpate and listen for carotid bruits to exclude carotid artery stenosis. This finding, along with a history of TIAs, are contraindications for carotid sinus massage. Massage one side of the neck at a time, *never both carotids at the same time!* Your patient's head should be turned to the left and the right carotid artery palpated high in the neck, at the angle of the jaw (where the carotid sinus is located). While listening with your stethoscope over the patient's chest (and/or recording the procedure with constant ECG monitoring), press this area firmly for 3–5 seconds at a time with either your index and middle fingers, or with your thumb. Stop the pressure immediately if a response is obtained. Do not use prolonged carotid sinus stimulation, since serious consequences (e.g., prolonged asystole) may occur. Repeat as necessary. It is important to apply sufficient pressure that will usually cause some discomfort to the patient (of which the patient should be warned).

When carotid sinus massage is not effective, it may mean that the exact spot at the angle of the jaw has not been located, and that you need to reposition your fingers or move to the left side. *Keep in mind, slowing (e.g., sinus tachycardia, atrial flutter-fibrillation) or conversion (e.g., supraventricular tachycardia) of the ventricular rate with carotid sinus pressure rules out the most serious arrhythmia, VT, which generally will not respond.* For patients being evaluated in a medical facility, adenosine can also be used as a diagnostic tool in differentiating tachycardias. Adenosine is the drug of choice (before verapamil or diltiazem) for converting AV nodal reentry tachycardia, since it blocks the AV node temporarily, breaks the reentrant circuit, and rapidly terminates SVT (but not most VT), helping to establish that the problem was an AV nodal reentry tachycardia. Worthy of mention, verapamil and diltiazem, by their myocardial depressant and peripheral vasodilatory effects, can produce hypotension and VF and be fatal when given to patients with VT.

Figure 22-2. Left. Technique of carotid sinus massage. The patient's head is tilted backward and to the left. The practitioner's hand applies pressure with the thumb to the carotid artery pulsation just under the angle of the right jaw. The procedure is monitored by listening with the stethoscope and/or by continuous ECG recording. **Right.** Effect of carotid sinus pressure on various tachycardias. (Courtesy of Dr. W. Proctor Harvey). **Note:**

- Gradual slowing and gradual return to former rate with sinus tachycardia.
- AV nodal reentrant tachycardia (AVNRT) abruptly stopped, followed by normal sinus rhythm.
- Atrial fibrillation. Rate originally irregular and rapid. Immediate slowing with irregular return to former rhythm.
- Prompt slowing with irregular "jerky" return to original 2:1 atrial flutter. The atria remain undisturbed.
- Paroxysmal atrial tachycardia (PAT) with block (not every P wave gets through in this tachyarrhythmia). Carotid pressure produces slowing. Note atrial waves easily identified.
- No effect whatsoever on ventricular tachycardia.

Sophisticated diagnostic and therapeutic modalities have revolutionized the approach to patients with arrhythmias. Antiarrhythmic drugs, and particularly catheter ablation techniques and implantable devices (e.g., pacemakers, ICD) have cured otherwise refractory and even life-threatening rhythm disturbances. The patient presenting with a tachyarrhythmia may be asymptomatic or have a range of symptoms from palpitations, lightheadedness, shortness of breath, and chest pain, to profound hemodynamic compromise or sudden cardiac death. Unfortunately, many arrhythmias occur intermittently, and patients may present to the practitioner after an episode has resolved. Nonetheless, clues

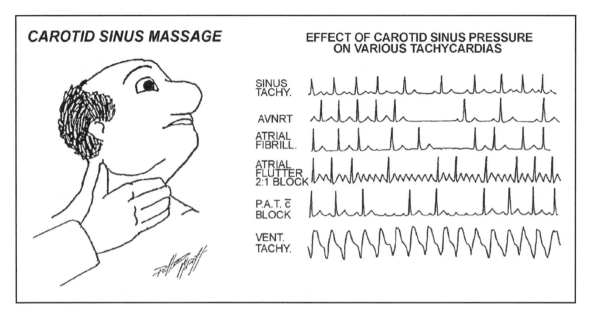

Figure 22-2 (Courtesy of W. Proctor Harvey, M.D.)

may be present on the ECG even if the arrhythmia is not present at the time. For example:

- A short PR interval and/or a delta wave suggests preexcitation (WPW) syndrome, which may be associated with AV reentrant arrhythmias and atrial fibrillation with rapid AV conduction over a bypass tract. (**Figure 3-55**).
- The presence of Q waves on the ECG raises the suspicion of CAD and a prior MI with ventricular tachyarrhythmias.
- LV hypertrophy with apical T wave inversions and pronounced septal Q waves (the septum in particular is hypertrophic in HOCM) suggest HOCM and VT/VF.
- RBBB with ST segment elevation in the right precordial leads provides a clue to *Brugada's syndrome* (**Figure 22-3**), where there is a susceptibility to VT/VF and sudden cardiac death.

Figure 22-3. Conventional precordial ECG leads in a patient with the Brugada syndrome. Note the ST segment elevation in leads V1-V3 along with a right bundle branch morphology in lead V1. These patients may develop ventricular tachycardia, ventricular fibrillation and sudden cardiac death.

Metabolic abnormalities (e.g., hypokalemia, hypomagnesemia, hypoxemia, hyperthyroidism), acute illness (e.g., CHF, anemia, infection), alcohol and caffeine intake, and certain prescription medications (e.g., digoxin, theophylline, antiarrhythmic therapy) and non-prescription drugs (e.g., decongestants, cocaine) may precipitate arrhythmias.

Certain arrhythmias (e.g., atrial fibrillation) may not be an acute problem but still warrant treatment to prevent

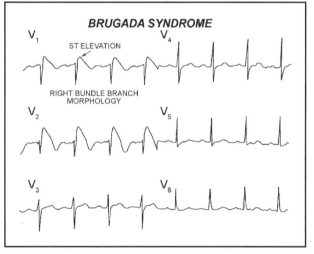

Figure 22-3

long-term complications (e.g., embolic stroke). Other arrhythmias (e.g., VT) can cause hemodynamic instability and may require aggressive treatment to prevent recurrences. An arrhythmia may be tolerated well and require no therapy in patients with structurally normal hearts, but may not be tolerated in patients with LV systolic or diastolic dysfunction or valvular heart disease. Patients with incessant, uncontrolled tachycardia, however, can develop a dilated cardiomyopathy as a result. The process may be reversible if the arrhythmia is successfully treated. These patients therefore require aggressive therapy.

Some arrhythmias are more likely to occur at times of high sympathetic tone (e.g., VT), others at times of high vagal tone (e.g., AV Nodal Reentry Tachycardia), or both (e.g., atrial fibrillation). The presence of symptoms is of paramount importance in the decision-making process regarding the treatment of an arrhythmia. Before institution of an antiarrhythmic agent, the risk of therapy versus the risk of the arrhythmia itself must be taken into account in each patient. The practitioner should not over-treat otherwise asymptomatic patients with non-sustained VT or PVCs in the absence of heart disease. Antiarrhythmic therapy may not be indicated in those cases and may even be harmful (i.e., adverse noncardiac and/or proarrhythmic side effects). Beta blockers may be helpful in symptomatic patients.

The basic rule for all therapeutic interventions is to decrease morbidity and mortality as well as improve the quality of life. The specific treatment modalities for extrasystoles and tachyarrhythmias include reassurance and observation (e.g., for benign extrasystoles), correction of precipitating factors (e.g. anxiety, caffeine, alcohol, hyperthyroidism, etc), and pharmacologic or other intervention to slow a rapid rate or convert it to a normal rhythm.

Figures 22-4 and 22-5 summarize the clinical approach to the more common tachyarrhythmias.

ATRIAL FIBRILLATION

Atrial fibrillation is the most common sustained supraventricular arrhythmia encountered in clinical practice, affecting an estimated 5.2 million Americans. The incidence increases with age, so that the lifetime risk for developing atrial fibrillation is nearly 25% for individuals over age 40. Modifiable risk factors for atrial fibrillation include hypertension, diabetes mellitus, obesity, alcohol consumption ("holiday heart"), and obstructive sleep apnea. Atrial fibrillation occurs with many forms of structural heart disease including mitral valve disease, CAD, dilated cardiomyopathy, CHF, atrial septal defect, as well as in other settings, e.g., hyperthyroidism, pericarditis, COPD (as well as with pulmonary medications, e.g., theophylline and beta-adrenergic agonists), and after cardiac surgery. Many patients with atrial fibrillation have no structural heart disease (i.e., "lone" atrial fibrillation, neurogenic atrial fibrillation). Occasionally it is familial. Atrial fibrillation can be classified into three main types: paroxysmal (lasts less than 7 days), persistent (does not terminate spontaneously but can be pharmacologically or electrically converted to sinus rhythm), or permanent. Clues to the diagnosis include the presence of palpitations, shortness of breath, dizziness, and chest pain. Some patients feel no different when fibrillating, while others sense and dread each attack. *Clinical problems relate to the hemodynamic effect of losing the "atrial kick", to an excessively rapid ventricular rate, and the risk of clot formation in the poorly contracting atria.* Complications of atrial fibrillation include the precipitation of CHF (tachycardia-induced cardiomyopathy) and systemic arterial embolism (e.g., stroke). The risk for

stroke is similar whether atrial fibrillation is paroxysmal, persistent, or permanent. If the ventricular rate is extremely rapid, hypotension and/or myocardial ischemia may also result. **Note:** when the ventricular rate of an irregular wide-complex tachycardia is >200 beats/min, always consider antegrade conduction through an accessory pathway (WPW syndrome), since the AV node does not conduct at rates >200/min.

The clinical findings of atrial fibrillation include a rapid, irregularly irregular rhythm with a pulse deficit (i.e., not all ventricular beats are palpable peripherally), absent A waves in the JVP, and a variable intensity of S1. Although an S3 may be present, an S4 is absent in all patients with atrial fibrillation, since the S4 is the consequence of normal atrial contraction toward the end of diastole. On the ECG, discrete P wave activity is absent and the QRS complexes occur irregularly.

Therapy options for atrial fibrillation include:

1. *Control ventricular rate,* even if the fibrillation itself is not corrected, with beta blockers (including IV esmolol, which has an ultra-short half life), calcium channel blockers (e.g., verapamil, diltiazem), or digoxin, which reduces symptoms and avoids a tachycardia-induced cardiomyopathy.

2. *Restore and maintain normal sinus rhythm* through *cardioversion* or *antiarrhythmic agents.* Cardioversion preserves AV synchrony, maintains cardiac output, reduces symptoms and may decrease risk of future thromboembolism. Cardioversion may be applied:
   - Urgently in unstable patients (ongoing angina, CHF, hypotension), or
   - Electively in stable patients, either electrically or with certain antiarrhythmic agents, e.g., the Class III agents, ibutilide (Corvert), amiodarone (Cordarone, Pacerone), sotalol (Betapace), and dofetilide (Tikosyn); the Class IA agents, e.g., procainamide (Pronestyl, Procan) and disopyramide (Norpace), or the Class IC agents, e.g., flecainide (Tambocor) and propafenone (Rythmol). Cardioversion should be considered in stable patients with atrial fibrillation if the rhythm disturbance has been present for <48 hours, or an LA thrombus has been ruled out (by TEE) or effectively treated (international normalized ratio [INR] of 2–3) with warfarin (Coumadin) for at least 3 weeks prior (and 4 weeks after) the procedure, to avoid the risk of an embolic stroke.

3. *Prevent thromboembolic complications.* Warfarin (Coumadin) prevents thromboembolism in high-risk patients, e.g., those with a prior TIA or stroke, valvular heart disease, CHF, hypertension, diabetes, and age >75 years. NOACS, e.g., dabigatran (Pradaxa), an

FIGURE 22-4

Clinical Approach to Common Arrhythmias

Arrhythmia	Predisposing Conditions	Treatment
Atrial premature contractions (premature impulse originates from ectopic foci in the atria)	Normal individual or due to anxiety, caffeine, alcohol, CHF, hypoxemia, electrolyte abnormality ($\downarrow$ K$^+$, $\downarrow$ Mg^{++})	Remove precipitating cause. Treatment rarely required. If symptomatic—β-blocker.
Sinus tachycardia (rapid impulse formation from the SA node)	Fever, pain, anemia, dehydration, CHF, hyperthyroidism, COPD, autonomic disorder (POTS).	Treat the underlying cause, e.g., pain, fever, anemia, anxiety, hypovolemia, CHF, beta-agonists. If symptomatic—β-blocker.
Supraventricular tachycardia —AV nodal reentrant tachycardia (AVNRT) (reentry using dual pathways in the AV node) —AV reciprocating tachycardia (AVRT) (reentry using accessory pathway)	Normal individual or due to preexcitation (WPW) syndrome.	Acutely–vagal maneuvers (abruptly converts to sinus rhythm or no effect at all). If unsuccessful, adenosine, verapamil, β-blocker. Cardioversion (if hemodynamically unstable). Avoid AV nodal blockers in WPW syndrome (can accelerate conduction via bypass tract and precipitate ventricular fibrillation). RF ablation is useful for preventing recurrence.
Atrial fibrillation (wavelets of activation in the atria irregularly passing down the AV node) **Atrial flutter** (macroreentry within the atria)	Idiopathic ("lone"), mitral valve disease, hypertension, pericarditis, hyperthyroidism, obstructive sleep apnea, COPD, alcohol, post cardiac surgery.	1. Slow the ventricular rate (β-blocker, verapamil, cardizem, digoxin). 2. Convert to sinus rhythm (after anticoagulation if chronic) with IV Ibutilide, Procainamide, Amiodarone, or orally with group IC, III, or IA agent. May require elective cardioversion (likelihood of success dependent on duration of atrial fibrillation and size of atria). 3. RF ablation for common type atrial flutter and atrial fibrillation (foci in or near pulmonary veins and posterior LA wall). If not successful, try AV node ablation and permanent pacemaker.
Multifocal atrial tachycardia (increased automatically at multiple sites in the atria)	Severe COPD	Treat underlying lung disease. Verapamil may be used to slow ventricular rate. K$^+$, Mg^{++} supplement. AV node ablation and permanent pacemaker.
Ventricular premature contractions (premature impulse originates from ectopic foci in the ventricle)	CAD, MI, cardiomyopathy, CHF, hypoxemia, $\downarrow$ K$^+$	May not require therapy. If symptomatic— β-blocker
Ventricular tachycardia (3 or more consecutive PVCs) —Monomorphic and polymorphic —Nonsustained VT: lasts $<$ 30 seconds —Sustained VT: lasts $>$ 30 seconds	CAD, MI, cardiomyopathy CHF, hypoxemia, $\downarrow$ K$^+$, arrhythmogenic RV dysplasia/cardiomyopathy, or idiopathic (i.e., no structural heart disease).	May not require therapy. If symptomatic— β-blocker. If unstable–electrical cardioversion. Acute–IV amiodarone, procainamide, lidocaine. Chronic prevention po Class IA, IB, IC, III drugs. Implantable cardioverter defibrillator in patients at high risk of sudden cardiac death. Idiopathic VT may respond to vagal maneuvers, adenosine, verapamil, and β-blocker (RV outflow tract VT), or verapamil, but not adenosine or β-blocker (LV fascicular VT), RF ablation can be curative.

Clinical Approach to Common Arrhythmias (*continued*)

Arrhythmia	Predisposing Conditions	Treatment
Torsades de pointes (A type of polymorphic VT in which QRS morphology twists around the baseline)	↑QT interval (congenital or drugs e.g., Class IA and III antiarrhythmics, tricyclic antidepressants, antibiotics (e.g., erythromycin, trimethoprim-sulfa), antihistamines (astemizole, terfenadine), hypokalemia, hypomagnesemia, antipsychotics (e.g., phenothiazines, haloperidol).	In acquired long QT, IV magnesium, overdrive pacing (which shortens QT interval), and IV isoproterenol (unless CAD present) which increases the heart rate. Drugs that ↑QT interval are contraindicated. In congenital long QT, β-blockers if symptomatic. Implantable cardioverter defibrillator if syncope or VT despite β-blocker therapy.

Clinical Clues to Wide Complex Tachycardia

Supraventricular Tachycardia	Ventricular Tachycardia
Irregularly irregular rhythm	AV dissociation (e.g., independent P waves, capture or fusion beats)
Typical RBBB or LBBB morphology	Atypical RBBB or LBBB morphology*
QRS <0.14 sec (RBBB) or <0.16 sec (LBBB)	QRS >0.14 sec (RBBB type) or >0.16 sec (LBBB Type)
History of SVT or WPW syndrome	Positive (or negative) QRS concordance in chest leads
QRS unchanged or slightly wider than in sinus rhythm	QRS axis −60° to −180°
	No response to carotid sinus massage
All or none response to carotid sinus massage	Presence of heart disease (prior MI, CHF, LV dysfunction)

Note: Assume all wide complex tachycardia is ventricular tachycardia until proven otherwise. The overall appearance of the patient and the hemodynamic stability of the rhythm do not reliably distinguish ventricular from supraventricular tachycardia. Termination of a wide complex tachycardia by physical maneuvers (e.g., carotid sinus massage, Valsalva) or medication (adenosine) is highly suggestive of SVT.

*Atypical BBB morphology includes a monophasic R wave or an initial R > r' in V1, and a small r and large S wave (r/S ratio < 1) in V6 (in RBBB-type VT); and an initial r wave > 30 msec, and the onset of QRS to the nadir of S wave (RS interval) > 60-100 msec with a notched or slurred S wave in V1, and a q wave in V6 (in LBBB-type VT).

oral direct thrombin inhibitor, and rivaroxaban (Xarelto), apixaban (Eliquis), and edoxaban (Savaysa), oral factor Xa inhibitors, are safe and effective alternatives to warfarin in patients with "nonvalvular" atrial fibrillation (i.e., without a mechanical valve or rheumatic MS) who have difficulty monitoring or controlling the PT/INR. Of note, aspirin, with or without clopidogrel (Plavix), is less effective than warfarin and the NOACs for the prevention of thromboembolic complications of atrial fibrillation.

4. *Consider AV nodal catheter ablation* with pacing for rate control, in patients refractory to medical therapy. *RF or cryo ablation for cure* by circumferential isolation of foci ("triggers") in or around the pulmonary veins along with linear ablation in the LA may be considered for patients who fail or do not tolerate at least one antiarrhythmic drug or as first-line therapy for select patients with recurrent symptomatic paroxysmal atrial fibrillation.

The first step in managing the patient with atrial fibrillation is to decide whether there is a high likelihood of safe conversion to normal sinus rhythm or whether the patient should be allowed to remain in atrial fibrillation. The decision is governed by the risk of thromboembolism, the severity of symptoms, and whether the patient is likely to maintain sinus rhythm.

Urgent synchronized electrical cardioversion is indicated in patients with rapid atrial fibrillation who are hypotensive or have angina, CHF, or other evidence of severe hemodynamic compromise. In general, a patient with recent onset atrial fibrillation and no evidence of left atrial enlargement has a greater chance of achieving and maintaining normal sinus rhythm. If atrial fibrillation has been present for <48 hours, rate control (e.g., with beta blockers, calcium channel blockers, digoxin) along with electrical cardioversion can be performed. Patients with long-standing atrial fibrillation (especially if due to mitral valve disease, hypertension, or advanced LV dysfunction) are least likely to maintain normal sinus rhythm after cardioversion, but often have the most to gain if successful (due to the importance of "atrial kick" to cardiac output). Most patients, therefore, merit at least one attempt at cardioversion.

If the arrhythmia is long-standing, and the patient is not a suitable candidate for cardioversion, treatment should focus on ventricular rate control, and long-term stroke prophylaxis. Patients who have been in atrial fibrillation for >48 hours are more likely to have atrial thrombi and may develop embolic stroke (2–5% of cases) with immediate electrical or pharmacologic cardioversion. Restoration of atrial mechanical function, not DC shock, causes ejection of clot from the LA appendage. Keep in mind that atrial thrombi are not evident on transthoracic echo, but they can be seen on TEE. If atrial fibrillation is present for >48 hours, or the TEE reveals thrombi, therapeutic oral anticoagulation with warfarin (target INR 2-3) or NOAC is recommended ≥ 3 weeks before cardioversion, and at least 4 weeks after cardioversion is attempted, since the longer the atrial fibrillation is present, the longer the atria are mechanically stunned after cardioversion.

It is estimated that antiarrhythmic drugs (other than amiodarone) are only about 50% successful in maintaining sinus rhythm after one year. Amiodarone is effective at preventing recurrent atrial fibrillation in 50–75% of patients. All antiarrhythmic medications are accompanied by a risk of proarrhythmia, particularly in those with CHF. At the present time, it appears that both therapeutic strategies (i.e., rate control vs. maintaining sinus rhythm) are of equal benefit.

For patients with recurrent paroxysms of atrial fibrillation but no underlying heart disease (so-called "lone atrial fibrillation"), Class IC agents, e.g., flecainide (Tambocor) and propafenone (Rythmol) are safe and effective. Class III agents, e.g., sotalol (Betapace), amiodarone (Cordarone, Pacerone), and dofetilide (Tikosyn) are also effective but there is a risk of torsades de pointes, particularly with sotalol and dofetilide, in vulnerable patients. Overall, the incidence of torsades with amiodarone has been less than previously suspected. Cardioversion with maintenance of sinus rhythm by antiarrhythmic agents all have potentially serious side effects. Rate control with AV nodal blocking agents (e.g., beta blockers, rate-slowing calcium channel blockers, digoxin) should be given first. As mentioned above, accepting chronic atrial fibrillation with appropriate rate control and long-term anticoagulation is a viable option in many patients. Once atrial fibrillation is established as a persistent rhythm and the ventricular rate controlled, symptoms often subside. AV nodal blocking agents, however, should not be used if WPW is present, since conduction down the accessory pathway may be *enhanced* and fatal ventricular fibrillation may result.

Stroke risk should always be considered when contemplating anticoagulation. Patients ≤60 years of age with "lone" atrial fibrillation (i.e., no risk factors) have an excellent prognosis with an extremely low risk (~1%/year) for embolic phenomena. The risk of stroke in these patients is similar to the risk of serious bleed on anticoagulation. Therapy in this group, therefore, should be directed toward relief of symptoms with rate control as the primary objective. Some recommend aspirin therapy to such patients although no convincing data supports this approach. On the basis of available information, it appears unlikely that most young patients with lone atrial fibrillation will benefit from chronic anticoagulation or antiarrhythmic therapy to prevent recurrences. In patients without structural heart disease, chemical conversion can be tried by using oral flecainide or propafenone as a one-dose trial ("pill in the pocket"). Chronic anticoagulation is indicated, however, in adults >60–65 years of age, particularly those who have additional stroke risk factors, e.g., CHF or LV systolic dysfunction, hypertension, diabetes, mitral valve disease, and history of prior embolic events, even if NSR is thought to be maintained since recurrent episodes of atrial fibrillation are often asymptomatic and can go undetected (i.e., "silent" atrial fibrillation). In patients with refractory symptomatic atrial fibrillation, or in those with persistently rapid rates, radiofrequency AV nodal ablation and permanent pacing may be considered. There is growing experience with RF ablation by circumferential isolation of foci ("triggers") in or around the pulmonary veins and linear ablation in the LA that initiate and perpetuate atrial fibrillation, following which sinus rhythm may be restored or maintained. Some patients with atrial fibrillation can be treated surgically to restore and maintain sinus rhythm by the "maze procedure", where multiple incisions are created in the atria to prevent reentry circuits at the time of cardiac surgery. To decrease stroke risk, obliteration of the LA appendage can be performed during the surgical "maze procedure". A percutaneous LA appendage occluder device, e.g., the Watchman, may be an effective alternative to reduce cardioembolic stroke in select patients with atrial fibrillation who are intolerant to anticoagulation.

* * *

Pearls:

- When evaluating the risk for stroke in atrial fibrillation, keep in mind the mnemonic "**CHADS-VASc**" (**C**HF, **H**ypertension, **A**ge ≥ 75, **D**iabetes, prior **S**troke or TIA, **V**ascular disease, **A**ge 65-74, and **S**ex **c**ategory [female]). Each risk factor is assigned 1 point except for prior stroke/TIA and age ≥ 75 years, which are assigned 2 points. Anticoagulation is recommended for a score ≥ 2. Anticoagulation should be withheld for~ 2-4 weeks after a large stroke, however, due to the risk of hemorrhagic conversion.

- When assessing the bleeding risk in atrial fibrillation, remember the mnemonic "**HAS-BLED**" (**H**ypertension, **A**bnormal renal/liver function, **S**troke, **B**leeding history or predisposition, **L**abile INR, **E**lderly [age >65], **D**rugs/Alcohol concomitantly [including antiplatelet agents and NSAIDs]).
- In patients with atrial fibrillation, "lenient" heart rate control (<110 beats/min at rest) may be as effective as "strict" heart rate control (<80 beats/min at rest) in preventing cardiovascular events.
- A narrow-complex supraventricular tachycardia (SVT) that has a regular heart rate of 150 beats/min is atrial flutter with 2:1 AV block, until proven otherwise.
- An irregularly irregular rhythm in a patient with COPD is more commonly *multifocal atrial tachycardia* (MAT) than atrial fibrillation. MAT is an irregular fast rhythm defined by the presence of three or more P waves of varying morphologies. (**Figures 3-45 and 3-46**). It may also be caused by hypokalemia or hypomagnesemia. MAT occurs most commonly in chronic lung disease but is also seen in patients with severe metabolic abnormalities or sepsis. Potassium and magnesium replacement may suppress the tachycardia. Rate-slowing calcium channel blockers (e.g., verapamil) may be useful for rate control. Medications causing atrial irritability (e.g., theophylline, inhaled albuterol) should be avoided if possible. AV nodal ablation with permanent pacing can be helpful if refractory to medical treatment.

* * *

SUPRAVENTRICULAR TACHYCARDIAS

Paroxysmal SVT occurs in individuals of all ages, and is often seen in otherwise healthy young adult females without underlying structural heart disease. *AV nodal reentrant tachycardia (AVNRT)* is the most common type of paroxysmal SVT, occurring in 50–60% of cases. The reentry circuit is located within the AV node with impulses traveling down the slow (α) pathway and then retrograde up the fast (β) pathway of the AV node (**Figure 3-54**). The atria and ventricles are depolarized simultaneously, and the P waves are hidden in the QRS complexes on the ECG. The episode usually begins and ends abruptly and may last seconds to several hours or longer. The QRS complexes are typically narrow.

AV reciprocating tachycardia (AVRT), which includes WPW, is the second most common form of paroxysmal SVT (30–40% of cases) and most commonly utilizes the normal AV pathway and an accessory bypass tract for antegrade and/or retrograde conduction (preexcitation [WPW] syndrome). About one half of patients with the WPW pattern on a routine ECG have periodic tachyarrhythmias, whereas the other half demonstrate no rhythm disturbances. In some patients with this syndrome, the characteristic ECG features (short PR interval, delta wave) occurs intermittently, or not at all. In these patients, the accessory pathway functions only in the retrograde direction (i.e., "concealed"), so that the QRS complexes are electrocardiographically normal.

Frequently, the first episode of AVNRT occurs before the age of 30 although it may start after the patient has reached 60 years of age. AVNRT is characterized by the sudden onset and offset of a regular tachycardia at rates of 150 to 250 beats per minute. Many attacks of paroxysmal SVT resolve spontaneously. If not, vagal maneuvers (e.g., Valsalva maneuver [with leg elevation and supine positioning], carotid sinus massage, breath holding, immersing the face in ice water) may terminate the attack. *Response to vagal maneuvers may be diagnostic since paroxysmal SVT is, with rare exception, the only tachycardia that can be broken and stay normal during these maneuvers.* Adenosine (Adenocard), a naturally occurring nucleoside with a very short half life, is useful for the treatment of paroxysmal SVT. If adenosine is not effective in terminating AVNRT, or if acute bronchospasm is present, IV verapamil (or diltiazem) is generally effective. IV adenosine and verapamil are equally effective in rapidly terminating paroxysmal SVT in >90% of cases. Verapamil should not be used as a diagnostic test, however, because it may precipitate ventricular fibrillation (VF) if the initial rhythm is VT. *AV nodal blocking agents (e.g., adenosine, beta blockers, calcium channel blockers, and digoxin) should be avoided in WPW, because they can lead to arrhythmia acceleration through the accessory pathway.* Extremely rapid ventricular rates are possible and may precipitate hemodynamic collapse and sudden death. (**Note:** IV procainamide, amiodarone, and ibutilide are the drugs of choice for controlling the rate of atrial fibrillation in patients with bypass tracts because they decrease conduction over the accessory pathway and are safe if antegrade accessory pathway conduction is present in atrial fibrillation.)

Prevention of frequent attacks of SVT can be achieved by beta blockers, calcium channel blockers (e.g., verapamil, diltiazem), and digoxin. Radiofrequency ablation of the abnormal reentrant circuit (or accessory pathway) has a >90% success rate. In atrial flutter, Class IA agents should not be given prior to the administration of AV nodal blocking agents, since 1:1 conduction through the AV node may result, thereby increasing the ventricular response.

A history of paroxysmal SVT in a young woman should lead you to consider three possibilities:

- SVT in an otherwise normal heart
- Underlying MVP
- The possibility of preexcitation (WPW) syndrome

When atrial fibrillation occurs with an extremely rapid ventricular response, consider the presence of an accessory pathway (as in WPW). Remember that abnormal Q waves can (and often are) mistaken as being caused by an acute MI in patients with WPW syndrome. When conduction occurs antegrade via the AV node and then returns retrograde up the accessory pathway, the QRS complexes during SVT appear normal and are not widened (so-called *orthodromic AV reentrant tachycardia*). (**Figure 3-55**). When antegrade conduction is through the accessory pathway, and retrograde conduction is through the normal pathway, the QRS complexes are maximally preexcited, so that they appear bizarre and widened (so-called *antidromic reciprocating tachycardia*) and may be confused with VT (**Figure 3-57**). Such cases of retrograde conduction respond best to procainamide (which prolongs the refractory period of the accessory pathway) or to electrical cardioversion. As previously discussed, AV nodal blocking agents, e.g., digitalis, beta blocker, and verapamil (although useful in rapid atrial fibrillation in the absence of WPW) should be avoided in WPW, since they may shorten the refractory period in the accessory pathway, further increase the ventricular rate, and precipitate ventricular fibrillation. Worthy of mention, continuous supraventricular tachycardia may produce LV systolic dysfunction (tachycardia-induced cardiomyopathy). Medical and/or electrophysiological (i.e., radiofrequency catheter ablation) control of the tachycardia can cause reversal of the cardiomyopathy.

VENTRICULAR TACHYCARDIA

Ventricular tachycardia is defined as three or more consecutive PVCs. It may produce cardiac arrest, syncope, mildly symptomatic hypotension, or no symptoms other than the sensation of tachycardia. Although some forms of VT can occur in younger patients without structural heart disease, most VT is associated with serious underlying heart disease and is either nonsustained (lasting less than 30 seconds) or sustained (lasting more than 30 seconds). (**Figure 3-50**). Common causes include myocardial ischemia, acute MI, dilated cardiomyopathy, hypertrophic cardiomyopathy, MVP, CHF, or digitalis toxicity. *Torsades de pointes,* a form of VT in which QRS morphology waxes and wanes ("twists") around the baseline (**Figure 3-48**), may occur spontaneously in hypokalemia or hypomagnesemia or after any drug that prolongs the QT interval. A wide complex tachycardia, usually between 140 and 220 beats/min on the ECG, along with AV dissociation (**Figure 3-50**), capture or fusion beats, and extreme axis deviation in a patient with underlying heart disease, acute ischemia, a history of MI, cardiomyopathy with a low EF, is a clue to VT, until proven otherwise. (**Note:** "Capture" beats are normal QRS complexes that appear amidst the wide, abnormal QRS complexes of VT, representing atrial waves that got through to the ventricles. A "fusion" beat is a QRS that partially appears, having fused with an abnormal QRS complex in VT. Both capture and fusion beats help confirm that the abnormal QRS complexes originate in the ventricles.) (**Figure 3-49**). Unlike paroxysmal SVT, many episodes of VT do not stop spontaneously. Even worse, there is a predisposition for VT to deteriorate into ventricular fibrillation (VF).

Treatment is directed at ending the bout of VT. If the VT is acute and hemodynamically stable, IV amiodarone (Cordarone), procainamide (Pronestyl), or lidocaine (Xylocaine) can be used. If IV administered medications do not produce immediate results, or if the patient is hemodynamically unstable (i.e., hypotension, CHF, or angina is present), immediate synchronized electrical cardioversion should be employed. In acute MI, prophylactic lidocaine is associated with a higher rate of asystole and a poorer outcome and is no longer recommended, except in treating patients with non-sustained VT. The management of torsades de pointes differs from that of other forms of VT. Class I or III antiarrhythmic agents, which prolong the QT interval, should be avoided (or withdrawn immediately if being used). Beta blockers, IV magnesium, along with correction of electrolyte abnormalities, e.g., hypokalemia and/or temporary pacing, can both break and prevent the rhythm disturbance.

The next step in treatment of VT is to prevent it from recurring. Options include medication, correction of an underlying problem, use of an implantable device, or surgical or catheter ablation procedures to eliminate the site in the LV or RV that is causing the VT. In post-MI patients, there is movement away from the use of most of the antiarrhythmic agents for the suppression of ventricular arrhythmias because of the increased risk of proarrhythmia (e.g., torsades de pointes). Beta blockers, however, have a beneficial effect on long-term outcome and have evolved as the drugs of choice; amiodarone also has good evidence in its favor. Amiodarone can also induce polymorphic VT ("torsades de pointes") although the drug has a lower incidence of pro-arrhythmic effects than other antiarrhythmic agents. Side effects (usually dose-related) of amiodarone include bluish-gray discoloration of the skin, thyroid dysfunction, pulmonary fibrosis (rarely, but occasionally irreversible), corneal microdeposits and liver abnormalities.

VT in the setting of acute ischemia or MI responds to treatment of the ischemia and does not necessarily require prolonged antiarrhythmic therapy. For chronic, recurrent, sustained VT, either implantable cardiac defibrillator (ICD) and/or antiarrhythmic therapy (guided by EPS studies) should be considered. A distinction must be made between suppression of PVCs (which is virtually useless) and control of VT or VF, which can prolong life. ICDs are most beneficial for patients with depressed LV function and life-threatening ventricular arrhythmias. Amiodarone is often used together with an ICD. Although the implanted device is the ultimate protection against sudden cardiac death, the drug prevents or reduces the number of serious arrhythmias that cause the device to fire, thus lengthening battery life and minimizing the psychological (and sometimes physical) effects of being "shocked" multiple times. Electrolyte abnormalities e.g., ↓ K$^+$, ↓ Mg^{++} (particularly with torsades de pointes), digitalis toxicity or pacemaker malfunction can be the cause of VT, and should be kept in mind and treated accordingly.

If sudden cardiac death occurs in the patient with CAD in the absence of an MI, the prognosis is paradoxically worse than if in the setting of an MI (since it suggests active ongoing ischemia). Urgent cardiac catheterization (with an eye toward revascularization to prevent another event) is warranted. ICD is indicated for cardiac arrest due to VT/VF that is not due to a transient or reversible cause. Another cause of sudden cardiac death is *Brugada's syndrome*, an autosomal dominant disorder most frequently associated with mutations in the sodium channel (*SCN5A*), followed by the L-type calcium channel (*CACNA1C*) genes. In affected patients (most commonly young Asian males) with syncope or cardiac arrest (due to polymorphic VT/VF), the ECG reveals RBBB with ST segment elevation in precordial leads V1 and V2. (**Figure 22-3**). Because antiarrhythmic drug therapy is thought to be ineffective, and the chance of recurrent syncope or sudden death is substantial (~35% within 24 months), implantation of an ICD is usually recommended for these patients.

* * *

Pearls:

Whether you are caring for a patient with an acute MI in the ED, a bypass patient in the cardiac intensive care unit, a hip replacement patient in the surgical intensive care unit, or a patient in your office, you need to correctly recognize and react promptly to common arrhythmias. The following clues may help you solve an arrhythmic mystery:

1. Gather all the facts on *history taking*.
    *   Symptoms that may prompt a search for an arrhythmia include palpitations, fatigue, shortness of breath, lightheadedness, syncope, or even sudden cardiac death (and a successful resuscitation).
    *   A history of CAD, prior MI, or CHF favors a diagnosis of VT over SVT in a patient with a wide complex tachycardia.
2. Use evidence from the *cardiac physical examination*.
    *   Analyze the *neck veins* for the presence or absence of A waves (atrial fibrillation), cannon A waves (PVCs, VT, complete heart block), or flutter waves (atrial flutter).
    *   Palpation of the *arterial pulse* establishes the rhythm and ventricular rate (at least of conductive beats). Keep in mind that not all ventricular contractions lead to a significant ejection of blood from the LV in patients

with atrial fibrillation and rapid ventricular response rates. Counting the number of palpable peripheral arterial pulsations may underestimate the actual ventricular rate (i.e., pulse deficit). The ECG should be used to calculate the true ventricular response rate.
    *   A laterally displaced apex, along with a dyskinetic LV impulse on *precordial palpation,* and S4 and S3 gallop sounds, denote the substrate for ventricular arrhythmias.
    *   *Auscultation of the heart* also establishes the ventricular rate and rhythm and the splitting and intensity of S1.
        —Variation in splitting of S1 suggests VT, complete heart block, or atrial fibrillation.
        —A loud S1 and a short PR interval occur in LGL syndrome (a form of preexcitation whereby a short accessory pathway connects the atria directly to the His-Purkinje system)
        —A faint S1 and a long PR interval are found in first degree AV block.
        —Abnormal splitting of S2 may occur with RBBB (wide physiologic split) or LBBB (paradoxical split).
    *   Cannon A waves, varying intensity of S1, multiple "staccato-like" sounds, and no response to carotid sinus massage, are clues to the diagnosis of VT.
3. The *ECG* is the cornerstone of the diagnosis.
    *   The evaluation of an arrhythmia may come about because an abnormality has been detected on ECG during a routine check-up.
    *   Compare the ECG with previous tracings. Prior tracings may reveal ectopic complexes (PACs, PVCs), and provide clues to the origin of the current arrhythmia.
    *   If there is an abrupt onset and termination of a regular narrow complex tachycardia, think of AVNRT.
    *   Wide complex tachycardia in the setting of structural heart disease is VT until proven otherwise.
    *   If there is a short PR interval and delta wave on a previous ECG, consider WPW as the possible reason for a "bizarre" tachyarrhythmia.
    *   In patients with atrial fibrillation, an excessively fast ventricular response (>250 beats/min) may be a clue to WPW syndrome and the presence of an accessory pathway (and the need to avoid digoxin, beta blockers, and calcium channel blockers, since any drug that blocks the AV node can accelerate the rhythm and precipitate VF). (**Figure 3-56**).
    *   The presence of AV dissociation, extremely wide QRS complexes with morphology not typical of RBBB or LBBB, QRS concordance (all QRS complexes in the same direction in

V1-V6), and fusion (or capture) beats in the setting of underlying heart disease (especially prior MI) are all clues favoring the diagnosis of VT over SVT with aberrancy (**Figure 22-5**).

- Atrial fibrillation, MAT and atrial flutter produce irregularly irregular QRS complexes. However, with MAT, P waves of 3 or more differing morphologies precede the QRS complexes. With atrial flutter, flutter waves ("sawtooth pattern") often are visible between the QRS complexes.
- Always keep in mind that when "P waves" are halfway between QRS complexes, there may be another P wave hiding in or near the QRS complex, and the rhythm represents some variety of SVT with 2:1 conduction. If the rate is >150 beats/min, think of atrial flutter with 2:1 block.
- If a regular tachycardia is present, observe the response to vagal maneuvers. SVT may revert back to NSR; VT generally will not. Postural modification to the Valsalva maneuver (lying flat with legs elevated at the end of the strain), may improve its effectiveness in reverting SVT.

* * *

BRADYARRHYTHMIAS AND CONDUCTION ABNORMALITIES

Bradyarrhythmias are common, especially in young, athletic individuals. They are usually due to increased vagal tone and do not require intervention. Abnormalities of conduction can occur between the sinus node and atrium, within the AV node, and in the intraventricular conduction pathways. Bradyarrhythmias due to these abnormalities may occur with aging and are usually due to idiopathic fibrosis in the conduction tissue (*Lenegre's disease)* or calcification of the cardiac skeleton (*Lev's* disease), CAD, cardiac trauma (postcardiac surgery/TAVR), tumors, infections (endocarditis, Chagas, Lyme), or other inflammatory or infiltrative disease (e.g., amyloid, sarcoid). Abnormalities of the cardiac conduction system may result in three general clinical syndromes:

- The *sick sinus syndrome* (which includes marked sinus bradycardia, sinoatrial exit block or arrest, and the so-called brady-tachy syndrome) (**Figure 3-47**)
- *AV nodal-His heart block* (**Figure 3-51**)
- *Intraventricular (bundle branch) block*

Patients with bradyarrhythmias and conduction abnormalities may be asymptomatic, or present with syncope, near-syncope, lightheadedness, worsening CHF or angina.

For the most part, management of bradyarrhythmias and conduction disturbances involves:

- Excluding self-limited causes (e.g., inferior MI, which causes transient ischemia of the AV node).
- Withdrawing bradycardia-inducing drugs (e.g., digoxin, beta blockers, rate-slowing calcium channel blockers).
- Administering intravenous atropine sulfate (an anticholinergic agent that blocks the vagal effect and thereby increases heart rate and enhances AV nodal conduction), or temporary pacing, if symptoms, e.g., dizziness, near-syncope or syncope, and angina pectoris, as well as hypotension, or frequent PVCs (due to the slow rhythm) are present.
- Deciding on the need for implantation of a permanent pacemaker. Asymptomatic sinus bradycardia, first degree AV block, and Mobitz type I second degree AV block often need no specific therapy. The presence of asymptomatic bifascicular block is not an indication for pacemaker therapy. A pacemaker may especially be indicated in symptomatic Mobitz type II second degree AV block, third degree heart block, chronic bifascicular or trifascicular block, or sick sinus syndrome. A pacemaker may also be indicated when there is a need to continue bradycardia-inducing drugs for other conditions.

* * *

Pearls:

- If on examining a *stable* patient you detect a regular sinus rhythm with a slow ventricular rate (i.e., sinus bradycardia in the 50's or 60's), think of two things: 1) the patient is a well-trained athlete or is physically conditioned (vagal tone) or 2) the patient might be taking a rate-slowing medication (e.g., beta-blocker, calcium channel blocker, amiodarone, clonidine, lithium). An *unstable* patient (e.g., acute inferior MI), on the other hand, may also have a slow heart rate. Keep in mind that timolol eye drops (a beta blocker) in the elderly may result in sufficient systemic absorption to slow the sinus node or unmask sinus node dysfunction. The medications your patient is receiving must always be considered when evaluating heart rate.
- The onset of AV conduction system disease (first, second, or third degree AV block) in a young patient with a flu-like illness and a rash, should raise the suspicion of *Lyme disease,* the leading tick-borne disease in the United States (caused by Borrelia burgdorferi, a spirochetal organism transmitted by the bite of the deer tick). Heart block usually resolves following treatment with antibiotics.

* * *

CHAPTER 23.   APPROACH TO THE PATIENT WITH ADULT CONGENITAL HEART DISEASE

Congenital heart defects occur in 8 out of every 1,000 live births. In general, the risk of congenital heart disease occurring in the offspring of an individual with an underlying congenital heart lesion is ~10–15%. Additional heart diseases that can be genetically transmitted include mitral valve prolapse, hypertrophic cardiomyopathy, dilated cardiomyopathy, Marfan's syndrome, long QT syndrome, and CAD. Until recently, practitioners rarely encountered adult patients with congenital heart disease in their daily practice. This is changing with the increased number of patients with previously undiagnosed or known congenital heart lesions who are reaching adulthood. By the time the practitioner sees the adult patient with congenital heart disease, many of the patients with cyanotic heart disease have either died or have had surgical correction of their lesions. Those who present with severe cyanosis resulting in clubbing of the fingers and toes have *Eisenmenger's syndrome* with severe pulmonary hypertension leading to a right-to-left shunt. Heart murmurs in these patients may be faint or absent, and the clinical picture is often overshadowed by the clinical findings of RV dilatation with or without signs of RV failure. Doppler-echo studies with agitated saline bubble contrast and/or cardiac catheterization may be required to help identify the location of the defect (e.g., ASD, VSD, PDA) through which the right-to-left shunt is occurring.

Most adults with previously undiagnosed and/or untreated congenital heart disease do not develop reversed (right-to-left) shunting and are acyanotic. Certain congenital lesions that were not apparent in early childhood, either because of the subtle nature of the defect or the close resemblance to innocent systolic murmurs, may be detectable in adulthood. These patients generally come later to the attention of the practitioner because of an abnormal clinical and/or laboratory finding. A comprehensive review of all of congenital heart disease is beyond the scope of this book. Acyanotic congenital heart lesions in adults that have not been altered by a surgical intervention, including bicuspid aortic valve, pulmonic valve stenosis, ASD and patent foramen ovale, VSD, coarctation of the aorta, and PDA, will be reviewed. The clinical approach to the patient who presents with Marfan's syndrome, and other inherited connective tissue disorders, e.g., Loeys-Dietz and Ehlers-Danlos syndromes, will also be discussed.

BICUSPID AORTIC VALVE

Aside from MVP (which itself is not due to a congenital malformation of the valve), the congenital bicuspid aortic valve is the most common congenital heart lesion in adults. It occurs in up to 2% of the population, predominantly in males, in a ratio of 3-4:1. Most bicuspid aortic valves usually function normally throughout early and mid-life, but eventually develop AS, AR, or both, as a result of turbulent flow that leads to leaflet injury, thickening, fibrosis, and calcification ("wear and tear").

Figure 23-1. Left. Schematic representation of the clinical spectrum of a congenital bicuspid aortic valve. **Right.** Auscultatory findings present with a congenital bicuspid aortic valve may vary from only an ejection sound (E) (no murmur) to a systolic murmur (SM), or a diastolic murmur (DM), or combinations of both. An S4 gallop is likely to be present with more severe degrees of valvular AS.

Progressive fibrocalcific thickening of a bicuspid valve accounts for nearly 50% of adult cases of symptomatic AS (syncope, exertional dyspnea, chest pain) requiring valve surgery. Bicuspid valves are the most common cause of isolated valvular AR. Sudden onset of acute severe AR can result from infective endocarditis. Detection of a bicuspid aortic valve is important, therefore, because of the risk of infective endocarditis and the need for meticulous oral hygiene and dental care. The clinical diagnosis is made by auscultating a short, grade 1-2/6 mid-systolic murmur (especially in a male) introduced by an aortic ejection sound (heard best over the aortic area and cardiac apex, not fluctuating in intensity with respiration), accompanied by a faint diastolic murmur of AR (**Figure 23-1**).

Figure 23-2. A middle aged man with congenital bicuspid aortic valve stenosis. Note the ejection sound (e) and systolic murmur (sm) well heard over the aortic area (ao). The ejection sound is a hallmark of a congenital bicuspid aortic valve and occurs with "doming" of the valve in early systole. The ejection sound and the systolic murmur are also generally well heard at the apex. The aortic ejection sound does not diminish in intensity with inspiration (as can occur with the pulmonic ejection sound). (Courtesy of Dr. W. Proctor Harvey).

A complication that appears to be unique to the congenital form of AS is aortic aneurysm and dissection with pathologic evidence of cystic medial necrosis in the aorta. The diagnosis of bicuspid aortic valve and the degree of AS and/or AR are usually confirmed by Doppler-echo (and cardiac catheterization when indicated) in most if not all cases. Cardiac catheterization is usually not necessary unless aortic balloon valvuloplasty or surgery is planned. Aortic repair should be considered when the aortic root diameter is > 5.0 cm (> 4.5 cm if undergoing AVR).

PULMONIC VALVE STENOSIS

Patients with pulmonic valve stenosis often have systolic murmurs and early systolic ejection sounds resembling those

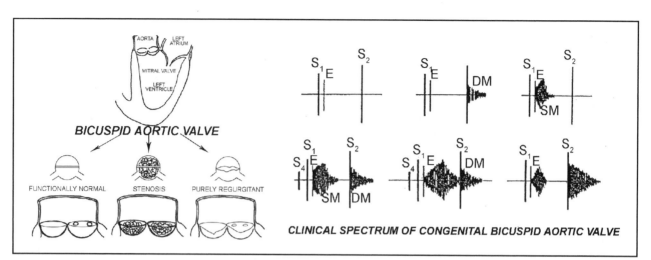

Figure 23-1 (Courtesy of W. Proctor Harvey, M.D.)

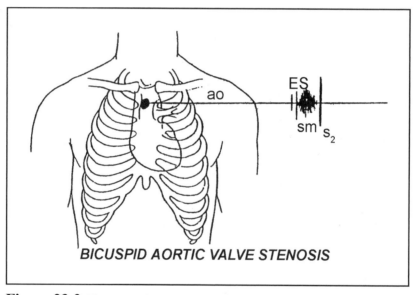

Figure 23-2 (Courtesy of W. Proctor Harvey, M.D.)

heard in patients with bicuspid aortic valves. Those with severe pulmonic stenosis usually are discovered in childhood and treated by pulmonary valvuloplasty. However, a number of patients escape detection and reach adulthood with surprisingly few symptoms. Adult patients with mild or moderate pulmonic stenosis are generally asymptomatic. When symptoms develop, patients with valvular pulmonic stenosis complain of exertional dyspnea and fatigue as a result of the inadequate rise in cardiac output during exercise. Eventually, effort-related chest pain (due to RV ischemia), syncope, and/or clinical findings of RV failure may develop when pulmonic stenosis becomes severe. On cardiac auscultation, patients with valvular pulmonic stenosis have a harsh systolic murmur loudest at the pulmonic area, accompanied by

an ejection sound that becomes faint or disappears with inspiration, along with a palpable systolic thrill. Signs of RV dilatation and hypertrophy are also noted on physical examination (e.g., a large A wave in the JVP, an RV parasternal impulse), ECG, and CXR (along with normal or reduced pulmonary vasculature). Doppler-echo (and cardiac catheterization) demonstrates a peak gradient across the pulmonic valve (mild: < 30 mmHg; moderate: 30-60 mmHg; severe: > 60 mmHg [or mean gradient > 40 mmHg]). Patients with mild pulmonic stenosis can be managed conservatively, while those who are symptomatic or with severe pulmonic stenosis are candidates for percutaneous balloon valvuloplasty. Antibiotic prophylaxis against infective endocarditis, however, is no longer required, even after valvuloplasty.

ATRIAL SEPTAL DEFECT AND PATENT FORAMEN OVALE

Atrial septal defect (ASD), particularly the ostium secundum type, which occurs in the region of the fossa ovalis in the mid portion of the interatrial septum, is the second most common type of congenital heart lesion diagnosed in adults. It is the most common congenital cardiac abnormality to escape detection until adulthood. It is more common in females than in males, by a ratio of 3:1. Many patients with ASD have few or no symptoms. With increasing age, a decrease in LV compliance (due to CAD, hypertension, or the aging effects on the myocardium) causes elevation of the LA pressure and increased left-to-right shunting through the ASD. This may lead to exertional dyspnea, fatigue, poor exercise tolerance, new onset palpitations (especially atrial fibrillation) and CHF. Other presentations in adults include peripheral or central nervous system emboli, due to paradoxical (from right side of heart to left) embolism. Endocarditis rarely occurs in patients with ASD (due to the low interatrial gradient); thus antibiotic prophylaxis is not necessary in the absence of associated higher risk lesions. Symptomatic ASDs should be closed to prevent pulmonary hypertension, the progression of right heart failure, and atrial arrhythmias (e.g., atrial fibrillation). In asymptomatic patients, open surgical repair or percutaneous catheter-based closure device techniques are recommended for patients with pulmonary to systemic blood flow ratios of 1.5:1 or greater (implying a significant left-to-right shunt).

The classic clinical clues to a secundum ASD include wide "fixed" splitting of S2, a systolic ejection murmur due to increased pulmonary flow (not due to flow through the ASD because there is almost no pressure gradient across the defect), and a low-pitched diastolic flow rumble across the tricuspid valve heard over the lower left sternal border. ECG findings of right axis deviation (left axis deviation with ostium primum ASD) with incomplete or complete RBBB (rSr′) in lead V1 (atrial fibrillation in older patients), along with CXR findings of dilated pulmonary arteries, increased pulmonary ("shunt") vascularity, and RV enlargement are also commonly present.

Figure 23-3. Atrial septal defect, secundum type (arrow). Auscultatory findings show wide "fixed" splitting of second heart sound (S2). In approximately one fourth of patients, there may be slight widening of the degree of splitting coincident with inspiration, though not becoming single with expiration. Also note the short early to mid systolic murmur. The absence of a systolic murmur practically rules out the diagnosis of ASD.

Since symptoms may be trivial or absent and physical signs can be subtle, the first clue to the diagnosis of ASD may come from a routine CXR (which shows increased pulmonary vascularity and RV enlargement) in an apparently healthy-appearing adult. Auscultatory findings of a systolic click (or clicks) and systolic MR murmur of MVP may be present since there is an association between ostium secundum ASD and MVP. Doppler-echo (particularly TEE) with agitated saline bubble contrast injection is diagnostic and permits assessment of the location and size of the defect along with RV and RA dilatation due to RV volume overload. Cardiac catheterization demonstrates an increase in oxygen saturation between the venae cavae and RV due to admixture of oxygenated blood from the LA (**Figure 5-25**) and reveals the ratio of pulmonary flow to systemic flow. Cardiac catheterization is usually unnecessary to confirm an ASD unless coexistent CAD is suspected before surgical repair or catheter-based device (double-disk prosthesis) closure is planned. Of note, septal tissue is absent in an ASD, which distinguishes it from a patent foramen ovale (PFO). A PFO (which is present in ~25% of the population), particularly those associated with an atrial septal aneurysm or a large interatrial shunt, may be responsible for a paradoxical embolism and cryptogenic stroke (especially in patients under age 55 years). Recent clinical trial data has shown that closure of the defect may offer a significant advantage over medical therapy (with aspirin, clopidogrel, or warfarin) in preventing recurrent cerebrovascular events in select patients, albeit at an increased risk of procedure-related atrial fibrillation.

VENTRICULAR SEPTAL DEFECT

In a ventricular septal defect (VSD), a persistent opening in the upper interventricular septum allows blood to travel from the high pressure LV into the low pressure RV. The subsequent natural history and pathophysiology depends on the size of the defect and the magnitude of the left-to-right shunt. In general, a significant lesion will usually present clinically with a holosystolic murmur, LV chamber enlargement or hypertrophy on the ECG, and an abnormal cardiac silhouette or pulmonary "shunt" vascularity on the CXR. In children, VSDs are the most common congenital malformation, but most of these patients who survive to adulthood without surgical correction will have spontaneous closure of the defect. The defects seen in adult life are of intermediate size, neither very large nor small enough to have closed spontaneously. Patients are typically asymptomatic, and the only abnormal physical finding is a loud, harsh, holosystolic murmur along the left sternal border, frequently accompanied by a palpable systolic thrill. The intensity of the murmur is no indication of the size of the defect. A small "pinhole" defect (the so-

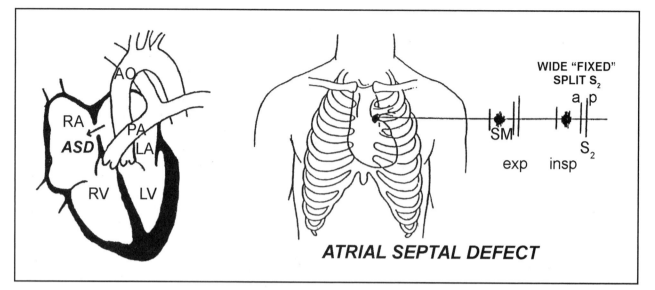

Figure 23-3 (Courtesy of W. Proctor Harvey, M.D.)

called *maladie de Roger*) may produce a palpable thrill. Echo-Doppler can visualize the defect, assess chamber size, the magnitude of shunting, and the pulmonary artery pressure. Cardiac catheterization confirms the diagnosis in all but the most trivial defects (**Figure 5-25**), and is usually unnecessary unless coexistent CAD is suspected before surgical repair. Although the most important risk associated with an uncorrected defect is endocarditis, antibiotic prophylaxis is no longer recommended due to the lack of conclusive evidence of benefit. Small left-to-right ventricular shunts in asymptomatic patients (i.e., pulmonary to systemic blood flow ratio of <1.5:1) do not require surgery. Large shunts should be repaired to prevent pulmonary hypertension or late heart failure. Some defects can be closed percutaneously.

Figure 23-4. Ventricular septal defect (arrow). Note that the systolic murmur (SM) of a VSD is louder along the left sternal border (LSB) than at the apex and is often associated with a palpable systolic thrill.

COARCTATION OF THE AORTA

Coarctation of the aorta is one of the causes of secondary hypertension. It usually is detected in childhood, but may be overlooked and present in adolescence or adulthood. It should be suspected when a young adult male presents with an elevated BP in the upper extremities (and diminished BP in the legs). It occurs five times more often in men than women and is associated with a congenital bicuspid aortic valve in 80% of cases. The most common location of the

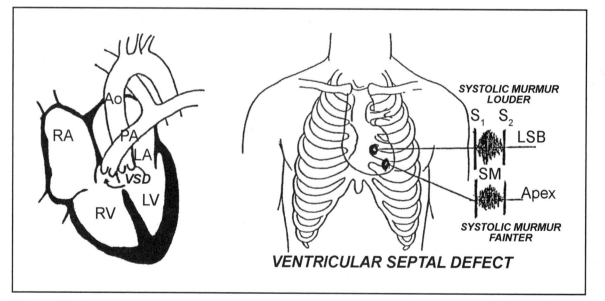

Figure 23-4 (Courtesy of W. Proctor Harvey, M.D.)

coarctation is in the descending aorta just distal to the origin of the left subclavian artery. Collateral circulation develops through the intercostal arteries and the branches of the subclavian arteries. Most patients are asymptomatic when diagnosed. The clinical clues are:

- Differential BP and pulses in the arms (high and strong) vs. the legs (lower and weak).
- Femoral pulsations are delayed in comparison with the radial (or brachial) pulse (the so-called radial-femoral delay) (**Figure 23-5**). However, when significant aortic regurgitation is present, the femoral pulses may be better felt than the radial, brachial, or carotid pulses.
- A systolic murmur (from obstruction) and continuous murmur (from collaterals) may be heard in the mid-upper back, especially over the spinous processes.
- The ECG may show LV hypertrophy and the CXR may reveal rib notching, a highly specific clue, due to enlargement of the collateral intercostal arteries. The CXR may also include a classic *"figure 3" sign* (**Figure 4-12**) beneath the aortic knob which represents dilatation of the aorta above and below the coarctation.
- Echo is useful to measure the pressure gradient across the obstruction and permits simultaneous assessment of associated findings, e.g., LV hypertrophy or a bicuspid aortic valve.
- MRI or aortic root angiography can delineate the coarctation and determine whether there are any collaterals.

Figure 23-5. Coarctation of the aorta (arrow). Arterial pulse and pressure recordings showing a contour that was also felt in the radial (left) and femoral (right) arterial pulses. Note the elevated systolic and pulse pressures in the ascending aorta and slow rate of rise and delayed peak below, in the descending aorta beyond the coarctation. (Courtesy of Dr. Gordon A. Ewy).

The indications for surgery in adults include symptoms (e.g., exertional dyspnea, headache, epistaxis, leg fatigue), proximal hypertension or LV hypertrophy in the presence of significant coarctation narrowing. These patients have an increased risk of aortic dissection (probably as a consequence of hypertension in association with intrinsic abnormalities of the aortic wall), CHF, a ruptured cerebral aneurysm of the circle of Willis, and infective endocarditis that may involve the coarctation or an associated bicuspid aortic valve. In most cases, surgical repair of the coarctation is recommended at the time of the diagnosis. Relief of the coarctation is indicated when there is proximal hypertension and the peak gradient exceeds 20 mmHg. Balloon dilatation with stent placement is a treatment option in the presence of a discrete narrowing, but is considered second-line therapy.

PATENT DUCTUS ARTERIOSUS

Patent ductus arteriosus (PDA), an abnormal communication between the descending aorta and pulmonary artery can also escape detection in childhood. It is associated with birth at high altitudes and maternal rubella. Patients with PDA may be asymptomatic or may complain of dyspnea on exertion and fatigue. The larger the left-to-right shunt, the more likely CHF will develop. Brisk, bounding pulses and a wide pulse pressure, resembling those seen with AR, may be noted. The

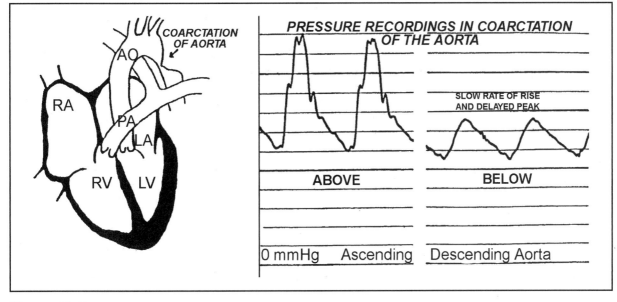

Figure 23-5

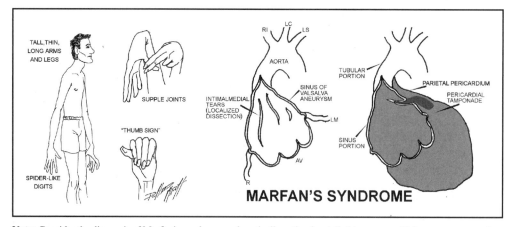

MARFAN'S SYNDROME

Note: Consider the diagnosis of Marfan's syndrome and aortic dissection in a tall, thin person with long arms, acute chest and back pain, a normal ECG, and a new aortic diastolic murmur (right sternal border > left).

Figure 23-6

most important clinical finding is a loud continuous systolic and diastolic ("machinery") murmur under the left clavicle (**Figure 2-81**). Pulmonary hypertension with reversed (right-to-left) shunting (Eisenmenger syndrome) may develop gradually over time. In those cases, the diastolic component of the murmur may disappear. Cyanosis and clubbing of the toes, but not the fingers ("differential cyanosis") may occur when poorly oxygenated blood from the pulmonary artery passes through the PDA into the descending aorta. The ECG may show LV hypertrophy, and the CXR may demonstrate increased pulmonary vascular markings along with an enlarged main pulmonary artery, ascending aorta, and LV, and occasionally calcification of the ductus. The diagnosis of PDA can be confirmed by Doppler-echo studies and cardiac catheterization. (**Figure 5-25**). The recommendation is for closure of even a small PDA (by surgical ligation or percutaneously) because of the risk of infective endocarditis.

MARFAN'S SYNDROME AND OTHER CONNECTIVE TISSUE DISORDERS

Marfan's syndrome is a genetically transmitted (autosomal dominant) connective tissue disorder characterized by ocular, musculoskeletal, and cardiovascular manifestations (e.g., aortic root dilatation and MVP). It is caused by mutations in the gene that codes for the structural protein fibrillin-1 (FBN1), which impairs the formation of microfibrils in elastin. Typically, these patients are tall and thin, with long, slender extremities, spider-like digits (arachnodactyly), hyperextensible joints, high-arched palate, and dislocated lenses. With patients with a typical body habitus and a positive family history, the diagnosis of Marfan's syndrome can be made. The aortic root dilatation may be isolated to the sinuses of Valsalva or may be fusiform and involve the entire ascending aorta. The complications of aortic disease include progressive AR, dissection, and rupture (**Figure 23-6**).

Figure 23-6. Marfan's syndrome. Left. Note tall, thin man with typical body habitus demonstrating disproportionately long arms and legs, spider-like digits, and supple joints. Also note marked protrusion of the thumb ("thumb sign"). Right. The pathology of the Marfan ascending aorta may lead to sudden death. In some cases (Left), the sinus portion of the ascending aorta is markedly dilated and the aorta has multiple intimal-medial tears. In other cases (right) the sinus of Valsalva aneurysm ruptures, causing pericardial temponade. (Courtesy of Dr. Bruce F. Waller).

Serial CXRs should be performed and if any question is found concerning the aorta, then either a CT scan or MRI may be performed to exclude aneurysm formation or dissection. Periodic echo evaluation of aortic root dilatation is key in the treatment of patients with Marfan's syndrome. Prophylactic aortic root repair is recommended when the aortic diameter exceeds 5.0–5.5 cm. Pregnancy is relatively contraindicated for women with Marfan's syndrome because of the high risk for aortic dissection. Prophylactic therapy with beta blockers is recommended to decrease the pressure load on the aorta, to reduce the risk of aortic dilatation, and to decrease the incidence of AR and dissection. Angiotensin receptor blockers may also have a role in preventing aneurysm formation by inhibiting transforming growth factor-β, a signaling molecule that regulates cellular proliferation and differentiation. Restriction from contact sports and vigorous physical exertion, especially isometric exercise and weight lifting, also protects against aortic dissection. With acute aortic dissection, aggressive surgical intervention frequently is required.

Other Marfan-like inherited connective tissue disorders, e.g., Loeys-Dietz syndrome (mutation in transforming growth factor β receptor), characterized by widely spaced eyes and a bifid uvula or cleft palate, and Ehlers-Danlos syndrome (defect in type III collagen), characterized by skin hyperelasticity and hypermobile joints, may also predispose to aortic aneurysm formation and dissection and warrant aggressive intervention.

CHAPTER 24.   APPROACH TO THE PATIENT WITH HEART DISEASE UNDERGOING NONCARDIAC SURGERY

Today's clinician is often asked to assess cardiovascular risk in patients undergoing noncardiac surgery to aid in their preoperative and postoperative management. Although the practitioner may be asked to "clear" the patient for surgery, it is important to emphasize that even the healthiest patient has some surgical risk and that the highest risk patient may actually need surgery the most. Of an estimated 25 million Americans undergoing noncardiac surgery each year, >6 million are at increased risk for developing postoperative cardiac complications (e.g., MI, CHF, cardiac death), depending on the type and severity of the underlying cardiac disease and the urgency and nature of the planned surgery (**Figures 24-1** and **24-2**). The role of the medical consultant includes clearly defining the patient's cardiac disease, evaluating the severity and stability of the condition, providing a surgical risk assessment (low, intermediate, or high), and recommending perioperative measures to reduce surgical risk.

PREOPERATIVE ASSESSMENT OF RISK

Clinical Predictors of Risk

In order to identify those patients at increased risk, it is important to perform a thoughtful preoperative clinical cardiovascular evaluation. A careful clinical history helps to determine whether or not the patient has had a prior coronary evaluation (including an adequate stress test or coronary angiogram) over the past several years, or has undergone previous coronary revascularization (PCI, CABG). There is compelling evidence that recent coronary revascularization confers protection against perioperative cardiac events. The history may also help to identify patients at particularly high risk. These include patients with a history of unstable angina pectoris, recent MI, decompensated CHF, severe symptomatic valvular heart disease (especially AS),

---

FIGURE 24-2

Surgery Specific Markers of Perioperative Risk

Risk	Surgery
High	Emergency, aortic or peripheral vascular, and extensive and prolonged operations with large volume shifts.
Intermediate	Orthopedic, urologic, thoracic, abdominal, carotid endarterectomy, and head and neck procedures.
Low	Cataract, breast, endoscopic procedures, superficial biopsy.

FIGURE 24-1

Clinical Markers of Increased Perioperative Cardiac Risk

Major	Intermediate	Minor
• Unstable coronary syndromes • Decompensated CHF • Significant arrhythmias (e.g., high grade AV block, VT, SVT with uncontrolled heart rate) • Severe valvular heart disease	• Mild angina pectoris • Prior MI • Compensated or prior CHF • Diabetes mellitus	• Advanced age • Abnormal ECG (e.g., LV hypertrophy, LBBB, ST-T abnormalities) • Rhythm other than sinus (e.g., atrial fibrillation) • Prior stroke • Uncontrolled hypertension • Low functional capacity

Source: Eagle KA, Brundage BH, Chaitman BR, et al: Guidelines for perioperative cardiovascular evaluation for Noncardiac surgery: Report of the American College of Cardiology (ACC)/ American Heart Association (AHA) Task Force on Practice Guidelines, *Circulation* 1996; 93:1278–1317.

significant or uncontrolled cardiac arrhythmias, or other comorbid conditions, e.g., diabetes mellitus, stroke, COPD, liver or kidney disease, and poor functional capacity (i.e., the diminished ability to climb stairs, do housework, perform regular exercise, etc.). In addition, a thorough physical examination may provide important clues such as jugular venous distention, pulsus alternans, S3 gallop, a displaced PMI (cardiomegaly), bibasilar rales, peripheral edema (indicating the presence of CHF), murmurs (valvular or congenital heart disease), and bruits (carotid artery and/or peripheral vascular disease). The preoperative ECG may reveal evidence of an underlying rhythm or conduction disturbance, abnormal Q waves denoting a prior MI, or LV hypertrophy secondary to valvular AS, HOCM or long-standing hypertension. The chest x-ray may reveal evidence of cardiomegaly, significant coronary or aortic calcification, and pulmonary vascular congestion.

Patients can generally be placed into low, intermediate, and high risk categories. Those at low risk do not require further workup. Those at intermediate risk should undergo some type of noninvasive diagnostic testing, e.g., stress (treadmill or pharmacologic) nuclear perfusion, or echo imaging study. Those at high risk should undergo more invasive diagnostic testing, e.g., coronary angiography, and surgery delayed (if possible) until the cardiovascular problem (i.e., decompensated CHF, severe CAD) is resolved. If your patient is going for emergency surgery, there is no need to stratify risk preoperatively. Pre and perioperative use of cardiac drugs, particularly beta blockers in patients with CAD, and those at increased risk of developing an arrhythmia may help to reduce postoperative cardiac complications. *Keep in mind, there is no data to support prophylactic PCI or CABG before noncardiac surgery just to "get the patient through the operation". Indications for revascularization are the same as if the patient were not going for surgery (e.g., ACS, refractory symptoms, large territory at risk).*

LOWER RISK: The absence of a history of angina, MI, CHF, or diabetes, for example, has been demonstrated to have a negative predictive value of >95% for left main or severe triple vessel CAD, and therefore these patients are at lower clinical risk for perioperative events. Physically active patients < age 70 who lack these high risk clinical markers, and patients who have had CABG surgery in the past 5 years or PCI 6 months to 5 years previously, who are free of clinical evidence of ischemia, may undergo noncardiac surgery without further testing. In addition, there is no convincing evidence that prophylactic cardiac catheterization and revascularization will reduce risk in patients with mild (CCS Class I or II) stable angina.

INTERMEDIATE RISK: Patients at intermediate risk (e.g., those with one or two clinical risk variables) may benefit from non-invasive testing (e.g., exercise and/or pharmacologic stress testing, accompanied by nuclear perfusion imaging or echo), if they have not already been previously conducted. The goal of noninvasive testing includes an accurate quantitation of the patient's functional capacity (i.e., cardiac reserve) and the assessment of the presence and degree of inducible ischemia, as well as LV function. For those unable to achieve a high workload during exercise (due to poor functional capacity) and who have significant ischemia identified by stress echo or nuclear imaging, along with transient LV dilatation (due to ischemic-induced LV dysfunction), the risk of postoperative cardiac complications (e.g., MI, death) increases dramatically. On the other hand, for those with a normal stress nuclear scan or echo, a low risk of cardiac complications exists.

In addition to prognostic value, noninvasive testing is indicated in selective patients if there is a reasonable chance that the test results will have substantive impact on the medical or surgical management, e.g., whether to perform invasive hemodynamic or TEE monitoring during surgery, administer anti-ischemic medical therapy, or perform preoperative coronary angiography with a consideration of myocardial revascularization (e.g., PCI, CABG) or even to cancel surgery.

HIGH RISK: In general, most patients with stable CAD can be assessed for risk from clinical information alone, without the need for any specialized cardiac testing. If the history is unreliable and/or clinical risk assessment unclear, provocative exercise or pharmacologic stress testing may be useful to help stratify risk. Patients who have severe angina (CCS Class III or IV angina—**Figure 1-9**) or an unstable clinical status (i.e., recent MI; increased frequency, severity or new angina; uncontrolled CHF, significant ventricular arrhythmias) are considered to be at high clinical risk (they have a high probability of left main or triple vessel CAD). These patients should be considered for further diagnostic evaluation and/or therapeutic intervention, including coronary angiography (the same indications as in the nonoperative setting) if they are appropriate candidates for coronary revascularization.

Surgery Specific Markers of Risk

The specific type of noncardiac surgery the patient is to undergo also influences the risk. Patients (particularly the elderly) who need emergency surgery are at 4–5 times greater risk than those undergoing elective surgery (because of the inability to completely evaluate or prepare them for surgery). In addition, patients undergoing vascular surgical procedures (especially abdominal aortic aneurysm repair) have nearly a 2–3 fold greater risk of postoperative cardiac events, primarily due to the high incidence of associated symptomatic or silent CAD, especially in those patients with diabetes mellitus. Patients scheduled for major intrathoracic, abdominal (intraperitoneal), or extensive surgery associated with large extra and intravascular fluid shifts and/or significant blood loss, as well as postoperative hypoxemia resulting from compromised ventilatory function, are also at increased risk (>5%). Those undergoing ophthalmologic (e.g., cataract), breast, endoscopic procedures, or superficial biopsy, are at the lowest risk (<1%). Cardiac complications from noncardiac surgery are usually noted on the second or third day postoperatively.

PERIOPERATIVE EVALUATION AND MANAGEMENT

In general, preoperative myocardial revascularization (e.g., PCI, CABG) is indicated in patients for whom it would be indicated even if there were no elective surgery, e.g., selected patients with very symptomatic CAD despite medical therapy, or those with strongly positive ECG exercise or pharmacological radionuclide or echo stress tests. Otherwise, no data exists to support doing prophylactic PCI or CABG before noncardiac surgery just to reduce the incidence of postoperative cardiac complications. Coronary stents are now being used in more than 90% of percutaneous coronary interventions. It is prudent to delay elective surgery for at least 4 weeks after bare metal stenting and 6 months or more after implantation of a drug eluting stent to allow complete endothelialization and to avoid the possibility of late stent thrombosis that may result from premature discontinuation of dual antiplatelet therapy (particularly ADP receptor blocker) prior to planned surgery.

Clinical experience indicates that patients with symptomatic valvular AS or MS severe enough to warrant surgical treatment should have valve surgery (or balloon valvuloplasty or TAVR as a temporizing step) before elective (or urgent) noncardiac surgery. Patients with severe AR or MR may benefit from afterload reduction and diuretic therapy to produce maximal hemodynamic stabilization before high risk surgery. The severity of valvular lesions should be determined prior to surgery to allow for appropriate fluid management and consideration of invasive intraoperative monitoring. Patients with mechanical heart valves or atrial fibrillation receiving oral anticoagulation at high thrombotic risk should be bridged with IV unfractionated or subQ low molecular weight heparin. Endocarditis prophylaxis is recommended for all patients with prosthetic heart valves.

Myocardial ischemia and MI, due to plaque rupture/thrombus, i.e., ACS (type 1) or supply-demand mismatch (type 2), may occur with a postoperative hypercoagulable state, surge in catecholamine levels, hemodynamic changes, hypoxemia, and fluid shifts. For high risk patients, administering β-blockers a week or more preoperatively and maintaining treatment uninterrupted as long as possible (especially in patients with CAD) may be helpful in reducing ischemia, postoperative

MI, and arrhythmias e.g., atrial fibrillation. These beneficial effects, however, may be off-set by an increased risk of bradycardia, hypotension, stroke and death, particularly if high dose β-blockers are administered acutely and careful dose titration and monitoring is not maintained. Most cardiac medications should be continued whenever possible through noncardiac surgery, including aspirin (in patients with coronary stents), antianginal, antihypertensive, and statin therapy. However, the routine use of perioperative aspirin (in unstented patients) and α-agonists, e.g., clonidine, is not recommended since recent evidence suggests the risk of major bleeding and hypotension, respectively, may outweigh the potential cardiac benefits.

Patients >50 years of age, particularly those with risk factors, or who have signs or symptoms suggestive of cardiac disease, should have a 12 lead ECG. A preoperative ECG not only helps to estimate cardiac risk, but also serves as a baseline, should cardiac problems develop in the postoperative period. It is important to document if any abnormalities exist before surgery in order to determine that they did not develop during or after surgery. Changes in the patient's clinical condition, ECG, or elevated troponin levels, may detect ischemic events, which can be painless during or after surgery. Given a patient with known CAD, a routine postoperative ECG (in the absence of symptoms) may help exclude the possibility of a silent MI. When the clinical evaluation indicates that the risk of noncardiac surgery is moderate but acceptable to the patient, aggressive medical therapy should be provided that is designed to stabilize the cardiac condition (i.e., control heart rate and blood pressure, reduce myocardial ischemia, and improve LV function). Elective surgery should be postponed at least 4–6 weeks after a recent MI. Patients with negative post-MI risk stratification, or those who have had successful reperfusion therapy with normal or near-normal LV function, and no spontaneous or inducible ischemia, may proceed with elective operation at 4–6 weeks after MI.

Patients with poor LV function, as may be manifested by symptoms and/or signs of CHF or a markedly reduced ejection fraction, on preoperative testing, are at increased risk of cardiac complications. CHF may develop postoperatively due to delayed mobilization of extravascular fluid (to the intravascular space), over-hydration, or undetected myocardial ischemia. CHF should be well controlled prior to all but emergent surgery. Consideration should be given, however, to holding diuretics, ACE inhibitors/ARBs before surgery since these agents may cause intraoperative hypotension and potentiate postoperative acute kidney injury. As increasingly complex surgical procedures are being performed in patients who are older and have more chronic diseases, a careful preoperative cardiac evaluation has become even more important. Proper perioperative assessment and management of patients undergoing noncardiac surgery requires careful teamwork among the practitioner, anesthesiologist, and surgeon.

CHAPTER 25. APPROACH TO THE PATIENT WITH NEOPLASTIC HEART DISEASE

An understanding of the effects of cancer and its treatment on the heart, so-called *cardio-oncology*, is an essential requisite for the effective management of patients with neoplastic heart disease. Although cardiac tumors are distinctly unusual, when they occur they may involve the endocardium or myocardium or infiltrate into the heart from the pericardium. Tumors of the heart may be primary or secondary, and either benign or malignant. This chapter will review the clinical approach to the most common primary and secondary tumors of the heart in adults and the effects of their treatment on the cardiovascular system. The clinical evaluation of malignant carcinoid syndrome, which may be associated with characteristic cardiovascular abnormalities (e.g., right heart failure, tricuspid and/or pulmonic valve disease) will also be discussed.

PRIMARY TUMORS OF THE HEART

Atrial Myxoma

The most common primary cardiac tumor in adults, comprising 30–50% of all cases, is the atrial myxoma. Myxomas are usually benign, characteristically arise from the interatrial septum, and grow into the left atrium, although 10% are malignant and 10% arise in other locations (e.g., right atrium, right or left ventricle). The tumor is usually solitary and commonly is attached to the chamber wall by means of a pedicle. Most left atrial myxomas are mobile. They slowly enlarge and interfere with normal mitral valve function, producing clinical findings that closely simulate rheumatic MS and/or MR. The patient with an atrial myxoma may be asymptomatic or present with clinical symptoms that fit into one or more of three categories: *cardiac* (dyspnea and syncope), *embolic* (acute vascular or neurologic deficit), and *constitutional* (fever, malaise, weight loss).

The patient with a myxoma may seek medical attention because of occasional lightheadedness (e.g., upon change in position) or dyspnea on exertion. LA myxomas often mimic the symptoms and signs of rheumatic mitral valve disease. However, there are some subtle clues that should arouse your index of suspicion to the presence of an LA myxoma:

- Absence of a history of rheumatic fever
- The unusually rapid progression of symptoms of dyspnea
- The occurrence of syncope
- Positional variation of symptoms or unexpected improvement of symptoms in a patient suspected of having rheumatic MS

- The finding on physical examination of a diastolic third heart sound ("*tumor plop*") with or without other findings of mitral valve disease
- Variability of the physical findings of mitral valve disease with changes in body position
- The occurrence of a TIA or stroke (due to embolism) in a young adult (especially those that are in normal sinus rhythm)
- The presence of constitutional symptoms, e.g., fever, weight loss, arthralgias, rash, pallor (secondary to anemia), elevated ESR, hyperglobulinemia (signs and symptoms suggestive of infective endocarditis)
- Signs of LA enlargement on the ECG or CXR

Keep in mind that an atrial myxoma may present with all of the features of endocarditis, including CHF, but a clue sometimes may be found in CHF that comes and goes, since CHF due to the destructive process of infective endocarditis rarely remits spontaneously. Any of these clinical clues should prompt you to consider the diagnosis of atrial myxoma and order further appropriate laboratory studies, e.g., echo (particularly TEE) and cardiac catheterization. Angiocardiography can diagnose myxoma by outlining a filling defect in the involved chamber. Surgical removal of the tumor is usually curative, eliminating symptoms and signs promptly and effectively. Careful attention should be directed to screening (filtering) tumor fragments from the blood to prevent systemic emboli. Although recurrences may occur (~5%), long-term follow-up after surgery reveals that most patients remain well.

The key to diagnosis is a careful history and physical examination aided by a high index of suspicion. The usual patient is a young, or middle-aged female, who complains of shortness of breath, fatigue and weight loss, at times accompanied by fever, dizziness or even syncope, which may follow changes in posture. Atrial myxoma may release emboli (20–45% of patients) due to thrombus on the surface of the tumor that may dislodge, or pieces of the tumor itself that may break loose and enter the systemic circulation. These embolic episodes may mimic systemic vasculitis or infective endocarditis. Evidence of peripheral emboli of unexplained origin may be one of the first clues that alert the clinician to the diagnosis. Occasionally, the diagnosis is first suggested by the pathologist's report of a myxomatous embolus removed at surgical embolectomy. On cardiac auscultation, a diastolic rumble at the apex or a systolic regurgitant murmur may suggest rheumatic mitral valvular disease. A diastolic third heart sound ("tumor plop"), which may resemble the opening snap of MS (although it is usually later in diastole than an OS and lower in pitch), is common and may be heard as the myxoma descends through the mitral valve. The degree of obstruction or interference with mitral valve function may vary with position. Changes in the murmur, both systolic and diastolic (as well as symptoms of dyspnea or syncope), may also be related to the patient's position. Episodic pulmonary edema may occur when the patient assumes an upright posture.

The ECG in atrial myxoma often displays abnormal P waves of left or right atrial enlargement. The chest x-ray may exhibit LA enlargement, pulmonary artery dilatation and RV prominence. The cardiac silhouette may, in fact, resemble that of rheumatic MS. Leukocytosis, anemia, and an elevated erythrocyte sedimentation rate (ESR) may be present. Disability, unlike rheumatic MS, often evolves quickly. The patient may progress from no symptoms to significant impairment in a few months. Such rapid deterioration of apparent MS is unusual, and should suggest atrial myxoma (as should syncope, which seldom accompanies rheumatic MS). Echo (particularly TEE) is extremely valuable for the detection of atrial myxoma.

Figure 25-1. Schematic diagram of 2D echocardiogram in left atrial myxoma. **Left.** Parasternal long axis view. Note the myxoma can be seen between the mitral valve leaflets. **Right.** Apical 4 chamber view. Note the large mobile tumor is attached by a narrow stalk or pedicle to the interatrial septum.

The presence of a mass lesion can be confirmed at cardiac catheterization, along with the hemodynamic pressure tracings, e.g., diastolic LV-LA pressure gradient, prominent V waves in PCWP that are similar to those seen in MS and/or MR respectively.

Myxomas may occur as part of the Carney complex, an autosomal dominant disorder associated with pigmentation abnormalities (e.g., blue nevi), schwannomas, and endocrine tumors.

Angiosarcoma

The most common malignant primary cardiac tumor in adults is angiosarcoma. These tumors arise on the right side of the heart from the endocardium or pericardium and can grow rapidly. The partient is usually a young or middle-aged male. Progressive CHF with cardiomegaly, cardiac arrhythmias, hemopericardium, and sudden cardiac death are common. Cardiac tumors may be discovered initially by transthoracic echo. TEE, CT, and/or cardiac MRI may further evaluate its location and the extent of its involvement in the heart. The role of PET in the evaluation of cardiac tumors is in evolution. Angiosarcomas are generally associated with a poor prognosis, as they have often spread too extensively for complete surgical resection. Palliative surgery, however, along with chemotherapy and radiation, may be helpful in select patients to relieve compressive or obstructive symptoms.

SECONDARY TUMORS OF THE HEART AND THE EFFECTS OF TREATMENT

Many malignant tumors metastasize to the heart or pericardium or infiltrate from the mediastinum or adjacent lung

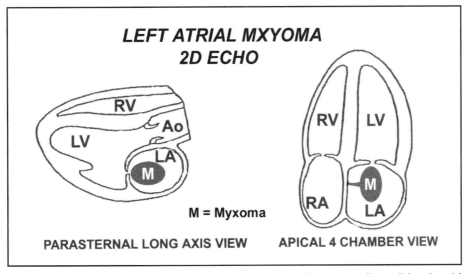

Note: Left atrial myxomas (M) most commonly appear as a mass attached by a narrow stalk or pedicle to the atrial septum. The mass can involve the mitral valve intermittently to cause a "tumor plop" that may clinically mimic mitral stenosis. Myxomas should be resected due to the risk of systemic embolization.

Figure 25-1

and/or pleura (the closer the noncardiac tumor is to the heart, the greater the likelihood of spreading to the heart). Some tumors (e.g., lung, breast, kidney, malignant melanoma, lymphoma, and acute leukemia) are especially prone to metastasize to the heart and are many times more frequent than primary tumors originating in the heart. In general, metastatic tumors of the heart account for ~95% of all cardiac tumors. Clues to infiltration of the myocardium may include cardiac arrhythmias, conduction disturbances, and unexplained CHF. Secondary neoplastic invasion of the pericardium is more common than invasion of the myocardium or endocardium. Symptoms and signs (e.g., chest pain, dyspnea, pericardial friction rub, elevated JVP, pulsus paradoxus), when present, usually relate to pericardial metastases and effusion. Cardiac tamponade may occur. A chest x-ray may reveal an enlarged cardiac silhouette produced by the effusion and lung fields that do not display pulmonary venous congestion. The ECG may reveal low voltage and occasional total electrical alternans (of the P, QRS, and T waves). Echo is valuable in establishing the presence of pericardial fluid. Therapy is palliative, consisting of pericardiocentesis (with or without the installation of chemotherapeutic or sclerosing agents into the pericardial space), or surgical creation (subxiphoid) of a pleural-pericardial window (which allows pericardial fluid to drain into the pleural space).

Treatment of the patient's underlying malignancy may cause further cardiac compromise. Cardiomyopathy, for example, may result from chemotherapy with the anthracycline agents e.g., doxorubicin (Adriamycin), particularly when combined with the monoclonal antibody trastuzumab (Herceptin). Anthracycline-related cardiomyopathy is dose-related and is not reversible. (and only rarely occurs at cumulative doses below 450 mg per square meter of body surface area). Thirty percent of individuals treated with >450–500 mg/m² develop CHF. Serial assessment of LV function (ejection fraction) by MUGA scan and/or echo has been used to monitor such therapy. The drug should be stopped if the LV ejection fraction shows a decrease of 10% or more or a decline to <50% during the course of therapy. Unlike anthracyclines, trastuzamab-related cardiomyopathy is not dose related and is reversible. Selected patients can be successfully rechallenged with the drug after recovery of LV function. Of note, cardioprotective strategies, e.g., use of liposomal doxorubicin, and agents, e.g., dexrazoxane, an iron chelator, reduce the risk of cardiotoxicity and may be considered in patients being treated with higher doses of anthracyclines. Standard CHF treatment should generally be initiated with the earliest detection of cardiotoxicity. The benefit of preventive β-blockers and/or ACE inhibitors/ARBs has recently been investigated with promising results; however, larger confirmatory studies are needed prior to use of these agents prophylactically.

Radiation therapy to the mediastinum can cause acute pericarditis and pericardial constriction, myocardial disease, valvular heart disease, electrical conduction disturbances, and CAD. CAD following radiation tends to involve the ostia of the left main and right coronary arteries. Because cigarette smoking, hyperlipidemia, and hypertension appear to increase the risk of radiation induced heart disease, the practitioner should screen for and reduce or eliminate these CAD risk factors in patients who have received cardiac irradiation.

CARCINOID SYNDROME

Carcinoid tumors are rare, slow growing neuroendocrine tumors that usually arise from the small intestine or appendix, with metastases to the liver. Secretion of serotonin (5-hydroxytryptamine), a potent vasoactive agent, is a feature of malignant carcinoid tumors. When the tumor is confined to the intestine, the serotonin it produces is inactivated by monoamine oxidase as it passes through the liver. However, when hepatic metastases develop, active serotonin may enter the systemic circulation producing the carcinoid syndrome. This is characterized by episodic or permanent (end-stage) violaceous flushing of the face, neck and upper chest, bronchoconstriction with wheezing, intestinal hypermotility with diarrhea, and eventually CHF and death. The serotonin and kinin peptides secreted by the tumor are responsible for many of the clinical manifestations of the disease, including the characteristic fibrotic right-heart lesions (e.g., pulmonic stenosis, tricuspid stenosis and regurgitation, and right heart failure).

Whenever a patient has evidence of right-sided heart failure or tricuspid and/or pulmonic stenosis/regurgitation (and little evidence of left-sided heart disease), always ask if he or she has experienced "flushing", abdominal discomfort, diarrhea, or wheezing (which result from serotonin excess). The right-sided cardiac findings can be confirmed by echo and should raise the suspicion of carcinoid syndrome. Once suspected, the diagnosis can be made by detecting large quantities of 5-hydroxyindoleacetic acid (a serotonin metabolite) in the urine. CT, MRI, and somatostatin receptor scanning (OctreoScan) will usually reveal metastases to the liver.

Treatment with somatostatin analogues e.g., octreotide (Sandostatin) or alpha interferon improves symptoms and survival but does not appear to improve valvular abnormalities. On occasion, valvular surgery may be required, in addition to conventional medical therapy for control of CHF.

CHAPTER 26.   APPROACH TO THE PATIENT WITH "FALSE" HEART DISEASE

PITFALLS IN THE CLINICAL RECOGNITION AND MANAGEMENT OF HEART DISEASE

Regrettably, many anxious and frightened, but otherwise healthy individuals today are carrying the stigma of "false" heart disease, along with its attendant and often tragic consequences. These include unnecessary restriction of activity, prejudice in insurability, increased psychologic stress, and inappropriate treatment resulting from an incorrect diagnosis due to misinterpretation of the patient's symptoms, physical signs, ECG, CXR and other diagnostic laboratory findings. Concern in the practitioner's mind regarding possible errors of omission often fosters such errors of commission. This chapter will provide the reader with an overview of some of the most common errors in cardiac diagnosis made in everyday clinical practice. A practical approach to differentiating normal (*physiologic*) from abnormal (*pathologic*) clinical findings in the well-trained athlete will also be discussed.

MISLEADING CLUES IN THE CLINICAL CARDIOVASCULAR EVALUATION

Misinterpretation of Symptoms and Signs

Many patients with normal hearts complain of "chest pain", "shortness of breath", and/or "palpitations". An incomplete, cursory analysis of patients with these symptoms may lead to a premature and often erroneous diagnosis of heart disease. For example, it is not unusual to see patients with chest pain of noncardiac origin (who also happen to have a so-called "abnormal" ECG) treated for years with medication based on the false diagnosis of "CAD". There are no "shortcuts" in the proper evaluation of this important symptom. CAD should be a diagnosis based on a careful detailed history, not a "waste basket" diagnosis made because no other cause is readily apparent.

Remember that symptoms identified as being associated with heart disease can also occur without any significant cardiovascular abnormality whatsoever. It is worthwhile to explain to your patient the types of chest pain that generally are not related to heart disease, e.g., fleeting, momentary, sharp, sticking, stabbing or knife-like pain, localized to the left inframammary region, lasting only seconds, or constant pain ("all the time"), unrelated to effort, aggravated by change in position or palpation. Your patient can

be reassured that these types of noncardiac chest pain are not signs of new or recurrent CAD. Dyspnea, characterized by a vague sensation of breathlessness, or a feeling of needing to take a good deep breath, not associated with physical effort, and punctuated by deep sighing respirations, often accompany noncardiac chest pain, and is a frequent manifestation of stress or emotional disturbance. Episodes of hyperventilation can sometimes cause symptoms similar to those of heart disease, e.g., chest discomfort, numbness and tingling of the fingers, lightheadedness, and shortness of breath that may even be misinterpreted as due to acute pulmonary edema. Reproducing the patient's symptoms by having him or her overbreathe confirms the diagnosis.

Lending further confusion to interpreting "shortness of breath" is the presence of rales. There is truth to the saying that most patients with rales do not have heart failure (and conversely, most patients with heart failure do not have rales). Rales are nonspecific for heart failure and are most often due to secretions in the airways in the presence of pulmonary disease. Likewise, edema of the lower extremities secondary to obesity or venous insufficiency may be wrongly attributed to CHF. During pregnancy, dyspnea and orthopnea, due to elevation of the diaphragm and gestational hormonal changes, lightheadedness, caused by decreased vena caval return to the heart (*supine hypotensive syndrome*), and palpitations (noted frequently as the heart rate increases) are common complaints in the absence of a cardiopulmonary abnormality.

Fatigue and palpitations commonly present in patients with heart disease can be seen in many illnesses, both organic and psychiatric (e.g., anxiety, depression). Normal individuals may have PACs and PVCs, particularly associated with fatigue, alcohol, tobacco and caffeine intake. Such individuals should be encouraged to alter their lifestyles and/or habits, but, ironically, often outlive those who label them as having heart disease. It is surprising how often patients with palpitations prove on ambulatory 24-hour ECG (Holter) monitoring to have normal sinus rhythm at the time of symptoms. Conversely, many patients with arrhythmias documented by Holter monitoring are quite oblivious to their presence.

Keep in mind that certain drugs currently being utilized in clinical practice have a large number of undesirable and/or potentially harmful side effects that can mimic symptoms and signs of cardiovascular disease. For example, syncope can be caused by antihypertensive medications and nitrates (postural hypotension), Class IA and Class III antiarrhythmic agents (polymorphic VT of the "torsades de pointes" variety), beta blockers (bradycardia), diuretics (cardiac arrhythmias due to hypokalemia and hypomagnesemia), calcium channel blockers (hypotension), and warfarin (blood loss). Other "cardiovascular" symptoms, e.g., cough (ACE inhibitors), shortness of breath (amiodarone), lethargy and fatigue (beta blockers) and fluid retention and/or peripheral edema (calcium channel blockers, beta blockers, steroids) may all be misdiagnosed as heart disease. Furthermore, although prompt relief from nitroglycerin is characteristic of angina, any smooth muscle constriction, e.g., esophageal spasm and even psychogenic causes, may also respond to its administration and thus at times provide a misleading clue. Fatigue, although a symptom of heart disease (low cardiac output), is far more often a consequence of depression.

Additional misleading clues may come from the cardiac physical examination. For example, a diagnosis of hypertension may be made and the patient treated for it simply because the blood pressure is elevated on a single reading. Furthermore, certain medications (e.g., NSAIDs, oral contraceptives, sympathomimetic agents) may all raise blood pressure. Keep in mind that improper blood pressure technique (e.g., using wrong blood pressure cuff size), measuring BP immediately after the patient is sitting instead of allowing at least five minutes of rest, or taking the BP within thirty minutes of a cigarette or ingestion of caffeine) may result in falsely elevated readings. Erroneous overestimates of BP may cause a normal individual to be labeled a hypertensive with significant economic, medical, and psychological repercussions. Unfortunately, the assumption that all heart murmurs (including an "innocent" murmur) represent valvular heart disease is being fostered nowadays by the incorrect correlation of overly sensitive Doppler-echo studies revealing minor amounts of "physiologic" valvular regurgitation (e.g., MR, TR, PR, AR), so-called "*echocardiographic heart disease*". In addition, echo has significant "false" positives in the diagnosis of MVP. This may lead the inexperienced clinician to diagnose valvular heart disease when, in fact, none is present.

Pregnancy is also associated with notable physical findings that might otherwise suggest underlying heart disease, including:

- Prominent JVP (due to increased plasma volume)
- Hyperdynamic PMI
- Lateral displacement of LV impulse (due to elevation and rotation of the heart by the gravid uterus)
- Palpable RV impulse
- Rapid heart rate
- Loud S1
- Wide splitting of S2

- Physiologic S3 (due to rapid ventricular filling in the volume overloaded state)
- Grade 1-2/6 systolic flow murmur ("innocent")
- Continuous murmurs (e.g., jugular venous hum, mammary souffle)
- Peripheral edema (due to vena caval compression)

Figure 26-1. Auscultatory findings in a pregnant woman. Note innocent early to mid systolic murmur (SM) over the 3rd left sternal border (3 L) and apex, an expected finding in a pregnant female. A normal physiologic third heart sound (S3) along with a jugular venous hum over the right supraclavicular fossa are also present. (Courtesy of Dr. W. Proctor Harvey).

Familiarity with the normal clinical findings of pregnancy is essential to the proper clinical cardiovascular evaluation of the gravid female.

Misinterpretation of ECG, CXR, and Diagnostic Laboratory Data

Over-interpretation of insignificant changes on the ECG (e.g., nonspecific ST-T wave abnormalities) may falsely label healthy patients as having heart disease.

Figure 26-2. 12 lead ECG tracing showing "poor R wave progression". The patient has no underlying heart disease. In a normal heart, the R waves should become gradually taller from leads V1-V6, with the R/S ratio >1 by lead V4. If the R waves remain small in leads V1-V3 (or V4), "poor R wave progression" is said to be present. This may be caused by an anteroseptal MI, COPD, LV hypertrophy, dilated cardiomyopathy, misplaced chest leads, clockwise rotation of the heart as well as represent a normal variant.

In childhood, the precordial T waves are commonly inverted in leads V1-V3, and their continued presence in young adults ("*persistent juvenile pattern*") is a common normal variant.

Figure 26-3. ECG tracing in a young marathon runner. Note the T wave may normally be inverted in the precordial leads ("juvenile T wave pattern").

Reversal of the arm leads, if not recognized, may lead to a spurious diagnosis of lateral wall MI.

Figure 26-4. 12 lead ECG tracing in a young asymptomatic technology student practicing ECG technique. This tracing represents an example of misplaced leads, i.e., right and left arm limb lead reversal. Note the negative P wave, QRS and T wave in lead I, which may mimic dextrocardia. However, in contrast to dextrocardia, there is normal R wave progression in the precordial leads.

Incorrect placement of the precordial leads may also lead to a false diagnosis of MI. In addition, QRS abnormalities (e.g., as may occur in patients with WPW syndrome)

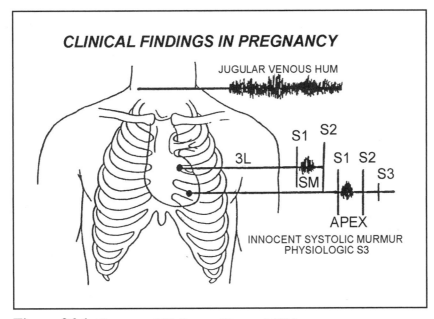

Figure 26-1 (Courtesy of W. Proctor Harvey, M.D.)

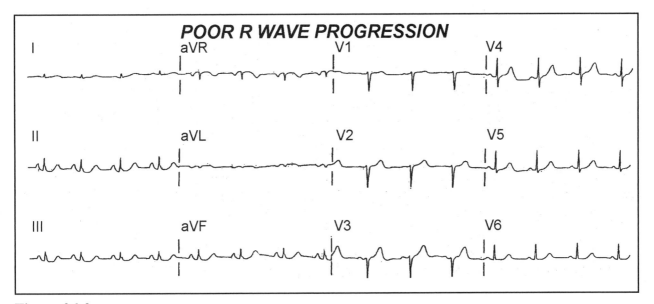

Figure 26-2

may also be misdiagnosed as an MI. Patient-related technical factors (e.g., muscle tremors and movement) may create artifacts that result in an incorrect diagnosis of arrhythmias that may lead to unnecessary interventions and treatment.

Figure 26-5. A motion artifact simulating ventricular tachycardia. This tracing "caught the attention" of the cath lab staff during a routine diagnostic study. Note the presence of the same movement artifact disturbing the arterial pulse tracing. Misinterpretation of ECG artifacts may result

in unnecessary therapeutic intervention (e.g., antiarrhythmic drugs, implantation of an ICD).

The over-reliance on computer interpretation of ECGs nowadays has also created a significant source of confusion. Over-diagnosis of normal or insignificant findings is not unusual and the astute clinician needs to be aware of these "variants" of normal.

Misleading clues may also arise from the CXR. An erroneous diagnosis of cardiomegaly, for example, is often

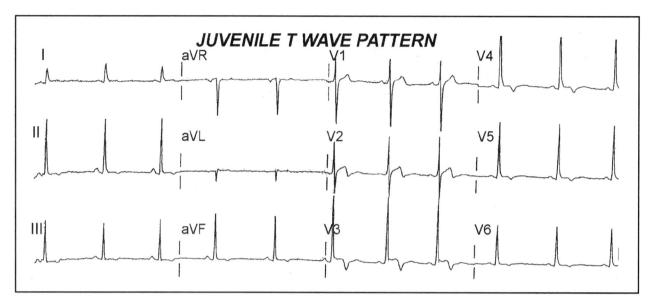

Figure 26-3

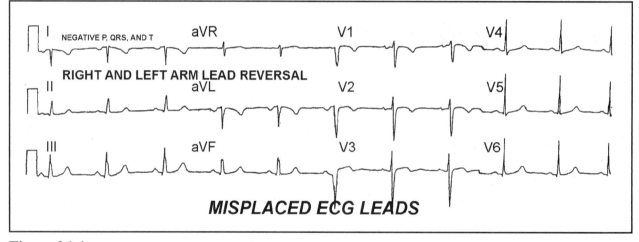

Figure 26-4

made when the apparent enlargement is in reality due to thoracic cage abnormalities, e.g., pectus excavatum, straight back ("pancake heart"), an epicardial fat pad, obesity, or poor technique, e.g., film taken during expiration with high diaphragms (i.e., "compresses the heart"), in supine or rotated position, or in a portable AP projection. An underpenetrated film may accentuate pulmonary vascular markings, thus heightening the illusion of cardiomegaly with LV failure. Also, the chest film may demonstrate a globally enlarged heart in endurance trained athletes (see below). The frequency of associated systolic heart murmurs, wide exaggerated splitting of S2, minor ECG abnormalities and parasternal movements (e.g., palpable pulmonary artery

and/or RV impulses) in the "straight back syndrome" frequently lead to the false impression of organic heart disease.

Virtually every variety of supraventricular and ventricular tachy/brady arrhythmias have been mimicked and consequently misdiagnosed as a result of artifacts registered during ambulatory ECG (Holter) monitoring (e.g., resulting from a loose or mechanical "stimulation" of an electrode, or failure of the battery or motor of the recorder, causing slowing of the tape speed).

Figure 26-6. An example of artifact on Holter monitor recording simulating sinus arrest. Note the loss of the U wave in the last beat on the upper strip. (Courtesy of

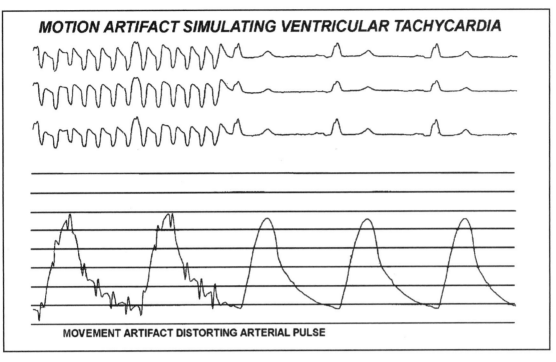

Figure 26-5

Dr. Bernard D. Kosowsky). The main cause of pseudo sinus arrest is disconnection of an electrode or, less commonly, fracture of a cable. Misinterpretation of these artifacts may lead to unnecessary pacemaker insertion.

Echocardiographic bowing of the mitral valve leaflets as well as "echo dropout" in the mid atrial septum, on the 2-D apical four chamber view, can lead to the "false positive" diagnosis of MVP and an atrial septal defect respectively. All too often, the report of the presence of valvular regurgitation, in the absence of any clinical evidence of such, may lead the clinician who is not familiar with the nuances of color Doppler echo, to think that there is significant pathology of the valves when, in fact, none exists. Unnecessary anxiety is thereby created for the patient (and practitioner), leading to additional unnecessary and expensive tests.

Exercise ECG stress testing may also yield "false positive" results especially in young asymptomatic females, or in the setting of hyperventilation or when nonspecific ST-T abnormalities on the resting ECG are present, which the practitioner may erroneously diagnose as CAD. Since false-positive tests often exceed true positives, leading to much patient anxiety and disability, exercise testing of asymptomatic individuals should be performed only for those at high risk (e.g., strong family history of premature CAD, or hyperlipidemia) or those with occupations that place them or others at special risk (e.g., airline pilots).

Nuclear imaging may further confuse the clinician by demonstrating perfusion defects due to attenuation artifacts (e.g., breast tissue, elevated diaphragm, obesity) when, in fact, none exist. Even coronary angiography (the "gold standard") may over-diagnose a clinically insignificant coronary lesion ("*oculostenotic reflex*") or falsely label a patient as having CAD when, in reality, catheter-induced spasm at the site of contact with the tip of the catheter may be the underlying "culprit". Such spasm creates coronary narrowings and can lead to incorrect treatment. Furthermore, certain disorders may alter laboratory test results. Skeletal muscle injury, along with vigorous exercise, for example, may increase cardiac enzymes (CK, CK-MB, troponin T) without evidence of myocardial ischemia and/or injury ("false positive").

THE ATHLETE'S HEART

Clinical evaluation of the well-trained athlete may present a challenge to the practitioner. Clinical findings that at first appear "abnormal" are not uncommon in healthy young athletes. You should be aware that intensive physical training may alter the cardiovascular system in such a way as to create pseudo-"abnormal" findings (the *"athletic heart syndrome"*). Common clinical examination findings in highly-trained athletes include:

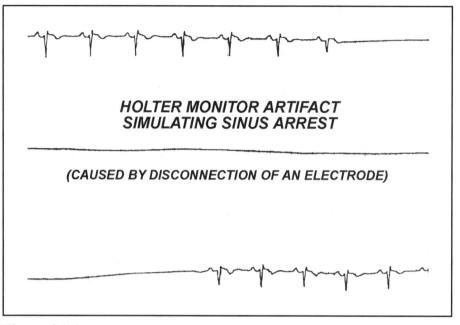

Figure 26-6

- Slow heart rate
- Grade 1-2/6 systolic murmur ("innocent")
- Wide splitting of S1
- Wide splitting of S2
- S3 and S4 gallop sounds
- Jugular venous hum

There are many variations of heart rate, rhythm, conduction, and alteration of both depolarization and repolarization that are considered to be within the range of "normal" in the well-trained athlete. Common "normal" resting ECG and ambulatory (Holter) ECG findings in the athlete include:

- Sinus bradycardia, sinus arrhythmia, and sinus pauses
- First degree AV block
- Second degree AV block of the Wenckebach type (from enhanced vagal tone)
- AV junctional escape rhythm
- Ectopic supraventricular and ventricular beats
- Vertical axis
- Right axis deviation
- Incomplete RBBB
- LV hypertrophy
- Minor ST-T wave changes
- "Pseudo" anterolateral wall ischemia
- Early repolarization changes

The chest x-ray and echocardiogram can also be affected in the athlete. Common "normal" radiographic and echo findings in the highly trained athlete include cardiomegaly, increased LV chamber size and wall thickness. Keep in mind that LV dilation is generally seen in endurance (isotonic or aerobic) trained athletes (e.g., runners and swimmers), and increases in LV thickness (usually <13 mm and symmetric) is predominantly seen in strength (isometric) trained athletes (e.g., weight lifters). In most cases, increased LV wall thickness due to athlete's heart regresses after cessation of training, although up to 20% of elite athletes have residual chamber enlargement.

As a rule, ST-T wave changes on the resting ECG in athletes tend to normalize during exercise. Stress testing, therefore, may help avoid the misdiagnosis of CAD. To avoid over-interpretation and inappropriate diagnosis of heart disease in these special individuals, the range of reported physiologic changes in the cardiovascular system in the athlete should be understood and correctly recognized.

The distinction between the athlete's heart and cardiac disease has important implications. The diagnosis of heart disease in an athlete may disqualify him or her from participation in competition. On the other hand, with certain cardiac conditions, participation in competitive athletics carries the risk for sudden death. Many of the conditions responsible for sudden cardiac death in the athlete can be suspected and even diagnosed by means of a thoughtful clinical evaluation. These conditions include *HOCM, Marfan's syndrome* with aortic aneurysm/dissection, *coronary anomalies, CAD, bicuspid valvular aortic stenosis, dilated cardiomyopathy, illicit drug use* (e.g., cocaine, anabolic steroids), *long QT syndrome, preexcitation (WPW)* and *Brugada's syndrome,* and potentially lethal *arrhythmias* (e.g., VT/VF), which can also occur as a result of blunt chest wall trauma (*commotio cordis*), even in the absence of underlying heart disease. The following are clues to pathology in athletes:

- A history of early or premature sudden death in a parent or close relative (suggests the possibility of HOCM, CAD, dilated cardiomyopathy, long QT syndrome, Marfan's syndrome, and *Arrhythmogenic Right Ventricular Dysplasia/Cardiomyopathy [ARVD/C]; a rare disorder of the RV myocardium that leads to progressive myocardial atrophy with fibrofatty tissue replacement*).
- A history of syncope or exercise-induced dizziness, exertional chest pain, shortness of breath, and palpitations (raises the suspicion of HOCM, valvular AS, congenital coronary anomalies, CAD).
- Since HOCM is responsible for ~50% of sudden deaths in athletes <30 years of age you should look closely for a family history of sudden cardiac death, a quick-rising arterial pulse, and a systolic murmur best heard at the lower left sternal border that decreases with squatting and increases with standing. The ECG is almost always abnormal. These findings should lead to further diagnostic tests (e.g., echo).
- A harsh systolic ejection murmur heard best at the second intercostal space radiating to the neck, accompanied by an ejection sound (also heard well at the apex) is a clue to the diagnosis of bicuspid valvular aortic stenosis.
- A tall, hyperflexible narrow-chested (pectus excavatum) young athlete (e.g., a basketball player) should raise the suspicion of Marfan's syndrome, which may be associated with aortic root dilatation and MVP.
- A careful search for the blowing high-frequency diastolic murmur of AR, louder along the right sternal border as compared to the left in the setting of severe chest pain radiating to the interscapular region, are clues to the diagnosis of aortic dissection.
- Subtle signs of CHF, e.g., decreased exercise tolerance, chronic dry cough when changing position, along with pulsus alternans, heart sound and/or murmur alternans and an S3 gallop provide clues to myocarditis or dilated cardiomyopathy.
- Arrhythmias, including SVT, atrial fibrillation or VT, can occur in patients with HOCM, dilated cardiomyopathy, ARVD/C, CAD, MVP, valvular AS, preexcitation (WPW) syndrome, long QT and Brugada's syndrome, as well as from the use of illicit and even over-the-counter drugs (e.g., decongestants and epinephrine-like medication, ephedra, Ma-huang) and "binge" alcohol intake.

- Left bundle branch block is not a common finding in trained athletes. Its presence should prompt a search for an underlying cause (e.g., dilated cardiomyopathy, CAD, valvular AS).
- Sudden death in the young athlete (<30 years of age) may be caused by congenital coronary anomalies, e.g., aberrant origin of the coronary artery (especially the left main or LAD) with passage of the vessel between the aorta and pulmonary artery. In the older athlete (>30 years of age) the most common cause of sudden cardiac death is atherosclerotic CAD. In this age group a careful history with close attention to the patient's complaint of chest discomfort is the best screening test for underlying CAD. This is particularly important when evaluating an older individual who exercises vigorously with the misconception that his or her training program will protect him or her from heart disease.

While controversy surrounds the routine use of ECG or echo as part of the preparticipation cardiovascular screening of athletes (due to the low prevalence of disease and high rate of false positive findings), the American Heart Association considers a targeted history and physical examination, designed to identify those conditions known to cause sudden cardiac death, to be the most practical and cost-effective approach. If any cardiovascular abnormality is detected or suspected on the initial evaluation, further testing can be obtained on an individual basis as needed.

IATROGENIC HEART DISEASE

The diagnostic process should always consider the possibility of a technical error in laboratory abnormalities (even considering the possibility of the wrong patient). It is important to check the name and date to be sure that it is the correct patient's report. Seasoned consultants cannot always erase the fear that has been engendered by an initial "false" diagnosis of heart disease. Many so-called "cardiac cripples" who have no disabling cardiac disease, but who suffer from irreversible cardiac neuroses, practitioner-induced, are "limping" their way through life maimed as a result of a wrong diagnosis or careless statement about their hearts (*"iatrogenic heart disease"*). Classifying a healthy patient as one with heart disease based on falsely positive clinical information or laboratory tests can cause much psychological harm and may lead to risks from unnecessary or inappropriate therapy. You should ask your patient to relate his or her perception of their problem to you in an attempt to "clear up" any misperceptions regarding their condition.

CHAPTER 27. APPROACH TO THE PATIENT WITH AN ACUTE CARDIAC EMERGENCY

The approach to the patient with an acute cardiac emergency requires astute evaluation and immediate intervention. This chapter will review the evaluation and treatment of the patient who presents with a sudden cardiac arrest, with a special emphasis on the basic and advanced cardiac life support measures used to preserve myocardial and cerebral viability, and treat potentially life threatening cardiac arrhythmias and shock.

GENERAL CONSIDERATIONS

Sudden cardiac death is generally defined as unexpected natural death from cardiac causes which occurs within one hour of the patient's collapse. Although sudden cardiac death may complicate a variety of cardiovascular diseases (e.g., HOCM; severe AS; dilated cardiomyopathy; MVP; prolonged QT, preexcitation [WPW], and Brugada's syndromes), coronary artery disease (with or without an acute MI) is by far the most common predisposing condition in patients with cardiac arrest. Regardless of the underlying etiology, cardiac arrest invariably results from one of the following rhythms:

- Ventricular fibrillation (VF)
- Pulseless ventricular tachycardia (VT)
- Pulseless electrical activity (PEA)
- Ventricular standstill (asystole)

The sudden collapse of an individual must be considered a cardiac arrest until proven otherwise. The approach to the patient involves the prompt and accurate recognition of a cardiac arrest, activation of the emergency response system (911 for out-of-hospital or "code blue" for in-hospital cardiac arrest), and rapid initiation of basic life support (BLS). The American Heart Association has issued updated guidelines on cardiopulmonary resuscitation (CPR) and emergency cardiac care. According to the guidelines, the BLS sequence of steps for trained rescuers has been changed from "A-B-C" (Airway, Breathing, Compressions) to "C-A-B" (Compressions, Airway, Breathing), to reflect our understanding of the positive impact on survival of early initiation of chest compressions, along with rapid Defibrillation (if pulseless VT and/or VF is present), often available via the use of automated external defibrillators (AEDs).

The key points to remember are the following:

- Cardiopulmonary resuscitation (CPR) comprises a series of steps aimed at the delivery of oxygenated blood to the heart and brain until spontaneous and effective circulation can be restored.
- Speed of diagnosis is critical. The chance of resuscitation diminishes (by ~ 7-10%) with each minute that has elapsed. Within 4 minutes of cardiac arrest, some cerebral damage is likely.
- Continuous chest compressions without assisted ventilation, i.e., cardiocerebral resuscitation (also known as "compression-only" or "hands-only" CPR) is an effective bystander approach to witnessed out-of-hospital cardiac arrest.
- A cardiac output of one fourth to one third can be achieved through external cardiac compression. Even these flow rates maintain adequate perfusion to the brain and other vital organs, thus preventing irreversible damage.
- Treat the *patient,* not the monitor.
- In patients with tachycardia or bradycardia who are hemodynamically stable, a 12 lead ECG can be helpful in making an accurate rhythm diagnosis and in guiding decisions regarding subsequent therapy.
- In patients with tachycardia who are hemodynamically unstable (manifested by hypotension, CHF, decreased level of consciousness, persistent chest pain), the decision to treat may need to be based on the presence or absence of heart sounds and/or pulses, or a single lead rhythm strip. In such cases, it is appropriate to treat a wide complex tachycardia as ventricular tachycardia until proven otherwise.
- The keys to the successful management of pulseless VT/VF are high quality CPR and early defibrillation (**Figure 27-1**).
- VF can usually be converted into a more stable rhythm when defibrillation occurs within the first few minutes (the "electrical phase"). Defibrillation alone (without chest compressions) is rarely successful when initiated after 4–5 minutes (the "circulatory phase").
- Defibrillator attempts should be preceded and followed by minimal interruptions in chest compressions.
- Survival rates for cardiac arrest are higher if the initial rhythm is "shockable" (pulseless VT/VF), the VF is "coarse", the arrest is "witnessed", and if it occurs "in-hospital" (especially in a monitored unit).
- The outcome from asystole and PEA is extremely poor despite treatment, with the exception of bradycardia due to hypoxemia from airway obstruction, hyperkalemia, drug overdose (e.g., digoxin,

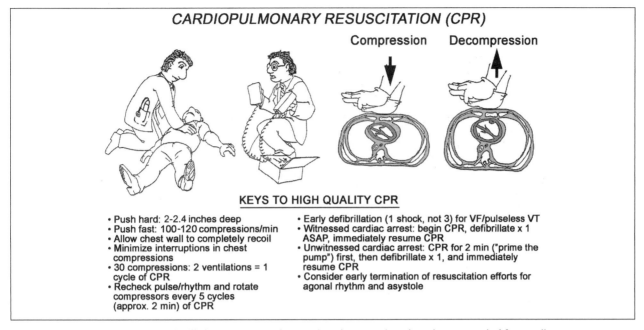

CARDIOPULMONARY RESUSCITATION (CPR)

Compression   Decompression

KEYS TO HIGH QUALITY CPR

- Push hard: 2-2.4 inches deep
- Push fast: 100-120 compressions/min
- Allow chest wall to completely recoil
- Minimize interruptions in chest compressions
- 30 compressions: 2 ventilations = 1 cycle of CPR
- Recheck pulse/rhythm and rotate compressors every 5 cycles (approx. 2 min) of CPR

- Early defibrillation (1 shock, not 3) for VF/pulseless VT
- Witnessed cardiac arrest: begin CPR, defibrillate x 1 ASAP, immediately resume CPR
- Unwitnessed cardiac arrest: CPR for 2 min ("prime the pump") first, then defibrillate x 1, and immediately resume CPR
- Consider early termination of resuscitation efforts for agonal rhythm and asystole

Note: High quality CPR and prompt defibrillation, when appropriate, are the only proven therapies to increase survival from cardiac arrest.

Figure 27-1

β-blocker, calcium channel blocker) or tamponade. Therefore, look for these reversible causes.

- After resuscitation of cardiac arrest, check for one of the following:
  - Reactive pupils, spontaneous respirations, and purposeful response to painful stimuli (signs associated with a high percentage of neurologic recovery).
  - Bilaterally dilated and fixed pupils (may be due to inadequate perfusion during cardiopulmonary resuscitation (CPR).
  - Unilateral pupil dilatation and unresponsiveness (which indicate a catastrophic central nervous system event and a dismal prognosis).
- Once a victim of cardiac arrest has been successfully resuscitated, consideration should be given to therapeutic hypothermia. Targeted temperature management (32–36° C in adults) and avoidance of hyperthermia may improve neurological outcomes and survival, and should be considered, along with urgent cardiac catheterization and PCI (if appropriate) in patients who remain comatose after resuscitation from cardiac arrest.

Survivors of cardiac arrest are at high risk for a recurrent episode if not evaluated and treated properly. Important information may be gained from interviewing the patient and/or the patient's family. A history of angina pectoris or a prior MI indicates that CAD is likely present. If the cardiac arrest is preceded by chest pain (either during exertion or at rest), this may indicate that acute myocardial ischemia or infarction is responsible for precipitating the malignant ventricular arrhythmia. A history of dyspnea on exertion in the weeks or months preceding the cardiac arrest suggests that dilated cardiomyopathy, HOCM, or valvular heart disease, e.g., AS, may be present. A family history of sudden death raises the suspicion of long QT syndrome, HOCM, and rarely MVP and WPW syndrome with extremely rapid ventricular rates conducted over the accessory pathway that may precipitate VF. A drug history is important to obtain. VT may occur as a complication of certain antiarrhythmic drugs (proarrhythmic effect with long QT interval and polymorphic VT ["torsades de pointes"]), and diuretic-induced hypokalemia and hypomagnesemia. A history of alcohol consumption may suggest alcohol-induced cardiomyopathy and acutely predispose the patient to VT.

Relevant physical examination findings to look for include signs of CHF (e.g., pulsus alternans, elevated JVP, S3 gallop), apical systolic click and/or murmur of MVP, quick rise pulse and systolic ejection murmur (louder with standing or Valsalva, fainter with squatting) of HOCM, and slow and delayed carotid artery pulse along with harsh, late peaking systolic ejection murmur of valvular AS. The ECG can also provide important diagnostic information. Specific abnormalities to look for include ST elevation and new Q waves of acute transmural MI, ST segment depression and T wave inversion of non ST elevation MI, a prolonged QT interval (long QT syndrome), a short PR interval and delta wave (WPW syndrome), a RBBB morphology with ST elevation in precordial leads V1-V2 (Brugada Syndrome), and an incomplete RBBB with a terminal notch in the QRS ("epsilon wave") and T wave inversion in V1-V3 (arrhythmogenic RV dysplasia/cardiomyopathy). The chest x-ray can be helpful in the evaluation of cardiac

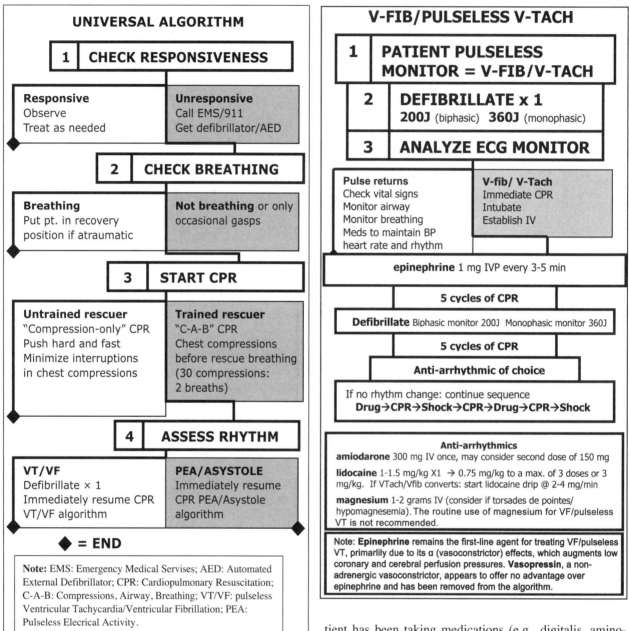

Figure 27-2

size and confirming the presence of CHF. The presence of intracardiac calcification may be helpful in the diagnosis of valvular heart disease (e.g., AS) or an LV aneurysm.

In the initial laboratory evaluation, particular attention should be directed toward the serum electrolyte concentrations (especially ↓ K^+, ↓ Mg^{++}) and serial determination of cardiac enzymes, e.g., CK-MB, and troponin (although these enzymes can be elevated after defibrillation and cardiopulmonary resuscitation). If the pa-

tient has been taking medications (e.g., digitalis, aminophylline) which could potentially precipitate a malignant ventricular arrhythmia, the serum levels of these drugs should be obtained. At times, it may be appropriate to order a toxicology screen if a drug overdose is suspected.

An echo-Doppler is often of great value in elucidating chamber size and function, along with the nature and severity of the patient's underlying structural heart disease (e.g., LV aneurysm, dilated cardiomyopathy, HOCM, AS, MVP). Radionuclide studies may also be helpful in select patients. Cardiac MRI is particularly valuable if arrhythmogenic RV dysplasia/cardiomyopathy (ARVD/C) is suspected. In most patients, cardiac catheterization is indicated either to elucidate the severity of struc-

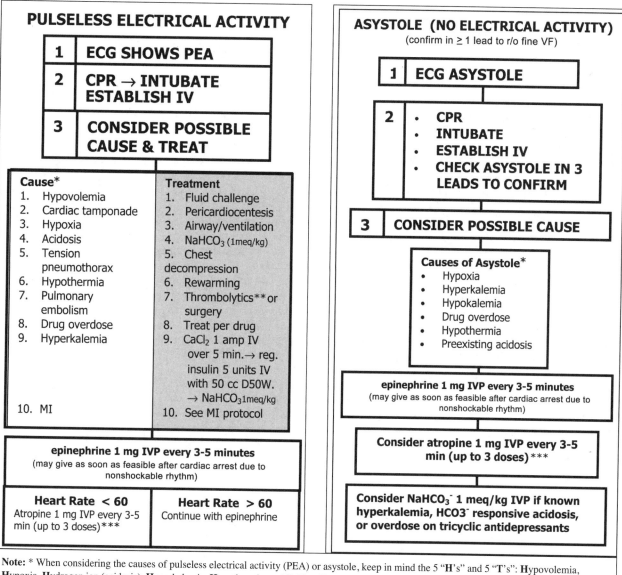

Figure 27-4

Figure 27-5

tural heart disease which has been found by clinical and noninvasive evaluation, or to rule out occult forms of structural heart disease (e.g., CAD, congenital coronary abnormality) in patients who are not found to have identifiable heart disease after clinical and noninvasive evaluation. Invasive electrophysiologic testing also plays an important role in the diagnostic evaluation and management of patients who survive cardiac arrest. Following cardiac catheterization and/or electrophysiologic testing, an ICD (with or without antiarrhythmic drug therapy), and/or PCI, or cardiac surgery (CABG, aneurysmectomy, or resection/ablation of arrhythmic foci) is often necessary.

The algorithms that follow provide an overview of the approach to the patient with potentially life threatening cardiac arrhythmias including VF, pulseless VT, PEA asystole (no electrical activity), bradycardia with pulses, tachycardia with pulses, as well as shock (**Figures 27-2 through 27-10**). The content of these protocols is based on the 2015 guidelines update on advanced cardiac life support (ACLS) established by the American Heart Association (AHA) and the Emergency Cardiac Care Committee.

Figures 27-2 through 27-11. Advanced Cardiac Life Support and Shock Algorithms. (Modified from Hancock, J. The Practitioner's Pocket Pal. MedMaster, Inc. 2012).

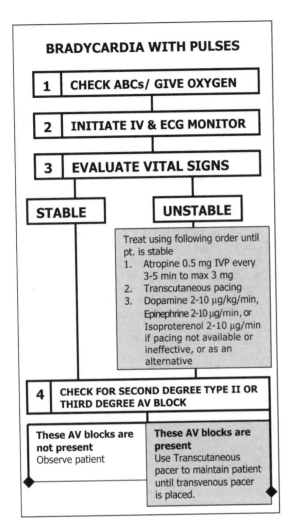

Figure 27-6

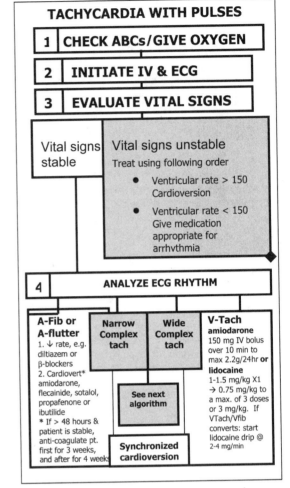

Figure 27-7

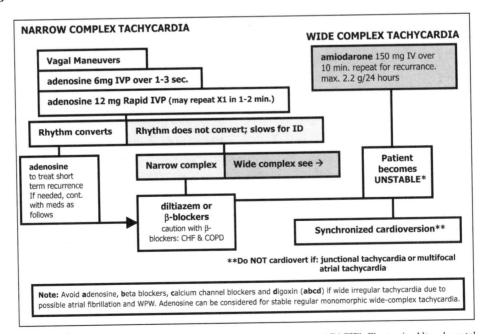

*Note: When evaluating if a patient is unstable, keep in mind the mnemonic "CASH": Chest pain, Altered mental status, Shortness of breath, and Hypotension.

Figure 27-8

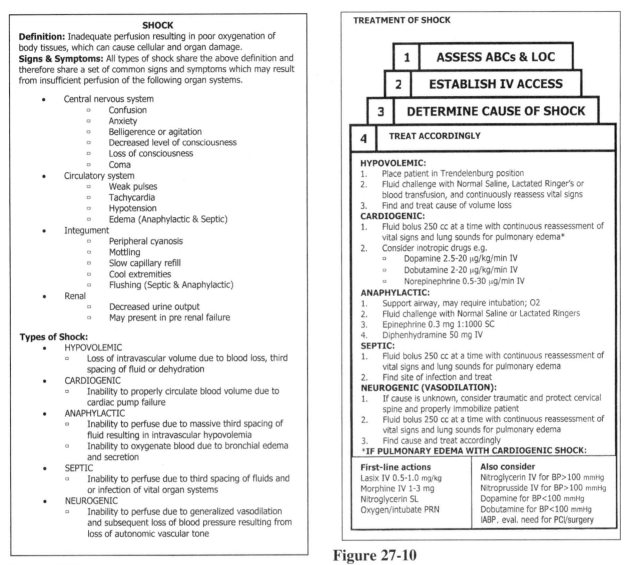

SHOCK

Definition: Inadequate perfusion resulting in poor oxygenation of body tissues, which can cause cellular and organ damage.

Signs & Symptoms: All types of shock share the above definition and therefore share a set of common signs and symptoms which may result from insufficient perfusion of the following organ systems.

- Central nervous system
  - Confusion
  - Anxiety
  - Belligerence or agitation
  - Decreased level of consciousness
  - Loss of consciousness
  - Coma
- Circulatory system
  - Weak pulses
  - Tachycardia
  - Hypotension
  - Edema (Anaphylactic & Septic)
- Integument
  - Peripheral cyanosis
  - Mottling
  - Slow capillary refill
  - Cool extremities
  - Flushing (Septic & Anaphylactic)
- Renal
  - Decreased urine output
  - May present in pre renal failure

Types of Shock:
- HYPOVOLEMIC
  - Loss of intravascular volume due to blood loss, third spacing of fluid or dehydration
- CARDIOGENIC
  - Inability to properly circulate blood volume due to cardiac pump failure
- ANAPHYLACTIC
  - Inability to perfuse due to massive third spacing of fluid resulting in intravascular hypovolemia
  - Inability to oxygenate blood due to bronchial edema and secretion
- SEPTIC
  - Inability to perfuse due to third spacing of fluids and or infection of vital organ systems
- NEUROGENIC
  - Inability to perfuse due to generalized vasodilation and subsequent loss of blood pressure resulting from loss of autonomic vascular tone

Figure 27-9

TREATMENT OF SHOCK

1	**ASSESS ABCs & LOC**
2	**ESTABLISH IV ACCESS**
3	**DETERMINE CAUSE OF SHOCK**
4	**TREAT ACCORDINGLY**

HYPOVOLEMIC:
1. Place patient in Trendelenburg position
2. Fluid challenge with Normal Saline, Lactated Ringer's or blood transfusion, and continuously reassess vital signs
3. Find and treat cause of volume loss

CARDIOGENIC:
1. Fluid bolus 250 cc at a time with continuous reassessment of vital signs and lung sounds for pulmonary edema*
2. Consider inotropic drugs e.g.
   - Dopamine 2.5-20 µg/kg/min IV
   - Dobutamine 2-20 µg/kg/min IV
   - Norepinephrine 0.5-30 µg/min IV

ANAPHYLACTIC:
1. Support airway, may require intubation; O2
2. Fluid challenge with Normal Saline or Lactated Ringers
3. Epinephrine 0.3 mg 1:1000 SC
4. Diphenhydramine 50 mg IV

SEPTIC:
1. Fluid bolus 250 cc at a time with continuous reassessment of vital signs and lung sounds for pulmonary edema
2. Find site of infection and treat

NEUROGENIC (VASODILATION):
1. If cause is unknown, consider traumatic and protect cervical spine and properly immobilize patient
2. Fluid bolus 250 cc at a time with continuous reassessment of vital signs and lung sounds for pulmonary edema
3. Find cause and treat accordingly

*IF PULMONARY EDEMA WITH CARDIOGENIC SHOCK:

First-line actions	Also consider
Lasix IV 0.5-1.0 mg/kg	Nitroglycerin IV for BP>100 mmHg
Morphine IV 1-3 mg	Nitroprusside IV for BP>100 mmHg
Nitroglycerin SL	Dopamine for BP<100 mmHg
Oxygen/intubate PRN	Dobutamine for BP<100 mmHg
	IABP, eval. need for PCI/surgery

Figure 27-10

HEMODYNAMIC RELATIONSHIPS OF DIFFERENT SHOCK STATES

	Hypovolemic Shock	Septic Shock	Cardiogenic Shock	Cardiac Tamponade	Pulmonary Embolism
Pulmonary Capillary Wedge Pressure	↓↓	↓↓	↑↑	↑	Normal or ↓
Pulmonary Vascular Resistance	Normal	Normal	Normal	Normal	↑
Pulmonary Artery Pressure	↓	Normal or ↓	↑	↑	↑
Cardiac Output	↓↓	↑	↓↓	↓	↓↓
Peripheral Vascular Resistance	↑↑	↓↓	↑	↑	↑
Right Atrial Pressure	↓	Normal or ↓	↑	↑	↑
Right Ventricular Pressure	↓	Normal or ↓	↑	↑	↑

Figure 27-11

Epilogue

Contemporary cardiology is replete with a myriad of "high-tech" diagnostic tools and therapeutic techniques that in many cases, seem to have eclipsed the essential role of clinical skills, particularly the cardiac history and physical examination, in the evaluation of the patient with heart disease. Indeed, in this age of advanced technology, it is not uncommon for a patient to be put through an extensive battery of tests and procedures without a careful medical history being taken, or even a stethoscope placed on the patient's chest. (**Figure E-1**).

Sophisticated high technology, however, is not a substitute for a solid foundation in clinical cardiology. When performed properly, the cardiac clinical examination, including cardiac auscultation, remains a rapid, accurate, and cost-effective clinical tool that often establishes the diagnosis, etiology, and severity of heart disease, forms the basis for further non-invasive and invasive testing and treatment when needed, and provides an added level of quality control by placing the interpretation of any additional laboratory tests in their proper perspective. Furthermore, by virtue of the "laying on of hands", the cardiac clinical exam helps establish the personal bond with the patient that fosters the close rapport, trust, and confidence so important to the privileged "doctor-patient" relationship (**Figure E-2**).

Despite the increasing reliance on modern technology, it is still true that the well trained clinician can derive a great deal of information about a patient's cardiovascular status by:

> ### *FIGURE E-2*
>
> ### The Cardiac Clinical Examination
>
> - Long and rich tradition in clinical medicine ("time-honored" art)
> - Rapid, accurate, and cost-effective clinical tool
> - Often establishes the diagnosis, etiology, and severity
> - Provides the basis for further non-invasive and invasive testing and treatment when needed
> - Keeps tests honest (quality control)
> - Value of "laying on of hands" (doctor-patient relationship)
> - Training and competence currently inadequate (disuse atrophy)

1) Taking a careful detailed history
2) Performing a skillful physical examination
3) Studying the electrocardiogram (ECG)
4) Reviewing the chest x-ray (CXR), and then, if necessary, by
5) Ordering appropriate diagnostic laboratory tests.

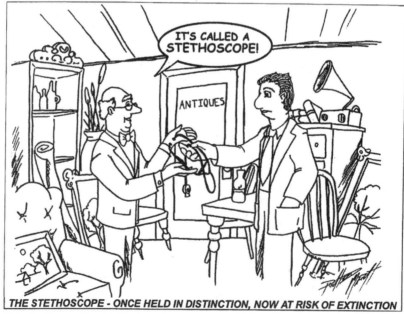

Note: In this age of hand-held echo and newer, more sophisticated imaging techniques, the "time-honored" art of cardiac auscultation is rapidly becoming a lost art, and the simple stethoscope a medical relic – an antique!

Figure E-1

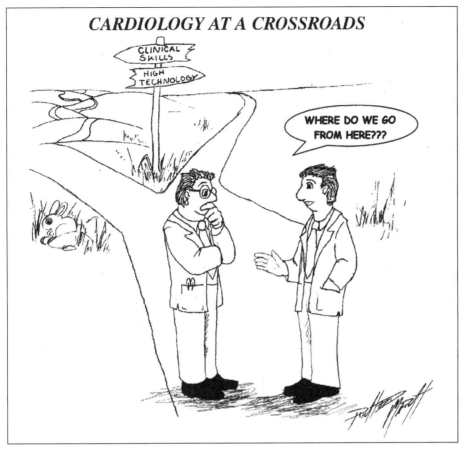

In today's era of technologic advances and cost containment, skillful use of the clinical, so-called "five finger" approach is the way to go! Figure E-3

This systematic and highly cost-effective "hands-on" approach to cardiovascular evaluation, referred to as the "five finger" approach, by legendary cardiologist, Dr. W. Proctor Harvey, is an excellent and efficient way to help today's practitioner with the difficult decisions he or she frequently faces in the clinical practice of medicine, i.e., when to employ the more elaborate and expensive technological advances in cardiac diagnosis and treatment, or when they can safely be held in reserve with confidence that the simpler, less costly clinical methods will suffice.

It should be emphasized that no test is perfect. Even in the best of hands, test results can be erroneous (i.e., "false positives" and "false negatives"), misleading, or conflicting, especially when multiple tests are employed. When ordering a diagnostic laboratory test, several key questions should be addressed:

1) Is the test needed to confirm (or refute) the diagnosis?
2) What additional information will the test provide?
3) Do the benefits justify the risk and cost?
4) Will the results influence your management decision?

Specialized laboratory tests are often expensive, time-consuming, and sometimes even risky. They may delay treatment, heighten the patient's (and physician's) anxiety, and may, at times, lead to additional unnecessary testing. If the treatment plan is the same regardless of the test results, then the test may not be necessary. Keep in mind that *not every patient needs every test*.

In this age of increasing technological sophistication, cost containment, and managed care, today's practitioners stand at the crossroads in cardiology in providing high quality cost-effective cardiac care. At no time in the history of medicine has the need been greater than it is today for the contemporary practitioner to learn and apply the "time-honored" clinical art of cardiac diagnosis. When used in conjunction with the latest scientific advances, skillful use of "low technology", including the clinical history and physical exam, leads to intelligent, cost-effective use of high technology, and ensures the best of medical, interventional, and surgical care for the cardiac patient. (**Figure E-3**) Remember, *hands before scans!*

Michael A. Chizner, M.D.

Selected Reading

ABRAMS J. *Synopsis of Cardiac Physical Diagnosis*. 2nd ed. Boston: Butterworth-Heinemann, 2001.

AL-KHATIB SM, STEVENSON WG, ACKERMAN MJ, et al. 2017 AHA/ACC/HRS Guideline for Management of Patients with Ventricular Arrhythmias and the Prevention of Sudden Cardiac Death: A Report of the American College of Cardiology Foundation / American Heart Association Task Force on Clinical Practice Guidelines and the Heart Rhythm Society. J Am Coll Cardiol, 2017

AMERICAN HEART ASSOCIATION. 2015 American Heart Association Guidelines Update for Cardiopulmonary Resuscitation and Emergency Cardiovascular Care. Circulation: 132 (18) supplement 2: S315–S573, 2015.

AMSTERDAM EA, WENGER NK, BRINDIS RG, et al. 2014 AHA/ACC Guideline for the Management of Patients with Non-ST-Elevation Acute Coronary Syndromes. A Report of the American College of Cardiology/American Heart Association Task Force on Practice Guidelines. J Am Coll Cardiol 130:e344–426, 2014.

ANDERSON JL, ADAMS CD, ANTMAN EM, et al. ACC/AHA 2007 Guidelines for the management of patients with unstable angina/non-ST-elevation myocardial infarction: Executive summary. A report of the American College of Cardiology/American Heart Association task force on practice guidelines. Circulation 116: 803–877, 2007.

ANTMAN EM, SABATINE MS, COLUCCI WS, GOTTO AM (eds). *Cardiovascular Therapeutics. A Companion to Braunwald's Heart Disease*, 4th ed. Philadelphia: Elsevier Saunders, 2013.

BRICKNER ME, HILLIS LD, LANGE RA. Congenital heart disease in adults: Parts I and II. N Engl J Med 342:256–263, 334–342, 2000.

CALHOUN DA, JONES D, TEXTOR S, et al. Resistant Hypertension: Diagnosis, Evaluation, and Treatment. A Scientific Statement from the American Heart Association Professional Education Committee of the Council for High Blood Pressure Research. Hypertension, 51:2008.

CHEITLIN MD, ARMSTRONG WF, AURIGEMMA GP, et al. ACC/AHA/ASE 2003 guideline update for the clinical application of echocardiography: summary article: a report of the American Heart Association Task Force on Practice Guidelines for the Clinical Application of Echocardiography. J Am Coll Cardiol 42:954–70, 2003.

CHIZNER MA (ed). *Classic Teachings in Clinical Cardiology: A Tribute to W. Proctor Harvey, M.D.* Cedar Grove, NJ: Laennec Publishing Inc., 1996.

CHIZNER MA. The diagnosis of heart disease by clinical assessment alone. Curr Probl in Cardiol 26:285–380, 2001.

CHIZNER MA. Cardiac auscultation: Rediscovering the lost art. Curr Prob Cardiol, 33:317–408, 32:2008.

CHIZNER MA. Bedside diagnosis of the acute myocardial infarction and its complications. Curr Prob Cardiol 7:1–86, 1982.

CONSTANT J. *Bedside Cardiology*. 5th ed. Philadelphia: Lippincott Williams and Wilkins, 1999.

CRAWFORD MH, BERNSTEIN SJ, DEEDWANIA PC, et al. ACC/AHA guidelines for ambulatory electrocardiography. A report of the American College of Cardiology/ American Heart Association Task Force on Practice Guidelines. J Am Coll Cardio 34:912–948, 1999.

DAJANI AS, TAUBERT KA, WILSON W, et al. Prevention of bacterial endocarditis: Recommendations by the American Heart Association. Circulation 96:358–366, 1997.

DON MICHAEL TA. *Auscultation of the Heart. A Cardiophonetic Approach*. New York: McGraw-Hill, 1998.

EPSTEIN AE, DIMARCO JP, ELLENBOGEN KA, et al. ACC/AHA/HRS 2008 Guidelines for Device-Based Therapy of Cardiac Rhythm Abnormalities: A Report of the American College of Cardiology/American Heart Association Task Force on Practice Guidelines. J Am Coll Cardiol 51:2085–2105, 2008.

EXECUTIVE SUMMARY OF THE THIRD REPORT OF THE NATIONAL CHOLESTEROL EDUCATION PROGRAM (NCEP), Expert Panel on Detection, Evaluation, and Treatment of High Blood Cholesterol in Adults (Adult Treatment Panel III). JAMA 285 (19):2486–2497, 2001.

FIHN SD, GARDIN JM, ABRAMS J, et al. 2012 ACCF/AHA/ACP/AATS/PCNA/SCA/STS Guideline for the Diagnosis and Management of Patients with Stable Ischemic Heart Disease. A report of the American College of Cardiology Foundation/American Heart Association Task Force on Practice Guidelines, and the American College of Physicians, American Association for Thoracic Surgery, Preventive Cardiovascular Nurses Association, Society for Cardiovascular Angiography and Interventions, and Society of Thoracic Surgeons. Circulation; 126:3097–3137, 2012.

FLEISHER LA, FLEISCHMANN KE, AUERBACH AD, et al. 2014 ACC/AHA Guideline on Perioperative Cardiovascular Evaluation and Management of Patients Undergoing Noncardiac Surgery. A Report of the American College of Cardiology/American Heart Association Task Force on Practice Guidelines. J Am Coll Cardiol 64:e77–137, 2014.

FOWLER NO. *Diagnosis of Heart Disease*. New York: Springer-Verlag Inc., 1991.

FUSTER V, HARRINGTON R, NARULA J (eds). *Hurst's The Heart*. 14th ed. New York: McGraw-Hill, 2017.

GAZES PC. *Clinical Cardiology: A Cost-Effective Approach*. 4th ed. NY: Chapman and Hall, 1997.

GIBBONS RJ, BALADY GJ, BEASLEY JW, et al. ACC/AHA Guideline for Exercise Testing: A report of the American College of Cardiology/American Heart Association Task Force on Practice Guidelines . J Am Coll Cardiol 30:260–311, 1997.

GOLDBERGER AL, GOLDBERGER ZD, SHVILKIN A. *Goldberger's Clinical Electrocardiography: A Simplified Approach*. 9th ed. Elsevier Saunders, 2018.

GOLDMAN L, BRAUNWALD E (eds). *Primary Cardiology*. Philadelphia: Saunders, 2003.

HARVEY WP, BEDYNEK J, CANFIELD DC. *Clinical Heart Disease: Clinical Auscultation and Physical Examination of the Cardiovascular System: Five Finger Approach*. Fairfield, NJ: Laennec Publishing Co., 2009.

HARVEY WP. *Cardiac Pearls*. Newton, NJ : Laennec Publishing Co., 1993.

HILLIS LD, LANGE RA, WINNIFORD MD, PAGE RL. *Manual of Clinical Problems in Cardiology with Annotated Key References*. Philadelphia: Lippincott Williams & Wilkins, 2003.

HILLIS LD, SMITH PK, ANDERSON JL, et al. 2011 ACCP/AHA Guideline for Coronary Artery Bypass Graft Surgery: A Report of the American College of Cardiology Foundation/American Heart Association Task Force on Practice Guidelines. Circulation 124:2610–2642, 2011.

HIRSCH AT, HASKAL ZJ, HERTZER NR, et al. ACC/AHA 2005 guidelines for the management of patients with peripheral arterial disease (lower extremity, renal, mesenteric, and abdominal aortic)—executive summary. J Am Coll Cardiol; 47(6):1239–1312, 2006.

HORWITZ LD, GROVES BM (eds). *Signs and Symptoms in Cardiology*. Philadelphia: JB Lippincott, 1985.

HURST JW. *Cardiovascular Diagnosis. The initial examination*. St. Louis: Mosby, 1993.

JAMES PA, OPARIL S, CARTER BL, et al. 2014 Evidence-Based Guidelines for the Management of High Blood Pressure in Adults. Report from the Panel Members Appointed to the Eighth Joint National Committee, JNC 8. JAMA, 311(5):507–520, 2014.

JANUARY CT, WANN LS, ALPERT JS, et al. 2014 AHA/ACC/HRS Guideline for the Management of Patients With Atrial Fibrillation: A Report of the American College of Cardiology/American Heart Association Task Force on Practice Guidelines and the Heart Rhythm Society: Executive Summary. J Am Coll Cardiol 64 (21): 2246-2280, 2014.

KENNY T. *The Nuts and Bolts of Cardiac Pacing*. 2nd ed. Wiley Blackwell, 2008.

KLOCKE FJ, BAIRD MG, LORELL BH, et al. ACC/AHA/ ASNC guidelines for the clinical use of cardiac radionuclide imaging: executive summary: a report of the American College of Cardiology/American Heart Association Task Force on Practice Guidelines. Circulation 108:1404–18, 2003.

KONSTAM M, DRACUP K, BAKER D, et al. Heart Failure: Evaluation and Care of Patients with Left Ventricular Systolic Dysfunction. Clinical Practice Guidelines No. 11. AHCPR Publication No. 94–0612. Rockville, MD, Agency for Health Care Policy and Research and the National Heart, Lung, and Blood Institute, Public Health Service, U.S. Department of Health and Human Services. June 1994.

LEVINE GN, BATES ER, BLANKENSHIP JC, et al. 2011 ACCF/AHA/SCAI Guideline for Percutaneous Coronary Intervention: A Report of the American College of Cardiology Foundation/American Heart Association Task Force on Practice Guidelines/Society for Cardiovascular Angiography and Interventions. Circulation 124:2574–2609, 2011.

LEVINE SA, HARVEY WP. *Clinical Auscultation of the Heart*. 2nd ed. Philadelphia: WB Saunders, 1959.

LILLY LS. *Pathophysiology of Heart Disease*. 6th ed. Philadelphia: Lippincott Williams & Wilkins, 2016.

LINZER M, YANG EH, ESTES NA III, et al. Diagnosis syncope: I. Value of history, physical examination, and electrocardiography. Clinical Efficacy Assessment Project of the American College of Physicians. Ann Intern Med 126:989, 1997.

MARCH SK. W. Proctor Harvey: A Master Clinician-Teacher's Influence on the History of Cardiovascular Medicine. Tex Heart Inst J 29:182-192, 2002.

MARCH SK. BEDYNEK JL JR, CHIZNER MA. Teaching cardiac auscultation: effectiveness of a patient-centered teaching conference on improving cardiac auscultatory skills. Mayo Clin Proc 80:1443-1448, 2005.

MARK DB, BERMAN DS, BUDOFF MJ, et al. 2010 Expert Consensus Document on Coronary Computed Tomographic Angiography: A Report of the American College of Cardiology Foundation Task Force on Expert Consensus Documents. J Am Coll Cardiol 55(23):2663–2699, 2010.

MARRIOTT HJL. *Bedside Cardiac Diagnosis*. Philadelphia: JB Lippincott, 1993.

MOSCUCCI M (ed). *Grossman and Baim's Cardiac Catheterization, Angiography and Intervention* 8th ed. Philadelphia: Lippincott Williams & Wilkins, 2014.

NISHIMURA RA, OTTO CM, BONOW RO, et al. 2014 AHA/ACC Guideline for the Management of Patients with Valvular Heart Disease: Executive Summary: A Report of the American College of Cardiology/American Heart Association Task Force on Practice Guidelines. J Am Coll Cardiol 63(22):2438–2488, 2014.

O'GARA PT, KUSHNER FG, ASCHEIM DD, et al. 2013 ACCF/AHA Guideline for the Management of ST Elevation Myocardial Infarction: Executive Summary: A Report of the American College of Cardiology Foundation/American Heart Association Task Force on Practice Guidelines. J Am Coll Cardiol: 61 (4): 485–510, 2013.

OPIE LH, GERSH BJ (eds). *Drugs for the Heart.* 8th ed. Philadelphia: Elsevier Saunders, 2013.

O'ROURKE RA, BRUNDAGE BH, FROELICHER VF, et al. American College of Cardiology/American Heart Association Expert Consensus Document on Electron Beam Computed Tomography from the Diagnosis and Prognosis of Coronary Artery Disease. J Am Coll Cardiol 36:326, 2000.

OTTO C (ed). *The Practice of Clinical Echocardiography.* 5th ed. Philadelphia: Elsevier Saunders, 2017.

PEPINE CJ, HILL J, LAMBERT C (eds). *Diagnostic and Therapeutic Cardiac Catheterization.* 3rd ed, Philadelphia: Lippincott Williams & Wilkins, 1998.

PERLOFF JK. *Physical Examination of the Heart and Circulation.* 3rd ed. Philadelphia: Saunders, 2000.

ROLDAN CA, ABRAMS J (eds): *Evaluation of the Patient With Heart Disease. Integrating the Physical Exam & Echocardiography.* Philadelphia: Lippincott Williams & Wilkins, 2002.

ROSENDORFF C (ed). 3rd ed. *Essential Cardiology. Principles and Practice.* New York: Springer Inc., 2013.

ROSENDORFF C, LACKLAND DT, ALLISON M, et al. Treatment of Hypertension in Patients with Coronary Artery Disease, A Scientific Statement from the American Heart Association, American College of Cardiology, and American Society of Hypertension. J Am Coll Cardiol 65 (18): 1998–2038, 2015.

RYAN TJ, ANTMAN EM, BROOKS NH, et al. 1999 update: ACC/AHA guidelines for the management of patients with acute myocardial infarction: Executive summary and recommendations: A report of the American College of Cardiology/American Heart Association Task Force on Practical Guidelines. J Am Coll Cardiol 34:890–911, 1999.

SCANLON PJ, FAXON DP, AUDET AM, et al. ACC/AHA guidelines for coronary angiography: A report of the American College of Cardiology/American Heart Association Task Force on Practice Guidelines. J Am Coll Cardiol 33:1756–1824, 1999.

SCHLANT RC, ADOLPH RJ, DIMARCO JP, et al. ACC/AHA guidelines for electrocardiography. A report of the American College of Cardiology/American Heart Association Task Force on Assessment of Diagnostic and Therapeutic Cardiovascular Procedures. J Am Coll Cardiol 19:473–481, 1992.

SEVENTH REPORT OF THE JOINT NATIONAL COMMITTEE ON PREVENTION, DETECTION, EVALUATION, AND TREATMENT OF HIGH BLOOD PRESSURE. The JNC 7 Report. JAMA; 289 (19): 2560–2572, 2003.

SMITH SC JR., BENJAMIN EJ, BONOW RO, et al. AHA/ACCF Secondary Prevention and Risk Reduction Therapy for Patients with Coronary and Other Atherosclerotic Vascular Disease: 2011 Update. Circulation 124; 2458–2473, 2011.

STONE NJ, ROBINSON J, LICHTENSTEIN AH, et al. 2013 ACC/AHA Guideline on the Treatment of Blood Cholesterol to Reduce Atherosclerotic Cardiovascular Risk in Adults. J Am Coll Cardiol 63(25):2889–2934, 2014.

TOPOL EJ (ed). 3rd ed. *Textbook of Cardiovascular Medicine.* Philadelphia: Lipincott Williams & Wilkins, 2007.

VANDEN BELT RJ, RONAN JA, BEDYNEK JL JR. *Cardiology: A clinical approach.* 2nd ed. Chicago: Yearbook Medical Publishers, 1987.

WAGNER GS, STRAUSS DG. *Marriott's Practical Electrocardiography.* 12th ed. Philadelphia: Lippincott Williams & Wilkins, 2014.

WALLER BF, HARVEY WP. *Cardiovascular evaluation of athletes.* Cedar Grove, NJ: Laennec Publishing, Inc., 1993.

WARNES CA, WILLIAMS RG, BASHORE TM, et al. AHA/ACC 2008 guidelines for the management of adults with congenital heart disease: a report of the American College of Cardiology/American Heart Association Task Force on practice guidelines. J Am Coll Cardiol 52:e 143-263, 2008.

WHELTON PK, CAREY RM, ARONOW WS, et.al. 2017 ACC/AHA Guidelines for the Prevention, Detection, Evaluation, and Management of High Blood Pressure in Adults. A report of the American College of Cardiology/American Heart Association Task Force on Clinical Practice Guidelines. Hypertension, 2017.

WILLERSON JT, COHN JN (eds.) *Cardiovascular Medicine,* 3rd ed. London: Springer-Verlag, 2007.

WILSON W, TAUBERT KA, GERWITZ M, et al. Prevention of Infective Endocarditis. Guidelines from the American Heart Association. A Guideline from the American Heart Association Rheumatic Fever, Endocarditis, and Kawasaki Disease Committee, Council on Cardiovascular Disease in the Young, and the Council on Clinical Cardiology, Council on Cardiovascular Surgery and Anesthesia, and the quality of Cae and Outcomes Research Interdisciplinary Working Group. Circulation 115: 2007.

YANCY C, JESSUP M, BOZKURT B, et al. 2013 ACCF/AHA Guideline for the Management of Heart Failure. A Report of the American College of Cardiology Foundation/American Heart Association Task Force on Practice Guidelines. Circulation, 128: 1810–1852, 2013.

ZIPES DP, DIMARCO JP, GILLETTE PC, et al. ACC/AHA guidelines for clinical intracardiac electrophysiologic and catheter ablation procedures. A report of the American College of Cardiology/American Heart Association Task Force on Practice Guidelines. J Am Coll Cardiol 26:555, 1995, Circulation 92:673–691, 1995.

ZIPES DP, LIBBY P, BONOW RO, MANN DL, TOMASELLI GF (eds) *Braunwald's Heart Disease. A Textbook of Cardiovascular Medicine.* 11th ed. Philadelphia: Elsevier Inc., 2019.

Index